Infections and Sepsis Development

Edited by Vincenzo Neri, Lixing Huang and Jie Li

Published in London, United Kingdom

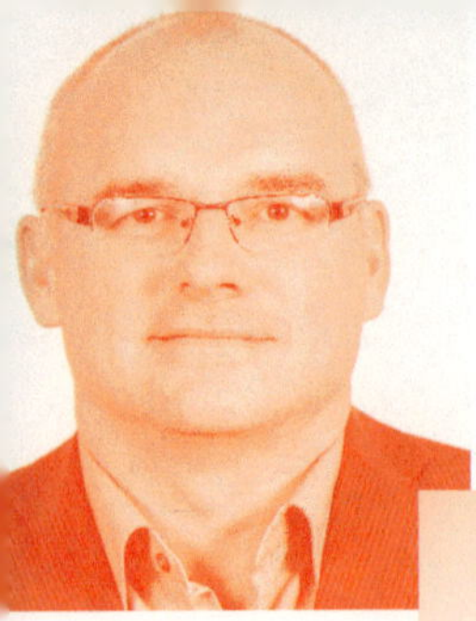

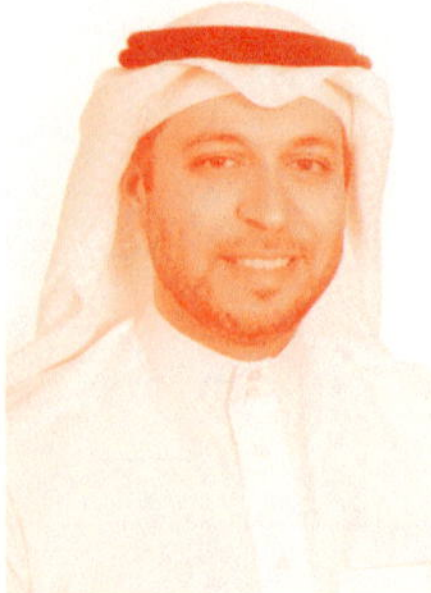

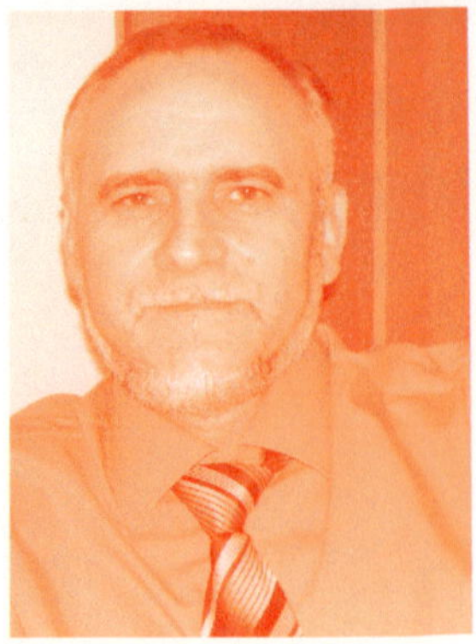

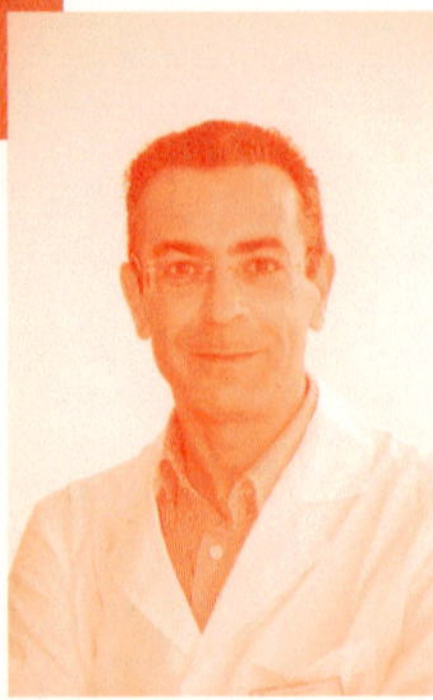

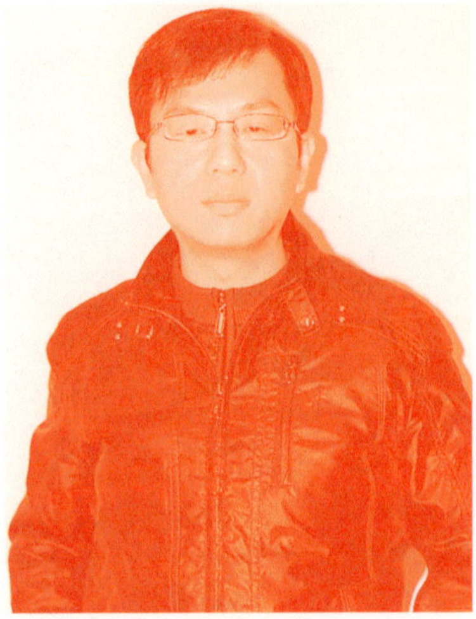

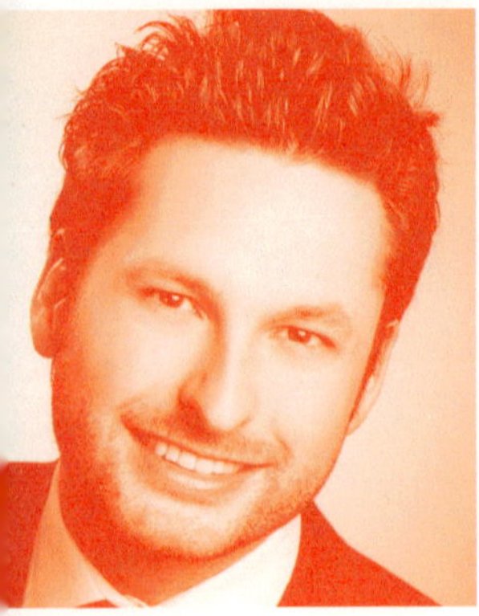

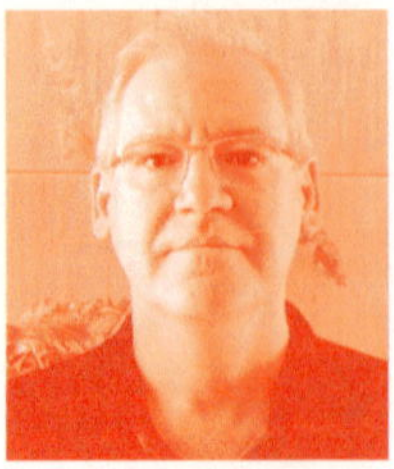

IntechOpen

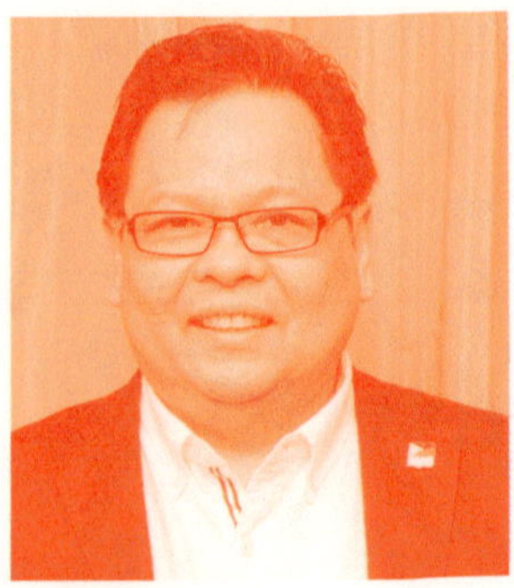

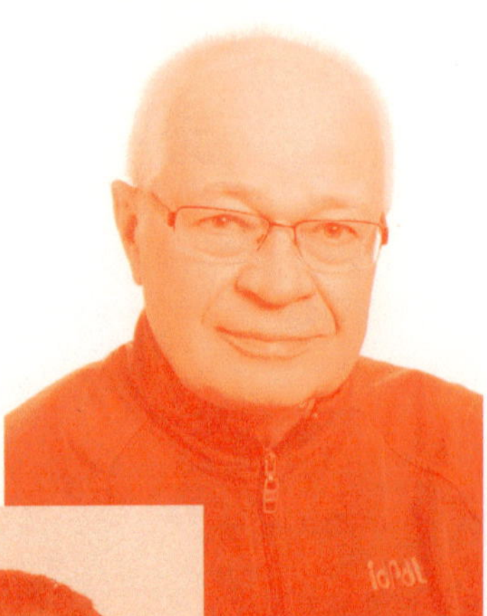

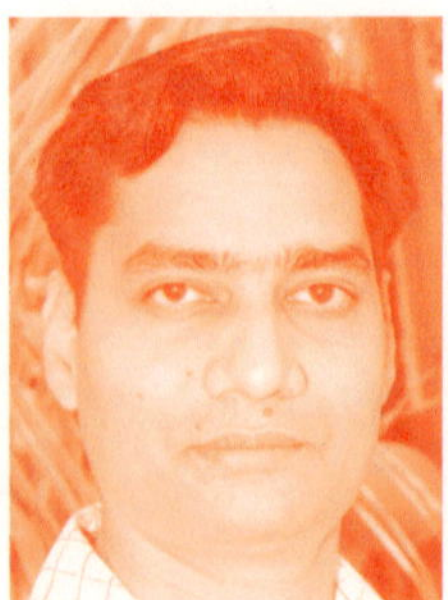

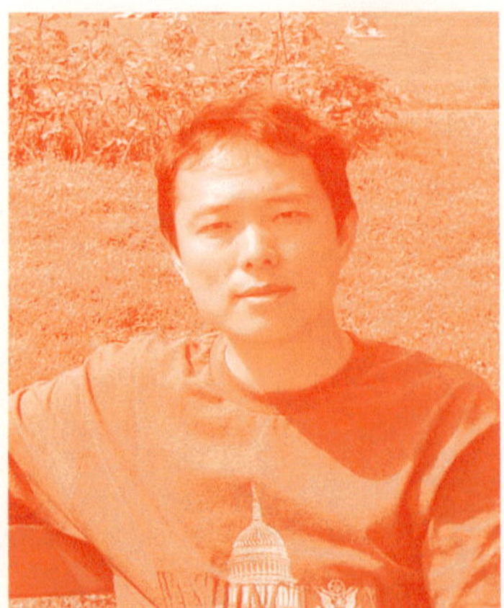

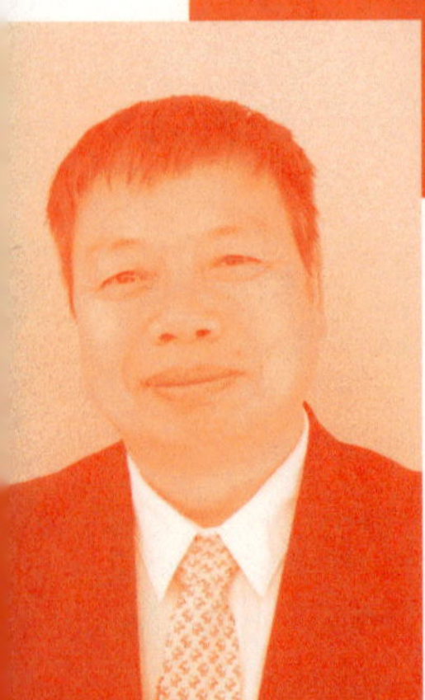

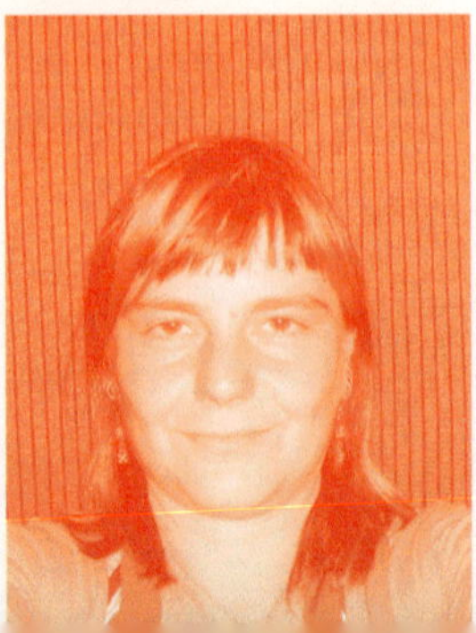

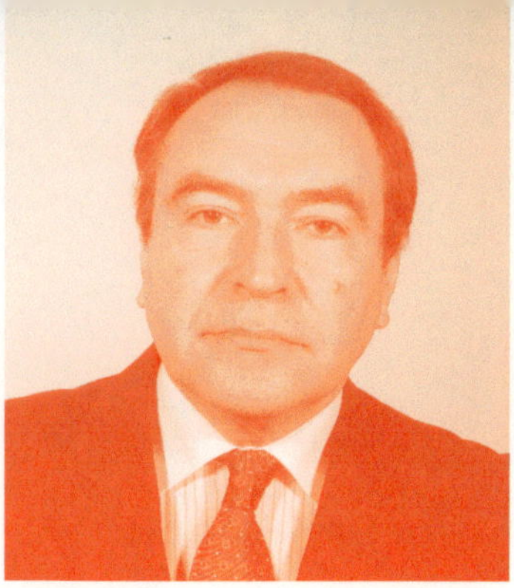

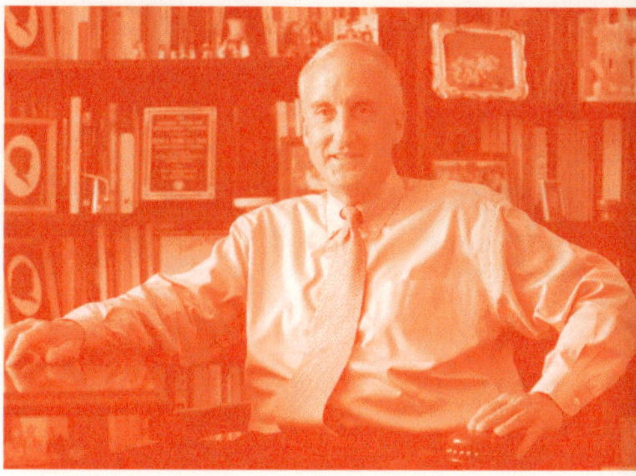

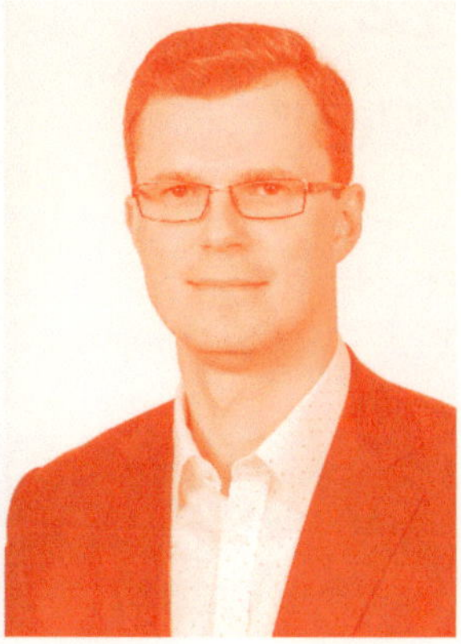

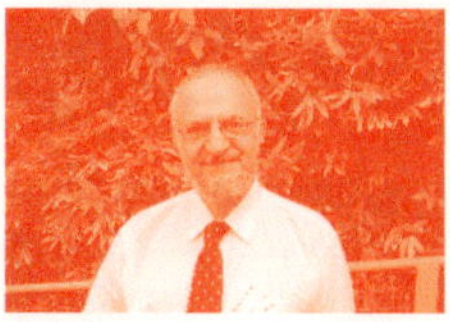

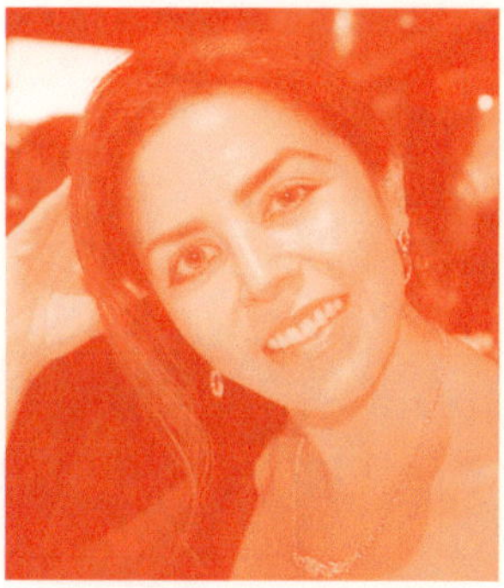

Supporting open minds since 2005

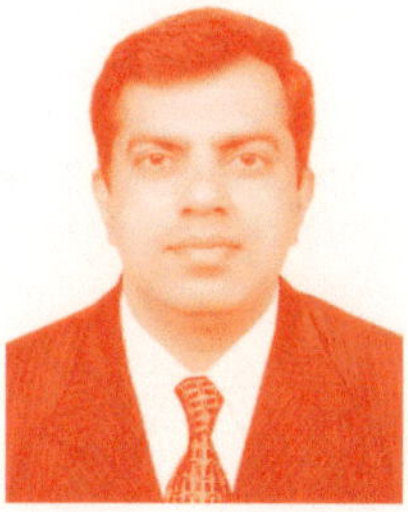

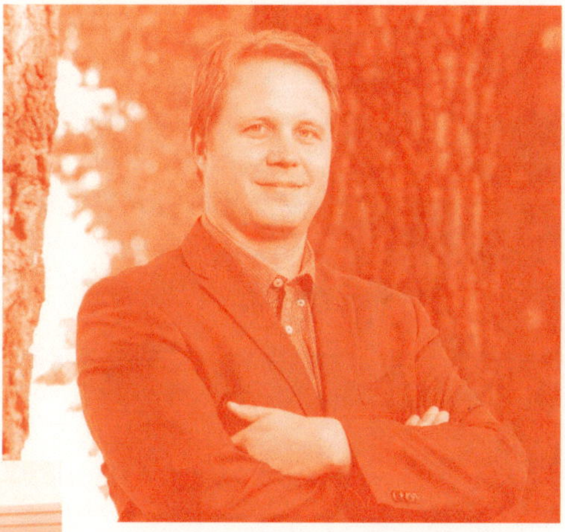

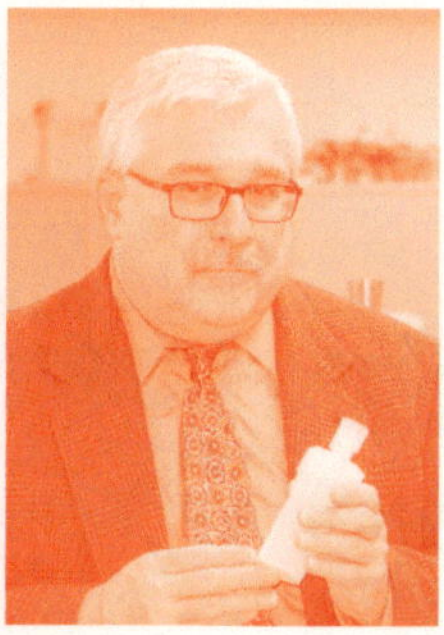

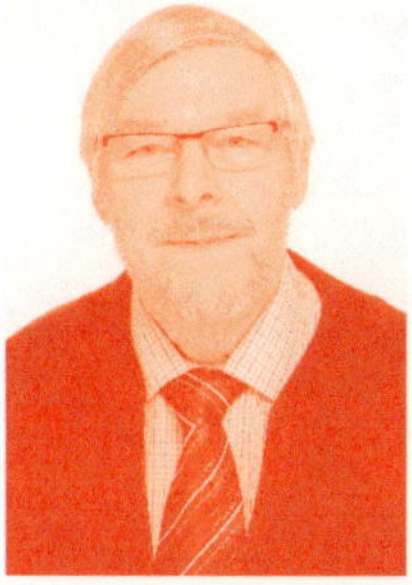

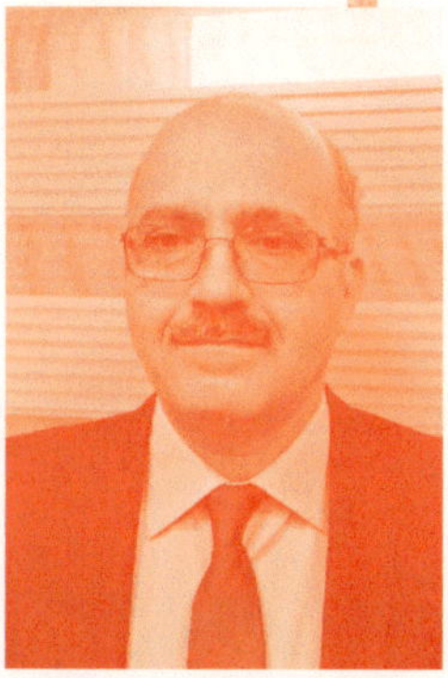

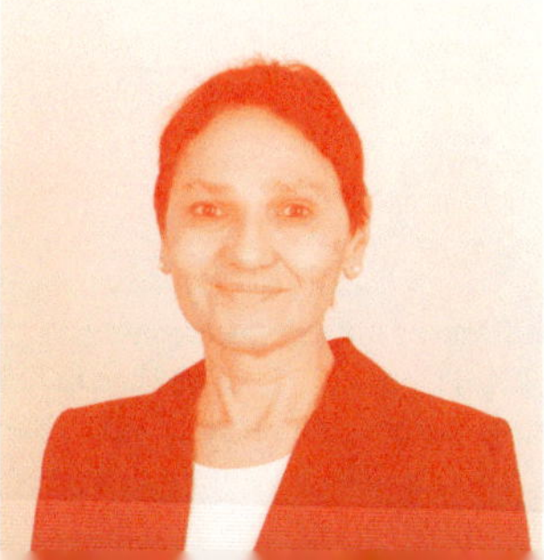

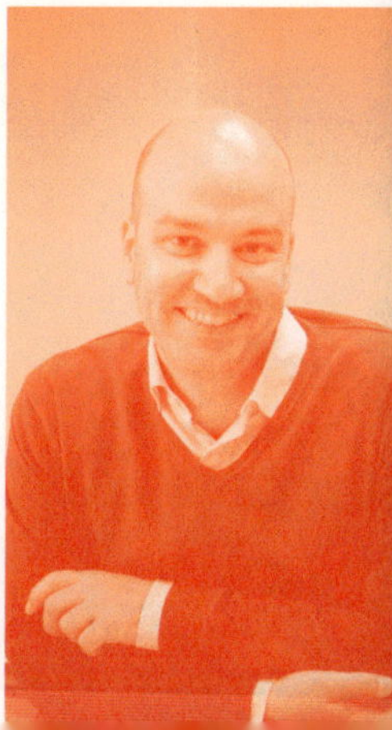

Infections and Sepsis Development
http://dx.doi.org/10.5772/intechopen.94701
Edited by Vincenzo Neri, Lixing Huang and Jie Li

Contributors
Velma Rebić, Mufida Aljičević, Sajra Vinčević-Smajlović, Damir Rebić, Marylise Duperthuy, Annabelle Mathieu-Denoncourt, Sean Giacomucci, Hafsa Lamrani Alaoui, Khalid Oufdou, Nour-Eddine Mezrioui, Robson Faria, Guilherme Teixeira, Lixing Huang, Qiancheng Gao, Youyu Zhang, Wei Xu, Qingpi Yan, Hethesh Chellapandian, Jeyachandran Sivakamavalli, A. Vijay Anand, Balamuralikrishnan Balasubramanian, Shivnarayan Patidar, Naimahmed Nesaragi, Nicolas Vogel, Ilker Uçkay, Tanja Huber, Zohair Al Aseri, Ferdinando Da Rin de Lorenzo, Grażyna Sygitowicz, Dariusz Sitkiewicz, Seyed Arad Senaobar Tahaei, Zoltán Mencser, Pál Barzó, Seyyed Ashkan Senobar Tahaei, Ahlem Trifi, Sami Abdellatif, Salah Ben Lakhal, Sameh Trabelsi, Tinni Trihartini Maskoen, Titik Setyawati, Ricky Aditya, Sachin M. Patil, Parag Patel, Rahmayati Rusnedy, Gulberk Ucar, Bercis Imge Ucar, Manuel Vélez-Gimón

First published in London, United Kingdom, 2021 by IntechOpen
IntechOpen is the global imprint of INTECHOPEN LIMITED, registered in England and Wales, registration number: 11086078, 5 Princes Gate Court, London, SW7 2QJ, United Kingdom
Printed in Croatia

British Library Cataloguing-in-Publication Data
A catalogue record for this book is available from the British Library

Additional hard and PDF copies can be obtained from orders@intechopen.com

Infections and Sepsis Development
Edited by Vincenzo Neri, Lixing Huang and Jie Li
p. cm.
Print ISBN 978-1-83969-457-8
Online ISBN 978-1-83969-458-5
eBook (PDF) ISBN 978-1-83969-459-2

For EU product safety concerns:
IN TECH d.o.o., Prolaz Marije Krucifikse Kozulić 3, 51000 Rijeka, Croatia, info@intechopen.com or visit our website at intechopen.com.

Meet the editors

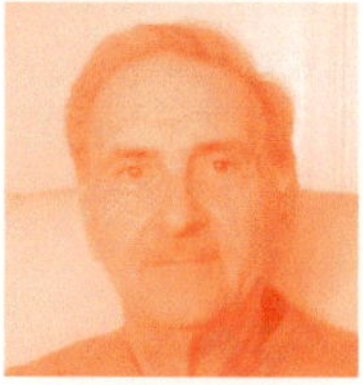

Vincenzo Neri has held numerous positions at the University of Foggia, Italy, including full professor, director of the Division of General Surgery, Residency School of General Surgery, and the Department of Surgical Sciences, and president of the Course of Degree of Medicine and Surgery. He is now retired. Dr. Neri graduated in Medicine and Surgery in 1970 and completed post-graduate training in General Surgery in 1975 and in Emergency Surgery in 1979 at the University of Bari, Italy. He received an MEd in University Health Science Pedagogy from the University Paris-Nord Bobigny in 1995. His clinical and research interest is hepatobiliary pancreatic surgery, with a focus on the management of acute pancreatitis and treatment of pancreatic and liver tumours. He has published several research papers, reviews, congress proceedings, and book chapters. During 1991–2016, he attended for short periods every year the Hepatobiliary Pancreatic Surgery Service of Beaujon Hospital, Universitè de Paris, Clichy. As part of the ERASMUS Program 2010–2011, Dr. Neri developed a seminar on "Cystic Tumours of the Pancreas" at Ghent University, Belgium. He is also a member of SIC, IHPBA, EASL, NESA, and SLS.

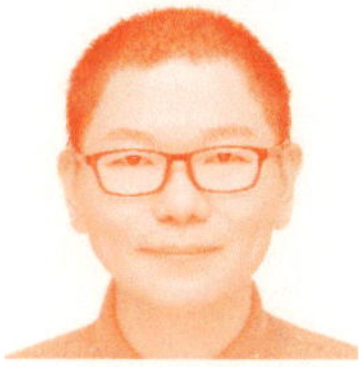

Dr. Lixing Huang is an associate professor at Jimei University, China. He is engaged in research of molecular mechanisms of bacterial pathogen-host interaction, including but not limited to applying dual RNA-seq and dual iTRAQ approaches to complex infection settings comprising bacterial pathogens, their hosts, and resident gut microbiota; the interplay between host cell microRNAs/proteins and bacterial infection; the impact of bacterial pathogens on host cell RNA metabolism; the effect of bacterial non-coding RNAs/proteins on key host intracellular pathways; and nutritional immunity, the struggle for nutrient metals between hosts and pathogens. He is the author of more than sixty research articles. He is also a member of the China Society of Fisheries (CSF) and the Chinese Society of Toxicology (CST).

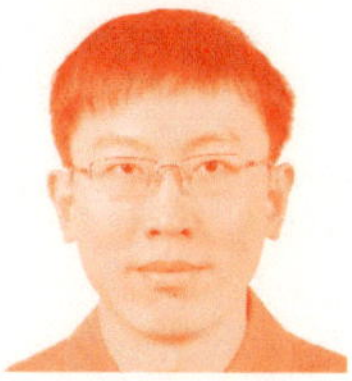

Dr. Jie Li is an Associate Professor and Research Fellow of the Yellow Sea Fisheries Research Institute, Chinese Academy of Fishery Sciences. He completed a Ph.D. at the Institute of Oceanology, the Chinese Academy of Science. His research is directed at the epidemiology and immunology of bacterial pathogens in farming fish, including but not limited to fish disease control, fish vaccine development, and pathogenicity mechanisms of fish pathogens. He is the author of ten research articles and a member of the China Society of Fisheries (CSF).

Contents

Preface

Infection is a common clinical condition that may cause local inflammation but, in some cases, can lead to systemic inflammation, with sepsis and organ dysfunction. The inflammatory response is a very complex course that is engendered by the harmful action of various agents, be they infectious, physical, or chemical, towards the host. The inflammatory response, in the biological perspective, should carry out a protective action of the organism, but this response produces several detrimental substances, such as proteolytic enzymes and oxygen metabolites. Usually, the system of host protection performs an effective action and avoids tissue damage. Nevertheless, in some cases, the protective resources are ineffectual or lost and the inflammatory response becomes harmful. Moreover, the tissue damage causes further inflammation with progressive worsening [1].

The clinical scenario of this "malignant inflammation" [2] develops in multiorgan dysfunction, which can progress to multiorgan failure because the final effect of inflammatory tissue damage is diffuse tissue hypoxia, which, if prolonged, causes irreversible cell changes. This is septic shock.

The clinical appearance of the first phase of systemic inflammation, Systemic Inflammatory Response Syndrome (SIRS), is represented by increased temperature, heart rate, respiratory rate, and white blood cell count. Organ dysfunction in Multiple Organ Dysfunction Syndrome (MODS) involves the lungs, kidneys, cardiovascular system, and central nervous system [3].

Septic shock can be evaluated as distributive shock, that is, vasodilatory shock. Distributive shock is based on the increase of intravascular space. In septic shock, especially with gram-negative bacteremia, the lipopolysaccharide endotoxin that comes from the gram-negative bacteria promotes the deliverance of effective vasodilators from damaged cell membranes. In the first phase of septic shock, the most evident clinical appearance is the vascular hyperdynamic state, followed, with the progression of the disease and the expanded intravascular space, by a low cardiac output state. The general clinical condition in distributive shock is insufficient tissue perfusion. In fact, general vasodilation causes a reduction of blood perfusion and tissue damage in the kidneys, brain, and heart. Moreover, in distributive/septic shock there is leakage of fluid from capillaries in the surrounding tissue [4].

The pathophysiology of septic shock is characterized not by altered tissue oxygenation but by cytopathic hypoxia, which is a defect in cellular oxygen availability. Consequently, the tissue level of oxygen can be increased in septic shock [5].

The first section of the book, "Therapeutic Control of Infectious Agents," includes contributions on this wide and complex topic. It provides updates on the bactericidal and bacteriostatic action of antibiotics and on the distribution and molecular detection of methicillin-resistant *Staphylococcus aureus*. It also discusses the therapeutic perspective of potential natural products from tropical fruits, empiric antimicrobial therapy in critically ill septic patients, and bacterial immunotherapy in treating chronic osteomyelitis. This section also includes some interesting studies on the epidemiology and bacterial characteristics of the bacteria *Vibrio cholerae*, including information on its prevalence, antimicrobial resistance, pathogenicity in suburban groundwater supplies of Marrakesh, secretome, and challenges in controlling vibriosis in shrimp farms.

The second section, "Specific Infectious Pathologies," examines diagnostic findings and therapeutic management of some pathological conditions with infective etiology, such as diabetic foot osteomyelitis and infections in neurosurgery.

The third section, "Sepsis Pathophysiology," evaluates some of the most important aspects of the pathophysiology and management of sepsis and septic shock. Topics covered in this section include early diagnosis of sepsis using machine learning; the pathophysiology of septic shock; intestinal barrier dysfunction, bacterial translocation, and inflammation; assessment and management of hypoperfusion in sepsis; sepsis-associated acute kidney injury; and atrial fibrillation during septic shock.

Vincenzo Neri
Department of Medical and Surgical Sciences – University of Foggia,
Foggia, Italy

Lixing Huang
Jimei University,
China

Jie Li
Chinese Academy of Fishery Sciences,
China

References

[1] Marino PL. Infection, inflammation and multiorgan injury. In Marino PL. The ICU Book. Lippincott, Williams, Wilkins. Philadelphia 2007; pagg. 737-747.

[2] Pinsky MR, Vincent JL, Deviere J et al. Serum cytokine levels in human septic shock: relation to multiple-system organ failure and mortality. Chest 1993;103:565-575.

[3] Alyesil C, Dogan NO, Ozturan IU et al. Distributive shock in the emergency department: sepsis, anaphylaxis, or capillary leak syndrome? Emerg Med 2017;52:e229-e231.

[4] Smith N, Lopez RA, Silberman M. Distributive shock (Updated 2021 Jul 26). StatPearls. Treausure Island (FL). Publishing 2021.

[5] Fink MP. Cytopathic hypoxia: mitochondrial dysfunction as mechanism contributing to organ dysfunction in sepsis. Crit Care Clin 2001;17:219-237.

Section 1

Therapeutic Control of Infectious Agents

Chapter 1

Bactericidal and Bacteriostatic Antibiotics

Sachin M. Patil and Parag Patel

Abstract

Of all the medications available to physicians worldwide, antibiotics play an essential role in inpatient and outpatient settings. Discovered in the early nineteenth century by Alexander Fleming, penicillin was the first antibiotic isolated from a mold. Dr. Gerhard Domagk developed synthetic sulfa drugs by altering the red dye used in chemical industries. Since then, multiple antibiotic classes have been discovered with varying antimicrobial effects enabling their use empirically or in specific clinical scenarios. Antibiotics with different mechanisms of action could be either bactericidal or bacteriostatic. However, no clinical significance has been observed between cidal and static antibiotics in multiple trials. Their presence has led to safer deep invasive surgeries, advanced chemotherapy in cancer, and organ transplantation. Indiscriminate usage of antibiotics has resulted in severe hospital-acquired infections, including nosocomial pneumonia, *Clostridioides difficile* infection, multidrug-resistant invasive bacterial infections, allergic reactions, and other significant side effects. Antibiotic stewardship is an essential process in the modern era to advocate judicial use of antibiotics for an appropriate duration. They play a vital role in medical and surgical intensive care units to address the various complications seen in these patients. Antibiotics are crucial in severe acute infections to improve overall mortality and morbidity.

Keywords: Sepsis, antibiotics, bactericidal, bacteriostatic, stewardship

1. Introduction

Antibiotic is a term used to define a chemical substance produced by one microorganism that stunts the metabolism and development of other organisms [1]. The antibiotic term was used initially for naturally acquired substances; however, now the term encompasses both natural and synthetic antimicrobial substances. Although penicillin was the first antibiotic isolated from the mold, it was superseded by sulfa drugs used by physicians to treat infections successfully [2]. Due to antibiotic use, the infectious disease death rate has declined from 280 per 100,000 to 60 per 100,000 in the 1950s [3]. A common belief is that cidal antibiotics are efficient than static antibiotics with no clinical evidence supporting it. Both cidal and static are invitro terms which, refer to the effect of antibiotic concentrations affecting bacterial growth at a predefined threshold. They cannot predict the infection outcome in vivo. Antibiotics targeting the organism's cell wall are mostly bactericidal, whereas those targeting protein syntheses are bacteriostatic. MIC (minimum inhibitory concentration) is the lowest antibiotic concentration, which prevents visible growth at 24 hours. MBC (minimum bactericidal concentration) is the minimal concentration of antibiotics that causes bacterial death. Breakpoints for antibiotic MIC's are set by the the European Committee on Antimicrobial Susceptibility Testing (EUCAST) and National Committee for Clinical and Laboratory Standards Institute (CLSI). A bactericidal antibiotic MBC is less than or equal to four folds above the MIC, accounting for a 1000-fold decline in bacterial density [4]. A bacteriostatic antibiotic achieves a > 1000-fold reduction at eight-fold above MIC or a 500-fold reduction in bacterial density at 4-fold above its MIC. They are still labeled as static despite the clear demonstration of bacterial killing. An antibiotic becomes more bactericidal as the MIC moves closer to the MBC. Bacteriostatic agents have an MBC to MIC ratio > than that for bactericidal antibiotics.

A systematic literature review revealed no confirmation that cidal agents are better than static agents [5]. In addition, there was no substantial difference in efficiency, including critically ill patients with severe infections and sepsis. Six trials demonstrated the superiority of static agent linezolid over cidal agents such as vancomycin [5]. A single trial showed the efficiency of cidal agent imipenem over tigecycline; however, the dose of tigecycline was small, and with increased appropriate dosing, the efficacy disappeared [6, 7]. A rapidly bactericidal agent such as daptomycin does not perform better than a slowly cidal agent such as vancomycin to treat right-sided infective endocarditis (IE) and staphylococcal bacteremia [8] . A synergistic combination of beta-lactam with aminoglycosides enhances the bactericidal effect with rapid blood clearance [9]. However, this synergistic combination has not improved clinical outcomes or mortality [10]. In the initial studies, static agents such as tetracyclines and macrolides were inferior to cidal agents in IE therapy [11]. This assumption can be erroneous as the static agents do not achieve adequate low blood concentrations to treat infective endocarditis effectively. A bacteriostatic antibiotic such as linezolid can attain sufficient bloodstream concentrations resulting in higher cure rates for IE [12]. Daptomycin, a rapidly bactericidal agent, is inferior to vancomycin in left-sided IE [13]. For an individual antibiotic to be effective, the importance of its pharmacokinetic-pharmacodynamic properties and attaining adequate drug levels at the infection site is substantial than static versus cidal properties used in predicting clinical efficacy. An intact immune system is critical for the efficacy of bacteriostatic agents, and bactericidal agents are preferred in immunosuppressed patients. Broad-spectrum agents cover many susceptible pathogens, whereas narrow-spectrum agents cover a limited number of pathogens. Broad-spectrum agents are used empirically in the therapy of lung and abdominal infections. Narrow-spectrum agents are used in a limited number of indications.

2. Bacteriostatic antibiotics

These include folate inhibitors (sulfonamides and trimethoprim) in **Table 1** (2A I), tetracyclines in **Table 2** (2A II), glycylcyclines in **Table 3** (2A III), macrolides in **Table 4** (2A IV), lincosamides in **Table 5** (2A V), oxazolidinones in **Table 6** (2A VI) and fusidic acid in **Table 7** (2A VII).

Dapsone can substitute sulfamethoxazole in the TMP-SMX combination for PCJ pneumonia in patients with allergies to sulfonamide antibiotics [89]. TMP-SMX is the drug of choice for Q-fever in pregnancy. An essential fact to remember is that TMP-SMX does not cover *pseudomonas* and should be avoided in streptococcal infections due to a higher incidence of resistance [90]. Iclaprim is a DHFR inhibitor with bactericidal activity against *methicillin-sensitive Staphylococcus aureus* (MSSA), *Methicillin-resistant* (MRSA), *beta-hemolytic Streptococcal spp,* and *Enterococcus*

Origin	Sulfonamides are sulfanilamide derivatives identical to para-aminobenzoic acid (PABA) required for folic acid synthesis in most bacteria. Trimethoprim is a synthetic derivative from trimethoxybenzyl-pyrimidine [14].
Mechanism of action	Sulfonamides antagonize PABA inclusion into dihydropteroate by its greater affinity for tetrahydropteroic acid synthetase in microorganisms resulting in decreased dihydrofolic acid, a substrate for dihydrofolate reductase (DHFR) [15, 16]. Trimethoprim is a potent bacterial inhibitor of DFR, preventing the formation of tetrahyrofolic acid needed for purine and deoxyribonucleic acid [14]. Thus, sulfonamides and trimethoprim together stop two consecutive steps essential in the folic acid synthesis. A combination of both is synergistic and bactericidal in trimethoprim and the sulfa ratio of 1:20 [17].
Routes	Sulfonamides are available in oral, intravenous (IV), topical, and ophthalmic formulations. Trimethoprim is available in oral and intravenous formulations.
Indication	Sulfonamides: Nocardiosis, Toxoplasmosis, Plasmodium falciparum malaria, Nongonococcal urethritis, Trimethoprim: Acute urinary tract infection (UTI), Recurrent UTI Trimethoprim and sulfamethoxazole (TMP-SMX): Above indications plus UTI, Skin and soft tissue infections (SSTI) due to *Staphylococcus aureus, Pneumocystis jiroveci* (PCJ) pneumonia, and prophylaxis, Melioidosis, Whipple disease, Alternative in Listeria meningitis
Resistance	Sulfonamides: Point mutations in folP gene modifying dihydropteroate synthetase resulting in decreased affinity for sulfonamide [18]. PABA binding site alteration due to F28L/T and P64S mutations [19]. Integrons sul1, sul2, and sul3 coding drug resistance enzymes [20]. Trimethoprim: Plasmid-mediated resistant DHFR enzyme
Pharmaco-kinetics	Sulfonamides: Well distributed throughout the body, and protein binding predicts the blood and tissue levels. It is metabolized in the liver (CYP2C9 & CYP3A4 hepatic enzyme system) and excreted via renal excretion. Chronic kidney disease results in decreased renal clearance [21]. It can interact with multiple other drugs resulting in increased serum levels and toxicity especially antiseizure medications.
Toxicity	Skin: Rashes, Steven-Johnson syndrome (SJS), Toxic epidermal necrolysis (TEN) [22, 23]. Blood: Anemia, agranulocytosis, thrombocytopenia, methemoglobinemia [24]. Renal: Hyperkalemia, Acute renal failure, Interstitial nephritis, Lactic acidosis [24–26]. Gastrointestinal (GI): Pseudomembranous colitis, Pancreatitis, and Fulminant liver failure [27–29]. Others: aseptic meningitis

Table 1.
2AI folate inhibitors: Sulfonamides & trimethoprim.

faecalis. It undergoes hepatic clearance, and dose adjustment is needed in hepatic impairment. Tissue penetration is excellent in the lungs. It is effective without a sulfa moiety so that it can be used in patients with sulfa allergy. The side effects include nausea, headache, fatigue, and QT interval prolongation. Currently, it is under trials for SSTI and nosocomial pneumonia [91, 92].

Doxycycline is the drug of choice in bioterrorism caused by *Bacillus anthracis*, *Yersinia pestis*, *Francisella tularensis*, *Coxiella burnetti*, and *Brucella spp* [93]. In the medical intensive care unit (MICU), tetracyclines are the drug of choice in acute sepsis due to cholera, ehrlichiosis, *stenotrophomonas* infections, rickettsial disease, anaplasmosis, and PID.

In sepsis, tigecycline is used in MDR infections as a last resort, and the federal drug authority (FDA) has placed a boxed warning about this death risk. It can also be used effectively at a higher dosage in MDR hospital-acquired pneumonia (HAP) and ventilator-associated pneumonia (VAP).

Origin	Tetracycline is derived from catalytic dehalogenation of chlortetracycline obtained from *Streptomyces rimosus* [30]. Doxycycline and Minocycline are semisynthetic derivatives of oxytetracycline.
Mechanism of action	Reversibly binds 30S ribosomal subunit of the bacteria and inhibits protein synthesis. In protozoa, it additionally binds to 70S ribosome and stops protein synthesis [30, 31].
Routes	Orally via capsules, tablets, syrups, and IV formulations.
Indication	Community-acquired bacterial pneumonia (CABP), MSSA &MRSA SSTI, Stenotrophomonas infections, *Helicobacter pylori* infection, Nongonococcal urethritis, Lyme disease, Rickettsial infections, Nocardiosis, Falciparum malaria, Cholera, Anaplasmosis, and Ehrlichiosis. Q fever, Brucellosis, Melioidosis, Acne vulgarism, the second line in syphilis, and a part of the combination regimen in pelvic inflammatory disease (PID).
Resistance	It is mediated mainly by active efflux pumps and ribosomal protection proteins. Other minor mechanisms include antibiotic enzymatic lysis, a decline in-wall permeability, and binding site alterations [32].
Pharmac-okinetics	Unlike tetracycline, food does not substantially alter doxycycline and minocycline absorption, and both have excellent bioavailability [33]. Lipid solubility determines the tissue and fluid levels of which minocycline > doxycycline > tetracycline. At higher doses, doxycycline reaches adequate levels in the cerebrospinal fluid (CSF) [34]. The clearance mechanism is via both renal (tetracycline) and hepatic (doxycycline and minocycline).
Toxicity/ Adverse effects	GI: pill-induced esophagitis, heartburn, epigastric pain, nausea, vomiting, acid reflux disorder [35]. Hepatotoxicity from IV tetracycline [36]. Skin: photosensitive rash and hyperpigmentation of body parts [37]. Nephrogenic diabetes insipidus: by demeclocycline [38]. Central Nervous System(CNS): Vestibular symptoms, Pseudotumor cerebri Teeth, and Bone: tooth staining, enamel hypoplasia, and diminished bone growth in premature infants exposed to tetracycline [39]. Hypersensitivity reactions: facial swelling, drug-induced lupus, anaphylaxis, urticaria [40]. Tetracyclines are teratogenic and reach the fetus via the placenta.

Table 2.
2A II tetracyclines.

Origin	Tigecycline is a semisynthetic derivative of minocycline developed against resistant organisms [41].
Mechanism of action	Its reversal binding to 30S ribosomes is stronger by five times, and ribosomal protection proteins do not affect it [42, 43].
Routes	Due to poor oral absorption, it is available in IV formulations.
Indication	Complicated SSTI, Complicated intraabdominal infections (cIAIs), CABP, Used as salvage therapy in critically ill patients when no other alternatives exist for multidrug-resistant infections (MDR).
Resistance	It is due to increased efflux pumps such as AcrAB and MexAB-OprM after detecting the drug [44]. *Pseudomonas* is intrinsically resistant due to MexXY efflux pump presence [45].
Pharmac-okinetics	Adequate tissue distribution was observed with a half-life of 37 to 67 hours and a plasma protein binding of about 80% [46]. No dose adjustment is required in renal impairment and mild to moderate hepatic impairment. Dose adjustment is needed for severe hepatic impairment. It is not removed by hemodialysis [47]. It is excreted by the liver and minimally by the kidney.
Toxicity/Adverse effects	GI: nausea, vomiting, transaminase elevation, acute pancreatitis. Others: infection, phlebitis, headache, dizziness, skin rash [47]. It is associated with increased mortality compared to other antibiotics used for the same indication. 13 clinical trials have validated this pooled analysis [48].

Table 3.
2A III glycylcyclines.

Origin	Erythromycin was obtained from *Streptomyces erythreus* present in the soil. Azithromycin and Clarithromycin are semisynthetic derivatives from erythromycin, which improve stability in gastric acid [49].
Mechanism of action	Macrolides bind to 23S ribosomal ribonucleic acid (rRNA), a subunit of the 50S subunit of the bacterial ribosome, and stop the RNA-based synthesis of proteins [50]. Bactericidal activity is seen against , *Hemophilus influenzae,* and *Streptococcus pneumoniae.*
Routes	It is available as oral liquid, tablet, capsule, IV, ophthalmic and topical preparations.
Indication	Erythromycin: used as an alternative to penicillin (PCN) in allergic patients. Treatment and preexposure prophylaxis in pertussis. Azithromycin: CABP, Pertussis, Trachoma, Chancroid, Babesiosis, *Mycobacterium avium complex* (MAC) infections, alternative for Lyme disease, sinusitis, pharyngitis, and acute otitis media. Clarithromycin: *Helicobacter pylori* infection, Nontubercular mycobacterial infection, *Campylobacter* enteritis, *MAC* infections
Resistance	50S ribosomal protein mutations or 23S rRNA receptor alterations confer resistance to macrolides (M), lincosamides (L), and streptogramin B (SB) (MLSB phenotype). *Erm* (erythromycin ribosome methylation) genes present on transposons or plasmids mediate this effect [51, 52].
Pharmac-okinetics	Erythromycin is metabolized by hepatic CYP3A cytochrome subclass of cytochrome 450 system. It is incompatible with other IV preparations [53, 54]. It follows total body water distribution [55] and persists in tissues longer than in blood. Oral azithromycin bioavailability is around 37% [56]. It is well distributed in tissues with levels > than in blood by 10 to 100 fold. It is excreted primarily unchanged via hepatic clearance into the feces. No dose adjustments are required for renal and hepatic impairment. Clarithromycin oral bioavailability is 55%, has excellent tissue distribution, and undergoes mainly hepatic clearance with 30% clearance vis the kidneys [50]. Dose adjustment is needed for renal failure only [57].
Toxicity/Adverse effects	Erythromycin: GI side effects (nausea, vomiting, and abdominal pain), Thrombophlebitis, Allergic reactions, Ototoxicity, Torsades de pointes. Clarithromycin and Azithromycin: GI side effects as above, Acute mania, Torsades de pointes, reversible cholestatic hepatitis [58–60].

Table 4.
2A IV macrolides.

Origin	Lincomycin is derived from *Streptomyces lincolnensis* present in the soil. Clindamycin is semisynthetically by chemically modifying lincomycin resulting in increased potency and bioavailability [61].
Mechanism of action	It binds to 50S ribosomal sites and inhibits protein synthesis, and competes with macrolides for the same site.
Routes	Available in IV, oral capsules and liquid solution, topical gel, foam or solution, and vaginal cream or suppository.
Indication	Gram-positive or anaerobic SSTI, acne vulgaris, part of the combination regimen against toxoplasmosis, falciparum malaria, and *Pneumocystis jiroveci* pneumonia.
Resistance	MLSB phenotype regulated by the ermA or ermC genes [62]. rRNA mutations, including the receptor site, 23S rRNA nucleotide methylation, and adenylation of clindamycin [51, 63–65].
Pharmac-okinetics	90% oral bioavailability with good tissue levels except in CSF [61, 66]. It is metabolized by the liver, and excretion occurs via feces and urine [67]. Dosing adjustment is needed in severe renal and hepatic impairment
Toxicity/Adverse effects	Cutaneous drug reactions in patients with (human leukocyte antigen)HLA-B*51:01 genotype including maculopapular eruptions, erythema multiforme, urticaria, drug rash with eosinophilia, and systemic symptoms (DRESS), SJS, TEN [68]. GI: diarrhea, pseudomembranous colitis by *Clostridioides difficile,* reversible transaminitis [69]. Others: agranulocytosis, thrombocytopenia, and neutropenia which are transient.

Table 5.
2A V lincosamides.

Two other newer tetracycline derivatives have been released Eravacycline, a fluorocycline, and Omadacycline, an aminomethylcycline., while omadacycline has been approved for SSTI and CABP. In contrast, Eravacycline has been approved for cIAI [94, 95]. Similar to tigecycline, neither of these agents cover pseudomonas.

Origin	Linezolid and Tedizolid are derived from 5-(halomethyl)-3-aryl-2-oxazolidinones (organic synthesis) by chemical modification. Unique structure with no cross-resistance seen.
Mechanism of action	Halts bacterial protein synthesis by binding to the V-domain of 23S RNA, a part of the 50S ribosomal unit [70]. Efficacy is proportional to the drug level area under the curve AUC/MIC ratio.
Routes	Available as oral tablets and IV formulations.
Indication	Linezolid: MSSA/MRSA nosocomial pneumonia, CABP, Gram-positive complicated and uncomplicated SSTI, *Vancomycin-resistant Enterococcus* (VRE) infections, Nocardiosis. Tedizolid: Gram-positive SSTI.
Resistance	It is <1% and due to 23S rRNA domain V region receptor site mutation, cfr (chloramphenicol-florfenicol resistance) ribosomal RNA methyltransferase, and optrA causing adenylation [71–73].
Pharmac-okinetics	Linezolid: oral bioavailability is 100%, excellent tissue distribution, and 31% plasma protein-bound [74]. It is oxidized and renally excreted. No dosage adjustment is needed. Tedizolid: oral bioavailability is 91% with adequate tissue distribution and 80% plasma protein-bound. It undergoes hepatic clearance with 20% excreted renally. No dosage adjustment is needed [75, 76].
Toxicity/Adverse effects	Blood: Thrombocytopenia, pancytopenia, pure red cell aplasia, and reversible myelosuppression [77]. Mitochondrial toxicity: lactic acidosis, peripheral and optic neuropathy [78–80]. Others: Serotonin syndrome with serotonergic medications, tooth and tongue discoloration, and hypoglycemia [78, 81, 82].

Table 6.
2A VI oxazolidinones.

Origin	It was derived from the fungus *Fusidium coccineum*.
Mechanism of action	It inhibits protein synthesis by preventing the translocation, elongation phase, and blocking the elongation factor G (EF-G) effect on the ribosome, making the bacteria susceptible to phagocytosis due to reduced surface proteins [83, 84]. It is active against MSSA, MRSA, *Coagulase-negative staphylococci*, *Clostridium spp*, *Peptostreptococcus*, and most anaerobes except for *Fusoabcterium spp*.
Routes	Available in oral, eye, topical, and IV formulations.
Indication	As a part of a combination regimen against staphylococcal SSTI and bone infections, especially with rifampin or beta-lactams.
Resistance	Chromosomal or plasmid-mediated mutations in the gene encoding the EF-G (fusA, fusB, fusC, and fusE).
Pharmac-okinetics	Newer film-coated tablets have better oral bioavailability, highly plasma protein-bound with adequate intracellular and tissue penetration [85, 86]. It undergoes hepatic metabolism and needs dose adjustment with hepatic impairment [87].
Toxicity/Adverse effects	Nausea, diarrhea, vomiting, and elevated bilirubin due to bile transport blockade. When used along with statin, the risk of rhabdomyolysis is observed after 20 to 30 days after therapy initiation [88].

Table 7.
2A VII fusidane (fusidic acid).

No dosing modification is needed for renal or hepatic impairment. They are teratogenic, and the anticoagulant dose needs adjustment when used concomitantly. A slightly increased mortality was observed in the CABP trial of omadacycline [94].

Azithromycin is an excellent choice for treating CABP caused by atypical organisms such as *Mycoplasma pneumoniae*, *Legionella* spp., *Chlamydia pneumoniae,* and *Coxiella burnetti.* An important fact is to remember the numerous interactions this class has with other medications, and also, it can prolong the QT interval resulting in ventricular tachyarrythmias.

When used in the therapy for staphylococcal infections, it is prudent always to perform a "D" test to identify any chance of inducible resistance. It is recommended not to use clindamycin as an empirical regimen against streptococcal infections due to a higher risk of resistance. Clindamycin can suppress the cyclosporine effect and can cause neuromuscular blockade.

Linezolid is an alternative for vancomycin in MRSA/MSSA pneumonia and is used in combination regimens for nosocomial pneumonia. It is an alternative in Nocardiosis and a part of combination regimens in the therapy of *Mycobacterium tuberculosis*, *Mycobacterium avium complex,* and *Mycobacterium abscessus complex*.

3. Bactericidal antibiotics

These include glycopeptides in **Table 8** (3A I), lipoglycopeptides in **Table 9** (3A II), lipopeptides in **Table 10** (3A III), aminoglycosides in **Table 11** (3A IV), quinolones in **Table 12** (3A V), penicillin in **Table 13** (3A VI), cephalosporins in **Table 14** (3A VII), beta-lactamase and beta-lactamase inhibitor combinations in **Table 15** (3A VIII), monobactams in **Table 16** (3A IX), carbapenems in **Table 17** (3A X), polymixins in **Table 18** (3A XI), epoxide in **Table 19** (3A XII), pleuromutilin in **Table 20** (3A XIII), rifamycins in **Table 21** (3A XIV) and metronidazole in **Table 22** (3A XV).

An increased risk of renal failure is observed when vancomycin is administered along with aminoglycosides and piperacillin-tazobactam [218, 219]. If a VRE strain susceptibility reveals sensitivity to teicoplanin, it should be avoided due to resistance emergence during therapy. When teicoplanin is used for IE, bone, and joint infections as a monotherapy, the recommendation is to keep serum levels close to 20 μg/mL and, if needed >30 μg/mL [220]. A higher AUC/MIC ratio is related to better clinical outcomes and decreased mortality with vancomycin therapy [221].

The lipoglycopeptides have a longer half-life and are currently undergoing trials for bacteremia, joint infections, osteomyelitis.

Retrospective data indicate higher cure rates and lower mortality when a higher dose (> 8 mg/kg/day) of daptomycin is used [222]. In the therapeutic failure of vancomycin therapy, a suggestion is to use a higher dose of daptomycin or combine it with a beta-lactam or aminoglycoside or TMP-SMX to increase its bactericidal activity. In VRE endocarditis with bacteremia, daptomycin with beta-lactam is an ideal combination to prevent the emergence of resistance [223, 224]. Due to lack of CNS penetration, it should not be used in the therapy for meningitis [225]. Daptomycin is inactivated by the pulmonary surfactant and is rendered ineffective in bronchoalveolar pneumonia but is adequate in hematogenous pneumonia [226]. In patients with chronic kidney disease and on dialysis, more frequent monitoring of CPK is ideal. CPK monitoring is a must if the patient is on statins for hyperlipidemia. It needs to be stopped if the CPK levels are >1000 units/L with clinical features of myopathy or > 2000 (ten times the upper limit) with no myopathy features [123].

Origin	Vancomycin was derived from *Amycolatopsis orientalis*. Teicoplannin was isolated from *Actinoplanes teichomyceticus*. Teicoplanin has not been approved in the United States as it did not offer any advantage over vancomycin.
Mechanism of action	Cell wall synthesis is stopped by inhibition of transpeptidation and disaccharide subunits incorporation into peptidoglycan.
Routes	Vancomycin is available in oral, IV, intrathecal, intraventricular, intraperitoneal, and intraocular formulations. Teicoplanin is available in oral, intramuscular, and IV formulations.
Indication	Vancomycin: Gram-positive and MRSA SSTI, MRSA bacteremia, MRSA native and prosthetic valve IE, Vancomycin sensitive Enterococcal IE, *Corynebacterium jeikeium* and *striatum* infections, MRSA meningitis, and ventriculitis, MRSA pneumonia, joint infections, and osteomyelitis. Pseudomembranous colitis by *Clostridioides difficile*, Febrile neutropenia, Pre-procedure surgical prophylaxis. Teicoplanin: MRSA bacteremia, Gram-positive and MRSA SSTI, Alternative for IE due to *Streptococci viridans* and *Enterococci*, Pseudomembranous colitis by Clostridioides difficile, Pre-procedure surgical prophylaxis.
Resistance	Vancomycin: mecA and mecC encode for a low-affinity penicillin-binding protein PBP2a and PBP2c. Some MRSA strains acquire the VanA gene from enterococci species. Enterococci with VanA, VanB, VanC, VanD, VanE, VanG, VanL, VanM and VanN genes encode a ligase assembling the last two amino acids or peptidoglycan precursors, resulting in a peptidoglycan precursor with less affinity for glycopeptides. Teicoplanin: All *Vancomycin intermediate Staphylococcus aureus* (VISA) strains are cross-resistant [96]. Enterococci containing the above Van genes render them resistant to it.
Pharmac-okinetics	Vancomycin: Oral intake results in minimal absorption. When given IV, efficacy is best indicated by 24 hour AUC/MIC ratio ≥ 400 associated with lower clinical failure [97]. Adequate CSF levels are seen in infection [98]. It is renally excreted with no tubular secretion or absorption, and creatinine clearance inversely affects its serum level. In obese patients, the dosing should be based on actual body weight instead of ideal weight due to increased distribution volume [99]. Therapy needs to be monitored with trough levels (correlate with AUC/MIC ratio) to prevent toxicity. Dose adjustment is needed with renal failure. Teicoplanin: Poor oral absorption, 90% bound to plasma protein, and highly bound in tissues. It reaches adequate concentrations in all tissues except for vitreous and CSF, even with infection. It undergoes renal clearance, and dosing adjustments are needed in renal failure. Trough levels ≥28 μg/mL are associated with hepatotoxicity. Monitoring not needed if dose used is <12 mg/kg/day. It has a long half-life of 83 to 168 hours [100].
Toxicity/Adverse effects	Frequently seen when the trough levels are ≥15 μg/mL with a treatment duration of >7 days [101]. Infusion-related reactions: red man syndrome, hypotension, and cardiac arrest. Others: Nephrotoxicity, Ototoxicity, Neutropenia, Thrombocytopenia, and DRESS [102–104]. Teicoplanin: Nephrotoxicity, fever, maculopapular rash, red man syndrome.

Table 8.
3A I glycopeptides.

Streptogramins are another class of lipopeptides rarely used currently. They are made up of two macrocyclic lactone peptolide components. They are labeled as streptogramin A, and streptogramin B. Quinupristin-Dalfopristin is a 30: 70 ratio IV formulation available for therapy. These components are bacteriostatic as dalfopristin ends protein synthesis by binding to 50S ribosomal unit and quinupristin prevents peptide elongation. Dalfopristin binding increases the affinity to quinupristin due to structural change resulting in synergistic bactericidal activity. It is currently used as an alternative for MSSA or streptococcal SSTI. It needs a central line for administration as it is an irritant and can cause thrombophlebitis [227].

Origin	Telavancin is a vancomycin derivative post alkylation [105]. Dalbavancin is a semisynthetic derivation from teicoplanin like glycopeptide, a fermentation product of Nonomuraea spp. Oritavancin is a semisynthetic derivation from lipoglycopeptide chloroeremomycin.
Mechanism of action	Telavancin: binds to peptidoglycan precursors, inhibits transglycosylation, and inhibits cell wall synthesis. It also disrupts cell wall homeostasis [106]. Dalbavancin: binds to peptidoglycan precursors with higher affinity and inhibits cell wall synthesis. Oritavancin: Binds to peptidoglycan precursors, stops transglycosylation, transpeptidation and inhibits cell wall synthesis. It disrupts the cell wall membrane [107].
Routes	Telavancin: available in IV formulations Dalbavancin: available in IV formulations Oritavancin: available in IV formulations
Indication	Telavancin: Acute gram-positive bacterial SSTI Dalbavancin: Acute gram-positive bacterial SSTI Oritavancin: Acute gram-positive bacterial SSTI in adults only
Resistance	Telavancin: VRE containing VanA gene are resistant to it [108]. Dalbavancin: is bacteriostatic against VISA strains, no activity against VanA but is active against VanB and VanC possessing bacterial strains. Oritavancin: VanZ gene and mutations in vanSB sensor gene ofthevanBcluster confer cross-resistance to teicoplanin and oritavancin [109].
Pharmac-okinetics	Telavancin: Tissue distribution is similar to vancomycin, 90% plasma protein bound, undergoes renal clearance and dose adjustment needed in renal failure [105]. It is recommended to avoid use in severe acute renal failure. Dalbavancin: High volume tissue distribution, plasma protein binding of 93%, and a half-life of 8 to 9 days. It undergoes primarily renal clearance with the remaining via feces. It requires dose modification in renal failure [110]. The best predictor of its activity is the 24-hour AUC/MIC. Oritavancin: High volume tissue distribution, plasma protein binding of 85–90%, and a half-life of 10 days. It gets intracellularly retained in the liver, kidneys, lungs, and lymphoid tissue, from where it is released slowly. No dosage adjustment is done for mild to moderate liver or renal impairment.
Toxicity/Adverse effects	Telavancin: prolongs the QTc interval, nephrotoxicity, nausea, vomiting, chills, and creatinine rise. It is teratogenic. Dalbavancin: pruritis, vomiting, nausea, infusion reactions, skin, and hypersensitive reactions. Oritavancin: nausea, headache, vomiting, diarrhea, mild transaminitis, hypersensitive reactions. Drug interactions can be seen as it inhibits cytochrome P450 enzymes.

Table 9.
3A II lipoglycopeptides.

Origin	Daptomycin is a lipopeptide antibiotic isolated from *Streptomyces roseosporus.*
Mechanism of action	It is an antimicrobial peptide of cation origin attaching to the cell wall in the presence of calcium, disrupting the cell wall structure by displacing the cell wall proteins and formation of an oligomer in the cell wall. This action is unalterable, causing impaired cell wall function and leakage of ions leading to cell death [111–113].
Routes	Available in only IV formulations
Indication	Acute SSTI by MSSA, MRSA, *Enterococcus faecalis*, streptococcal species (as an alternative in glycopeptide therapy failure or intolerance or higher MRSA vancomycin MIC. Acute MSSA, MRSA bacteremia, and right-sided endocarditis [114].
Resistance	Cell wall changes with increased fluidity, net positive charge, and lack of depolarization or permeability decreased phosphatidylglycerol, leading to daptomycin resistance. Multiple genes are involved in this, including mprF, yycFG, vraSR, dlt, rpoB, rpoC, pgsA, and cls [115–118].

Pharmac-okinetics	It has a long half of 7.3 to 9.6 hrs with a small distribution volume and is highly bound to plasma proteins (90% - 93%) [119, 120]. It gets excreted via the renal system unchanged. Dose adjustment is needed in acute renal failure and dialysis patients. It has poor penetration into CSF [121]. It is inactivated by the pulmonary surfactant leading to ineffectiveness against bronchioalveolar pneumonia. It exerts a dose-dependent postantibiotic effect longer than vancomycin [122].
Toxicity/Adverse effects	Higher doses (>8 mg/kg/day) results in elevation of serum creatinine phosphokinase (CPK) levels with no muscle cell lysis or fibrosis [123]. CPK level monitoring during therapy is a must. Peripheral neuropathy with paraesthesia and dysesthesia. Acute eosinophilic pneumonia (after ten days of therapy)

Table 10.
3A III lipopeptides.

Origin	Aminoglycoside with the name ending in mycin is derived from *Streptomyces* [124]. Aminoglycoside with the name ending in micin is derived from *Micromonospora spp.* Fermentation products: Neomycin, Gentamicin, Kanamycin Semisynthetic derivatives: Amikacin, Netilmicin
Mechanism of action	Cationic aminoglycosides bind to the anionic lipopolysaccharides and disrupt their structure resulting in cell wall leaks and altered permeability. Once in the cytosol, it binds reversibly to ribosomal decoder acceptance site on 16S reverse transfer RNA portion of messenger RNA (mRNA), a 30S subunit of prokaryotic ribosomes. This decreases the mRNA translocation and translation stopping protein synthesis [125–128]. They demonstrate the postantibiotic effect, synergistic behavior with other antibiotics, and concentration-dependent effect.
Routes	Available in IV and oral formulations.
Indication	Empirical therapy of aerobic gram-negative bacilli (GNB) including *Pseudomonas spp*. As a part of a combination therapy for HAP, *Enterococcal* bacteremia, and IE due to *enterococcus* and *streptococcus spp*. Acute urinary tract infection and cystic fibrosis exacerbations. Preoperative prophylaxis in gastrointestinal and genitourinary procedures.
Resistance	Altered cell wall membrane with diminished interaction, active efflux pumps resulting in lesser concentration in the cytosol [129, 130]. Decreased ribosomal binding due to mutation or methylation of the binding site [131]. Inactivation of the aminoglycosides by phosphorylation, adenylation, and nucleotidation [132]. Induce biofilm formation [133].
Pharmac-okinetics	Plasma protein binding is low, highly soluble in water, with distribution resembling extracellular fluid compartments [134, 135]. Appropriate concentrations are attained in all body fluids except for CSF and vitreous humor [136–138]. They undergo renal clearance unchanged with minimal excretion via feces [139]. Dose adjustment is needed in renal failure.
Toxicity/Adverse effects	Nephrotoxicity Ototoxicity includes both cochlear and vestibular Neuromuscular blockade

Table 11.
3A IV aminoglycosides.

Due to the lack of active intrinsic electron transport chain and cell membrane potential difference, the anaerobic bacteria are resistant to aminoglycosides. *Enterococci* are intrinsically resistant to aminoglycosides [228]. Once-daily dosing is effective as traditional multiple doses, decreases the risk of ototoxicity and nephrotoxicity, is straightforward, and is economical towards resources and time [229]. This dosing pattern does not decline neuromuscular function in sick intubated patients but needs evaluation in cystic fibrosis, meningitis, and osteomyelitis caused by aerobic gram-negative bacilli [230–232]. The once-daily dose should be used

Origin	Initially derived as a byproduct of chloroquine synthesis, the newer quinolones are semisynthetic with chemical modifications to increase their efficacy and absorption.
Mechanism of action	Inhibit deoxyribonucleic acid (DNA) synthesis by inhibiting DNA gyrase and topoisomerase IV. It also leads to hydroxy radicals, damaging the bacterial cellular molecules causing bacterial cell death [140, 141].
Routes	Available as oral, IV, and eye drop formulations
Indication	Acute cystitis, Acute uncomplicated, and cUTI. Acute Bacterial prostatitis, Sexually transmitted disease, PID, *Chlamydiae trachomatis*, *Hemophilus ducreyi*. Acute bacterial gastroenteritis due to *Shigella spp*, *Campylobacter jejuni*, Cholera, Typhoid, *Nontyphoidal Salmonellae* gastroenteritis in specific patients. Acute intraabdominal infections, Spontaneous bacterial peritonitis (SBP). Acute CABP, Acute bronchitis, Aspiration pneumonia, Lung abscess, HAP, *stenotrophomonas* infections. Acute osteomyelitis, Acute native and prosthetic joint infections, SSTI. MDR pulmonary tuberculosis, Nontuberculous mycobacterial infections, GNB susceptible organisms causing meningitis, Prophylaxis in neutropenic patients.
Resistance	Chromosomal gene mutations alter DNA gyrase, and topoisomerase IV decreases cell membrane permeability. Plasmid-mediated genes enabling acetylation and efflux pumps decreasing efficacy.
Pharmac-okinetics	Excellent oral bioavailability and food can alter absorption [142]. Plasma protein binding is low except for delafloxacin and gemifloxacin. Tissue distribution is excellent, with above serum levels seen in bile, prostate, kidney, lung, and stool [143]. Levofloxacin and moxifloxacin attain adequate CSF penetration [144]. Levofloxacin, ofloxacin, ciprofloxacin undergo renal clearance, whereas moxifloxacin undergoes hepatic metabolism. Dose adjustment is needed in renal insufficiency [145].
Toxicity/Adverse effects	GI: vomiting, nausea, abdominal discomfort, diarrhea, *Clostridioides difficile* associated diarrhea [146]. CNS: headache, dizziness, mood changes, peripheral neuropathy [147, 148]. Skin: allergy and skin reactions such as maculopapular rash, phototoxicity [149, 150]. Others: hypoglycemia, prolongs QT interval, increased risk of aortic aneurysm and dissection, retinal detachment, tendinitis with arthropathy [151–155].

Table 12.
3A V quinolones.

Origin	PCN was isolated from *Penicillium chrysogenum* in 1928 by Alexander Fleming [156]. Chemical modifications created numerous semisynthetic PCNs. Natural PCNs: PCN V, PCN G. Penicillinase resistant PCN: Methicillin. Nafcillin, Oxacillin. Aminopenicillins: Amoxicillin, Ampicillin. Carboxypenicillins: Ticarcillin and Carbenicillin. Ureidopenicillins: Piperacillin, Azlocillin and Mezlocillin.
Mechanism of action	PCNs bind to multiple PBP simultaneously, stopping the cell wall synthesis and creating hydroxy radicals that permanently damage the cell. PCNs do not affect dormant bacteria [141, 157].
Routes	Oral, IV, and intramuscular (IM) formulations are available.
Indication	IV PCN G is the antibiotic of choice for PCN susceptible strains causing pneumococcal and meningococcal meningitis, streptococcal IE, and neurosyphilis. Benzathine PCN is used in syphilis treatment and for rheumatic fever prophylaxis. Oral PCN V or G or Benzathine PCN are used to stop outbreaks of streptococcal infection. Intrapartum prophylaxis with PCN is used at membrane rupture or at labor to prevent *Streptococcal agalactiae* infections in colonized patients. PCNase resistant PCNs are the agent of choice for MSSA infections and an alternative to treat streptococcal infections. AminoPCNs treat UTI, Upper and lower airway infections, Gastroenteritis, IE, Meningitis by susceptible non-beta- lactamase organisms. IV ampicillin is the treatment of choice for *Enterococcus faecalis* IE and other infections. Amoxicillin is a part of the combination regimen against *Helicobacter pylori.* Oral amoxicillin or ampicillin are used as prophylaxis in asplenic

	or agammaglobulinemia patients to prevent infections by capsulated organisms. Ampicillin-sulbactam is the drug of choice for aspiration pneumonia. Piperacillin-tazobactam is an antipseudomonal and is also used for necrotizing fasciitis, susceptible GNB infections.
Resistance	Presence of beta-lactamase [158]. Alteration of cell membrane permeability with a decreased intracellular entry (absence of porin) [159]. Presence of efflux pumps [159]. Synthesis of PBP with decreased affinity for the beta-lactam [160].
Pharmac-okinetics	PCNs vary in their oral absorption and plasma protein binding. The tissue distribution is more than adequate in most tissues. The primary route of excretion is via the renal system, whereas some undergo biliary excretion too.
Toxicity/Adverse effects	Hypersensitivity reactions: rash, anaphylaxis, exfoliative dermatitis, allergic vasculitis, SJS, and TEN [161]. GI: nausea, vomiting, diarrhea, Clostridioides difficile associated diarrhea, liver function test abnormality with oxacillin in patients with HLA-B 5701 [162, 163]. Hematological: neutropenia [164]. Renal: Nephrotoxicity, allergic interstitial nephritis [165]. CNS: Myoclonic seizures.

Table 13.
3A VI penicillin (beta-lactams).

Origin	Semisynthetic derivatives of Cephalosporin C isolated from *Acremonium chrysogenum* [166]. First-generation: cefazolin, cephalexin, and cefadroxil. Second generation: cefprozil and cefuroxime, cephamycin: cefoxitin Third generation: cefdinir, cefditoren, cefixime, cefotaxime, cefpodoxime, ceftazidime, ceftibuten, ceftriaxone. Fourth generation: Cefepime, Cefpirome. Fifth-generation: Ceftaroline, ceftobiprole. Siderophore cephalosporins: Cefiderocol.
Mechanism of action	They bind to PBPs and stop transpeptidation and block the cell wall synthesis resulting in a bactericidal effect with a postantibiotic effect [167]. MRSA active cephalosporins bind to PBP2A, whereas the other cephalosporins bind to PBP1A&B in gram negatives [168]. Cephalosporins active against gram-positive organisms bind to PBP 2&3 (186). Cefiderocol binds to iron and enters the bacteria via siderophores into the periplasmic space and binds to PBP in addition to being a poor substrate for efflux pumps [169].
Routes	First, second and third generations are available in oral and parenteral (IV/IM) formulations. The fourth and fifth-generation are available in IV formulations. Fifth-generation are available in IV formulations. Siderophore cephalosporins: available in IV formulations.
Indication	First-generation: oral therapy for MSSA and *Streptococcal* SSTI outpatient, susceptible *Streptococcal* SSTI, MSSA IE, the prophylactic antibiotic of choice for prosthesis implantation and surgical procedures with a high risk of infection except for intraabdominal procedures. Second generation: as a part of a combination regimen for PID (cefoxitin), nontuberculous mycobacterial infection (cefoxitin), cefuroxime for acute otitis media, pharyngitis, maxillary sinusitis, and an alternative for Lyme disease [170, 171]. Third generation: treatment of susceptible GNB bacilli induced SSTI, Prosthetic joint infection (PJI), CABP, cUTI, and peritonitis [172]. Empirical therapy for CABP, acute bronchitis, and meningitis. IM single dose for Neisseria gonorrhea and chancroid [173]. Lyme disease and an alternative for PCN allergic patients with syphilis, typhoid fever, and shigellosis [174, 175]. Monotherapy for *Streptococcal* IE [176]. Ceftazidime is the drug of choice for susceptible *Pseudomonas spp* infections, including CNS [177]. Fourth generation: antibiotic of choice for infections caused by AmpC (Class C beta-lactamases) inducible resistant organisms [178]. Febrile neutropenia monotherapy or a part of a combination regimen [179]. Empirical therapy in severe CABP, HAP by *Pseudomonas spp* or resistant *Enterobacteriaceae* [180]. It is an alternative for susceptible GNB meningitis, bacteremia, SSTI, PJI and cUTI. Fifth-generation: Ceftaroline used for MRSA pneumonia, CABP, SSTI, HAP, and in combination with daptomycin for daptomycin resistant MRSA infections [181–183]. Ceftobiprole also is an alternative for *Pseduomonal spp* infections. Siderophore cephalosporins:

	approved for use in cUTI by *Enterobacterales & P. aeruginosa*, HAP, and VAP by the *Enterobacterales, P. aeruginosa, and Acinetobacter baumannii complex* [169].
Resistance	Beta-lactamase hydrolyzes the antibiotic. Cell wall membrane changes alter the entry of antibiotics through the lipopolysaccharide layer. Efflux pumps removing the antibiotic from the periplasmic space. PBP changes to alter antibiotic binding.
Pharmac-okinetics	The first three generations are water-soluble and come in oral and parenteral formulations, whereas the fourth and fifth-generation are parenteral only. Distribution is dependent on their lipid solubility and plasma protein binding. They reveal higher serum concentrations and lower tissue levels. The third and fourth generations attain adequate CNS concentrations. Most of them undergo renal clearance except for ceftriaxone and cefoperazone, which undergo biliary excretion. Probenecid inhibits tubular secretion of cephalosporins and increases their half-life. Renal failure will need a dose adjustment. Ceftriaxone dose is adjusted with simultaneous renal and hepatic impairment [184]. Cefiderocol is excreted renally and needs renal dose adjustment [185].
Toxicity/Adverse effects	Hypersensitivity reactions: immunoglobulin E (IgE)-mediated reactions occur in <1 in 100,000 patients; fever, rash, eosinophilia, serum sickness, and anaphylaxis are seen. Cross-reaction frequency is ≤1%. Hematology: eosinophilia, neutropenia (prolonged use), anemia, thrombocytopenia, hypoprothrombinemia, impaired platelet aggregation, hemolytic anemia (ceftriaxone). Nephrology: allergic interstitial nephritis GI: nausea, vomiting, diarrhea, *Clostridioides difficile* infection, biliary pseudolithiasis (ceftriaxone), transaminitis. CNS: seizures, encephalopathy Others: fever, disulfiram-like reaction, phlebitis.

Table 14.
3A VII cephalosporins.

Combinations	Augmentin = Amoxicillin + Clauvulinic acid in an 2:1, 4:1,7:1 ratio (isolated from *Streptomyces clavuligerus* [186]. Unasyn = Ampicillin + Sulbactam in an 2:1 ratio Sulperazone = Cefoperazone + Sulbactam in an 1:1 ratio Zosyn = Piperacillin + Tazobactam in an 8:1 ratio Zerbaxa = Ceftolazone + Tazobactam in a 2:1 ratio Avycaz, Zavicefta = Ceftazidime + Avibactam in a 4:1 ratio Vabomere = Meropenem + Vaborbactam in a 1:1 ratio
Mechanism of action	Clavulanic acid: is potent and inhibits class A beta-lactamase and some extended-spectrum beta-lactamases (ESBL). Sulbactam: is a broad-spectrum inhibitor than clavulanic acid but less potent (inhibits class A beta-lactamases). Tazobactam: spectrum is similar to sulbactam but is more potent. Avibactam: inhibits class A beta-lactamases, including ESBL, *Klebsiella pneumoniae* carbapenemase (KPC), class C, and some class D beta-lactamases. It does not stop Metall0beta-lactamases (MBL). Vaborbactam: inhibits class A beta-lactamases including ESBL, KPC, class C beta-lactamases with no effect on MBL and class D beta-lactamases.
Routes	Augmentin: available orally and IV formulations. Unasyn: available in IV formulations Sulperazone: available in IV formulations Zosyn: available in IV formulations Zerbaxa: available in IV formulations Avycaz, Zavicefta: available in IV formulations Vabomere: available in IV formulations
Indication	Augmentin: acute otitis media, acute sinusitis, outpatient CABP by susceptible organisms with a higher dose, diabetic foot infection, SSTI, human or animal bites. Unasyn: as a part of a combination regimen against MDR *Acinetobacter baumannii* infection, SSTI, cIAIs, and obstetric and gynecological infections. Sulperazone: treatment of *A. baumannii* infection Zosyn: treatment of pneumonia, SSTI, cIAIs, febrile neutropenia, and polymicrobial infections [187]. Zerbaxa: indicated in cUTI, cIAIs, and Carbapenemase resistant *Pseudomonas aeruginosa* infections. Avycaz, Zavicefta: indicated in cUTI, cIAIs, HAP, and KPC *Enterobacteriaceae* infections. Vabomere: indicated in KPC *Enterobacteriaceae* infections and cUTI.
Resistance	Augmentin: plasmid-mediated beta-lactamase TEM-1 and OXA-1 (Oxacillin beta-lactamases) [188]. Unasyn: cephalosporinase, ESBL, and carbapenemase production by resistant strains. Sulperazone: cephalosporinase, ESBL, and carbapenemase

	production by resistant strains. Zosyn: ESBL and carbapenemase production by resistant strains. Zerbaxa: carbapenemase production KPC, OXA, ESBL, and MBL by resistant strains. Avycaz, Zavicefta: porin mutations, efflux pumps, and MBL. Vabomere: coproduction of KPC and class B or D beta-lactamases, porin mutations, and efflux pumps [189].
Pharmacokinetics	Augmentin: well absorbed orally and undergoes renal clearance with dosing adjustment needed in renal impairment. It does not penetrate CSF but reaches therapeutic levels in the peritoneum, bile, tonsils, and middle ear. Unasyn: renally cleared and dose adjustment needed in renal insufficiency. Levels in peritoneal and intestinal fluids are the same as in serum with minimal CSF penetration. Sulperazone: available in IV formulations Zosyn: renally cleared and will need a dose adjustment and minimal CSF penetration. Zerbaxa: renally cleared and will need a dose adjustment. Avycaz, Zavicefta: gets excreted renally unchanged, and dosage adjustment is a must when creat clearance is <50 mL/min. Vabomere: the majority of the drug undergoes renal clearance so that it will need dose adjustment with renal insufficiency.
Toxicity/Adverse effects	Augmentin: skin reactions, delayed hypersensitivity, diarrhea, and nausea. Unasyn: occasional transaminitis and similar reactions as seen with ampicillin Sulperazone: occasional transaminitis and similar reactions as seen with ampicillin. Zosyn: platelet dysfunction, immune thrombocytopenia, allergic reactions, renal failure, Clostridioides difficile infection [190, 191]. Zerbaxa: headache, nausea, diarrhea, *Clostridioides difficile* infection Avycaz, Zavicefta: anxiety, nausea, vomiting, and constipation. Vabomere: phlebitis, headache, diarrhea, and infusion site reactions.

Table 15.
3A VIII beta-lactamase inhibitors and beta-lactam combinations.

Origin	It is a semisynthetic derivation of a biochemical substance isolated from *Chromobacterium violaceum*.
Mechanism of action	It avidly binds to PBP3 of aerobic GNB, inhibiting cell wall synthesis resulting in death [192]. It remains active against all class B beta-lactamases and the majority of class A and D beta-lactamases. It is destroyed by KPC, ESBLs, and AmpC beta-lactamases if present in a larger quantity.
Routes	Available in IV formulations.
Indication	As an alternative in susceptible aerobic GNB infections in patients with beta-lactam allergy. As a part of a combination regimen against MBL producing GNB infections.
Resistance	It is via efflux pumps and alterations to the PBP3 binding site [193].
Pharmacokinetics	Orally it is absorbed poorly with 56% plasma protein binding after IV administration. Excellent tissue distribution with CSF penetration. Excretion is renally, and dose adjustment is needed in renal impairment and severe hepatic impairment.
Toxicity/Adverse effects	Nausea, vomiting, diarrhea, rash, phlebitis [194]. Crossreaction with other beta-lactams is rare even in patients with anaphylaxis to other beta-lactams.

Table 16.
3A IX monobactams.

cautiously in IE patients [176]. Inhaled aminoglycosides used in conjunction with a beta-lactam reveal better clinical outcomes [233]. For endophthalmitis and intracranial infections, they need to be administered locally (direct intravitreal injection, intraventricular administration). Aminoglycoside combination regimens diminish the emergence of resistant strains to the companion antibiotic and aminoglycoside. The synergistic antibiotic effect is observed when aminoglycoside is combined with an anti-cell wall antibiotic (beta-lactam). This combination is effective in the therapy of MSSA, enterococci, *pseudomonas spp*, and *Streptococcal viridans* infections but not in MRSA infections.

Origin	They are semisynthetic derivatives from thienamycin, an antibiotic isolated from *Streptomyces cattleya*. The human renal enzyme dehydropeptidase breaks down imipenem and is combined with cilastatin which inhibits this enzyme.
Mechanism of action	They gain entry into the periplasmic space via porins located on the cell wall and avidly bind to the PBPs 1a, 1b, 2, 4, and also to PBP3 minimally. This stops the cell wall synthesis and leads to the death of the bacteria. They are inactive against organisms producing MBL or class B beta-lactamases such as *Stenotrophomonas maltophilia* and *Elizabethkingia meningoseptica*. Ertapenem has minimal activity against *Pseudomonas* and *Acinetobacter* spp. Imipenem is partially active against *Enerococcus faecalis* [195].
Routes	IV formulations: Imipenem. Meropenem, Ertapenem, Doripenem. Oral formulations: Tebipenem in Japan.
Indication	Treatment of bacterial meningitis, *Pseudomonas spp*, and ESBL bacterial infections. An alternative choice for infections caused by AmpC organisms. Treatment of infections such as bacteremia, cUTI, cIAI, HAP, SSTI, nocardiosis, and actinomycosis.
Resistance	Beta-lactamase synthesis breaks down carbapenem such as KPC, OXA, and MBL. Decreased cell wall entry due to porin mutations or lack of porins. Efflux pumps. Alterations in PBPs site resulting in less avid binding of the carbapenem.
Pharmac-okinetics	Poor oral absorption except for Tebipenem. Plasma protein binding, if higher, leads to a longer half-life (Ertapenem) and once-daily dosing. Tissue distribution and penetration are excellent, including CSF [195]. Excretion is via the renal route, and dose adjustments are needed in renal impairment. Only imipenem undergoes destruction by dehydropeptidase.
Toxicity/Adverse effects	Phlebitis, nausea, vomiting, headache, diarrhea, rash, and *Clostridioides difficile* infection. Seizures, especially with imipenem. Interact with valproic acid and lead to subtherapeutic valproate levels [196]. Potential crossreactivity exists between PCN and cephalosporins; a negative PCN skin test makes it safer to administer a carbapenem [197].

Table 17.
3A X carbapenems.

Origin	Polymixin B is semisynthetically derived from a biochemical product from *Bacillus polymyxa*. Polymixin E (Colistin) is semisynthetically derived from a biochemical product from *Bacillus colistinus*. It is commercially available in an inactive prodrug methanesulfonate (CMS) which is converted to colistin invivo.
Mechanism of action	It is a surface-active agent with both lipophilic and lipophobic subunits which infiltrate the outer cell membrane of GNB. Then they interact with the phospholipids electrostatically, resulting in cell membrane destruction. They bind avidly to lipid A portion of lipopolysaccharide and stop its endotoxin effect [198].
Routes	Polymixin B: available in oral, IV/IM, and topical formulations. Polymixin E: available in oral, IV/IM, inhalation, and topical formulations.
Indication	Polymixin B favored over CMS in all infections except in UTI. Oral preparations are used for intestinal decontamination. Administered intraventricularly for GNB meningitis. Inhaled CMS for infections in Cystic fibrosis. Parenteral administration for severe systemic infections caused by MDR GNB, including VAP.
Resistance	Resistance is mediated via the plasmid-mediated MCR-1, MCR-2, and MCR-3, which alter the lipopolysaccharide structure and prevent polymixin binding [199]. Cross-resistance between the polymyxins is complete [200].
Pharmac-okinetics	They are poorly absorbed, and post IV administration, the distribution to the biliary tract, CSF, joint and pleural fluid is low. CMS undergoes renal clearance, so the dose needs to be adjusted in renal impairment. Both colistin and polymyxin undergo nonrenal clearance (Unknown exact mechanism) after extensive tubular reabsorption with no need for renal dose adjustment [201].

Toxicity/Adverse effects	Dose-related nephrotoxicity is frequent with colistin than polymyxin B seen as renal impairment often reversible on stopping the medication. Dose-related neurotoxicity manifesting as neuromuscular blockade resulting in muscular weakness, apnea, and respiratory failure. This effect can be augmented on concurrent administration with aminoglycosides. Peripheral neuropathy of extremities and perioral paraesthesia [202].

Table 18.
3A XI polymixins.

Origin	It was isolated from the soil bacteria *Streptomyces fradiae*.
Mechanism of action	It inhibits phosphoenolpyruvate synthetase, an enzyme needed to synthesize N-acetylmuramic acid, an essential component of cell wall formation, thus inhibiting cell wall formation. Its bactericidal effect is broad, covering resistant gram-negative and gram-positive microorganisms [203, 204].
Routes	Available in IV and oral formulations. Only oral formulation is currently approved.
Indication	The oral form has been approved for uncomplicated UTI due to susceptible strains of *Escherichia coli* and *Enterococcus faecalis*. IV formulation has been used in a combination regimen against deep-seated infections due to MDR organisms.
Resistance	Modification of phosphoenolpyruvate synthetase enzyme, porin mutations, and some carbapenemases such as OXA. No cross-resistance to other antimicrobial classes.
Pharmac-okinetics	It undergoes renal clearance with dose adjustment needed in renal impairment. Higher doses are associated with bradycardia [205].
Toxicity/Adverse effects	Hypernatremia, hypokalemia, hypocalcemia, and phlebitis.

Table 19.
3A XII epoxide (fosfomycin).

Origin	It is isolated from the fungus *Pleurotus mutilus.*
Mechanism of action	It inhibits protein synthesis by binding to 23SrRNA part of the 50S ribosome subunit. Its activity against gram-positive organisms is potent invitro (MSSA/MRSA/*Streptococcal spp*). Its spectrum of bactericidal effects is broad, covering both gram-positive and negative respiratory pathogens.
Routes	Available in both oral and IV formulations.
Indication	It is approved for CABP therapy in patients >18 years old by both IV and oral formulations.
Resistance	Mutations in the 23S rRNA and methylation of the target site preventing Lefamulin from 23S rRNA binding [206].
Pharmac-okinetics	It undergoes hepatic clearance by cytochrome CYP3A and can lead to interactions. Dose adjustment is needed in hepatic impairment and none in renal failure.
Toxicity/Adverse effects	Infusion site reactions, phlebitis, headache, nausea, diarrhea, and QT prolongation [207].

Table 20.
3A XIII pleuromutilin (lefamulin).

Plazomicin is a semisynthetic aminoglycoside derived from sisomicin. It is potent against MDR GNB, especially the ones with carbapenemase. It has been approved currently for the treatment of complicated UTI (cUTI) by aerobic

Origin	Rifampin was semisynthetically obtained from rifamycin SV isolated from *Amycolatopsis mediterranei*. Similarly, Rifabutin, Rifapentine, and Rifaximin are semisynthetic modifications.
Mechanism of action	Rifamycins bind avidly to DNA-dependent RNA polymerase and block RNA synthesis.
Routes	Rifampin: available in oral and IV formulations. Rifabutin, Rifapentine, Rifaximin: available in oral formulations.
Indication	Rifampin: Antitubercular therapy for active tuberculosis. Treatment of Nontubercular mycobacterial infections due to *Mycobacterium leprae* (*M. leprae*), *Mycobacterium avium-intracellulare* (MAC), *Mycobacterium kansasii*. Combination therapy for synergistic antistaphylococcal effect and antibiofilm effect in PJI, chronic osteomyelitis, and SSTI. Therapy for resistant *Streptococcus pneumoniae* strains causing CNS infections and *Enterococcal* hip and knee PJI. Therapy for severe *legionella* infection along with a macrolide. As a part of combination therapy of *Rhodococcus equi* infections in immunosuppressed patients. As a part of combination therapy of MDR GNB infections. Brucellosis and complicated Bartonella infection antimicrobial therapy. Chemoprophylaxis in Meningococcal meningitis and Active *Hemophilus influenzae* infection close contacts. Rifabutin: As an alternative to rifampin in the treatment of tuberculosis and MAC infection. Rifapentine: As a part of the short regimen for latent tuberculosis therapy, Rifaximin: Hepatic encephalopathy treatment, Alternative for travelers diarrhea and recurrent Clostridioides difficile infection. It is an alternative for GI invasive pathogens *Salmonella*, *Shigella*, *Campylobacter*, and *Escherichia coli*.
Resistance	*rpoB* gene mutations result in decreased binding of rifamycins to RNA polymerase [208]. Decreased cellular uptake of rifampin. Mutations in the *arr* gene lead to ribosylation of rifamycins and decreased binding [209].
Pharmac-okinetics	Rifampin: excellent oral bioavailability with broad tissue and fluid distribution, including brain [210]. It undergoes hepatic clearance, enterohepatic circulation with biliary excretion, and minimal renal excretion. Dosage adjustment is needed in hepatic impairment. It induces hepatic enzyme CYP3A resulting in drug interactions, especially with protease inhibitors. Rifabutin: is more lipid-soluble with a long half-life and extensive tissue distribution, including CSF. Its metabolites post hepatic metabolism undergo renal clearance, so dose adjustment is needed with hepatic and renal impairment. Hepatic enzyme induction is minimum. Protease inhibitors increase their levels. Rifapentine: Food increases its bioavailability, and it is more potent with a longer half-life. Intracellular concentrations are higher than rifampin with minimal CSF penetration. It undergoes hepatic clearance with induction of hepatic enzymes CYP3A4 and protease inhibitors decrease its absorption [211]. Rifaximin: Oral absorption is minimal, and 97% of the drug gets excreted in stools. It can induce cytochrome P450 3A4, but it is not seen as the systemic levels are minimal [212]. No dosage adjustment is required.
Toxicity/Adverse effects	Rifampin: type 1 hypersensitivity reactions, flu-like syndrome, hemolysis, thrombocytopenia, acute interstitial nephritis with tubular necrosis, mild transaminitis with increased risk of hepatotoxicity with isoniazid [213], and red-orange discoloration of body fluids. Rifabutin: polyarthralgia, leukopenia, and uveitis [214]. Rifapentine:flu-like syndrome, hyperuricemia, hemolysis, and renal failure. Rifaximin: neutropenia.

Table 21.
3A XIV rifamycins.

gram-negative bacilli. It is synergistic with other beta-lactams, especially zosyn cefepime and doripenem [234]. The main side effects are tinnitus, headache, dizziness, and mild to moderate drowsiness.

Delafloxacin, a newer quinolone, has MRSA activity and can be used in native and prosthetic joint infections as an oral pill.

Origin	It is a semisynthetic derivative of azomycin isolated from a *streptomyces* bacterium. Tinidazole, Secnidazole and Ornidazole are the other semisynthetic derivatives.
Mechanism of action	It enters the cell passively and then gets an electron transferred to its nitro group, creating a free radical which is cytotoxic and interacts with DNA (prodrug to an active drug). This change enhances the drug gradient in the cell by increased uptake. The active drug oxidizes DNA damaging it and block DNA synthesis [215].
Routes	Available in oral capsules, tablets, topical gels, creams, lotion, vaginal gel, suspension, and IV formulations.
Indication	Treatment of parasitic infections such as trichomoniasis, symptomatic GI *Dientamoeba fragilis* infection, Giardiasis, mild to moderate *Clostridioides difficile* infection, anaerobic infections of CNS, lung, abdomen, Skin, gynecologic, oral, dental, bone, and joint. As a part of a combination regimen against *Helicobacter pylori.* As an alternative agent recommended for surgical prophylaxis in intraabdominal, head, and neck cancer, urology surgery for patients intolerant or allergic to beta-lactams [216]. Prophylaxis perioperatively in obstetric and gynecologic procedures [217].
Resistance	Decreased uptake of the antibiotic. Active drug efflux pumps. Reduced activation of the prodrug (↓nitroreductase enzymes). Inactivation of the antibiotic (nim-encoded nitroimidazole reductase). Altered DNA repair [215].
Pharmac-okinetics	Oral bioavailability is close to 100%, with a more considerable volume of distribution attaining excellent concentrations in tissue, body fluids, abscess, and CSF [10]. It undergoes hepatic clearance and enterohepatic circulation with some amount being excreted renally with no change. Dosage adjustment is needed in hepatic impairment.
Toxicity/Adverse effects	Common ones include nausea, metallic taste, dry mouth, diarrhea, vaginal candida infection, CNS side effects on prolonged therapy (aseptic meningitis, encephalopathy, ataxia, seizure). Rare serious events include ototoxicity, Stevens-Johnson syndrome, pancreatitis [10].

Table 22.
3A XV metronidazole.

PCN skin tests are inaccurate in predicting skin reactions. In PCN or cephalosporin allergy patients, the clinical decision to use a different cephalosporin is decided by the severity of the reaction and the cephalosporin to be used. In patients with no severe reactions, a cephalosporin with a different side chain can be used. It is recommended not to use a cephalosporin in case of a severe reaction [235]. Cephalosporins are not active against atypical organisms responsible for CABP. An initial study disclosed increased mortality with cefepime than other cephalosporins compared to a beta-lactam plus beta-lactamase inhibitor (BLI), which was not observed in a more extensive meta-analysis [236, 237]. Cefepime is not recommended to be used in ESBL infections [238]. Siderophore cephalosporins Cefiderocol are active against all beta-lactamases and carbapenemase enzymes [239]. It is also active against the GNB lactose-non fermenters by its affinity for the PBP3.

Zosyn should not be used to treat ESBL infections with bacteremia due to higher mortality observed in trials compared to meropenem [240, 241].

Most *Burkholderia cepacia, Stenotrophomas maltophilia*, *Acinetobacter baumannii* strains are resistant to aztreonam.

Lactose-non fermenters such as *Stenotrophomonas maltophilia, B. cepacia,* and *Elizabethkingia meningoseptica* are intrinsically resistant to all carbapenems due to intrinsic MBL synthesis. Similarly, *Enterobacteriaceae* containing KPC (*Klebsiella pneumoniae*), OXA (*A. baumannii*), or acquired MBL are resistant to carbapenems. They are an ideal choice for polymicrobial infections as they also cover MSSA. *Pseudomonas aeruginosa* resistance to carbapenems is primarily due to porin mutations and efflux pumps than the carbapenemase. Porin mutations affect the imipenem, whereas the efflux pumps affect the meropenem and doripenem [242, 243]. The duration of therapy for lactose-non fermenters causing VAP is controversial, as a shorter duration of seven days is associated with an increased recurrence rate [244].

Compared to other antimicrobial classes, polymixins have been associated with poorer outcomes, but this appears to be a poor application of prior suboptimal dose adjustments based on the newer pharmacokinetics and pharmacodynamics data [245, 246]. Polymixin combination regimens should be used as a last resort in the absence of any alternative antimicrobial regimen.

Extreme consideration should be given to the possible drug interactions when rifamycins are used clinically due to their ability to induce the hepatic cytochrome system.

4. Antibiotics in ICU

Antimicrobial prescription in the intensive care unit has three essential ideals to be followed: the correct time when to initiate the antimicrobial, what dose to be used, and how long the antimicrobial should be used. Initiate empirical regimen as early as possible once the infection is suspected to prevent poor clinical outcomes [247]. Trials reveal a positive association between earlier antimicrobial use and mortality in sepsis and septic shock [248]. 2016 surviving sepsis guidelines recommend administering appropriate antimicrobial therapy within one hour of sepsis and septic shock recognition based on the moderate quality of evidence [249]. The empirical regimen should be based on the clinical presentation and associated risk factors. The dose used should be based on the antimicrobial pharmacokinetics, and antibiotics are labeled as either time-dependent (beta-lactams), concentration-dependent (aminoglycosides and daptomycin), and concentration-dependent with time dependence (fluoroquinolones, linezolid) [250].

For time-dependent antimicrobials, the best way to achieve efficacy is a continuous infusion to keep the drug levels above the MIC for a longer time [251]. For concentration-dependent antimicrobials, once-daily higher doses are adequate as they demonstrate postantibiotic effect with reduced adverse events [252]. It is prudent to increase the antimicrobial dosage in patients with augmented renal clearance (burns, trauma, febrile neutropenia) to increase the antimicrobial dosage to achieve the target drug levels [253]. De-escalation of antibiotics is done via three different methods. First, once empirical therapy is initiated, follow the pending culture results, and on day three, when the antimicrobials have reached adequate therapeutic levels, the regimen can be de-escalated to a narrower spectrum based on the patient's culture results and clinical diagnosis. Second, in patients with negative culture results, which is a common finding in ICU patients, the de-escalation process is unclear. For example, in patients treated for HAP who are clinically improving with negative sputum cultures for MRSA and *P. aeruginosa*, antibiotics covering these organisms can be stopped as per guidelines [254]. The third mechanism uses the empirical regimen for the shortest duration possible for a better clinical outcome [255]. This recommendation is based on expert opinion than clinical data.

Recent guidelines based on multiple trials conducted on the VAP antimicrobial therapy duration suggest using the treatment for seven days than 14 days [256]. However, they also recommend following the improvement in clinical, imaging, and laboratory parameters to decide the duration of therapy judiciously. Seven days of VAP therapy was associated with an increased recurrence of infections among lactose-non fermenter GNB such as Pseudomonas and Acinetobacter spp. [244].

Similarly, in MRSA and MSSA pneumonia, the duration is decided by the clinical picture, and most often, it is more than seven days and closer to 14 days.

Antibiotic use in the intensive care unit (ICU) usually follows two different thought processes. One way is to use a single or limited number of antimicrobials as workhorse agents as empirical therapy for infections which carries an inherent risk of resistance emergence via selective pressure (antibiotic homogeneity). This was initiated to control resistance. Another way is to select the antibiotics based on clinical presentation and comorbid risk factors associated with decreased resistance (antibiotic heterogeneity). This is a newer initiation in managing resistance. It is recommended to use antibiotic heterogeneity as much as possible to prevent antimicrobial resistance emergence [257]. Antibiotic stewardship is a must in this modern era for better clinical outcomes, prevent antibiotic adverse events and resistance using local data, reduce the costs by selecting the correct antibiotic dose duration and route. An ideal stewardship team should include an infectious disease consultant, clinical microbiologist, infectious disease trained clinical pharmacist. The current guidelines recommend two strategies to attain this objective. First, reduce the future antibiotic use by auditing institutional antimicrobial usage with feedback to the prescribers. Second, it is ideal to restrict certain antimicrobials to prevent inappropriate usage and decrease institutions' economic burden. Measures taken to enhance the ICU staff education boosts the stewardship process and increases its acceptance among health care workers.

5. Conclusion

Antibiotic resources are finite and need to be managed judiciously with principles based on antimicrobial stewardship. Management of sick patients in ICU will need timely appropriate antimicrobial adjustments based on new laboratory results and clinical parameters. It seems reasonable to utilize a stewardship team to support the intensivist in the ICU for better outcomes. It seems appropriate to extend the stewardship program to progressive care units or step-down units where antimicrobial utilization is greater than the floors. Education of the ICU staff and positive feedback to antibiotic prescribers can change prescription behavior from antibiotic homogeneity to antibiotic heterogeneity to prevent the emergence of MDR organisms.

Acknowledgements

"None, this manuscript preparation did not need external funds."

Conflict of interest

"We, the authors declare no conflict of interest."

Notes/thanks/other declarations

"A special thanks to the editor for allowing us to author this manuscript.

Acronyms and abbreviations

MIC	Minimum inhibitory concentration
MBC	Minimum bactericidal concentration
CLSI	Clinical and Laboratory Standards Institute
EUCAST	European Committee on Antimicrobial Susceptibility Testing
IE	Infective endocarditis
PABA	Para-aminobenzoic acid
DHFR	Dihydrofolate reductase
IV	Intravenous
UTI	Urinary tract infection
TMP-SMX	Trimethoprim and sulfamethoxazole
SSTI	Skin and soft tissue infections
PCJ	Pneumocystis jiroveci
foiP	Dihydrofolate reductase encoding gene
SJS	Steven-Johnson syndrome
TEN	Toxic epidermal necrolysis
GI	Gastrointestinal
MSSA	Methicillin-sensitive *S. aureus*
MRSA	Methicillin-resistant *S. aureus*
CABP	Community-acquired bacterial pneumonia
PID	Pelvic inflammatory disease
CSF	Cerebrospinal fluid
CNS	Central Nervous System
MICU	Medical intensive care unit
cIAIs	Complicated intraabdominal infections
MDR	Multidrug-resistant
FDA	Federal drug authority
HAP	Hospital-acquired pneumonia
VAP	Ventilator-associated pneumonia
rRNA	ribosomal ribonucleic acid
PCN	Penicillin
MAC	*M. avium* complex
MLSB	Macrolide Lincosamide and streptogramin B
Erm	Erythromycin ribosome methylation
HLA	Human leukocyte antigen
DRESS	Drug rash with eosinophilia and systemic symptoms
AUC	Area under the curve
VRE	Vancomycin-resistant Enterococcus
optrA	Adenylation coding gene
EF-G	Elongation factor G
fusA	Elongation factor G coding gene
PBP	Penicillin-binding protein
mecA&C	Methicillin resistance encoding gene
Van	Vancomycin resistance encoding gene
VISA	Vancomycin intermediate *S. aureus*
CPK	Creatinine phosphokinase
mRNA	messenger RNA
GNB	Gram-negative bacillus
cUTI	Complicated UTI
DNA	Deoxyribonucleic acid
SBP	Spontaneous bacterial peritonitis

IM	Intramuscular
PJI	Prosthetic joint infection
IgE	Immunoglobulin E
BLI	Beta-lactamase inhibitor
ESBL	Extended-spectrum beta-lactamases
KPC	*K. pneumoniae* carbapenemase
MBL	Metallo-beta-lactamase
OXA	Oxacillin beta-lactamases
AmpC	Class C beta-lactamses
CMS	Methanesulfonate
MCR	Lipopolysaccharide encoding gene
rpo	RNA polymerase rifamycin binding target encoding gene
arr	Methytransferase encoding gene

Author details

Sachin M. Patil* and Parag Patel
University of Missouri, Columbia, MO, USA

*Address all correspondence to: drssmp1@gmail.com

References

[1] Waksman SA. What is an antibiotic or an antibiotic substance? Mycologia. 1947;39(5):565-9.

[2] Northey EH. The sulfonamides and allied compounds. Journal of the American Pharmaceutical Association. 1948;37(8):338-.

[3] Armstrong GL, Conn LA, Pinner RW. Trends in infectious disease mortality in the United States during the 20th century. JAMA. 1999;281(1):61-6.

[4] Pankey GA, Sabath LD. Clinical relevance of bacteriostatic versus bactericidal mechanisms of action in the treatment of Gram-positive bacterial infections. Clin Infect Dis. 2004;38(6): 864-70.

[5] Wald-Dickler N, Holtom P, Spellberg B. Busting the Myth of "Static vs Cidal": A Systemic Literature Review. Clin Infect Dis. 2018;66(9):1470-4.

[6] Freire AT, Melnyk V, Kim MJ, Datsenko O, Dzyublik O, Glumcher F, et al. Comparison of tigecycline with imipenem/cilastatin for the treatment of hospital-acquired pneumonia. Diagn Microbiol Infect Dis. 2010;68(2):140-51.

[7] Ramirez J, Dartois N, Gandjini H, Yan JL, Korth-Bradley J, McGovern PC. Randomized phase 2 trial to evaluate the clinical efficacy of two high-dosage tigecycline regimens versus imipenem-cilastatin for treatment of hospital-acquired pneumonia. Antimicrob Agents Chemother. 2013;57(4):1756-62.

[8] Fowler VG, Jr., Boucher HW, Corey GR, Abrutyn E, Karchmer AW, Rupp ME, et al. Daptomycin versus standard therapy for bacteremia and endocarditis caused by *Staphylococcus aureus*. N Engl J Med. 2006;355(7):653-65.

[9] Korzeniowski O, Sande MA. Combination antimicrobial therapy for *Staphylococcus aureus* endocarditis in patients addicted to parenteral drugs and in nonaddicts: A prospective study. Ann Intern Med. 1982;97(4):496-503.

[10] Falagas ME, Matthaiou DK, Bliziotis IA. The role of aminoglycosides in combination with a beta-lactam for the treatment of bacterial endocarditis: a meta-analysis of comparative trials. J Antimicrob Chemother. 2006;57(4): 639-47.

[11] Finland M. Current status of therapy in bacterial endocarditis. J Am Med Assoc. 1958;166(4):364-73.

[12] Mancino P, Ucciferri C, Falasca K, Pizzigallo E, Vecchiet J. Methicillin-resistant *Staphylococcus epidermidis* (MRSE) endocarditis treated with linezolid. Scand J Infect Dis. 2008;40(1): 67-73.

[13] Kanafani Z, Boucher H, Fowler V, Cabell C, Hoen B, Miro JM, et al. Daptomycin compared to standard therapy for the treatment of native valve endocarditis. Enferm Infecc Microbiol Clin. 2010;28(8):498-503.

[14] Bushby SR, Hitchings GH. Trimethoprim, a sulphonamide potentiator. Br J Pharmacol Chemother. 1968;33(1):72-90.

[15] Woods DD. The Relation of p-aminobenzoic Acid to the Mechanism of the Action of Sulphanilamide. Br J Exp Pathol. 1940;21(2):74-90.

[16] Brown GM. The biosynthesis of pteridines. Adv Enzymol Relat Areas Mol Biol. 1971;35:35-77.

[17] Grose WE, Bodey GP, Loo TL. Clinical pharmacology of intravenously administered trimethoprim-sulfamethoxazole. Antimicrob Agents Chemother. 1979;15(3):447-51.

[18] Swedberg G, Castensson S, Skold O. Characterization of mutationally altered dihydropteroate synthase and its ability to form a sulfonamide-containing dihydrofolate analog. J Bacteriol. 1979; 137(1):129-36.

[19] Shin HW, Lim J, Kim S, Kim J, Kwon GC, Koo SH. Characterization of trimethoprim-sulfamethoxazole resistance genes and their relatedness to class 1 integron and insertion sequence common region in gram-negative bacilli. J Microbiol Biotechnol. 2015;25 (1):137-42.

[20] Watanabe T. Infective heredity of multiple drug resistance in bacteria. Bacteriol Rev. 1963;27:87-115.

[21] Wen X, Wang JS, Backman JT, Laitila J, Neuvonen PJ. Trimethoprim and sulfamethoxazole are selective inhibitors of CYP2C8 and CYP2C9, respectively. Drug Metab Dispos. 2002; 30(6):631-5.

[22] Chertow GM, Seifter JL, Christiansen CL, O'Donnell WJ. Trimethoprim-sulfamethoxazole and hypouricemia. Clin Nephrol. 1996;46 (3):193-8.

[23] Mittmann N, Knowles SR, Koo M, Shear NH, Rachlis A, Rourke SB. Incidence of toxic epidermal necrolysis and Stevens-Johnson Syndrome in an HIV cohort: an observational, retrospective case series study. Am J Clin Dermatol. 2012;13(1):49-54.

[24] Ho JM, Juurlink DN. Considerations when prescribing trimethoprim-sulfamethoxazole. CMAJ. 2011;183(16): 1851-8.

[25] Garvey JP, Brown CM, Chotirmall SH, Dorman AM, Conlon PJ, Walshe JJ. Trimethoprim-sulfamethoxazole induced acute interstitial nephritis in renal allografts; clinical course and outcome. Clin Nephrol. 2009;72(5):331-6.

[26] Hemstreet BA. Antimicrobial-associated renal tubular acidosis. Ann Pharmacother. 2004;38(6):1031-8.

[27] Kouklakis G, Mpoumponaris A, Zezos P, Moschos J, Koulaouzidis A, Nakos A, et al. Cholestatic hepatitis with severe systemic reactions induced by trimethoprim-sulfamethoxazole. Ann Hepatol. 2007;6(1):63-5.

[28] Trivedi CD, Pitchumoni CS. Drug-induced pancreatitis: an update. J Clin Gastroenterol. 2005;39(8):709-16.

[29] Sembera S, Lammert C, Talwalkar JA, Sanderson SO, Poterucha JJ, Hay JE, et al. Frequency, clinical presentation, and outcomes of drug-induced liver injury after liver transplantation. Liver Transpl. 2012;18 (7):803-10.

[30] Duggar BM. Aureomycin; a product of the continuing search for new antibiotics. Ann N Y Acad Sci. 1948;51 (Art. 2):177-81.

[31] Dahl EL, Shock JL, Shenai BR, Gut J, DeRisi JL, Rosenthal PJ. Tetracyclines specifically target the apicoplast of the malaria parasite Plasmodium falciparum. Antimicrob Agents Chemother. 2006;50(9):3124-31.

[32] Thaker M, Spanogiannopoulos P, Wright GD. The tetracycline resistome. Cell Mol Life Sci. 2010;67(3):419-31.

[33] Smith C, Woods CG, Woods MJ. Absorption of minocycline. J Antimicrob Chemother. 1984;13(1):93.

[34] Yim CW, Flynn NM, Fitzgerald FT. Penetration of oral doxycycline into the cerebrospinal fluid of patients with latent or neurosyphilis. Antimicrob Agents Chemother. 1985;28(2):347-8.

[35] Hey H, Jorgensen F, Sorensen K, Hasselbalch H, Wamberg T. Oesophageal transit of six commonly

used tablets and capsules. Br Med J (Clin Res Ed). 1982;285(6356):1717-9.

[36] Schultz JC, Adamson JS, Jr., Workman WW, Norman TD. Fatal Liver Disease after Intravenous Administration of Tetracycline in High Dosage. N Engl J Med. 1963;269: 999-1004.

[37] Smith K, Leyden JJ. Safety of doxycycline and minocycline: a systematic review. Clin Ther. 2005;27 (9):1329-42.

[38] Perks WH, Walters EH, Tams IP, Prowse K. Demeclocycline in the treatment of the syndrome of inappropriate secretion of antidiuretic hormone. Thorax. 1979;34(3):324-7.

[39] Cohlan SQ. Teratogenic Agents and Congenital Malformations. J Pediatr. 1963;63:650-9.

[40] Knowles SR, Shapiro L, Shear NH. Serious adverse reactions induced by minocycline. Report of 13 patients and review of the literature. Arch Dermatol. 1996;132(8):934-9.

[41] Sum PE, Lee VJ, Testa RT, Hlavka JJ, Ellestad GA, Bloom JD, et al. Glycylcyclines. 1. A new generation of potent antibacterial agents through modification of 9-aminotetracyclines. J Med Chem. 1994;37(1):184-8.

[42] Bauer G, Berens C, Projan SJ, Hillen W. Comparison of tetracycline and tigecycline binding to ribosomes mapped by dimethylsulphate and drug-directed Fe2+ cleavage of 16S rRNA. J Antimicrob Chemother. 2004;53(4): 592-9.

[43] Bergeron J, Ammirati M, Danley D, James L, Norcia M, Retsema J, et al. Glycylcyclines bind to the high-affinity tetracycline ribosomal binding site and evade Tet(M)- and Tet(O)-mediated ribosomal protection. Antimicrob Agents Chemother. 1996;40(9):2226-8.

[44] Visalli MA, Murphy E, Projan SJ, Bradford PA. AcrAB multidrug efflux pump is associated with reduced levels of susceptibility to tigecycline (GAR-936) in *Proteus mirabilis*. Antimicrob Agents Chemother. 2003;47(2):665-9.

[45] Dean CR, Visalli MA, Projan SJ, Sum PE, Bradford PA. Efflux-mediated resistance to tigecycline (GAR-936) in *Pseudomonas aeruginosa* PAO1. Antimicrob Agents Chemother. 2003;47 (3):972-8.

[46] Muralidharan G, Micalizzi M, Speth J, Raible D, Troy S. Pharmacokinetics of tigecycline after single and multiple doses in healthy subjects. Antimicrob Agents Chemother. 2005;49(1):220-9.

[47] Frampton JE, Curran MP. Tigecycline. Drugs. 2005;65(18): 2623-35; discussion 36-7.

[48] McGovern PC, Wible M, El-Tahtawy A, Biswas P, Meyer RD. All-cause mortality imbalance in the tigecycline phase 3 and 4 clinical trials. Int J Antimicrob Agents. 2013;41(5): 463-7.

[49] Bahal N, Nahata MC. The new macrolide antibiotics: azithromycin, clarithromycin, dirithromycin, and roxithromycin. Ann Pharmacother. 1992;26(1):46-55.

[50] Piscitelli SC, Danziger LH, Rodvold KA. Clarithromycin and azithromycin: new macrolide antibiotics. Clin Pharm. 1992;11(2): 137-52.

[51] Leclercq R, Courvalin P. Resistance to macrolides and related antibiotics in *Streptococcus pneumoniae*. Antimicrob Agents Chemother. 2002;46(9):2727-34.

[52] Edelstein PH. Pneumococcal resistance to macrolides, lincosamides, ketolides, and streptogramin B agents: molecular mechanisms and resistance

phenotypes. Clin Infect Dis. 2004;38 Suppl 4:S322-7.

[53] Ludden TM. Pharmacokinetic interactions of the macrolide antibiotics. Clin Pharmacokinet. 1985;10(1):63-79.

[54] Amsden GW. Macrolides versus azalides: a drug interaction update. Ann Pharmacother. 1995;29(9):906-17.

[55] Osono T, Umezawa H. Pharmaco kinetics of macrolides, lincosamides and streptogramins. J Antimicrob Chemother. 1985;16 Suppl A:151-66.

[56] Schentag JJ, Ballow CH. Tissue-directed pharmacokinetics. Am J Med. 1991;91(3A):5S-11S.

[57] Hardy DJ, Guay DR, Jones RN. Clarithromycin, a unique macrolide. A pharmacokinetic, microbiological, and clinical overview. Diagn Microbiol Infect Dis. 1992;15(1):39-53.

[58] Katapadi K, Kostandy G, Katapadi M, Hussain KM, Schifter D. A review of erythromycin-induced malignant tachyarrhythmia–torsade de pointes. A case report. Angiology. 1997; 48(9):821-6.

[59] Chandrupatla S, Demetris AJ, Rabinovitz M. Azithromycin-induced intrahepatic cholestasis. Dig Dis Sci. 2002;47(10):2186-8.

[60] Shaffer D, Singer S, Korvick J, Honig P. Concomitant risk factors in reports of torsades de pointes associated with macrolide use: review of the United States Food and Drug Administration Adverse Event Reporting System. Clin Infect Dis. 2002; 35(2):197-200.

[61] McGehee RF, Jr., Smith CB, Wilcox C, Finland M. Comparative studies of antibacterial activity in vitro and absorption and excretion of lincomycin and clinimycin. Am J Med Sci. 1968;256(5):279-92.

[62] Siberry GK, Tekle T, Carroll K, Dick J. Failure of clindamycin treatment of methicillin-resistant *Staphylococcus aureus* expressing inducible clindamycin resistance in vitro. Clin Infect Dis. 2003; 37(9):1257-60.

[63] Matzov D, Eyal Z, Benhamou RI, Shalev-Benami M, Halfon Y, Krupkin M, et al. Structural insights of lincosamides targeting the ribosome of *Staphylococcus aureus*. Nucleic Acids Res. 2017;45(17):10284-92.

[64] Poehlsgaard J, Pfister P, Bottger EC, Douthwaite S. Molecular mechanisms by which rRNA mutations confer resistance to clindamycin. Antimicrob Agents Chemother. 2005;49(4):1553-5.

[65] Leclercq R, Brisson-Noel A, Duval J, Courvalin P. Phenotypic expression and genetic heterogeneity of lincosamide inactivation in Staphylococcus spp. Antimicrob Agents Chemother. 1987;31 (12):1887-91.

[66] Panzer JD, Brown DC, Epstein WL, Lipson RL, Mahaffey HW, Atkinson WH. Clindamycin levels in various body tissues and fluids. J Clin Pharmacol New Drugs. 1972;12(7):259-62.

[67] DeHaan RM, Metzler CM, Schellenberg D, Vandenbosch WD. Pharmacokinetic studies of clindamycin phosphate. J Clin Pharmacol. 1973;13(5): 190-209.

[68] Yang Y, Chen S, Yang F, Zhang L, Alterovitz G, Zhu H, et al. HLA-B*51:01 is strongly associated with clindamycin-related cutaneous adverse drug reactions. Pharmacogenomics J. 2017;17(6):501-5.

[69] Bartlett JG. Historical perspectives on studies of *Clostridium difficile* and *C. difficile* infection. Clin Infect Dis. 2008; 46 Suppl 1:S4-11.

[70] Moellering RC. Linezolid: the first oxazolidinone antimicrobial. Ann Intern Med. 2003;138(2):135-42.

[71] Long KS, Vester B. Resistance to linezolid caused by modifications at its binding site on the ribosome. Antimicrob Agents Chemother. 2012;56 (2):603-12.

[72] Diaz L, Kiratisin P, Mendes RE, Panesso D, Singh KV, Arias CA. Transferable plasmid-mediated resistance to linezolid due to cfr in a human clinical isolate of *Enterococcus faecalis*. Antimicrob Agents Chemother. 2012;56(7):3917-22.

[73] Wang Y, Lv Y, Cai J, Schwarz S, Cui L, Hu Z, et al. A novel gene, optrA, that confers transferable resistance to oxazolidinones and phenicols and its presence in *Enterococcus faecalis* and *Enterococcus faecium* of human and animal origin. J Antimicrob Chemother. 2015;70(8):2182-90.

[74] Roger C, Roberts JA, Muller L. Clinical Pharmacokinetics and Pharmacodynamics of Oxazolidinones. Clin Pharmacokinet. 2018;57(5):559-75.

[75] Zhanel GG, Love R, Adam H, Golden A, Zelenitsky S, Schweizer F, et al. Tedizolid: a novel oxazolidinone with potent activity against multidrug-resistant gram-positive pathogens. Drugs. 2015;75(3):253-70.

[76] Flanagan S, Minassian SL, Passarell JA, Fiedler-Kelly J, Prokocimer P. Pharmacokinetics of Tedizolid in Obese and Nonobese Subjects. J Clin Pharmacol. 2017;57(10): 1290-4.

[77] Gerson SL, Kaplan SL, Bruss JB, Le V, Arellano FM, Hafkin B, et al. Hematologic effects of linezolid: summary of clinical experience. Antimicrob Agents Chemother. 2002;46 (8):2723-6.

[78] Narita M, Tsuji BT, Yu VL. Linezolid-associated peripheral and optic neuropathy, lactic acidosis, and serotonin syndrome. Pharmacotherapy. 2007;27(8):1189-97.

[79] De Vriese AS, Coster RV, Smet J, Seneca S, Lovering A, Van Haute LL, et al. Linezolid-induced inhibition of mitochondrial protein synthesis. Clin Infect Dis. 2006;42(8):1111-7.

[80] Barnhill AE, Brewer MT, Carlson SA. Adverse effects of antimicrobials via predictable or idiosyncratic inhibition of host mitochondrial components. Antimicrob Agents Chemother. 2012;56(8):4046-51.

[81] Nagel S, Kohrmann M, Huttner HB, Storch-Hagenlocher B, Schwab S. Linezolid-induced posterior reversible leukoencephalopathy syndrome. Arch Neurol. 2007;64(5):746-8.

[82] Refaat M, Hyle E, Malhotra R, Seidman D, Dey B. Linezolid-induced lingua villosa nigra. Am J Med. 2008;121 (6):e1.

[83] Harvey CL, Knight SG, Sih CJ. On the mode of action of fusidic acid. Biochemistry. 1966;5(10):3320-7.

[84] Gemmell CG, O'Dowd A. Regulation of protein A biosynthesis in *Staphylococcus aureus* by certain antibiotics: its effect on phagocytosis by leukocytes. J Antimicrob Chemother. 1983;12(6):587-97.

[85] Taburet AM, Guibert J, Kitzis MD, Sorensen H, Acar JF, Singlas E. Pharmacokinetics of sodium fusidate after single and repeated infusions and oral administration of a new formulation. J Antimicrob Chemother. 1990;25 Suppl B:23-31.

[86] Wise R, Pippard M, Mitchard M. The disposition of sodium fusidate in man. Br J Clin Pharmacol. 1977;4(5): 615-9.

[87] Godtfredsen WO, Jahnsen S, Lorck H, Roholt K, Tybring L. Fusidic

acid: a new antibiotic. Nature. 1962;193:987.

[88] Deljehier T, Pariente A, Miremont-Salame G, Haramburu F, Nguyen L, Rubin S, et al. Rhabdomyolysis after co-administration of a statin and fusidic acid: an analysis of the literature and of the WHO database of adverse drug reactions. Br J Clin Pharmacol. 2018;84(5):1057-63.

[89] Safrin S, Finkelstein DM, Feinberg J, Frame P, Simpson G, Wu A, et al. Comparison of three regimens for treatment of mild to moderate Pneumocystis carinii pneumonia in patients with AIDS. A double-blind, randomized, trial of oral trimethoprim-sulfamethoxazole, dapsone-trimethoprim, and clindamycin-primaquine. ACTG 108 Study Group. Ann Intern Med. 1996;124(9):792-802.

[90] Feikin DR, Dowell SF, Nwanyanwu OC, Klugman KP, Kazembe PN, Barat LM, et al. Increased carriage of trimethoprim/sulfamethoxazole-resistant *Streptococcus pneumoniae* in Malawian children after treatment for malaria with sulfadoxine/pyrimethamine. J Infect Dis. 2000;181(4):1501-5.

[91] Huang DB, O'Riordan W, Overcash JS, Heller B, Amin F, File TM, et al. A Phase 3, Randomized, Double-Blind, Multicenter Study to Evaluate the Safety and Efficacy of Intravenous Iclaprim Vs Vancomycin for the Treatment of Acute Bacterial Skin and Skin Structure Infections Suspected or Confirmed to be Due to Gram-Positive Pathogens: REVIVE-1. Clin Infect Dis. 2018;66(8):1222-9.

[92] Andrews J, Honeybourne D, Ashby J, Jevons G, Fraise A, Fry P, et al. Concentrations in plasma, epithelial lining fluid, alveolar macrophages and bronchial mucosa after a single intravenous dose of 1.6 mg/kg of iclaprim (AR-100) in healthy men. J Antimicrob Chemother. 2007;60(3):677-80.

[93] Brouillard JE, Terriff CM, Tofan A, Garrison MW. Antibiotic selection and resistance issues with fluoroquinolones and doxycycline against bioterrorism agents. Pharmacotherapy. 2006;26(1):3-14.

[94] Zhanel GG, Esquivel J, Zelenitsky S, Lawrence CK, Adam HJ, Golden A, et al. Omadacycline: A Novel Oral and Intravenous Aminomethylcycline Antibiotic Agent. Drugs. 2020;80(3):285-313.

[95] Lee YR, Burton CE. Eravacycline, a newly approved fluorocycline. Eur J Clin Microbiol Infect Dis. 2019;38(10):1787-94.

[96] Hiramatsu K. Vancomycin-resistant *Staphylococcus aureus*: a new model of antibiotic resistance. Lancet Infect Dis. 2001;1(3):147-55.

[97] Moise-Broder PA, Forrest A, Birmingham MC, Schentag JJ. Pharmacodynamics of vancomycin and other antimicrobials in patients with *Staphylococcus aureus* lower respiratory tract infections. Clin Pharmacokinet. 2004;43(13):925-42.

[98] Ricard JD, Wolff M, Lacherade JC, Mourvillier B, Hidri N, Barnaud G, et al. Levels of vancomycin in cerebrospinal fluid of adult patients receiving adjunctive corticosteroids to treat pneumococcal meningitis: a prospective multicenter observational study. Clin Infect Dis. 2007;44(2):250-5.

[99] Grace E. Altered vancomycin pharmacokinetics in obese and morbidly obese patients: what we have learned over the past 30 years. J Antimicrob Chemother. 2012;67(6):1305-10.

[100] Wilson AP. Clinical pharmacokinetics of teicoplanin. Clin Pharmacokinet. 2000;39(3):167-83.

[101] van Hal SJ, Paterson DL, Lodise TP. Systematic review and meta-analysis of vancomycin-induced nephrotoxicity associated with dosing schedules that maintain troughs between 15 and 20 milligrams per liter. Antimicrob Agents Chemother. 2013;57(2):734-44.

[102] Geraci JE, Heilman FR, Nichols DR, Wellman WE. Antibiotic therapy of bacterial endocarditis. VII. Vancomycin for acute micrococcal endocarditis; preliminary report. Proc Staff Meet Mayo Clin. 1958;33(7): 172-81.

[103] Elyasi S, Khalili H, Dashti-Khavidaki S, Mohammadpour A. Vancomycin-induced nephrotoxicity: mechanism, incidence, risk factors and special populations. A literature review. Eur J Clin Pharmacol. 2012;68(9): 1243-55.

[104] Von Drygalski A, Curtis BR, Bougie DW, McFarland JG, Ahl S, Limbu I, et al. Vancomycin-induced immune thrombocytopenia. N Engl J Med. 2007;356(9):904-10.

[105] Van Bambeke F. Glycopeptides in clinical development: pharmacological profile and clinical perspectives. Curr Opin Pharmacol. 2004;4(5):471-8.

[106] Higgins DL, Chang R, Debabov DV, Leung J, Wu T, Krause KM, et al. Telavancin, a multifunctional lipoglycopeptide, disrupts both cell wall synthesis and cell membrane integrity in methicillin-resistant *Staphylococcus aureus*. Antimicrob Agents Chemother. 2005;49 (3):1127-34.

[107] Zhanel GG, Schweizer F, Karlowsky JA. Oritavancin: mechanism of action. Clin Infect Dis. 2012;54 Suppl 3:S214-9.

[108] Goldstein EJ, Citron DM, Merriam CV, Warren YA, Tyrrell KL, Fernandez HT. In vitro activities of the new semisynthetic glycopeptide telavancin (TD-6424), vancomycin, daptomycin, linezolid, and four comparator agents against anaerobic gram-positive species and Corynebacterium spp. Antimicrob Agents Chemother. 2004;48(6):2149-52.

[109] Zeng D, Debabov D, Hartsell TL, Cano RJ, Adams S, Schuyler JA, et al. Approved Glycopeptide Antibacterial Drugs: Mechanism of Action and Resistance. Cold Spring Harb Perspect Med. 2016;6(12).

[110] Marbury T, Dowell JA, Seltzer E, Buckwalter M. Pharmacokinetics of dalbavancin in patients with renal or hepatic impairment. J Clin Pharmacol. 2009;49(4):465-76.

[111] Hobbs JK, Miller K, O'Neill AJ, Chopra I. Consequences of daptomycin-mediated membrane damage in *Staphylococcus aureus*. J Antimicrob Chemother. 2008;62(5):1003-8.

[112] Muller A, Wenzel M, Strahl H, Grein F, Saaki TNV, Kohl B, et al. Daptomycin inhibits cell envelope synthesis by interfering with fluid membrane microdomains. Proc Natl Acad Sci U S A. 2016;113(45):E7077-E86.

[113] Muraih JK, Pearson A, Silverman J, Palmer M. Oligomerization of daptomycin on membranes. Biochim Biophys Acta. 2011;1808(4):1154-60.

[114] Sharma M, Riederer K, Chase P, Khatib R. High rate of decreasing daptomycin susceptibility during the treatment of persistent *Staphylococcus aureus* bacteremia. Eur J Clin Microbiol Infect Dis. 2008;27(6):433-7.

[115] Ernst CM, Staubitz P, Mishra NN, Yang SJ, Hornig G, Kalbacher H, et al. The bacterial defensin resistance protein MprF consists of separable domains for lipid lysinylation and antimicrobial

peptide repulsion. PLoS Pathog. 2009;5 (11):e1000660.

[116] Mehta S, Cuirolo AX, Plata KB, Riosa S, Silverman JA, Rubio A, et al. VraSR two-component regulatory system contributes to mprF-mediated decreased susceptibility to daptomycin in in vivo-selected clinical strains of methicillin-resistant *Staphylococcus aureus*. Antimicrob Agents Chemother. 2012;56(1):92-102.

[117] Cafiso V, Bertuccio T, Spina D, Purrello S, Campanile F, Di Pietro C, et al. Modulating activity of vancomycin and daptomycin on the expression of autolysis cell-wall turnover and membrane charge genes in hVISA and VISA strains. PLoS One. 2012;7(1):e29573.

[118] Bertsche U, Weidenmaier C, Kuehner D, Yang SJ, Baur S, Wanner S, et al. Correlation of daptomycin resistance in a clinical *Staphylococcus aureus* strain with increased cell wall teichoic acid production and D-alanylation. Antimicrob Agents Chemother. 2011;55(8):3922-8.

[119] Benvenuto M, Benziger DP, Yankelev S, Vigliani G. Pharmacokinetics and tolerability of daptomycin at doses up to 12 milligrams per kilogram of body weight once daily in healthy volunteers. Antimicrob Agents Chemother. 2006;50(10):3245-9.

[120] Dvorchik BH, Brazier D, DeBruin MF, Arbeit RD. Daptomycin pharmacokinetics and safety following administration of escalating doses once daily to healthy subjects. Antimicrob Agents Chemother. 2003;47(4):1318-23.

[121] Cottagnoud P, Pfister M, Acosta F, Cottagnoud M, Flatz L, Kuhn F, et al. Daptomycin is highly efficacious against penicillin-resistant and penicillin- and quinolone-resistant pneumococci in experimental meningitis. Antimicrob Agents Chemother. 2004;48(10): 3928-33.

[122] Hanberger H, Nilsson LE, Maller R, Isaksson B. Pharmacodynamics of daptomycin and vancomycin on *Enterococcus faecalis* and *Staphylococcus aureus* demonstrated by studies of initial killing and postantibiotic effect and influence of Ca2+ and albumin on these drugs. Antimicrob Agents Chemother. 1991;35(9):1710-6.

[123] Figueroa DA, Mangini E, Amodio-Groton M, Vardianos B, Melchert A, Fana C, et al. Safety of high-dose intravenous daptomycin treatment: three-year cumulative experience in a clinical program. Clin Infect Dis. 2009; 49(2):177-80.

[124] Wright GD, Berghuis AM, Mobashery S. Aminoglycoside antibiotics. Structures, functions, and resistance. Adv Exp Med Biol. 1998;456: 27-69.

[125] Hurwitz C, Rosano CL, Landau JV. Kinetics of loss of vibility of *Escherichia coli* exposed to streptomycin. J Bacteriol. 1962;83:1210-6.

[126] Martin NL, Beveridge TJ. Gentamicin interaction with *Pseudomonas aeruginosa* cell envelope. Antimicrob Agents Chemother. 1986;29 (6):1079-87.

[127] Walter F, Vicens Q, Westhof E. Aminoglycoside-RNA interactions. Curr Opin Chem Biol. 1999;3(6):694-704.

[128] Lynch SR, Puglisi JD. Structural origins of aminoglycoside specificity for prokaryotic ribosomes. J Mol Biol. 2001; 306(5):1037-58.

[129] Hocquet D, Vogne C, El Garch F, Vejux A, Gotoh N, Lee A, et al. MexXY-OprM efflux pump is necessary for a adaptive resistance of *Pseudomonas aeruginosa* to aminoglycosides. Antimicrob Agents Chemother. 2003;47(4):1371-5.

[130] Mao W, Warren MS, Lee A, Mistry A, Lomovskaya O. MexXY-

OprM efflux pump is required for antagonism of aminoglycosides by divalent cations in *Pseudomonas aeruginosa*. Antimicrob Agents Chemother. 2001;45(7):2001-7.

[131] Magnet S, Blanchard JS. Molecular insights into aminoglycoside action and resistance. Chem Rev. 2005;105(2): 477-98.

[132] Bush K, Miller GH. Bacterial enzymatic resistance: beta-lactamases and aminoglycoside-modifying enzymes. Curr Opin Microbiol. 1998;1 (5):509-15.

[133] Hoffman LR, D'Argenio DA, MacCoss MJ, Zhang Z, Jones RA, Miller SI. Aminoglycoside antibiotics induce bacterial biofilm formation. Nature. 2005;436(7054):1171-5.

[134] Barza M, Brown RB, Shen D, Gibaldi M, Weinstein L. Predictability of blood levels of gentamicin in man. J Infect Dis. 1975;132(2):165-74.

[135] Bailey DN, Briggs JR. Gentamicin and tobramycin binding to human serum in vitro. J Anal Toxicol. 2004;28 (3):187-9.

[136] Rodriguez V, Stewart D, Bodey GP. Gentamicin sulfate distribution in body fluids. Clin Pharmacol Ther. 1970;11(2): 275-81.

[137] Rahal JJ, Jr., Hyams PJ, Simberkoff MS, Rubinstein E. Combined intrathecal and intramuscular gentamicin for gram-negative meningitis. Pharmacologic study of 21 patients. N Engl J Med. 1974; 290(25):1394-8.

[138] Baum J. Infections of the eye. Clin Infect Dis. 1995;21(3):479-86; quiz 87-8.

[139] Wilson TW, Mahon WA, Inaba T, Johnson GE, Kadar D. Elimination of tritiated gentamicin in normal human subjects and in patients with severely impaired renal function. Clin Pharmacol Ther. 1973;14(5):815-22.

[140] Wang JC. DNA topoisomerases. Annu Rev Biochem. 1996;65:635-92.

[141] Kohanski MA, Dwyer DJ, Hayete B, Lawrence CA, Collins JJ. A common mechanism of cellular death induced by bactericidal antibiotics. Cell. 2007;130(5):797-810.

[142] Dudley MN. Pharmacokinetics of Fluoroquinolones. Quinolone Antimicrobial Agents2003. p. 113-32.

[143] Tamai I, Yamashita J, Kido Y, Ohnari A, Sai Y, Shima Y, et al. Limited distribution of new quinolone antibacterial agents into brain caused by multiple efflux transporters at the blood-brain barrier. J Pharmacol Exp Ther. 2000;295(1):146-52.

[144] Alffenaar JW, van Altena R, Bokkerink HJ, Luijckx GJ, van Soolingen D, Aarnoutse RE, et al. Pharmacokinetics of moxifloxacin in cerebrospinal fluid and plasma in patients with tuberculous meningitis. Clin Infect Dis. 2009;49(7):1080-2.

[145] Stass H, Buhrmann S, Mitchell A, Kubitza D, Moller JG, Kribben A, et al. The influence of continuous venovenous haemodialysis on the pharmacokinetics of multiple oral moxifloxacin administration to patients with severe renal dysfunction. Br J Clin Pharmacol. 2007;64(6):745-9.

[146] Lode H, Rubinstein E. Adverse Effects. Quinolone Antimicrobial Agents2003. p. 405-19.

[147] Norrby SR. Central Nervous System Toxicity. Quinolone Antimicrobial Agents2003. p. 461-5.

[148] Etminan M, Brophy JM, Samii A. Oral fluoroquinolone use and risk of peripheral neuropathy: a

pharmacoepidemiologic study. Neurology. 2014;83(14):1261-3.

[149] Ball P, Mandell L, Patou G, Dankner W, Tillotson G. A new respiratory fluoroquinolone, oral gemifloxacin: a safety profile in context. Int J Antimicrob Agents. 2004;23(5): 421-9.

[150] Iannini P, Mandell L, Patou G, Shear N. Cutaneous adverse events and gemifloxacin: observations from the clinical trial program. J Chemother. 2006;18(1):3-11.

[151] Hypoglycemia and hyperglycemia with fluroroquinolones. Med Lett Drugs Ther. 2003;45(1162):64.

[152] Yap YG, Camm AJ. QT Prolongation with Quinolone Antimicrobial Agents. Quinolone Antimicrobial Agents2003. p. 421-40.

[153] Pasternak B, Inghammar M, Svanstrom H. Fluoroquinolone use and risk of aortic aneurysm and dissection: nationwide cohort study. BMJ. 2018; 360:k678.

[154] Etminan M, Forooghian F, Brophy JM, Bird ST, Maberley D. Oral fluoroquinolones and the risk of retinal detachment. JAMA. 2012;307(13): 1414-9.

[155] Stahlmann R. Effects on Connective Tissue Structures. Quinolone Antimicrobial Agents2003. p. 441-9.

[156] Fleming A. On the antibacterial action of cultures of a penicillium, with special reference to their use in the isolation of B. influenzae. 1929. Bull World Health Organ. 2001;79(8):780-90.

[157] Giesbrecht P, Kersten T, Maidhof H, Wecke J. Staphylococcal cell wall: morphogenesis and fatal variations in the presence of penicillin. Microbiol Mol Biol Rev. 1998;62(4):1371-414.

[158] Queenan AM, Bush K. Carbapenemases: the versatile beta-lactamases. Clin Microbiol Rev. 2007;20 (3):440-58, table of contents.

[159] Tomas M, Doumith M, Warner M, Turton JF, Beceiro A, Bou G, et al. Efflux pumps, OprD porin, AmpC beta-lactamase, and multiresistance in *Pseudomonas aeruginosa* isolates from cystic fibrosis patients. Antimicrob Agents Chemother. 2010;54(5):2219-24.

[160] Zapun A, Contreras-Martel C, Vernet T. Penicillin-binding proteins and beta-lactam resistance. FEMS Microbiol Rev. 2008;32(2):361-85.

[161] Yates AB. Management of patients with a history of allergy to beta-lactam antibiotics. Am J Med. 2008;121(7): 572-6.

[162] Slimings C, Riley TV. Antibiotics and hospital-acquired *Clostridium difficile* infection: update of systematic review and meta-analysis. J Antimicrob Chemother. 2014;69(4):881-91.

[163] Maraqa NF, Gomez MM, Rathore MH, Alvarez AM. Higher occurrence of hepatotoxicity and rash in patients treated with oxacillin, compared with those treated with nafcillin and other commonly used antimicrobials. Clin Infect Dis. 2002;34(1):50-4.

[164] Andersohn F, Konzen C, Garbe E. Systematic review: agranulocytosis induced by nonchemotherapy drugs. Ann Intern Med. 2007;146(9):657-65.

[165] Appel GB, Neu HC. The nephrotoxicity of antimicrobial agents (first of three parts). N Engl J Med. 1977;296(12):663-70.

[166] Bo G. Giuseppe Brotzu and the discovery of cephalosporins. Clin Microbiol Infect. 2000;6 Suppl 3:6-9.

[167] Waxman DJ, Strominger JL. Penicillin-binding proteins and the

mechanism of action of beta-lactam antibiotics. Annu Rev Biochem. 1983;52: 825-69.

[168] Fontana R, Cornaglia G, Ligozzi M, Mazzariol A. The final goal: penicillin-binding proteins and the target of cephalosporins. Clin Microbiol Infect. 2000;6 Suppl 3:34-40.

[169] Simner PJ, Patel R. Cefiderocol Antimicrobial Susceptibility Testing Considerations: the Achilles' Heel of the Trojan Horse? J Clin Microbiol. 2020;59 (1).

[170] Peterson HB, Galaid EI, Zenilman JM. Pelvic inflammatory disease: review of treatment options. Rev Infect Dis. 1990;12 Suppl 6:S656-64.

[171] Nadelman RB, Luger SW, Frank E, Wisniewski M, Collins JJ, Wormser GP. Comparison of cefuroxime axetil and doxycycline in the treatment of early Lyme disease. Ann Intern Med. 1992;117 (4):273-80.

[172] Trenholme GM, Schmitt BA, Nelson JA, Gvazdinskas LC, Harrison BB, Parkhurst GW. Comparative study of three different dosing regimens of cefotaxime for treatment of gram-negative bacteremia. Diagn Microbiol Infect Dis. 1989;12(1): 107-11.

[173] Workowski KA, Bolan GA, Centers for Disease C, Prevention. Sexually transmitted diseases treatment guidelines, 2015. MMWR Recomm Rep. 2015;64(RR-03):1-137.

[174] Augenbraun M, Workowski K. Ceftriaxone therapy for syphilis: report from the emerging infections network. Clin Infect Dis. 1999;29(5):1337-8.

[175] Shane AL, Mody RK, Crump JA, Tarr PI, Steiner TS, Kotloff K, et al. 2017 Infectious Diseases Society of America Clinical Practice Guidelines for the Diagnosis and Management of Infectious Diarrhea. Clin Infect Dis. 2017;65(12):1963-73.

[176] Baddour LM, Wilson WR, Bayer AS, Fowler VG, Jr., Tleyjeh IM, Rybak MJ, et al. Infective Endocarditis in Adults: Diagnosis, Antimicrobial Therapy, and Management of Complications: A Scientific Statement for Healthcare Professionals From the American Heart Association. Circulation. 2015;132(15):1435-86.

[177] Fong IW, Tomkins KB. Review of *Pseudomonas aeruginosa* meningitis with special emphasis on treatment with ceftazidime. Rev Infect Dis. 1985;7(5): 604-12.

[178] Sanders CC. Cefepime: the next generation? Clin Infect Dis. 1993;17(3): 369-79.

[179] Freifeld AG, Bow EJ, Sepkowitz KA, Boeckh MJ, Ito JI, Mullen CA, et al. Clinical practice guideline for the use of antimicrobial agents in neutropenic patients with cancer: 2010 update by the infectious diseases society of america. Clin Infect Dis. 2011;52(4):e56-93.

[180] Bartlett JG, Dowell SF, Mandell LA, File TM, Jr., Musher DM, Fine MJ. Practice guidelines for the management of community-acquired pneumonia in adults. Infectious Diseases Society of America. Clin Infect Dis. 2000;31(2):347-82.

[181] Noel GJ, Bush K, Bagchi P, Ianus J, Strauss RS. A randomized, double-blind trial comparing ceftobiprole medocaril with vancomycin plus ceftazidime for the treatment of patients with complicated skin and skin-structure infections. Clin Infect Dis. 2008;46(5): 647-55.

[182] Nicholson SC, Welte T, File TM, Jr., Strauss RS, Michiels B, Kaul P, et al. A randomised, double-blind trial comparing ceftobiprole medocaril with

ceftriaxone with or without linezolid for the treatment of patients with community-acquired pneumonia requiring hospitalisation. Int J Antimicrob Agents. 2012;39(3):240-6.

[183] Werth BJ, Sakoulas G, Rose WE, Pogliano J, Tewhey R, Rybak MJ. Ceftaroline increases membrane binding and enhances the activity of daptomycin against daptomycin-nonsusceptible vancomycin-intermediate *Staphylococcus aureus* in a pharmacokinetic/pharmacodynamic model. Antimicrob Agents Chemother. 2013;57(1):66-73.

[184] Bennett WM, Aronoff GR, Morrison G, Golper TA, Pulliam J, Wolfson M, et al. Drug prescribing in renal failure: dosing guidelines for adults. Am J Kidney Dis. 1983;3(3): 155-93.

[185] Katsube T, Wajima T, Ishibashi T, Arjona Ferreira JC, Echols R. Pharmacokinetic/Pharmacodynamic Modeling and Simulation of Cefiderocol, a Parenteral Siderophore Cephalosporin, for Dose Adjustment Based on Renal Function. Antimicrob Agents Chemother. 2017;61(1).

[186] Reading C, Cole M. Clavulanic acid: a beta-lactamase-inhiting beta-lactam from *Streptomyces clavuligerus*. Antimicrob Agents Chemother. 1977;11 (5):852-7.

[187] Gin A, Dilay L, Karlowsky JA, Walkty A, Rubinstein E, Zhanel GG. Piperacillin-tazobactam: a beta-lactam/beta-lactamase inhibitor combination. Expert Rev Anti Infect Ther. 2007;5(3):365-83.

[188] Stapleton P, Wu PJ, King A, Shannon K, French G, Phillips I. Incidence and mechanisms of resistance to the combination of amoxicillin and clavulanic acid in *Escherichia coli*. Antimicrob Agents Chemother. 1995;39 (11):2478-83.

[189] Dhillon S. Meropenem/ Vaborbactam: A Review in Complicated Urinary Tract Infections. Drugs. 2018;78 (12):1259-70.

[190] Fass RJ, Copelan EA, Brandt JT, Moeschberger ML, Ashton JJ. Platelet-mediated bleeding caused by broad-spectrum penicillins. J Infect Dis. 1987; 155(6):1242-8.

[191] Arnold DM, Kukaswadia S, Nazi I, Esmail A, Dewar L, Smith JW, et al. A systematic evaluation of laboratory testing for drug-induced immune thrombocytopenia. J Thromb Haemost. 2013;11(1):169-76.

[192] Sykes RB, Wells JS, Parker WL, Koster WH, Cimarusti CM. Aztreonam: discovery and development of the monobactams. N J Med. 1986;Spec No: 8-15.

[193] Jorth P, McLean K, Ratjen A, Secor PR, Bautista GE, Ravishankar S, et al. Evolved Aztreonam Resistance Is Multifactorial and Can Produce Hypervirulence in *Pseudomonas aeruginosa*. mBio. 2017;8(5).

[194] Ramsey C, MacGowan AP. A review of the pharmacokinetics and pharmacodynamics of aztreonam. J Antimicrob Chemother. 2016;71(10): 2704-12.

[195] Zhanel GG, Wiebe R, Dilay L, Thomson K, Rubinstein E, Hoban DJ, et al. Comparative review of the carbapenems. Drugs. 2007;67(7): 1027-52.

[196] Mori H, Takahashi K, Mizutani T. Interaction between valproic acid and carbapenem antibiotics. Drug Metab Rev. 2007;39(4):647-57.

[197] Romano A, Viola M, Gueant-Rodriguez RM, Gaeta F, Valluzzi R, Gueant JL. Brief communication: tolerability of meropenem in patients with IgE-mediated hypersensitivity to

penicillins. Ann Intern Med. 2007;146 (4):266-9.

[198] From AH, Fong JS, Good RA. Polymyxin B sulfate modification of bacterial endotoxin: effects on the development of endotoxin shock in dogs. Infect Immun. 1979;23(3):660-4.

[199] Liu YY, Wang Y, Walsh TR, Yi LX, Zhang R, Spencer J, et al. Emergence of plasmid-mediated colistin resistance mechanism MCR-1 in animals and human beings in China: a microbiological and molecular biological study. Lancet Infect Dis. 2016;16(2):161-8.

[200] Bergen PJ, Forrest A, Bulitta JB, Tsuji BT, Sidjabat HE, Paterson DL, et al. Clinically relevant plasma concentrations of colistin in combination with imipenem enhance pharmacodynamic activity against multidrug-resistant *Pseudomonas aeruginosa* at multiple inocula. Antimicrob Agents Chemother. 2011;55 (11):5134-42.

[201] Sandri AM, Landersdorfer CB, Jacob J, Boniatti MM, Dalarosa MG, Falci DR, et al. Population pharmacokinetics of intravenous polymyxin B in critically ill patients: implications for selection of dosage regimens. Clin Infect Dis. 2013;57(4): 524-31.

[202] Falagas ME, Kasiakou SK. Toxicity of polymyxins: a systematic review of the evidence from old and recent studies. Crit Care. 2006;10(1):R27.

[203] Kahan FM, Kahan JS, Cassidy PJ, Kropp H. The mechanism of action of fosfomycin (phosphonomycin). Ann N Y Acad Sci. 1974;235(0):364-86.

[204] Michalopoulos AS, Livaditis IG, Gougoutas V. The revival of fosfomycin. Int J Infect Dis. 2011;15(11):e732-9.

[205] Wenzler E, Ellis-Grosse EJ, Rodvold KA. Pharmacokinetics, Safety, and Tolerability of Single-Dose Intravenous (ZTI-01) and Oral Fosfomycin in Healthy Volunteers. Antimicrob Agents Chemother. 2017;61 (9).

[206] Paukner S, Riedl R. Pleuromutilins: Potent Drugs for Resistant Bugs-Mode of Action and Resistance. Cold Spring Harb Perspect Med. 2017;7(1).

[207] Prince WT, Ivezic-Schoenfeld Z, Lell C, Tack KJ, Novak R, Obermayr F, et al. Phase II clinical study of BC-3781, a pleuromutilin antibiotic, in treatment of patients with acute bacterial skin and skin structure infections. Antimicrob Agents Chemother. 2013;57(5):2087-94.

[208] Ramaswamy S, Musser JM. Molecular genetic basis of antimicrobial agent resistance in *Mycobacterium tuberculosis*: 1998 update. Tuber Lung Dis. 1998;79(1):3-29.

[209] Floss HG, Yu TW. Rifamycin-mode of action, resistance, and biosynthesis. Chem Rev. 2005;105(2): 621-32.

[210] Donald PR. Cerebrospinal fluid concentrations of antituberculosis agents in adults and children. Tuberculosis (Edinb). 2010;90(5): 279-92.

[211] Burman WJ, Gallicano K, Peloquin C. Comparative pharmacokinetics and pharmacodynamics of the rifamycin antibacterials. Clin Pharmacokinet. 2001;40(5):327-41.

[212] Jiang ZD, Ke S, Palazzini E, Riopel L, Dupont H. In vitro activity and fecal concentration of rifaximin after oral administration. Antimicrob Agents Chemother. 2000;44(8):2205-6.

[213] Ohno M, Yamaguchi I, Yamamoto I, Fukuda T, Yokota S, Maekura R, et al. Slow N-acetyltransferase 2 genotype affects the

incidence of isoniazid and rifampicin-induced hepatotoxicity. Int J Tuberc Lung Dis. 2000;4(3):256-61.

[214] Griffith DE, Brown BA, Girard WM, Wallace RJ, Jr. Adverse events associated with high-dose rifabutin in macrolide-containing regimens for the treatment of *Mycobacterium avium* complex lung disease. Clin Infect Dis. 1995;21(3):594-8.

[215] Lofmark S, Edlund C, Nord CE. Metronidazole is still the drug of choice for treatment of anaerobic infections. Clin Infect Dis. 2010;50 Suppl 1:S16-23.

[216] Bratzler DW, Dellinger EP, Olsen KM, Perl TM, Auwaerter PG, Bolon MK, et al. Clinical practice guidelines for antimicrobial prophylaxis in surgery. Am J Health Syst Pharm. 2013;70(3):195-283.

[217] Norman WV. Metronidazole prophylaxis before surgical abortion: retrospective review of 51 330 cases. J Obstet Gynaecol Can. 2012;34(7): 648-52.

[218] Cosgrove SE, Vigliani GA, Fowler VG, Jr., Abrutyn E, Corey GR, Levine DP, et al. Initial low-dose gentamicin for *Staphylococcus aureus* bacteremia and endocarditis is nephrotoxic. Clin Infect Dis. 2009;48 (6):713-21.

[219] Hammond DA, Smith MN, Li C, Hayes SM, Lusardi K, Bookstaver PB. Systematic Review and Meta-Analysis of Acute Kidney Injury Associated with Concomitant Vancomycin and Piperacillin/tazobactam. Clin Infect Dis. 2017;64(5):666-74.

[220] Wilson AP, Gruneberg RN, Neu H. A critical review of the dosage of teicoplanin in Europe and the USA. Int J Antimicrob Agents. 1994;4 Suppl 1:1-30.

[221] Men P, Li HB, Zhai SD, Zhao RS. Association between the AUC0-24/MIC Ratio of Vancomycin and Its Clinical Effectiveness: A Systematic Review and Meta-Analysis. PLoS One. 2016;11(1): e0146224.

[222] Moore CL, Osaki-Kiyan P, Haque NZ, Perri MB, Donabedian S, Zervos MJ. Daptomycin versus vancomycin for bloodstream infections due to methicillin-resistant *Staphylococcus aureus* with a high vancomycin minimum inhibitory concentration: a case-control study. Clin Infect Dis. 2012;54(1):51-8.

[223] Britt NS, Potter EM, Patel N, Steed ME. Comparative Effectiveness and Safety of Standard-, Medium-, and High-Dose Daptomycin Strategies for the Treatment of Vancomycin-Resistant Enterococcal Bacteremia Among Veterans Affairs Patients. Clin Infect Dis. 2017;64(5):605-13.

[224] Chuang YC, Lin HY, Chen PY, Lin CY, Wang JT, Chen YC, et al. Effect of Daptomycin Dose on the Outcome of Vancomycin-Resistant, Daptomycin-Susceptible *Enterococcus faecium* Bacteremia. Clin Infect Dis. 2017;64(8): 1026-34.

[225] Riser MS, Bland CM, Rudisill CN, Bookstaver PB. Cerebrospinal fluid penetration of high-dose daptomycin in suspected *Staphylococcus aureus* meningitis. Ann Pharmacother. 2010;44 (11):1832-5.

[226] Pertel PE, Bernardo P, Fogarty C, Matthews P, Northland R, Benvenuto M, et al. Effects of prior effective therapy on the efficacy of daptomycin and ceftriaxone for the treatment of community-acquired pneumonia. Clin Infect Dis. 2008;46(8): 1142-51.

[227] Delgado G, Jr., Neuhauser MM, Bearden DT, Danziger LH. Quinupristin-dalfopristin: an overview. Pharmacotherapy. 2000;20(12): 1469-85.

[228] Moellering RC, Jr. The Garrod Lecture. The enterococcus: a classic example of the impact of antimicrobial resistance on therapeutic options. J Antimicrob Chemother. 1991;28(1):1-12.

[229] Gilbert DN. Meta-analyses are no longer required for determining the efficacy of single daily dosing of aminoglycosides. Clin Infect Dis. 1997; 24(5):816-9.

[230] Wong J, Brown G. Does once-daily dosing of aminoglycosides affect neuromuscular function? J Clin Pharm Ther. 1996;21(6):407-11.

[231] Zabner R, Quinn JP. Antimicrobials in cystic fibrosis: emergence of resistance and implications for treatment. Semin Respir Infect. 1992;7 (3):210-7.

[232] de Groot R, Smith AL. Antibiotic pharmacokinetics in cystic fibrosis. Differences and clinical significance. Clin Pharmacokinet. 1987;13(4):228-53.

[233] Ghannam DE, Rodriguez GH, Raad, II, Safdar A. Inhaled aminoglycosides in cancer patients with ventilator-associated Gram-negative bacterial pneumonia: safety and feasibility in the era of escalating drug resistance. Eur J Clin Microbiol Infect Dis. 2009;28(3):253-9.

[234] Landman D, Kelly P, Backer M, Babu E, Shah N, Bratu S, et al. Antimicrobial activity of a novel aminoglycoside, ACHN-490, against *Acinetobacter baumannii* and *Pseudomonas aeruginosa* from New York City. J Antimicrob Chemother. 2011;66 (2):332-4.

[235] Zagursky RJ, Pichichero ME. Cross-reactivity in beta-Lactam Allergy. J Allergy Clin Immunol Pract. 2018;6(1): 72-81 e1.

[236] Paul M, Yahav D, Fraser A, Leibovici L. Empirical antibiotic monotherapy for febrile neutropenia: systematic review and meta-analysis of randomized controlled trials. J Antimicrob Chemother. 2006;57(2): 176-89.

[237] Kim PW, Wu YT, Cooper C, Rochester G, Valappil T, Wang Y, et al. Meta-analysis of a possible signal of increased mortality associated with cefepime use. Clin Infect Dis. 2010;51 (4):381-9.

[238] Tamma PD, Rodriguez-Bano J. The Use of Noncarbapenem beta-Lactams for the Treatment of Extended-Spectrum beta-Lactamase Infections. Clin Infect Dis. 2017;64(7):972-80.

[239] Wright H, Bonomo RA, Paterson DL. New agents for the treatment of infections with Gram-negative bacteria: restoring the miracle or false dawn? Clin Microbiol Infect. 2017;23(10):704-12.

[240] Rodriguez-Bano J, Navarro MD, Retamar P, Picon E, Pascual A, Extended-Spectrum Beta-Lactamases-Red Espanola de Investigacion en Patologia Infecciosa/Grupo de Estudio de Infeccion Hospitalaria G. beta-Lactam/beta-lactam inhibitor combinations for the treatment of bacteremia due to extended-spectrum beta-lactamase-producing *Escherichia coli*: a post hoc analysis of prospective cohorts. Clin Infect Dis. 2012;54(2): 167-74.

[241] Tamma PD, Han JH, Rock C, Harris AD, Lautenbach E, Hsu AJ, et al. Carbapenem therapy is associated with improved survival compared with piperacillin-tazobactam for patients with extended-spectrum beta-lactamase bacteremia. Clin Infect Dis. 2015;60(9): 1319-25.

[242] Trias J, Nikaido H. Outer membrane protein D2 catalyzes facilitated diffusion of carbapenems and penems through the outer membrane of

Pseudomonas aeruginosa. Antimicrob Agents Chemother. 1990;34(1):52-7.

[243] Davies TA, Marie Queenan A, Morrow BJ, Shang W, Amsler K, He W, et al. Longitudinal survey of carbapenem resistance and resistance mechanisms in Enterobacteriaceae and non-fermenters from the USA in 2007-09. J Antimicrob Chemother. 2011;66(10):2298-307.

[244] Chastre J, Wolff M, Fagon JY, Chevret S, Thomas F, Wermert D, et al. Comparison of 8 vs 15 days of antibiotic therapy for ventilator-associated pneumonia in adults: a randomized trial. JAMA. 2003;290(19):2588-98.

[245] Oliveira MS, Prado GV, Costa SF, Grinbaum RS, Levin AS. Ampicillin/sulbactam compared with polymyxins for the treatment of infections caused by carbapenem-resistant Acinetobacter spp. J Antimicrob Chemother. 2008;61 (6):1369-75.

[246] Shields RK, Nguyen MH, Chen L, Press EG, Potoski BA, Marini RV, et al. Ceftazidime-Avibactam Is Superior to Other Treatment Regimens against Carbapenem-Resistant *Klebsiella pneumoniae* Bacteremia. Antimicrob Agents Chemother. 2017;61(8).

[247] Kollef MH. Inadequate antimicrobial treatment: an important determinant of outcome for hospitalized patients. Clin Infect Dis. 2000;31 Suppl 4:S131-8.

[248] Ferrer R, Martin-Loeches I, Phillips G, Osborn TM, Townsend S, Dellinger RP, et al. Empiric antibiotic treatment reduces mortality in severe sepsis and septic shock from the first hour: results from a guideline-based performance improvement program. Crit Care Med. 2014;42(8):1749-55.

[249] Rhodes A, Evans LE, Alhazzani W, Levy MM, Antonelli M, Ferrer R, et al. Surviving Sepsis Campaign: International Guidelines for Management of Sepsis and Septic Shock: 2016. Crit Care Med. 2017;45(3):486-552.

[250] Blot SI, Pea F, Lipman J. The effect of pathophysiology on pharmacokinetics in the critically ill patient–concepts appraised by the example of antimicrobial agents. Adv Drug Deliv Rev. 2014;77:3-11.

[251] Beumier M, Casu GS, Hites M, Wolff F, Cotton F, Vincent JL, et al. Elevated beta-lactam concentrations associated with neurological deterioration in ICU septic patients. Minerva Anestesiol. 2015;81(5):497-506.

[252] Vogelman B, Craig WA. Kinetics of antimicrobial activity. J Pediatr. 1986; 108(5 Pt 2):835-40.

[253] Udy AA, Roberts JA, Boots RJ, Paterson DL, Lipman J. Augmented renal clearance: implications for antibacterial dosing in the critically ill. Clin Pharmacokinet. 2010;49(1):1-16.

[254] American Thoracic S, Infectious Diseases Society of A. Guidelines for the management of adults with hospital-acquired, ventilator-associated, and healthcare-associated pneumonia. Am J Respir Crit Care Med. 2005;171(4):388-416.

[255] Hayashi Y, Paterson DL. Strategies for reduction in duration of antibiotic use in hospitalized patients. Clin Infect Dis. 2011;52(10):1232-40.

[256] Kalil AC, Metersky ML, Klompas M, Muscedere J, Sweeney DA, Palmer LB, et al. Management of Adults With Hospital-acquired and Ventilator-associated Pneumonia: 2016 Clinical Practice Guidelines by the Infectious Diseases Society of America and the American Thoracic Society. Clin Infect Dis. 2016;63(5):e61-e111.

[257] Burke JP, Pestotnik SL. Antibiotic use and microbial resistance in intensive care units: impact of computer-assisted decision support. J Chemother. 1999;11 (6):530-5.

Chapter 2

Distribution and Molecular Detection of Methicilin-Resistant *Staphylococcus aureus*

Velma Rebić, Mufida Aljičević, Sajra Vinčević-Smajlović and Damir Rebić

Abstract

Isolation of *Staphylococcus aureus* is quite common in both the general population and hospital environment. The heterogeneity of the disease and the unique ability of *S. aureus* to develop resistance to the most recently discovered antibacterial drugs points to its ability to adapt and survive in different conditions. CA-MRSA is different from hospital strains of MRSA by its epidemiological, phenotypic and genotypic characteristics. The emergence of MRSA in the community suggests the need for a new approach to managing the indications and the certification of staphylococcal infections, with special emphasis on the selection of empiric antibiotic therapy. In the study, we analised of MRSA from 4341 samples taken from patients from the general population of Sarajevo Canton in the six-month period of follow-up processed at the Public Health Institute of Sarajevo Canton. We determined the epidemiological characteristics of the isolated strains. Methicillin resistance was determined by phenotypic methods. The following molecular methods were used for the confirmation of methicillin resistance: determination of the mecA gene, PFGE profile, genetic type of MRSA being determined by spa typing, the distribution of SCCmec types being examined, and the detected gene for PVL. The study stresses the need for national monitoring of spreading of the existing epidemic strains, as well as the monitoring of emergence of new strains which would enable the inclusion of our country in the international network of monitoring bacterial resistance.

Keywords: infection, CA-MRSA, phenotypic, antimicrobial susceptibility

1. Introduction

The first isolation of Staphylococci was carried out by Alexander Ogston during the investigation of the septicemia and wound infection bacteria in 1880, the microscopical examination of 88 pus specimens revealed the presence of Gram-positive cocci (*S. aureus*) [1]. In clinical observations, the most important species of Staphylococcus genus are *Staphylococcus aureus* and *Staphylococcus epidermids*, further falling into categories based on their coagulase activity. *S. aureus* is coagulase positive, expressing several virulence factors supporting host immune response evasion. *S. epidermidis* being coagulase negative, usually less virulent, able to avoid the host immune system by forming and resulting in its hiding in a biofilm [2]. *Staphylococcus aureus* (SA) represents one of the most important microorganisms that are part of the normal micro flora in humans, with ability to cause very serious infections in certain conditions. Approximately 20–30% of the general human population is persistently colonized with SA. Primary and natural reservoir of *S. aureus* is the asymptomatic carriage by humans, using the anterior nasal mucosa as the main ecological niche. The risk of subsequent infection increases as the colonization provides a reservoir open to bacteria introduction as host defences are breached [3]. Adding to humans and domestic animals, livestock and fomites can also serve as joint reservoirs, providing this bacterial pathogen with dramatic relevance in human and veterinary medicine. *Staphylococcus aureus* can cause a wide variety of infections in range from common, mild skin and soft tissue infections to hematogenous infections with multi organ injuries. *Staphylococcus aureus* is infamous for its ability to become resistant to antibiotics, resulting in issues with treatment of these infections due to the resistance development, especially with methicillin-resistant SA [4]. The virulence of *S. aureus* is multifactorial due to the combined actions of a variety of virulence factors that facilitate tissue adhesion, immune evasion, and host cell injury [5]. These virulence factors involve both structural, such as surface adhesins which provide adherence to host tissues, and secreted factors, such as enzymes, that convert host tissue into nutrients. Anyway, a lot more significant is the secretion of a variety of pyrogenic toxins also known as superantigens; the Panton–Valentine leukocidin (PVL) and toxic shock syndrome toxin-1 (TSST-1) as most remarkable [6].

1.1 Methicillin-resistant *Staphylococcus aureus*

Methicillin-Resistant *Staphylococcus aureus* (MRSA) should be taken into accounted for great concern. It is the cause of bacterium infections in various parts of body. As it develops resistance to usually prescribed antibiotics, its treatments becomes more difficult than with most strains of *Staphylococcus aureus*. MRSA is sometimes called a super bug. Methicillin-resistant *Staphylococcus aureus* (MRSA), or multidrug-resistant *S. aureus*, first described in the United Kingdom in the early 1960s, are *S. aureus* strains which developed resistance through natural selection process to all available penicillins and other β-lactam antimicrobial drugs. Methicillin resistant *Staphylococcus aureus* (MRSA) being one of the most important hospital pathogens, becomes responsible for community infection in patients without previous health-care contact at the end of the last century. Worldwide, it is mainly responsible for a broad spectrum of nosocomial and community associated infections and cause of endemic and epidemic infections in many parts of the world. Methicillin resistance in S.aureus developed through the acquisition of the mecA gene located on mobile genomic island designated staphylococcal chromosome cassette mec (SCCmec) by methicillin-susceptible S.aureus [7]. The mecA gene is primary cause for the synthesis of a novel penicillin-binding protein known as penicillin-binding protein 2a, that decreased binding affinity for penicillin and cephalosporins. It follows that MRSA strains are resistant to all ß-lactam antibiotics. In the beginning, MRSA was susceptible to nonbeta lactam antibiotics. Later, namely, from the late 1979s to this day, new strains of MRSA resistant to multi-non- ß-lactam agents including aminoglycosides, with only vancomycin left as an antibiotic of last resort for treating MRSA infections, appeared. These strains, also described as epidemic MRSA (EMRSA or HA-MRSA), have had the capacity to spread extensively causing serious infections worldwide and mostly among in-hospital patients [8].

1.2 What is community-associated MRSA?

During 1990s, in Western Australia, a new MRSA type appeared and it was causing infections in the community of younger and healthy people without previously reported history of hospital admission or medical treatment [9]. These types of MRSA strains were described as community-acquired, community-originated, community-associated, or community-onset MRSA (CA-MRSA). HA-MRSA and CA-MRSA belong to different genetic lineages. While CA-MRSA strains are usually sensitive to antibiotics other than beta-lactams and contain staphylococcal cassette chromosome SCCmec type IV, V or VII, HAMRSA are generally multidrug-resistant and harbour larger SCCmec type I, II or III [10]. MRSA pathogenicity is related to extensive arsenal of virulence factors and toxins. The most common and probably important is the Panton-Valentine leukocidin (PVL) toxin being lethal to neutrophils and associated with skin and soft tissue infections as well as severe necrotizing pneumonia. Huge number of CA-MRSA clones have developed on every continent [11]. Notably, these CA-MRSA strains, initially, were associated with community-onset (CO) infections, have been entering hospitals and may be replacing the conventional HA-MRSA strains with significant clinical and public health implications [12]. However, CA-MRSA penetration is still mostly undefined due to lack of thorough exploration of in large number of hospitals as well as knowledge of the risk factors involved in nosocomial transmission of CA-MRSA compared with HA-MRSA [13]. The prevalence of in vitro resistance to non-β-lactam antimicrobial agents could be increasing among MRSA strains related to community transmission. MRSA typing is an essential component of an overall follow up system of describing epidemiological trends and control strategies for infections. Contemporary challenges for MRSA typing are focused on choosing the most appropriate technique in terms of efficiency, reliability, ease of performance and cost included. The phenotypic methods in general are prone easier performance, interpretation, cost efficiency and wide availability, and less discrimination. The genotypic methods are rather expensive and technically demanding, however more discriminatory. Latest technologies that involve sequencing of various genes are emerging as highly applicable with wide throughput typing systems. Still there is no consensus regarding the single best method for typing of MRSA strains [14]. Pulsed-field gel electrophoresis (PFGE) has become the 'gold standard' for genotyping method of MRSA for over a decade, and it has been used widely for local outbreak investigation, long-term surveillance of MRSA infections at regional and national levels and for international comparisons [7]. Recently, in Europe, harmonization efforts to standardize the PFGE typing protocol of MRSA as well as to enable multicentric comparison of PFGE data have been made. The macro restriction analysis of chromosomal DNA using PFGE is a reference method for *Staphylococcus aureus* typing and can be combined with other methods [15].

1.3 Detection and diagnosis of MRSA strains

Identifying the causative organism can be challenging in treatment *Staphylococcus aureus* infection, especially for resistant strains. Traditional culture and susceptibility testing for MRSA lasts between 48 and 72 h, taking a 16- to 24-h incubation and 16 to 24 h more in completing the susceptibility tests. Latest progress in molecular and nonmolecular testing methods greatly reduced the time needed to detect MRSA [16]. These rapid and sensitive screening assays could contribute to infection control and reducing overall costs. With a rapid test,

Bauer et al. [17] observed bacteremia patients diagnosed with MRSA had a shorter length of stay and lower hospital costs, and for patients with MSSA, the switch from empiric to targeted therapy was 1.6 days shorter. Use of rapid molecular diagnostic tests rather than conventional methods is also related to a significantly lower mortality risk for patients with bloodstream infections (odds ratio (OR) [95% CI] 0.66 [0.54–0.80]), including those caused by Gram-positive organisms (OR [95% CI] 0.73 [0.55–0.97]). Combining rapid molecular testing with an antibiotic stewardship program will be able to lower the mortality risk [18]. Individual hospitals in decision making about the tests used should consider the specificity, sensitivity, price, turnaround time, and expertise, necessary for each test [16, 19]. Modification to the traditional culture method is the use of chromogenic agar, producing a colour reaction in the bacterial cultures. These media also contain antibiotics where only resistant bacteria is able to grow. According to this, MRSA can be detected in 20 to 26 h [16]. In clinical practice, the use of chromogenic media has been seen to shorten the time to aimed MRSA treatment by 12 h [20]. Another innovation in MRSA detection is the development of real-time polymerase chain reaction (PCR) tests with the ability to detect genes specific to *S. aureus*. In making difference in MRSA strains from MSSA or methicillin resistant coagulase-negative staphylococci, PCR methods are aimed at a part of DNA where the MRSA-specific SCCmec gene meets the *S. aureus* orfX gene. The PCR tests are usually performed directly on samples taken from blood or a nasal or wound swab, and results can be available within 1 to 3 h [16]. In clinical practice, generally, the turnaround times from taking samples to complete results are generally longer due to the length of time needed to transport samples, conduct the test, and send the results. As a rule, the overall time is usually much shorter with PCR-based assays than with chromogenic media culture [21]. Moreover, PCR tests showed pooled estimates for sensitivity and specificity of 92.5 and 97.0%, respectively, in the meta-analysis described earlier. In addition, the sensitivity of PCR has been notably higher than the one on chromogenic media, and the specificity was significantly higher than the one on traditional culture [19]. In relation to MRSA detection by chromogenic agar, PCR shortened the overall time of patient isolation as well as number of days patients were inadequately isolated during their hospital stay [21].

2. Aims

- To determine the prevalence and distribution of methicillin-resistant *Staphylococcus aureus* from different patient samples in general population of Canton Sarajevo, Bosnia and Herzegovina

- To determine epidemiological characteristics of isolated strains

- To evaluate isolated MRSA with phenotypic methods: disc diffusion test (DD), E-test, latex agglutination test with antibodies to penicillin-binding protein 2a (PBP2a), and a selective chromogenic medium

- To determine the presence of mecA gene in isolated outpatient strains

- To determine the genetic profile of MRSA strains by DNA Fingerprints by Pulsed-field Gel Electrophoresis (PFGE) and spa-typing test methods

- To evaluate the distribution of SCCmec types

- To determine the prevalence of Panton-Valentine leukocidin (PVL) -positive *Staphylococcus aureus* strains
- To estimate infection and colonization risk of outpatient MRSA strains

3. Materials and methods

Samples taken from January to August 2015 were collected from 4,341 patient samples admitted to the Laboratory of Institute of Public Health of Sarajevo Canton, Bosnia and Herzegovina (B&H) and they showed a total number of 653 methicillin-resistant *Staphylococcus aureus*, that is, out of 2279 found *Staphylococcus aureus* strains, 653 were methicillin-resistant *Staphylococcus aureus.* Those samples included nose swabs, throat, ear, eye, umbilicus swabs, wound and skin swabs. All MRSA isolates collected were identified by standard microbiological methods based on the demonstration of deoxyribonuclease, bound coagulase (rabbit plasma, bioMerieux, France) and free coagulase (Slidex Staph Plus, bioMerieux, France) [22]. Antibiotic susceptibility determination used the agar disk diffusion method in compliance with the guidelines of the Clinical Laboratory Standards Institute [23, 24]. The following twelve antibiotics were tested to the susceptibility of the *S. aureus* isolates: sulfamethoxazole-trimethoprim, oxacillin, cefoxitin, erythromycin, clindamycin, linezolid, ciprofloxacin, tetracycline, fusidic acid, rifampicin, vancomycin and gentamicin. Multiplex PCR was used for testing those MRSA strains for the presence of the mecA gene. Molecular analysis of the SCCmec cassette was conducted using a method earlier depicted by Oliveira et al. [25], with certain modification indicated by Budimir et al. [26]. Presence of the gene for PVL was found by use of PCR primers previously accounted for by Lina et al. [27]. In addition, all of these isolates passed analysis for epidemiological relatedness by pulsed-field gel electrophoresis (PFGE). Macrorestriction of chromosomal DNA used the restriction enzyme SmaI analysis, complying with previously described procedure. DNA fragments were separated using a CHEF-DR III electrophoresis system (Bio-Rad laboratories, Hercules, California, USA) at 6.0 V/cm for 2O h, with pulse times ramped from 5 s to 40 s. Gels used with ethidium bromide staining and they were photographed under UV illumination. PFGE patterns analysis was done by using GelCompare software (Applied Maths, Ghent, Belgium) according to the Tenover et al. scheme [28]. Isolates with indistinguishable band patterns were assigned to the same PFGE pattern type. Isolates that differed by ≤ three fragments were considered to be subtypes closely related i.e. of a given clonal group. The dendrogram was produced by use of 0, 5% optimization, a 3% band tolerance and the unweighted pair group method with arithmetic averages based on Dice coefficients.

4. Results

Out of the total number of isolates, the largest number of isolates included in our research was isolated from the nasal or nasopharyngeal swab (41%), while 35% isolates were found in a skin swab samples. There was 1% isolates isolated from the umbilical swab and sputum sample, and 2% from an abscess puncture sample and conjuctival swab.

Based on the analysis of data from the epidemiological questionnaire, we estimated the distribution of examinees by gender. Out of a total of 100 subjects included in the study, 49 (49%) were male and 51 (51%) female and there was no statistically significant difference in the percentage of the particular sex. The average age of the respondents was 10.9 ± 18.7 years.

Prior to the start of the study, 59% of subjects had hospital treatment according to the anamnestic data, but there was no statistically significant difference in the groups with and without hospital treatment in the year before the start of this study. Out of the 59 examinees who were hospitalized, 86.4% were hospitalized in the maternity hospital, while a significantly smaller number was hospitalized in orthopedics (5.1%), pediatrics (3.4%), dermatology, gynecology and surgery (1.7%).

Antibiotic usage within 12 months before the follow-up period was recorded in 32% of examinees, while 68% of them did not recieve therapy in that period, which is statistically significant. Out of the group of examinees who were taking antibiotics, 34.4% recieved amoxicillin and clavulanic acid, 18.8% recieved fourth-generation cephalosporins and sulfethoxazole-trimethoprim, while only 6.3% recieved macrolides.

MRSA was present in only 3% examinees out of those who had previosly documented MRSA strains (one year before this study). 6.0% of examinees included in the study had surgical procedure at the same time, while 94% of examinees didn't have surgery.

Epidemiological data are a significant variable for differentiating CA and HA MRSA. Therefore, variables that may have influenced the transmission and development of staphylococcal infections have been included in the epidemiological questionnaire. None of the subjects had been on dialysis therapy, nor had they been placed in a nursing home for 12 months prior to our study. 10% of examinees stated that they own a pet (80% own a dog as a pet and 20% a cat as a pet).

Out of total number of examinees, 8.0% of examinees had previous contact with a MRSA infected patients, 13% were involved in sports and 2.0% of examinees used an invasive /orthopedic device.

4.1 Microbiological analysis of the strains

During the follow-up period, out of a total of 4341 examined patient samples, 2279 *Staphylococcus aureus* were isolated, out of which 653 were methicillin-resistant SA. The prevalence of *Staphylococcus aureus* was 52.5% and the prevalence of MRSA was 28.7%.

We selected a representative sample of 100 strains, eliminating the "copy" strains (strains from the same patient at different places and those that are repeated), by random selection, trying to monitor the dynamics and even representation throughout the months of the study period).

4.2 Results of antibiotic susceptibility testing

In our study, 100 strains were tested for susceptibility to 12 antibiotics. Antibiotics that were tested include antibiotics that are therapeutically important for staphylococci, as well as other antibiotics that are known to be resistant to them as a marker for a virulent clone, such as fusidic acid.

All MRSA isolates were resistant to the β-lactam antibiotics tested, i.e. penicillin, oxacillin, and cefoxitin, 68% of MRSA strains were resistant to erythromycin, 5% to clindamycin, 5% to gentamicin and 4% to ciprofloxacin. All isolates were susceptible to sulphamethoxazole-trimethoprim, rifampicin, fusidic acid, linezolid and vancomycin (**Table 1**).

Based on the antibiogram, all examined strains were divided into 5 profile groups. Group A was represented in 32%, group B in 62%, group C 4%, group D 1% and 1% group E. (**Table 2**).

	Resistant	Sensitive
Penicillin	100 (100%)	0
Oxacillin	100 (100%)	0
Cefoxitin	100 (100%)	0
Erythromycin	68 (68%)	32 (32%)
Clindamycin	5 (5%)	95 (95%)
Sulphamethoxazole- trimethoprim	0	100 (100%)
Rifampicin	0	100 (100%)
Fusidic acid	0	100 (100%)
Gentamicin	5 (5%)	95 (95%)
Ciprofloxacin	4 (4%)	96 (96%)
Linezolid	0	100 (100%)
Vankomycin	0	100 (100%)

Table 1.
Antimicrobial susceptibility patterns (N = 100).

Groups	Profile groups
A	resistant to penicillin, oxacillin and cefoxitin; sensitive to erythromycin, clindamycin, sulphamethoxazole-trimethoprim, rifampicin, fusidic acid, garamycin, ciprofloxacin, linezolid and vancomycin
B	resistant to penicillin, oxacillin, cefoxitin and erythromycin; sensitive to clindamycin, sulphamethoxazole-trimethoprim, rifampicin, fusidic acid, garamycin, ciprofloxacin, linezolid and vancomycin
C	resistant to penicillin, oxacillin, cefoxitin, erythromycin, clindamycin, garamycin, ciprofloxacin; sensitive to sulphamethoxazole-trimethoprim, rifampicin, fusidic acid, linezolid and vancomycin
D	resistant to penicillin, oxacillin, cefoxitin, erythromycin, clindamycin; sensitive to sulphamethoxazole-trimethoprim, rifampicin, fusidic acid, garamycin, ciprofloxacin, linezolid and vancomycin
E	resistant to penicillin, oxacillin, cefoxitin, and garamycin; sensitive to erythromycin, clindamycin, sulphamethoxazole-trimethoprim, rifampicin, fusidic acid,ciprofoxacin, linezolid and vancomycin

Table 2.
Profile groups based on the antibiogram.

4.3 Results of phenotypic methods in MRSA detection

In our study, conventional phenotypic methods were used to detect MRSA isolates: disk diffusion oxacilin test and disk diffusion cefoxitin test. To confirm the MRSA isolates, a latex agglutination test with antibodies to PBP2a, a selective chromogenic medium, ChromID MRSA, and an E test were used to determine the value of the minimum inhibitory concentration for oxacillin.

Oxacillin disk diffusion and cefoxitin disk diffusion tests, due to their accuracy and economic acceptability, have proven to be good options for the detection methicillin resistance of S.aureus. The results of this study indicate a previously proven fact that the latex agglutination test, ChromID MRSA, and E test, due to their high sensitivity and specificity, play a significant role as confirmatory tests for the detection of methicillin resistance.

All phenotypic methods that were used had 100% sensitivity as well as specificity, except for the DD cefoxitin and DD oxacillin tests, 98.9 and 96.8.

4.4 Molecular analysis of tested strains

4.4.1 MecA gene detection

Reduced sensitivity or resistance to oxacillin or cefoxitin was found in all isolates, including the study by phenotypic methods. After detection of MRSA isolates by phenotypic methods, all isolates were subjected to molecular methods that tested the presence of the mecA gene.

All tested isolates were positive for the mecA gene. The control mecA positive strains used in our study are MRSA isolates described in the Methods section. One of the isolates used is COL and the other is WIS.

COL is an MRSA strain isolated for the first time in 1965 in Great Britain, known as a representative of the Archaic clone, whose characteristics are: SCCmec type I, ccr AB 1, sequential type (ST) 4.

WIS is an MRSA isolate native to Australia, SCCmec type V, possesses ccrC.

4.4.2 Spa-typing test results

As previously described in the Introduction to Spa Typing, the polymorphic region X consists of a variable number of 24 base pairs of repeating fragments. From a total of 100 strains examined, we selected a representative sample of 29 strains that underwent spa-typing. Seven different spa types were discovered: t008, t919, t041, t1179, t2187, t2674 and t10807. The most common type was t008 (55.2%).

4.4.3 SCCmec typing

We analysed and subjected 100 isolates to SCCmec typing. The obtained amplification products differ in molecular weight, and the typing result is obtained by visual comparison with the control strains. SCCmec loci of control strains were also amplified in each reaction cycle. A marker was applied to each individual gel, with a range of DNA fragments of 100-1500pb. The PCR products of the control strains were electrophoretically parallel separated. Each amplification cycle in which no corresponding PCR product was obtained in the control strains was repeated, as well as PCR reactions and electrophoresis of isolates that could not be typed with this method.

The distribution of SCCmec types is shown in **Figure 1**. The most prevalent SCCmec element was type IV (86%), followed by SCCmec I (4%) and SCCmec type

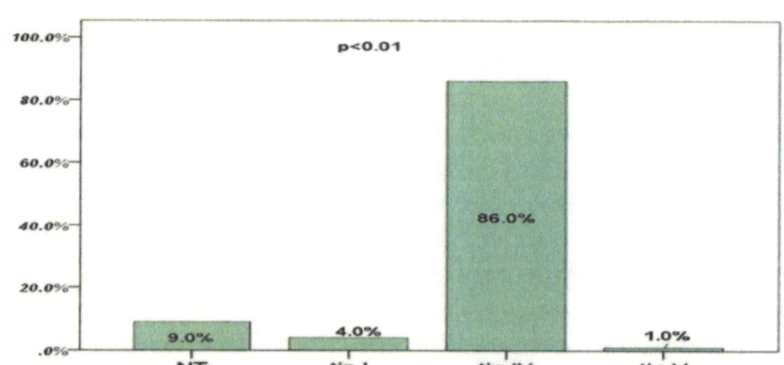

Figure 1.
SCCmec types distribution among MRSA isolates. Note: NT- non-typeable.

V (1%). Non-typical strains were found in 9.0% of cases. No isolates with SCCmec III were found during this analysis. Chi-square test was used for the analysis of categorical variables.

4.4.4 Determination of the presence of the PVL gene

Using the primers and amplification cycle conditions described in the Method section, 100 isolates were tested for the presence of the PVL toxin gene. MW2 strain, MRSA strain isolated in 1998 in the USA, SCCmec type IV, ST131 was used as a positive control strain.

Positive expression of PVL gene was found in 24.0% of isolates, while 76% showed a statistically significant higher negative expression of PVL gene.

The current prevalence of CA MRSA PVL positive isolates was 0.05% and the periodic prevalence was 0.037%.

Common to all positive PVL MRSA isolates is SCCmec type IV and the fact that they are outpatient isolates.

4.4.5 Results of PFGE analysis

Results PFGE - electrophoretic profiles of isolates.

Pulsed field electrophoresis after the splitting of chromosomal DNA by the restriction enzyme SmaI yielded clearly separated DNA fragments that were visualized by UV light illumination after staining with ethidium bromide and photographed with a Polaroid camera.

Figure 2 shows a photograph of electrophoretic gels that are part of the results obtained by this analysis. The number of fragments greater than 10 for each isolate is visible, the minimum of the bands to which the comparison standards described in the Methods section can be applied. **Figure 2** is a representation of a PFGE electrophoretic gel after cleavage with SmaI enzyme and separation in an electric field and staining with ethidium bromide.

M means a lambda marker, and genotyped strains are numbered 1–20. Blank fields 7 and 12 mean that the isolation probably failed in the first attempt and we repeated these isolates.

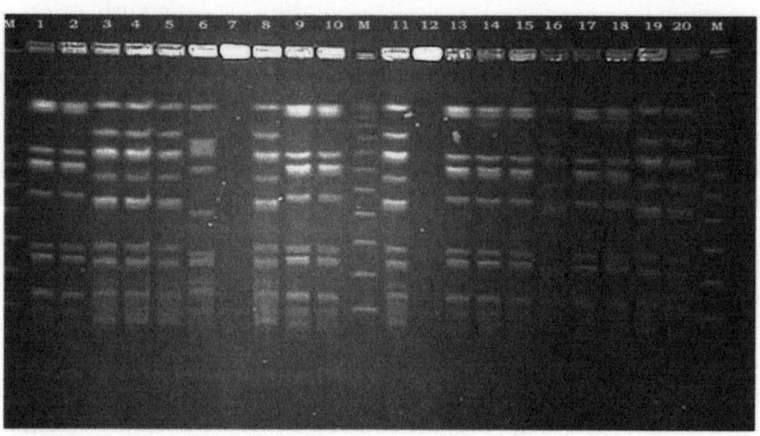

Figure 2.
Representative PFGE patterns of MRSA strains isolated from population included in the study, after splitting enzyme SmaI and separation in an electric field and staining with ethidium bromide.

Determination of PFGE groups using dendrogram percentage similarity:

The photos were scanned and stored in the database of the computer software system GelCompar. Each individual strip was subjected to a normalization procedure, in which, for each individual photograph, the size of the fragments was compared with the same molecular standard found on each gel in the electrophoretic reaction.

After normalization and entering basic data into the database, a dendrogram of similarity percentage was made, using Dice coefficient from PFGE data, using a limit value of ≥80%, with a tape tolerance of 3% and an optimization parameter of 0.5%.

In the PFGE profile analysis of the isolates with the computer system GelCompar, the isolates fell into five similarity groups: A-E. The largest number of isolates (87%) belonged to one of two groups: C (60%) and D (27%).

Group A includes 3 isolates, described as SCCmec type IV. There were no PVL positive isolates in this group.

Group B included four isolates, with three isolates being SCCmec type I, while one was SCCmec type IV. There were no PVL positive isolates in this group.

Group C represents the largest group in the PFGE analysis, including 60 isolates, and all isolates of this group belonging to SCCmec type IV. In this group, 28.33% (17) of isolates were PVL positive.

Group D includes 27 isolates, three of which were nontypeable, and the rest of the isolates belong to SCCmec type IV. In this group, only two isolates were PVL positive.

Group E included 3 isolates, SCCmec types I, IV and V. These three isolates were not PVL positive.

Three PFGE types were singletons, that is, not similar to any of the other strains, two of which are SCCmec IV, while one is nontypeable.

5. Discussion

Staphylococcus aureus is one of the most important and adaptable human pathogens, causing most often skin and soft tissue infections, although it can cause any organ and organic system infection as well as infections related to toxin production [29]. Colonisation is important step in pathogenesis of infections caused by *S. aureus*. Approximately 20–30% of overall population is persistently colonised by *S. aureus*, with verified colonisation at nasal mucosa [30]. This study microbiologically analyses 4341 different biological specimens from out of hospital respondents. *Staphylococcus aureus* is isolated in 2279 specimens, with prevalence of 52,5%. Out of 2279 identified *Staphylococcus aureus*, methicillin resistance was shown in 653 isolates proved by use of phenotype methods, thus MRSA prevalence was 28,7%. Considering the use of MRSA prevalence as an indicator of success in conducting infection control programme, there are series of data from various geographical areas that point to high variability of MRSA prevalence in the whole world. European research show high variability in MRSA prevalence results. Thus, percentage of MRSA in Scandinavian countries and Netherlands is less than 1%, while prevalence in Spain is more than 50% [31]. At latest, growth of bacterial isolates number resistant to methicillin becomes serious clinical and epidemiological problem. Introducing methicillin into clinical practice in 1961, MRSA soon becomes one of the main intra-hospital problems around the world. Nowadays, MRSA still holds primate in hospital environment, and in the last few years in out of hospital environments as well. Namely, in the nineties of the last century, the problem of out of hospital MRSA (Community-acquired methicillin-resistant *Staphylococcus aureus* or CA-MRSA) arises, in many features different from hospital MRSA strains. *Staphylococcus aureus* resistant to methicillin is placed highly in modern microbiology and infection control procedures. Recent studies show change in microbiology of MRSA as well as its limitation to hospital environment so the infection can appear in general population [29]. CA-MRSA strains become important health issue connected with high morbidity and mortality in general population [32].

In our study, we selected representative sample of 100 MRSA strains, eliminating "copy" strains (strains of the same patient from different places and those repeated ones), by random choice method, trying to follow the dynamics and equal representation through individual months of research period. In our study, 41% cases confirmed presence of the pathogen in the nasal, and 35% samples isolated *S.aureus* in skin smear. Creech et al. confirmed colonisation of nasal mucosa in paediatric cases with *S.aureus* in 35% cases, and in 9% cases they bore nasal MRSA [33]. Male sex was positive to MRSA in 49%, while females were positive in 51% of analysed MRSA specimens. In Farr et al. study [34] has shown that females were highly represented in verified CA-MRSA infections. The same study shows the greatest number of out of hospital infections in females aged 18–44. In our study average age was 10,9 (±18,7). Those results could be explained by high number of new-borns analysed in our research. Anamnestic data in epidemiology questionnaire about eventual hospitalisation within a year prior to beginning of the study has shown that 59% of respondents had been hospitalised at some clinical department, while the greatest percentage had been hospitalised at maternity department of the clinic (86.4%), adding to the data of high new-borns representation in the research. However, the German study done at in-hospital and out-of-hospital patients showed high prevalence of CA-MRSA in patients with hospitalisation data or prolonged stay at special purpose facilities (nursing homes) [35]. According to the definition of CDC, as well as numerous modifications of the definition, there are epidemiological circumstances among risk factors in appearance of out-of-hospital MRSA infection. Having that in mind, we analysed series of general prior data and the analysis followed the criteria for differentiating in-hospital from out-of-hospital MRSA. The data showed that only 6% of respondents had undergone surgeries in the prior year, while 2% of positive respondents have used some invasive apparatus. Pets had earlier been identified as the source and transmitters of MRSA infections to humans in contact [36].

Analysing data of epidemiological questionnaire it shows that 10% of the respondents keep a pet, 3% have had documented MRSA infection before, 8% have had contact with MRSA carrier, while 13% practiced collective sports. Resistance development becomes issue of priority, and the follow up system for resistance measurement in relevant data, according to which antibiotics would be given by recommendations to lower the resistance, e.g. try to stop or slow down the development of new resistance, has been established.

Data on resistance in the close by environment have to be basis for empirical therapy development, so it can be more successful in every single patient treatment, as well as efficient in spreading resistant types in the community.

For those reasons it is necessary to have local epidemiological data on sensitivity of out-of-hospital strains and specific hospital close at hand, due to variation of bacterial resistance level between hospital centres in different countries, between centres of the same country, as well as between hospital wards and departments of the same centre.

Staphylococcus aureus is a microorganism that developed resistance mechanisms to all antibiotics available for treating infections caused by staphylococci. The most important among those antibiotics that *S. aureus* developed resistance to, are the ones indispensable in therapy schemata for infection caused by staphylococci treatment and resistance mechanisms that mark antibiotics era. Penicillin as the medicine of first choice for staphylococci infection treatment is almost abandoned, while the remaining number of isolates sensitive to penicillin activity is 20% by some studies [37].

According to the data extracted by isolate testing in disc – diffusion method, resistance to penicillin, methicillin (oxacilin) and cefoxitin showed all MRSA strains. Among isolates of the collection, resistance to vancomycin, linezolid, rifampicin, sulfamectasole – trimethoprim and fusidine acid was not shown. For vancomycin the sensitivity out of inhibition zone less than 14 mm in disc – diffusion method according to CLSI standards was not confirmed [38].

Resistance to macrolides is 68%, while to clindamycin it is significantly less and in amount of only 5%.

Resistance to gentamicin is 5% while to ciproflaxcin is 4%.

It is well-known that great percentage of hospital MRSA strains is resistant to quinolone, in total 90%. Similar results are gathered in in the research in the area of Republic of Croatia (91%), where the progressive test to quinolone has been followed in the last 20 years [39].

In the world resistance phenomenon among *S.aureus* strains context, exact and early assessment of resistance is of key importance in infection caused by *S.aureus* prognosis.

Although many phenotype methods have been developed to achieve fast methicillin resistance detection, lack of these methods is lessened sensitivity, which in the end cannot ensure appropriate and timely treatment of all patients infected by MRSA.

Several studies have shown that revelation of *mec*A gene is the "golden standard" method for diagnosing MRSA in microbiological laboratories [40].

However, not all laboratories, especially in transition countries such as ours is, have the necessary equipment and educated stuff for establishing molecular techniques. Thus, the need for fast, exact and economically profitable identifying MRSA strains by phenotype methods appeared [41].

As for disc diffusion tests for MRSA detection, sensitivity of oxacilin disc diffusion test and cefoxitin disc diffusion test was 100%, while specificity was 96% and 98%.

Rao Venkatakrishna et al. also found high sensitivity and specificity of oxacilin DD and DD Cefoxitin test in MRSA detection [42].

Chromogenic surface use (ChromID) has shown 100% specificity and sensitivity. Morris et al. in their study compared chromogenic surfaces and showed sensitivity for ChromID 93% [43].

In some authors' studies [44] E-test in MRSA detection has been used as the golden standard and its advantages in the sense of conducting, as well as precision that approaches those of molecular methods PCR, *mec*A detection, have been proven. In our study we have also shown 100% sensitivity and specificity for E-test. Also, for latex agglutination test we have confirmed identical results. Ahmad has proven superiority of the test as the alternative method MRSA detection in his study [45].

After conducting phenotype methods, we have examined MRSA strains by molecular typing methods, and by analysis of data gathered in that way, we have come to interesting clinical and epidemiological findings.

With all isolates included in the research after detecting methicillin resistance by phenotype methods, they were subjected to molecular methods by which the presence *mec*Agene was tested. All examined isolates were positive to *mec*Agene, according to the claim that for *mec*Agene identification, polymerase chain reaction (PCR) is considered the golden standard [40].

By method *spa*-typing, developed by Freney et al. [46], based on sequencing polymorph region X gene protein A *Staphylococcus aureus* (*spa*), we typed 29 out of our 100 types. We had seven various *spa*-types, from which the most represented t008 16/29 (52,2%), t1179 5/29 (17,2%), t10807 3/29 (10,3), t2674 2/29 (69%), t041 1/29 (3,4%), t919 1/29 (3,4%), t2187 1/29 (3,4%). If we compare it with relative global frequency of appearance for single *spa*-types by Ridom Spa Basa, we can notice that t008 is globally represented in 6,32%. Spa t008 is present in the countries such as Australia, Austria, Bulgaria, Canada, Croatia, Check Republic, Denmark, Estonia, Finland, Germany, Hungary, Israel, Norway, Poland, Portugal, Spain, Great Britain, Switzerland and Sweden. The *spa* type is found in sequence types ST-8, ST-247, ST-250 and ST-254, and placed in CC8, Northern German MRSA, USA300 ORSA IV and Archaic/Iberian clonal complex.

In this study t041 was represented 3,4%, while globally it is less represented with only 0,31% (Austria, Belgium, B&H, Croatia, Check Republic, Denmark, France, Germany, Hungary, Island, Ireland, Italy, Netherlands, Norway, Slovenia, Sweden and Switzerland), in sequence types ST-111 i ST-228, placed in CC5 and Southern German MRSA clonal complexes.

Representation of t919 in our study is the same as t041 (3,4%), and it appears in Austria, Germany, Norway and Sweden, with globally significantly less representation of 0,01%.

In our study we had four, so far unknown, *spa* types, and it can be explained by polymorph region X consisting of 24 base pairs of repeating fragments.

In our analysis the SCC*mec* results of typification have shown dominance of SCC*mec* type IV (86%), typical for out-of-hospital population. It is necessary to emphasize there is appearance trend for SCC*mec* type IV inside hospital population, with the tendency of shifting SCC*mec* type I and dominant Iberian clone so far characteristic for in-hospital environment. SCC*mec* typing of strains included in our research we have proven that da SCC*mec* type I is seen in total of 4% strains, while SCC*mec* type V is seen in very small percentage (1%) in the examined strains. Valsesia et al. [47] have recently confirmed that SCC*mec* type IV and V was registered in examined population in the amount of 87% cases, while SCC*mec* type I and II appeared only sporadically, and SCC*mec* type III was completely absent in out-of-hospital population. In our analysis we have not confirmed any case of SCC*mec* type II or III. Those results are in accordance with our results, except that SCC typing of strains included in the study has not shown presence of SCC*mec* type V types.

Previous studies have indicated that HA-MRSA infections are mainly caused by multiresistant strains carrying SCC*mec* type I, II or III, but rarely SCC mec type IV. On the other hand, CA-MRSA strains carrying SCC*mec* type IV, V or VII, are usually sensitive to majority of un-β-lactam antibiotics, although series of studies indicate spreading CA-MRSA strains in hospital centres and consequently taking place of traditional HA-MRSA strains [48, 49].

Our study indicates possible existence of new combinations of SCC*mec* fragments and ccr genes evolving by recombining already described segments, and by completely new SCC*mec* types, due to genome *S.aureus* susceptibility to dynamic changes, changes of genetic parts inside the species as well as species typical for *S.aureus.* This conclusion is based on presence of 9% atypical strains.

In our collection of strains subjected to molecular analysis, all MRSA isolates have been tested to presence Panton-Velentine leukocidin (PVL) toxin. Number of PVL-positive MRSA was 23 isolates, while one isolate was atypical.

Some studies in which virulence factors with PVL of in-hospital and out-of-hospital MRSA were examined at the same time and it is discovered that less than 5% MRSA isolates are SCCmec I, II and III PVL positive, while 40–90% MRSA

SCCmec type IV contains PVL gene. [50]. CA-MRSA can represent serious problem for public health due to distribution of strains with potential to produce PVL toxin. Presence of genes coding Panton-Valentine leukocidin is important marker of virulence as well as determinant of clinical consequences of infections caused by PVL positive types which are far heavier than PVL negative *S. aureus* infections. Cocchi et al. [51] in their study showed the transmission of PVL -positive CA-MRSA, member of Southwest Pacific clone (SWP) with epidemic capacity. The same study shows transmission from father with recurrent skin and subcutaneous tissue infections, over mother with nasal colonisation, to their child with symptoms of necrotising pneumonia. These data indicated that recurrent skin infections, usually not given great clinical importance, can represent serious threat in development of severe clinical picture of the carrier with possibility of further transmission PVL positive causer.

However, the role of positive MRSA strains in predicting possible severe clinical manifestations for the carrier still remains undefined.

CA-MRSA is linked to the production of Panton-Valentin leukocidin. Probably the PVL is direct virulence factor in staphylococci necrotising pneumonia [52], while its role in skin and soft tissues infection remains controversy.

There is epidemiological connection between MRSA and PVL, especially in the USA where USA300 clone dominates which is PVL positive. But counterargument to the attitude, at the same time confirming still undefined role of PVL as virulence marker in prediction of clinical infection manifestations, is the fact that there are several types PVL negative with the same clinical outcome that this toxin cannot be taken as universal marker of CA-MRSA. In the conducted analysis on 100 MRSA isolates, it is confirmed that 23 isolates SCCmec type IV containing gene z PVL, one atypical isolate while there were 76 PVL negative isolates of various SCCmec types, but with dominance of type IV. By examining isolates origin we established that 11 PVL positive PVL isolates were from skin area, 8 from nasal mucosa, 2 from pustule smear, while others were represented by 1 PVL positive isolates from different corporal regions (sound conductor, wound smear).

In Great Britain, according to the National Reference Laboratory data, genes coding PVL are present in less than 2% of clinical isolates *S. aureusa*, whether MSSA or MRSA [52]. While PVL is currently accepted as important factor for *S. aureus* virulence, the latest research give preference to alternative virulence factors such as arginine catabolic mobile element (ACME), α toxin, regulatory genes coding expression, and newly described peptides.

PVL role is still very important, primarily due to fact it represents important marker in screening virulent *S.aureus* strains.

PFGE is genetic typing method used as means of molecular – epidemiological study of genetic variants of *S. aureus* and other numerous bacterial pathogens. For its highly discriminating capacity PFGE is considered golden standard for local epidemics of bacterial infections [53]. Combination of molecular typing methods (PFGE, mecA, SCC*mec* and MLST) with epidemiological and clinical data enable revelation of MRSA groups and their appearance, thus ensuring application of rational, appropriate, infection control measures [54]. Also, this study has enabled detection of MRSA groups in limited geographical area by applying methods of molecular typing so it can represent basis for similar studies on broad area and enable application of this region into European MRSA infection control network.

Comparing PFGE analysis results, by criteria of Tenover et al.(28), applying cut-off similarities 80%, our study has shown that most of the isolates is classified into two larger groups, indicating clonal connection and genetic similarity of isolates. Dendogram contains 5 groups, marked alphabetically from A to E.

PFGE analysis of profile isolates by computer system GelCompar isolates are grouped in similarity groups, inside which similarity between isolates is 80% and more. Thus we had results in five groups, marked alphabetically from A to E. Most of the isolates fell into two most numerous groups, C and D.

Group A contains 3 isolates, falling into SCC*mec* type IV. This group had no PVL positive isolates.

Group B contains four isolates, with 3 isolates belonging to SCCmec type I, while one belongs SCC*mec* type IV. This group does not have PVL positive isolates.

Group C contains 60 isolates, and represents the most numerous group in our PFGE analysis. All isolates of the group belong to SCC*mec* type IV. This group had 28,33% (17) PVL positive isolates.

Group D has had 27 isolates, three of them atypical and the rest of them also fall into SCC*mec* type IV. In this group only two isolates were PVL positive.

Group E has had 3 isolates, belonging to SCC*mec* type I, IV and V. These three isolates were not PVL positive.

Three PFGE types are single genotypes, with two of them SCC*mec* IV, while one is atypical.

Among mostly used definitions CA-MRSA that take into account epidemiological data, as well as genetic origin of isolates are modified definitions of the CDC. In cases of suspicion to CA-MRSA the first step is to eliminate any connection to hospitals and hospital system, because the connection for such isolates places them into HA-MRSA species [55].

Due to the fact it is necessary to have molecular analysis for the types aiming to avoid classifying MRSA strains into CA or HA MRSA strains based on epidemiological data, for it might lead to possibility of crosswise mistakes.

Concerning the received results indicating presence of isolates SCC*mec* type IV and with respondents of paediatric age with positive epidemiological data of hospital environment contact, traditional division to in-hospital and out-of-hospital MRSA is questionable and demands further revision.

Prevalence of "real" CA MRSA strains in general population broadly varies in different geographical areas. In meta analysis, Salgado et al. [56], showed prevalence in amount of 1,3% for MRSA colonisation in community. However, it must be pointed out that most of the people colonised by MRSA strains, had risk factors connected to hospitalisation.

After excluding these patients prevalence of "real" CA-MRSA colonised was 0,2%, responding to the prevalence of the study (0,13%).

About presence of CA MRSA in Bosnia and Herzegovina there is not enough data. There are several genotyping isolate methods *S.aureus* for epidemiological research. However, Harbarth et al. [57] still give advantage to molecular methods of MRSA identification comparing to standard cultivation methods. Anyway, length of the procedure and the need for specialised laboratories still represents limiting factor for broad use of molecular analysis.

Earlier reports on CA-MRSA strains describes appearance of new strains in patients with the lack of traditional epidemiological risk factors for MRSA infection and/or colonisation. Those patients with CA-MRSA infection are very often of younger age, with minimum comorbidities and negative epidemiological data of hospital environment contact, comparing to patients with infections caused by HA-MRSA strains. Furthermore, different socio-economic characteristics related to CA-MRSA infections, including ethnical background and socio-economic status.

Recently, [58] however, with the growth of CA-MRSA prevalence, epidemiological difference between these and HA-MRSA types became less defined, concerning numerous reports of hospital epidemics caused by CA-MRSA types.

CA-MRSA is more often defined as cause of infections arising at hospital environment and infections connected to hospital environment. On the other hand, hospital clones are described as cause of infections in general population, indicating the fact that some clones are capable of successful barrier crossing between hospitals and general population [59].

In spite of its clinical importance, multicentric research of the entire area of Bosnia and Herzegovina for prevalence and epidemiology of MRSA as the cause of infections in general population, has not been conducted. This imposes the necessity for national monitoring of spreading and presence of these types.

6. Proposal for algorithm of treatment CA-MRSA infection

The first choice for empirical antimicrobial medication depends on MRSA prevalence in the community, type and severity of infection. Vancomycin should be prescribed in cases of severe infections [60], while microbiological data is available, in areas where similar infections of outpatient MRSA strains were documented. Also, it is necessary to prescribe vancomycin in cases when it is known that patient had been colonised by MRSA strain, or is intravenous addict or when MRSA infection risk factors are included. In the last ten years skin and soft tissue infections caused by CA-MRSA have reached epidemic level. The key in their treatment is surgical care, incision and drainage, in avoiding further tissue destruction; with empirical application of antibiotics modified according to microbiological findings. In the areas of low prevalence CA-MRSA and in treatment of mild infections therapy should be started with some penicillin antibiotics resistant to penicillinase or the first generation of cephalosporins [61]. The carrier selection, if undertaken, is important in process of hospitalisation, in the open community it is impossible to be carried out. However, the follow up for discharged patients and control of their laboratory diagnostics with MRSA sensitivity examination, is more important than ever before. Screening can reduce MRSA incidence during hospitalisation admission process. MRSA eradication or decolonisation by topical application of mupirocin or cotrimaxazole are used with various success, and some studies show that sulfamethoxazole-trimethoprim in available oral antibiotics has the fastest bacteria impact [62]. Due to fast resistance development, decolonisation of all known carriers is not recommended [63].

Due to high morbidity and mortality connected to staphylococci isolates coding PVL, the selection of carriers and decolonisation by muciprocin is recommended with people having recurring abscesses despite antimicrobial therapy and their contacts if they have MRSA isolated in nasal vestibule.

PVL toxin and better understanding of toxin role in pathogenesis of CA-MRSA infections can have therapy implications. Some studies have shown that intravenous immunoglobulin use has benefits in positive treatment outcomes in shock therapy [64]. PVL neutralisation as well as other toxins by intravenous immunoglobulin is shown in vitro [65]. Based on the prevalence CA-MRSA of 0,13%, where none of the isolates caused severe infection, we estimate that empirical therapy for outpatient pneumonia treatment does not need any modification by adding antibiotics with impact on MRSA isolate, such as vancomycin.

6.1 Detection algorithm/treatment of outpatient MRSA

Having in mind the fact that in the world and Europe number of outpatient MRSA increases, in diagnostic and therapeutic approach it must be taken into account that it is MRSA strain.

Good sampling and choice for microbiological testing, (smear, wound aspirate in the case of localised infection and blood in the case of system infection), fast detection of MRSA in microbiological laboratory, as well as the result of sensitivity to adequate nonbetalactam antibiotics may contribute to adequate infection treatment and timely measure taking in infection control, aiming at reducing spreading of very adaptable outpatient MRSA strains in ambulances and hospital environment.

Diagnosis CA-MRSA infection should be considered with seriously ill young people who previously had had symptoms similar to influenza, pneumonia disease with hemoptysis symptoms, high febrility, leucopenic and and hypotensive. Those symptoms are signal to life threatening infection, necrotising pneumonia, and septic shock and, in consequence, even death outcome.

Important ways of presenting CA-MRSA infections are skin infection, with developing abscess, furuncle, carbuncle, without drainage infections progress to fasciitis, deep infections of soft tissues, after which, in case of recovery, tissue deformities are left.

Epidemiological definition and connection to hospital stay lose in importance because it is not unusual for typical CA-MRSA to cause epidemics in hospital wards [66].

As the first step in successful treatment the selection of suitable sample for microbiological testing is recommended. In cases of severe skin and subcutaneous tissue infections taking abscess aspirates or deep subcutaneous change will also have therapeutic effect.

In case of suspicion to necrotic pneumonia, blood sample usually contains cause, while sample from respiratory system is desirable.

For cause diagnostics of mild skin change, it is enough to take skin smear. Depending on sat down of infection, for sampling, standard rules of microbiological testing apply.

For treatment outcome it is important to apply suitable antimicrobial medication and in the case of suspicion to MRSA infection the confirmation is of extreme value.

With application of antistaphylococci antibiotics, penicillin or cephalosporin, skin and subcutaneous tissue infection and fascia it is necessary to surgically treat, incise and debride abscess.

By standard processes of isolation and detection of *S.aureus*, after which the testing is undertaken for isolates sensitivity to oxacilin/cephoxitin and the result due is in 48 hours later.

A lot better time frame is given by molecular MRSA detection based on PCR method. The latest PCR methods do not use amplification mecA as proof for MRSA, because there is a possibility of getting falsely positive results by amplification *mec*A gene coagulaze-negative staphylococci contaminating the sample. IDI-MRSA (Infecto Diagnostic, Canada), GenoType MRSA Direct (Hain Lifescience, Germany), detect part of orfX gene, specific For*s. aureus* and adjacent part of SCC*mec* chromosome region. In that way one PCR reaction detects MRSA in unsterile samples. Results are available in 24 hours.

Small number of routine laboratories in Bosnia and Herzegovina have molecular methods available, and they are limited to great and reference centres.

Also, the method by which MRSA diagnostics time can be significantly shorter, is method of latex agglutination by which PBP2a is detected (BioMerieux, France). Method does not require special equipment and stuff training, antigen extraction is simple, results relevant [67]. The method's purpose is not for detection MRSA coding *mec*A gene, which is not prominent, because such test is falsely negative.

Detection of virulent CA-MRSA strains is also important for application of measures for spreading prevention during admission to hospital [68] of the patient with CA MRSA infection and stay with seriously ill patients to which infection can have a fatal outcome. Some authors suggest selection of patients in intensive care units aiming at improving treatment [69]. During patient treatment with infection CA-MRSA, it is necessary to undertake prevention measures for spreading isolates, and avoid using common objects with other patients. It is considered that relatively great number of epidemic infections CA-MRSA is caused just by transmitting pathogens over objects of common use (soaps, towels...).

Transmission of out-of-hospital MRSA to laboratory employees is registered. Wagenvoort et al. [70] as well as to the doctor who resuscitated child with necrotic pneumonia caused by CA-MRSA [71] strain so it takes utmost care in treating this transmissible, more often described pathogen.

At this moment, MRSA strains as causes of epidemic should be typed in single hospitals or reference laboratories to establish whether they are CA-MRSA or HA-MRSA strains, for larger group of patients and stuff can represent risk that could demand new control strategies for CA-MRSA strains. New strategies can include screening the hospital stuff, enhanced follow up for cases with the infection beginning in hospital and out-of-hospital environment and vice versa. They would, also, include improved prevention and infection control measures in general population, focusing on MRSA in contaminated area [72].

Periodical examination of antimicrobial sensitivity profile of MRSA strains (cause of infection), in combination with representative isolate set typing of specific area, is useful to ensure necessary empirical therapy, having in mind that appearance CA-MRSA in certain parts of the world brought changes in empirical therapy of staphylococci infections.

Reference laboratories should periodically continue representative isolate sets typing to ensure adequate follow up of MRSA trends, as well as appearance of new types.

For complete estimation of their epidemiology, MRSA infections should be characterised as:

1. Caused by HA-MRSA or CA-MRSA strains.

2. Infections acquired in hospital or out of hospital environment.

3. Infections beginning in general population or in health care facilities [73].

7. Conclusions

- Prevalence *Staphylococcus aureus* in Sarajevo Canton is 52.5%, and methicilin resistance of *Staphylococcus aureus* is 28,7%.

- Phenotype methods in MRSA detection have high specificity and sensitivity, available commercially and can provide broad span application in laboratories as routine methods. However, they lack possibility of differentiating hospital from out of hospital MRSA.

- Differentiating HA and CA MRSA with epidemiological and phenotype isolate characteristics is possible only with molecular method application.

- MRSA strains in typing by spa-typing as follows: the most common type is t008 type (55.2%), than t1179 (17.2%) and t10807 (10.3%). Comparing relative global frequency of single type appearance of spa-types on Ridem Spa Server, t008 is globally the most registered type. New spa – types discovered in this study are t1179, t2187, t2674 and t10807.

- Prevalence of CA MRSA in six months period of follow up in geographical area of Sarajevo Canton in the amount 0,13%, while prevalence of CA MRSA PVL positive types is 0,037%.

- From total number of typed MRSA strains, 24% of them was PVL positive. Most of PVL positive isolates was resistant to beta lactam and macrolide antibiotics.

- Comparing PFGE genetic profile MRSA isolates were classified into 5 similarity groups, in which two of them are dominant, groups C and D, containing 60% and 27% isolates. Group C had 28,33% PVL positive types, while group D had only 2 PVL positive isolates.

- The greatest number of MRSA isolates, 84% has SCCmec type IV speaking on behalf of very high representation of out of hospital MRSA. SCCmec type I is present in 4%, while type V was present in only 1% isolates. Atypical isolates were 9%, while 95,8% PVL positive isolates fell into SCCmec type IV.

- The goal of every centre for microbiological diagnostics is to improve and speed up diagnostics of MRSA positive patients for treatment personalisation, and efficient spreading prevention of CA MRSA in hospital and out of hospital population.

- Results of the study, conducted in the most densely populated area of Bosnia and Herzegovina, indicate high level of MRSA prevalence.

- Standardization of national laboratory work is necessary, clinical as well as public health in testing antimicrobial bacteria sensitivity, due to transfer of patients between institutions, communication between institutions and follow up resistance development. For reduction of resistance level it is necessary to control spending and supervising, and prescribing antibiotic medications, in medicine and in veterinary and food industry.

- This study emphasizes the need for national monitoring of spreading existing types, as well as emerging of new strains thus enabling inclusion of our country into international network of follow up for resistant bacteria.

Author details

Velma Rebić[1*], Mufida Aljičević[1], Sajra Vinčević-Smajlović[1] and Damir Rebić[2]

1 Faculty of Medicine, Department of Medical Microbiology, University of Sarajevo, Bosnia and Herzegovina

2 Clinic for Nephrology, University Clinical Center of Sarajevo, Bosnia and Herzegovina

*Address all correspondence to: velmarebic@yahoo.com

References

[1] Lakhundi S, Zhang K. Methicillin-resistant *Staphylococcus aureus*: molecular characterization, evolution, and epidemiology. *Clin Microbiol* Rev. 2018;31(4).8,9

[2] (Tong SYC, Davis JS, Eichenberger E, Holland TL, Fowler VG. Staphylococcus aureus Infections: Epidemiology, Pathophysiology, Clinical Manifestations, and Management. *Clin Microbiol Rev*. 2015; 28 (3): p.603-661. doi: 10.1128/cmr.00134-14 . | Open in Read by QxMD)

[3] Rebić V, Budimir A, Aljicević M, Mahmutović Vranić S, Rebić D. Panton-Valentine leukocidin and staphylococcal cassette chromosome mec characterization of community acquired methicillin-resistant *Staphylococcus aureus*. Cent Eur J Public Health. 2019 Mar;27(1):58-63. doi:

[4] Udo EE. Community-acquired Methicillin-resistant *Staphylococcus aureus*: the new face of an old foe? Med Princ Pract. 2013;22(1):20-9. 3. Moellering RC Jr. MRSA: the first half century. J Antimicrob Chemother. 2012;67(1):4-11.

[5] Powers M, Wardenburg J. Igniting the fire: *Staphylococcus aureus* virulence factors in the pathogenesis of sepsis. PLoS Pathog. 2014; 10:e1003871 doi: 10.1371/journal.ppat.1003871 PMID: 24550724

[6] Krishna S, Miller L. Host–pathogen interactions between the skin and *Staphylococcus aureus*. Curr Opin Microbiol. 2012; 15:28-35 doi: 10.1016/j.mib.2011.11.003 PMID: 22137885

[7] Stryjewski ME, Corey GR. Methicillin-Resistant *Staphylococcus aureus*. An Evolving Pathogen. Clin Infect Dis. 2014; 58(1): 10-19

[8] Rebić V , Budimir A , Aljicevic M , Bektas S, Mahmutovic Vranić S, and Rebic D. Typing of Methicillin Resistant *Staphylococcus aureus* Using DNA Fingerprints by Pulsed-field Gel Electrophoresis. ACTA INFORM MED. 2016 AUG;24(4): 248-252 doi: 10.5455/aim.2016.24.248-252).

[9] Udo EE, Pearman JW, Grubb WB. Genetic analysis of community isolates of methicillin-resistant *Staphylococcus aureus* in Western Australia. J Hosp Infect. 1993; 25: 97-108.

[10] Loewen K, Schreiber Y, Kirlew M, Bocking N, Kelly L. Community-associated methicillin-resistant *Staphylococcus aureus* infection: Literature review and clinical update. Can Fam Physician. 2017 Jul; 63(7):512-520. Erratum in: Can Fam Physician. 2017 Aug; 63(8):596. PMID: 28701438; PMCID: PMC5507223.

[11] Mediavilla JR, Chen L, Mathema B, Kreiswirth BN. Global epidemiology of community-associated methicillin resistant *Staphylococcus aureus* (CA-MRSA). Curr Opin Microbiol. 2012; 15(5): 588-95

[12] Otter JA, Yezli S, French GL. Impact of the suspending medium on susceptibility of meticillin-resistant *Staphylococcus aureus* to hydrogen peroxide vapour decontamination. J Hosp Infect. 2012; 82(3): 213-5

[13] Popoola BO, Denloye OO, Iyun OI. Influence of parental socioeconomic status on caries prevalence among children seen at the university college hospital, Ibadan. Ann Ib Postgrad Med. 2013; 11(2): 81-6

[14] Mehndiratta PL, Bhalla P. Typing of Methicillin resistant *Staphylococcus aureus*: a technical review. Indian J Med Microbiol. 2012; 30(1): 16-23.

[15] Struelens MJ, Hawkey PM, French GL, Witte W, Tacconelli E.

Laboratory tools and strategies for methicillin-resistant *Staphylococcus aureus* screening, surveillance and typing: state of the art and unmet needs. Clin Microbiol Infect. 2009; 15(2): 112-9

[16] Palavecino EL. Rapid methods for detection of MRSA in clinical specimens. Methods Mol Biol. 2014;1085:71-83

[17] Bauer KA, West JE, Balada-Llasat J-M, Pancholi P, Stevenson KB, Goff DA. An antimicrobial stewardship program's impact. Clin Infect Dis. 2010;51:1074-80

[18] Timbrook TT, Morton JB, McConeghy KW, Caffrey AR, Mylonakis E, LaPlante KL. The effect of molecular rapid diagnostic testing on clinical outcomes in bloodstream infections: a systematic review and meta-analysis. Clin Infect Dis. 2017;64:15-23.

[19] Luteijn JM, Hubben GA, Pechlivanoglou P, Bonten MJ, Postma MJ. Diagnostic accuracy of culture-based and PCR-based detection tests for methicillin-resistant *Staphylococcus aureus*: a meta-analysis. Clin Microbiol Infect. 2011;17:146-54.

[20] Nicolsen NC, LeCroy N, Alby K, Martin KE, Laux J, Lin FC, et al. Clinical outcomes with rapid detection of methicillin-resistant and methicillinsusceptible *Staphylococcus aureus* isolates from routine blood cultures. J Clin Microbiol. 2013;51:4126-9.

[21] Polisena J, Chen S, Cimon K, McGill S, Forward K, Gardam M. Clinical effectiveness of rapid tests for methicillin resistant *Staphylococcus aureus* (MRSA) in hospitalized patients: a systematic review. BMC Infect Dis. 2011;11:336.54]

[22] Murray PR. Manual of Clinical Microbiology, 8th edn. American Society for Microbiology Press, Washington, D. C., 2003.

[23] Clinical and Laboratory Standards Institute Performance standards for antimicrobial susceptibility testing. Sixteenth informational supplement: CLSI M100-S16 (M2): Vol.27:No 1; 2006.

[24] Villanova PA. Susceptibility to mupirocin and fusidic acid was determined using methods recommended by the British Society for Antimicrobial therapy British Society for Antimicrobial Chemotherapy. BSAC methods for antimicrobial susceptibility testing. Version 5, 2006

[25] Oliveira DC, de Lencastre H. Multiplex PCR strategy for rapid identification of structural types and variants of the mec element in methicillin-resistant *Staphylococcus aureus*. Antimicrob Agents Chemother. 2002; 46: 2155-61.

[26] Budimir A, Deurenberg RH, Plecko V, Vink C, Kalenic S, Stobberingh EE. Molecular characterization of methicillin-resistant *Staphylococcus aureus* bloodstream isolates from Croatia. J Antimicrob Chemother. 2006; 57(2): 331-4

[27] Lina G, Piemont Y, Godail-Gamot F, et al. Involvement of Panton-Valentine leukocidin-producing *Staphylococcus aureus* in primary skin infections and pneumonia. Clin Infect Dis. 1999; 29: 1128-32.

[28] Tenover FC, Arbeit RD, Goering RV, Mickelsen PA, Murray BE, Persing DH, et al. Interpreting chromosomal DNA restriction patterns produced by pulsed-field gel electrophoresis: criteria for bacterial strain typing. J Clin Microbiol. 1995; 33: 2233-9.

[29] Boucher H, Miller LG, Razonable RR. Serious Infections Caused by Methicillin–Resistant

Staphylococcus aureus.Clin Infect Dis.2010;51(2):183-97

[30] Mulcahy ME, Geoghegan JA, Monk IR, O'Keeffe KM, Walsh JE, Fost TJ. (2012)Nasal colonisation by *Staphylococcus aureus* Depends upon Clumping Factor B Binding to the Squamous Epithelial Cell Envelope Protein Loricrin. PloS Pathog 8(12):e1003092.doi:10.13

[31] Budimir A, Bošnjak Z, Kalenić S. Methicilin-rezistentni *Staphylococcus aureus* (MRSA) u Hrvatskoj.Croat Journal of Infection.2012;32(2):59-66

[32] Okesola AO.Community-acquired methicillin-resistant *Staphylococcus aureus* - a reviw of literature. Afr J Med Med Sci.2011;40(2):97-107

[33] Creech CB , Kernodle DS, Alsentzer A, Wilson C, Edwards KM. Increasing rates of nasal carriage of methicillin-resistant *Staphylococcus aureus* in healthy children.Pediatric Infect Dis J.2005; 24:617-21

[34] Farr AM, Marx MA, Weiss D, Nash D. Association of neighborhood-level factors with hospitalization for community-associated methicillin-resistant *Staphylococcus aureus*, New York City, 2006: a multilevel observational study. BMC Infect Dis. 2013;13;13:84. doi: 10.1186/1471-2334-13-84

[35] Kupfer M, Jatzwauk L, Monecke S, Möbius J, Weusten A. MRSA in a large German University Hospital: Male gender is a significant risk factor for MRSA acquisition.GMS Krankenhhyg Interdiszip. 2010;21;5(2). doi: 10.3205/dgkh000154

[36] Weese JS, Dick H, Willey BM, McGeer A, Kreiswirth BN, Innis B, i sur. Suspected transmission of methicillin-resistant *Staphylococcus aureus* between domestic pets and humans in veterinary clinics and in the household. Vet Microbiol.2006;115(1-3):148-55

[37] Chambers HF, DeLeo FR. Waves of resistance: *Staphylococcus aureus* in the antibiotic era. Nat Rev Microbiol.2009;7:629-641

[38] Clinical and laboratory standards institute, N., Performace Standards for Antimicrobial Susceptibility Testing; Sixteenth Informational Supplement. CLSI document M-100. Wayne, Pennsilvanya, USA. 2006;26(3):182

[39] Kalenić S, Payerl PM, Palčevski VV, Horvatić J, Meštrović T, Baršić B, i sur. Smjernice za prevenciju, kontrolu i liječenje infekcija koje uzrokuje meticilin-rezistentni *Staphylococcus aureus* (MRSA). Liječ Vjesn.2008;130(1):7-32

[40] Adaleti R, Nakipoglu Y, Karahan ZC, Tasdemir C, Kaya F. Comparison of polymerase chain reaction and conventional methods in detection methicillin-resistant *Staphylococcus aureus*. J Infect Dev Ctries. 2008;2(1):46-50.

[41] Kirshnan PU, Miles K, Shetty N. Detection of methicillin and mupirocin resistance in *Staphylococcus aureus* isolates using conventional and molecular methods: a descriptive study from a burns unit with high prevalence of MRSA. J Clin Patho.2002;55(10):745-8

[42] Venkatakrishna RI, Kishore BG, Manohar KS et al.Detection of Methicillin Resistance in *Staphylococcus aureus*:Comparison of disc diffusion and MIC with mecA gene detection by PCR.Int J Pharm Bio Sci.2011;1(4):518-21

[43] Morris K, Wilson C, Wilcox MH. Evaluation of chromogenic meticillin-resistant *Staphylococcus aureus* media: sensitivity versus turnaround time. J Hosp Infect.2012;81(1):20-4

[44] Sasirekha B, Usha MS, Amruta AJ, Ankit S, Brinda N, Divya R, I sur. Evaluation and Comparison of Different Phenotypic Tests to Detect Methicillin Resistant *Staphylococcus aureus* and their Biofilm Production. International J PharmTech Research 2012;4(2):532-41

[45] Ahmad S. Detecting methicillin resistance in *Staphylococcus aureus*: comparison of different phenotypic methods and the polymerase chain reaction.Br J Biomed Sci.2013;70(3):93-6

[46] Frenay HM, Bunschoten AE, Schouls LM, van Leeuwen WJ, Vandenbroucke-Grauls CM, Verhoef J, i sur. Molecular typing of methicillin-resistant *Staphylococccus aureus* on the basis of protein A gene poymorphism. Eur J Clin Microbiol Infect Dis.1996;15:60-4.

[47] Valsesia G, Rossi M, Bertschy S, Pfyffer GE. Emergence of SCC*mec* type IV and SCC*mec* type V methicillin-resistant *Staphylococcus aureus* containing the Panton-Valentine leukocidin genes in a large academic teaching hospital in central Switzerland: external invaders or persisting circulators? J Clin Microbiol. 2010;48(3):720-7

[48] Strandén A, Frei R, Adler H, Flückiger U, Widmer A. Emergence of SCC*mec* type IV as the most common type of methicillin-resistant *Staphylococcus aureus* in a university hospital. Infection.2009;37:44-8

[49] Rossney A S, Herra CM, Brennan GI, Morgan PM, O'Connell B. Evaluation of the Xpert methicillin-resistant *Staphylococcus aureus* (MRSA) assay using the GeneXpert real-time PCR platform for rapid detection of MRSA from screening specimens. J Clin Microbiol.2008;46:3285-90

[50] Wannet WJ, Spalburg E, Heck ME, Pluister GN, Tiemersma E, Willems RJ, i sur. Emergence of virulent methicillin-resistant *Staphylococcus aureus* strains carrying Panton –Valentin leucocidin genes in The Netherlands. J Clin Microbiol.2005;43(7):3341-5

[51] Cocchi P, Taccetti G, Montagnani C, Campana S, Galli L, Braggion C, i sur. Evidence of transmission of a Panton-Valentine leukocidin-positive community-acquired methicilline-resistant *Staphylococcus aureus* clone:a femily affair. Clin Microbiol Infec.2013;19(12):1158-62.

[52] Health Protection Agency (HPA) Working Group.Guidance on the diagnosis and management of PVL-associated *Staphylococcus aureus* infections (PVL-SA) in England,2th Edition. 2008

[53] Udo EE. Community-Acquired Methicillin-Resistant *Staphylococcus aureus*: The New Face of an Old Foe? Med Princ Pract. 2013;22(1):20-9

[54] Velazquez-Meza ME, Vazquez-Larios R, Hernandez DAM, Rivera ME. Pulsed Field Gel Electrophoresis in Molecular Typing and Epidemiological Detection of Methicillin Resistant *Staphylococcus aureus* (MRSA). In Tech; 2012

[55] Struelens MJ, Denis O, Rodrigueze-Villalobos H.Microbiology of nosocomial infections: progress and challenges. Microbes Infect.2004;6(11):1043-8

[56] Salgado CD, Farr BM, Calfee DP. Community-acquired methicillin-resistant *Staphylococcus aureus*: a meta-analysis of prevalence and risk factor. Clin Infect Di.2003;36:131-139

[57] Harbarth S, Masuet-Aumatell C, Schrenzel J, Francois P, Akakpo C, Renzi G, i sur. Evaluation of rapid screening and pre-emptive contact isolation for detecting and controling

methicillin-resistant *Staphylococcus aureus* in critical care: an interventional cohort study. Crit Care.2006;10:R25

[58] Williamson DA, Roberts SA, Ritchie SR,Coombs GW, Thomas MG, Hannaford O, i sur. Clinical and Molecular Epidemiology of Methicillin-Resistant *Staphylococcus aureus* in New Zealand:Rapid Emergence of Sequence Type 5(ST5)-SCC*mec*-IV as the Dominant Community-Associated MRSA Clone.PloS One.2013;8(4):e62020

[59] Espadinha D, Faria NA, Miragaia M, Lito LM, Melo-Cristino J, de Lancastre H, i sur. Extensive Dissemination of Methicillin-Resistant *Staphylococcus aureus* (MRSA) between the Hospital and the Community in a Country with a High Prevalence of Nosocomial MRSA. PLoS One. 2013;8(4): e59960. doi:10.1371/journal.pone.0059960

[60] Budimir A, Kalenić S. Izvanbolnički meticilin-rezistentni *Staphylococcus aureus*-molekularna evolucija, karakteristike i značenje. Liječ Vjesn. 2007;129:355-63

[61] Scheurich D, Woeltje K. Skin and soft tissue infections due to CA-MRSA. Mo Med.2009;106(4):274-6

[62] Kaka AS, Rueda AM, Shelburne SA, Hulten K, Hamill RJ, Musher DM. Bactericidal activity of orall available agents against methicillin-resistant *Staphylococcus aureus*. J Antimicrob Chemother.2006;58:680-3.

[63] Coates T, Bax R, Coates A. Nasal decolonization of *Staphylococcus aureus* with mupirocin: strenghts, weaknesses and future prospect. J Antimicrob Chemother.2009;64:9-15

[64] Zetola N, Francis JS, Nuermberger EL, Bishai WR. Community-acquired methicillin-resistant *Staphylococcus aureus*: an emerging threat. Lancet Infect Dis.2005;5:275-86

[65] Dumitrescu O, Badiou C, Bes M, Reverdy ME, Vandenesch F, Etienne J. Effect of antibiotics, alone and in combination, on Panton-Valentine leukocidin production by a *Staphylococcus aureus* reference strain. Clin Microbiol Infect.2008;14:384-8

[66] Otter JA, French GL. Community-associated meticillin-resistant *Staphylococcus aureus* strains as a cause of healthcare-associated infection. J Hosp Infect.2011;79:189-93

[67] Budimir A, Plečko V, Presečki Stanko A, Tripković V, Rebrović B, Kalenić. Brza identifikacija meticilin-rezistentnih sojeva *Staphylococcus aureus* (MRSA).Liječ Vjes. 2003;125:159-60

[68] Mediavilla JR, Chen L, Mathema B, Kreiswirth BN. Global epidemiology of community-associated methicillin resistant *Staphylococcus aureus* (CA-MRSA).Curr Opin Microbiol.2012;15(5):588-95

[69] Abdallah SA, Al-Asfoor KK, Salama MF, Al-Awadi BM. Prospective Analysis Methicillin-resistant *Staphylococcus aureus* and risk Factors. J Glob Infect Dis. 2013;5(1):19-25

[70] Wagenvoort JH, De Brauwer EI, Gronenschhild JM, Toenbreker, Bonnemayers GP, Bilkert-Mooiman MA. Laboratory-acquired meticillin-resistant *Staphylococcus aureus* (MRSA) in two microbiology laboratory technicians. Eur J Clin Microbiol Infect Dis.2006;25(7):470-2

[71] Chalumneau M, Bidet P, Lina G, Mokhtari M, Andre MC, Gendtel D, i sur. Transmission of Panton-Valentine Leukocidin-Producing *Staphylococcus aureus* to a Physician during Resuscitation of a Child. Clin Infect Dis.2005;41:29-30

[72] Otter ja, French Gl. Molecular epidemiology of community-associated meticillin-resistant *Staphylococcus aureus* in Europe. Lancet Infect Dis.2010;10:227-39

[73] Otter JA, French GL. Community-associated meticillin-resistant *Staphylococcus aureus*: the case for a genotypic definition.J Hosp Infect. 2012;81(3):143-8.

Chapter 3

Potential Natural Product from Tropical Fruits: A Mixture Young Coconut Fruit and Kaffir Lime Fruit as Immunonutrition for the Treatment of Sepsis by Lipopolysaccaride *Escherichia coli* (Infectious Disease)

Rahmayati Rusnedy

Abstract

The high number of cases reported of antibiotic resistance use and mortality due to gram-negative sepsis, triggered the development of natural agents to be used in the prevention and treatment of sepsis. Studies continue to be developed on the use of tropical fruits such as coconut fruit and kaffir lime fruit which contain high antioxidants and many potential compounds. Recent experimental data has proven that the high antioxidant activity found in the coconut fruit mixture, namely processed fruit flesh and coconut water and added kaffir lime juice, can be used as an immunonutrition agent that can improve body physiology and can increase the survival rate of test animals from endotoxemia lipopolysaccharide induced by Eschercia coli intraperitoneally. This chapter provides an overview of the potential of natural products that can be used as immunonutrition preparations. Finally, this provides information showing the importance of the intake of immunonutrition in conditions of sepsis infection.

Keywords: sepsis, natural product, immunonutrition, coconut fruit, kaffir lime

1. Introduction

Infectious diseases are diseases caused by the entry of one of four types of microbes, namely viruses, bacteria, protozoa or fungi that are harmful (pathogens). Of the millions of types of microbes that exist, only about 1,400 are pathogenic in humans, but critically only 150 have the ability to transmit from human to human and have the potential to cause epidemics [1].

Sepsis is a severe infection, and when the body is exposed to infection it will affect all organs of the body and many organs can affect it. Infection can come from the respiratory cavity, digestive tract, and wounds. When the human immune system drops, the body cannot overcome the infection and the infection will circulate throughout the body so that our body will respond to inflammation to fight the bacteria cause death [2].

By definition, sepsis is divided into several conditions, namely bacteremia or fungimia, infection, sepsis, severe sepsis and septic shock [3]. Sepsis is divided into several stages based on the body's response to infection, ranging from fever and leukocytosis to hypotension and impaired function of several organs [4]. Although almost any microorganism can be associated with sepsis and septic shock, the most common pathogenic etiologies are gram-positive bacteria (40%): *Staphylococcus aureus*, *Streptococcus pneumoniae*, Staphylococcus coagulase negative, and Enterococcus. Meanwhile, gram-negative bacteria (38%): *Escherichia coli* and *Pseudomonas aeruginosa* were the most frequently isolated bacteria in sepsis [3].

The biggest cause of sepsis is gram-negative bacteria (−) with a percentage of 60–70% of cases being the main cause of death in intensive care units, although antibiotics are new, mortality due to gram-negative sepsis remains high. This is because gram-negative bacteria tend to be more resistant to antimicrobial agents than gram-positive bacteria, due to the additional protection provided by the outer membrane [5]. This is why antibiotic resistance is now a public health problem worldwide involving a broad spectrum of microorganisms and different classes of antibiotics, including multidrug-resistant bacteria [6]. Therefore, it is very important to find new drugs to overcome this problem.

Sepsis infection produces various products that can stimulate immune cells. These cells will be stimulated to release inflammatory mediators. The product that plays an important role in sepsis is lipopolysaccharide (LPS). LPS or endotosin glycoprotein complex is the main component of the outer membrane of gram-negative bacteria. Lipopolysaccharides stimulate tissue inflammation, fever and shock in infected patients [7].

Sepsis is also defined as an irregular host response caused by infection and associated with severe microvascular, hemodynamic, metabolic, endocrine, and immune disorders, causing life-threatening organ dysfunction, characterized by a severe inflammatory response to systemic infection caused by pathogenic microorganisms. In severe cases, sepsis can lead to death with multiple organ failure as the main cause [7]. The catabolic response during acute sepsis severely depletes the body's nutritional resources, generates large amounts of cellular waste products and is in dire need of adequate nutrition [8].

Sepsis is characterized by early massive catabolism, loss of lean body mass and increased hypermetabolism that lasts for months to years. Insufficient nutrition and immune dysfunction did not have a synergistic effect on mortality in critically ill septic patients but it is expected that well-fed patients with normal immune function have the best chance of survival. Immunocompetent patients who are undernourished have the worst prognosis. Early nutrition should seek to correct micronutrient/vitamin deficiencies, provide adequate protein and moderate non-protein calories and well-nourished patients produce endogenous energy [9].

From a pathophysiological perspective, sepsis is often regarded as a syndrome that progresses from an initial inflammatory and hypermetabolic state to a more protracted state, characterized by lymphocyte exhaustion, apoptosis, and reduced capacity of monocytes and macrophages to release pro-inflammatory cytokines and trigger secondary infection [10] and cellular metabolic processes undergo fundamental changes without returning to normal homeostasis [11]. The degree of inflammation and immune suppression varies between individuals and is determined by host-(genetic heterogeneity, age, and comorbidities), pathogen-(burden, type, and virulence), and therapy-related factors (time, adequacy) [12].

Since ancient times, humans have used plants to treat common infectious diseases and some of these traditional medicines are still included as part of the habit of treating various diseases. Chemicals from natural products facilitate a large number of several bioactive secondary metabolites that have been found to fight infectious diseases [1].

Natural products are secondary metabolites or chemical compounds produced by living organisms and which have bio-activity, can be useful against microbes originating from microorganisms that make secondary metabolites can be produced into drugs. The superiority of plants as a resource for the discovery of anti-infective drugs, and the latest technology allows a wider line of investigation. Natural plant products represent a promising and largely untapped source of new chemical entities from which new anti-infectives can be discovered [13].

2. Immunonutrition for infectius disease and sepsis

The natural defenses of the human body depend on the integrity of the immune system which is responsible for curbing the course of pathogens and their complications. The immune system is divided into two types, innate and adaptive, each of which is responsible for responding to initial and repeated infections. Both types of immune systems rely on the use of mediators such as enzymes, pro-inflammatory cytokines, antibodies, and reactive oxygen and nitrogen species to combat many disease processes. The synthesis and functionality of these mediators depend on the individual immunonutrient components [14].

Immunonutrition is the term given to nutritional interventions that regulate immune and inflammatory responses. This is done by administering a formula containing a range of immunonutrients in greater amounts than is normally found in food. Some of the more commonly used immunonutrients include arginine, glutamine, branched-chain amino acids, omega-3, 6 and 9 fatty acids, trace metals (eg zinc, copper, iron), and nucleotides or antioxidants [15, 16]. The main targets of these immunonutrients involve mucosal barrier function, cellular defenses, and local or systemic inflammation [17].

Previous research has shown a close relationship between nutritional deficiencies and impaired immune function. The correlation between malnutrition and infection is particularly pronounced in less immunocompetent groups, such as young children and the elderly, who are prone to higher rates of respiratory and gastrointestinal diseases. One study determined that enteral glutamine administration reduced the incidence of moderate to severe sepsis and pneumonia in premature infants and critically ill patients. Other studies have shown that zinc supplementation at physiological levels for 1–2 months enhances immune response, decreases the incidence of infection, and ultimately improves survival [14].

In contrast, patients who have undergone surgery, trauma, or infection may experience the deleterious effects of a prolonged systemic inflammatory response because of the greater need for metabolic and essential nutrients. They may even experience compensatory immunosuppression as a result of chronic inflammation [4]. Many studies have shown that various combinations of immunonutrients can provide appropriate metabolic support for patients experiencing complications from malnutrition associated with illness, while effectively reducing infection rates and length of hospital stay. In addition, other immunonutrients such as proteins, vitamins, trace metals, and enzymes exhibit antioxidant properties that limit the extent of tissue damage and reduce the possibility of carcinogenesis [14, 18].

Nutritional therapy refers to the administration of nutrients with certain beneficial actions (eg for antioxidant effects) specifically aimed at immune defense mechanisms and to inhibit excessive proinflammatory responses during the catabolic phase of a disease [19, 20]. Future research on immunonutrition should be multidisciplinary and on a larger scale to further validate the great benefits of immunonutrition, while providing data on optimal mixes and doses for use in different groups of patients [17, 21, 22].

Immunonutrition therapy is an effort to reduce or eliminate potential pathogens and toxins, fulfill nutritional intake and act as antioxidants that can modulate natural and adaptive immune defense mechanisms in patients with critical illnesses such as sepsis. The concept of nutritional support in an effort to modulate immune function is known as immunonutrition (Immune-enhancing diets or Immuno-modulating diets) which is a therapeutic approach to pathological changes in adaptive and natural immunity, which arise secondary to inflammation and systemic infection through the administration of immunonutrients [23, 24]. The most relevant nutritional therapy in septic patients is the intake of the amino acids glutamine and arginine, fatty acids, selenium, and vitamin C [8].

Micronutrients are nutrients that the body needs to carry out body functions. The amount is less than 100% g per day and consists of vitamins and minerals. It cannot be synthesized in the body. Research in the United States states that the prevalence of sepsis tends to increase by 8.7% every year. In sepsis, nutrition is one of the important components that can promote the success of treatment. Micronutrients, especially fat-soluble vitamins, are toxic if the amount exceeds the body's ability to accept them. Although there are guidelines and mutual agreement on the use of sepsis, it is still necessary to pay attention to micronutrients that have the potential to have adverse effects. In the case of sepsis, micronutrients also determine the success of treatment because of the redistribution of vitamins and trace elements from circulation to tissues that play a role in protein formation and the immune system. Micronutrient supplementation is considered to reduce mortality. However, the toxicity of fat-soluble micronutrients still needs to be watched out for if the dose is excessive [25].

The role of micronutrients in metabolic processes is to maintain the function of body tissues. Hypermetabolism causes an increase in the production of Reactive Oxygen Species (ROS) as a result of an increase in oxidative metabolism that can damage cells, especially unsaturated fatty acids found in cell membranes and nucleus. Micronutrients also play a role in helping the body neutralize the negative effects of free radicals [26].

3. Young coconut fruit and kaffir lime fruit as immunonutrition for the treatment of sepsis by Lipopolysaccaride *Escherichia coli* (infectious disease) through antioxidant activity

Young hybrid coconut (*Cocus nucifera* L.) and kaffir lime (*Citrus hystrix*) contain antioxidant compounds that are used as immunonutrient agents. A study has been conducted on a test dosage form of 100 mg/kgbw/day made from a mixture of young coconuts with a concentration of 20% flesh with added coconut water and 1 ml of kaffir lime juice, assessed as having the potential to be developed as an immunonutrient agent in sepsis in mice. White male induced sepsis with *Escherichia coli* Lipopolysaccharide through the antioxidant activity of the phytonutrients contained in the test preparation. Based on the antioxidant activity test of the preparations KJ1, KJ2 and KJ3, which are test preparations added with 1 ml of kaffir lime juice, it turns out to be able to increase the antioxidant activity of the preparations when compared to preparations that are not given additional kaffir lime juice, namely preparations K1, K2 and K3. This is closely related because of the effect of adding kaffir lime to the process of inhibiting rancidity or rancidity. The test preparation was KJ1 from 15% young coconut flesh with coconut water and 1 ml of kaffir lime juice was added. KJ2 of young coconut flesh 20% with coconut water and added 1 ml of kaffir lime juice. KJ3 from young coconut flesh 25% with coconut water and added 1 ml of kaffir lime juice. Next K1 of young coconut flesh 15% with coconut water. K2 of young coconut flesh 20% with coconut water. K3 from young coconut flesh 25% with coconut water [27].

The rancidity of processed coconut meat can be overcome by adding ingredients that contain antioxidants, one of which is kaffir lime juice. The effect of the addition of kaffir lime (*Citrus hystrix*) on the process of inhibiting rancidity or rancidity arising from the oxidation of unsaturated fatty acids contained in processed coconut meat [28].

The presence of antioxidant content in the test preparation of a mixture of meat and coconut water with the addition of kaffir lime juice is thought to act as a cofactor that plays a role in the immune response, especially as an enzyme catalyst and antioxidant [8].

Antioxidants play an important role in minimizing cellular damage due to increased production of reactive oxygen and nitrogen species (eg, oxidative stress). Antioxidant defense systems include enzymes (e.g., superoxide dismutase, glutathione peroxidase), trace elements (e.g., selenium, zinc), vitamins (e.g., vitamins C, E, beta-carotene), sulfhydryl group donors (e.g., glutathione), and glutamine. Critical illness is associated with deficits in circulating antioxidants due to sepsis-induced redistribution from blood to tissues and decreased nutrient intake [29].

The resulting decrease in antioxidant potential increases cellular oxidative injury (particularly lipid peroxidation). A number of clinical studies have explored the potential benefits of supplementation with antioxidants. Combinations and doses of single antioxidants vary widely. Heyland *et al*. conducted a meta-analysis of clinical studies of trace elements and vitamin supplements in critically ill patients. They concluded that trace elements and vitamins that support antioxidant function, particularly high doses of selenium (either alone or in combination with other antioxidants), are safe and may be associated with reduced mortality. However, the optimal combination and dose of micronutrients remains to be determined [30].

4. Coconut fruit (*Cocus nucifera* L.)

Exploration of the potential wealth of crops in all respects one of which is coconut. The coconut, *Cocos nucifera* L., is a cultivated tree for its various uses, primarily for its nutritional and medicinal values. In addition, coconut is an environmentally friendly plant that allows coexistence with multi-species plants. This enriches soil fertility and is quite suitable for organic farming if the crop is grown in suitable inter-spaces. Due to its various uses in the present and the future, this plant has very bright potential.

The versatile coconut tree is a source of various chemical compounds that are responsible for various activities, especially activities for treatment or health. Recently, modern medicinal research has confirmed the many health benefits of various coconut products in various forms. Therefore, extensive investigations are needed to exploit its therapeutic uses for fighting disease. A drug development program must be carried out to develop modern drugs with their compounds isolated from coconut. Modern drugs need to be developed after extensive investigation of their bioactivity, mechanism of action, pharmacotherapy, after standardization and appropriate clinical trials. As the global scenario changes towards the use of non-toxic plant products used for traditional medicine, the development of modern medicines from Cocus nucifera must be emphasized for the control of various diseases. Coconut that absorbs extraordinary potential needs special attention from its scientific fraternity to emerge as a milestone in the medical science history of this millennium because of its various medicinal uses. Further evaluation needs to be carried out on *C. nucifera* to explore hidden areas and their practical clinical applications, which can be used for the welfare of mankind.

Coconut (*Cocos nucifera* L.,) is a cultivated tree for its various uses, mainly for its nutritional and medicinal value. Various coconut products include young coconut water, copra, coconut oil, raw kernel, coconut cake, coconut shell, coconut shell and products made from wood, coconut leaves, coir pith and others. All parts of the coconut can be used in the daily life of people in traditional coconut growing areas. It is a unique source of various natural products for the development of medicines against various diseases and also for the development of industrial products. The fruit parts such as coconut hump and young coconut water have various medicinal properties such as antibacterial, antifungal, antiviral, antiparasitic, antidermatophyte, antioxidant, hypoglycemic, hepatoprotective, immunostimulant. Coconut water and coconut kernels contain microminerals and nutrients that are important for human health, therefore coconuts are used as food by people around the world, especially in tropical countries [31].

Coconut (*Cocos nucifera* L.) is a plant that is commonly found in tropical areas, especially Indonesia. Green coconut water, which is technically endosperm fluid, is formed in small amounts in the third month of seed development and reaches the highest amount in the eighth month and decreases after the seeds have matured [32].

Young coconut fruit is one of the unique tropical plant products because in addition to the flesh component that can be consumed directly, the fruit water component can also be drunk directly without going through processing. This uniqueness is supported by the physical properties and chemical composition of coconut meat and water, so that this product is very popular with consumers, both children and adults. In addition to having high economic value, young coconut fruit has a fairly good nutritional composition, including fatty acids and essential amino acids that are needed by the body. Meanwhile, coconut water, apart from being a fresh drink, also contains various minerals, vitamins and sugars as well as essential amino acids so that it can be categorized as a highly nutritious soft drink and can cure various diseases. However, for some consumers, consuming coconut water is only considered as a drink to relieve thirst. While the flesh is only as a complement after drinking the water. Compared to other soft drinks, coconut water which contains good nutrition can be categorized as a highly nutritious, hygienic and natural drink and has been proven to cure various diseases [33].

Coconut water contains macronutrients in the form of carbohydrates, fats and proteins as well as micronutrients in the form of vitamins and minerals. The vitamins contained in coconut water are vitamin B (B1, B2, B3, B5, B7, B9 and B12) and vitamin C and Nitrogen (N), Phosphorus (P), Potassium (K), Calcium (Ca) and Magnesium (Mg), whose levels decrease during maturity [34].

Coconut fruit (*Cocos nucifera* L.) contains high concentrations of polyphenols, and health-promoting phytonutrients. The content of components of phenolic compounds that are antioxidants (vitamin E from the monophenol group and phenolic acid from the polyphenol group) [35].

Young coconut flesh has a high nutritional composition, including fatty acids and essential amino acids that are needed by the body. While coconut water contains a variety of minerals, vitamins and sugars as well as essential amino acids, high nutritional value. Young coconuts contain amino acid components such as Glutamate (GLU) 14.50%; 4.02% of water and young coconut flesh, Arginine

(ARG) 12.75%; 2% of water and young coconut flesh, lauric acid 31.10% of young coconut flesh and vitamin C 2.2–3.4 mg/100 ml of young coconut water [33].

Barlina [36] has conducted research on the addition of young coconut meat (B1) 15%, (B2) 20% and (B3) 25% in the preparation of coconut drink powder. In addition, young coconut water is an endosperm fluid which is an excellent natural soft drink. It has a calorific value of 17.4/100 g. Coconut water contains B vitamins namely nicotinic acid B3 (0.64 g/mL), pantothenic acid B5 (0.52 g/mL), biotin (0.02 g/mL), riboflavin B2 (<0.01 g/mL).), folic acid (0.003 g/mL), trace amounts of thiamine B1 and pyridoxine B6 [37]. In addition, coconut water contains sugar, sugar alcohol, vitamin C, folic acid, free amino acids, phytohormones (auxin, 1, 3-diphenylurea, cytokinins), enzymes (acid phosphatase, catalase, dehydrogenase, diastase, peroxidase, RNA polymerase) and growth driving factor [38].

Coconut water, also known as coconut juice, is a natural refreshing drink common in the tropics [31, 39, 40], serving as a suspension of the coconut endosperm during the core phase of its development. Then, the endosperm matures and settles on the coconut shell during the cellular phase. Mature fruit has much less liquid than immature young coconuts. The health benefits of coconut water include: boosting the immune system, detoxifying and fighting viruses and helping cleanse the digestive tract [41]. The water from this coconut is a clear, colorless, sweet, natural drink that has a slightly sour taste. Decades of research has shown that coconut water is a rich source of nutrients, including essential amino acids (lysine, leucine, cystine, phenylalanine, tyrosine, histidine, and tryptophan), palmitic and oleic acids, vitamins and minerals [40–43]. Other minerals such as iron, zinc, copper and manganese are available at adequate levels [41, 44].

The free amino acid, L-arginine (30 mg/dL) is present in young coconut water which significantly reduces the formation of free radicals. Young coconut water also contains vitamin C (15 mg/100 mL) which significantly reduces lipid peroxidation when exposed to rats [45].

Young coconut water contains electrolytes that are very rich in inorganic ions such as K (290 mg%), Na (42 mg%), Ca (44 mg%), Mg (10 mg%), P (9.2 mg%) and others [46]. The concentration of these electrolytes in young coconut water produces an osmotic pressure similar to that observed in blood [9] and does not affect plasma coagulation. The high amount of K in coconut water has been reported to lower blood pressure [45]. The ethanolic extract of *C. nucifera* endocarp was found to have vasorelaxant and antihypertensive effects, via the production of nitric oxide in an endothelial-dependent concentration and manner, due to direct activation of the nitric oxide/guanylate cyclase pathway, stimulation of muscarinic receptors and/or via the cyclooxygenase pathway [47].

Young coconut water has many medicinal properties, according to Effiong *et al* [47], including a good drink for cholera patients because of its salt and albumen content; check for urinary tract infections, and diarrhea. The most abundant and powerful medium-chain saturated fatty acid (MCFA) in coconut is lauric acid, which accounts for nearly 50% of coconut fat content. MCFA and its derivatives such as monoglycerides (MG) found in coconut are effective in destroying a wide variety of lipid-coated bacteria by destroying their lipid membranes. For example, it is effective against bacteria that can cause heartburn, sinusitis, cavities, food poisoning, and urinary tract infections. Monoglycerides, particularly Monolaurin, have been used to protect the composition of intravenously adjustable oil-in-water emulsions against the growth of Escherechia coli (*E. coli*), *Pseudomonas aeruginosa* (*P. aeruginosa*), *Staphylococcus aureus* (*S. aureus*) and *Candida albicans* (*C. aeruginosa*). albicans). The 1.25 mM monolaurin emulsion in citrate-lactate buffer at pH 4 to 5 resulted in a > 6 to 7-log10 reduction in the number of Salmonella spp. and *E. coli* within 10 minutes [48]. Lauric acid, which is also present in breast milk, helps protect nursing infants from harmful pathogens [49], as contained in many other important medicinal plants which have antibacterial properties [50, 51]. *C. nucifera* is also very good against different pathogenic bacteria that cause several life-threatening infections in humans [52].

5. Kaffir lime fruit (Citrus Hystric DC.)

Antioxidant production is a control mechanism of the tissue to balance the concentration of ROS. Endogenous antioxidants such as glutathione, pyruvate, and lycopene are produced by the body to deal with the effects of oxidative stress. If the concentration of endogenous antioxidants is insufficient or unbalanced, exogenous antioxidants need the help of exogenous antioxidants. Exogenous antioxidants can be obtained from various sources such as synthetic antioxidants (vitamin E and Vitamin C) and natural antioxidants derived from plants [53].

Kaffir lime (*Citrus hystrix*) is a plant that grows in Indonesia, Malaysia, and Thailand. Citronelal, a monoterpenoid compound that has strong antioxidant activity so that it can be used as an alternative to exogenous antioxidants [54].

Kaffir lime is a fruit that is known to the public as a food source and used as herbal medicine with very high antioxidant activity, so it is widely used in daily needs [55]. Plants of the Citrus genus are known to be rich in polyphenols [56], considered to be one of the antioxidant resources containing sufficient amounts of ascorbic acid/vitamin C, tocopherols, flavonoids, −carotene and other phenolic compounds [57–60]. Polyphenols and flavonoids are good electron donors with their antioxidant power varies from one compound to another [61, 62].

6. Nutrition related to immune function

Along with the development of science and technology, nutrients that are known to have immunomodulating effects are prebiotics, proteins/amino acids, fats/fatty acids, vitamins and minerals.

6.1 Protein amino acids related to immune function contained in coconut fruit for the treatment of infectious diseases and sepsis

The protein contained in the flesh of young coconuts contains 15 types of amino acids, 10 of which include essential amino acids. The ten essential amino acids are threonine (THR), tyrosine (TYR), methionine (MET), valine (VAL), phenylalamine (PHE), ileucine (ILE), leucine (LEU), lysine (LYS), histidine (HIS). and arginine (ARG). HIS and ARG are not essential for adults, but essential for children. In addition, the amino acid content of Glutamate (GLU) in all types of coconut ranged from 3.59–4.02%, which was the highest compared to other types of amino acids. Thus, consuming young coconut flesh in addition to being able to fulfill some of the essential amino acid needs while at the same time obtaining GLU amino acids where these amino acids are important nutrients in infectious conditions [33].

Glutamine (GLU) has many roles in the immune system. Glutamine supplementation has been reported to have multiple benefits, including increasing nitrogen retention and reducing muscle cell mass loss, enhancing immune function, thereby reducing the risk of infection and maintaining organ glutamine. Glutamine is an essential nutrient for enterocytes and immune cells through its antioxidant and cytoprotective effects. Glutamine maintains the protective function of the gut, provides antioxidant and cytoprotective effects, stimulates nucleotide synthesis, maintains the killing of neutrophil bacteria, and increases the proliferation and secretion of lymphocytes and macrophages. Intense immune activity and/or hypercatabolism, as occurs in burns, trauma and sepsis, is associated with increased glutamine consumption and a drastic decrease in plasma glutamine concentrations. Loss of glutamine concentration during the body's defense processes can lead to severe impairment of immune function. Hypoglutaminemia is an independent predictor of mortality and/or poor clinical outcome in critically ill patients [63, 64].

Glutamine is the most common free amino acid in the body with various involvements in gluconeogenesis, ammoniagenesis in the kidney, and the integrity of the intestinal mucosa. Glutamine is also conditionally important during catabolic conditions as it provides oxidative energy for cell division, increases antioxidant production, and acts as a major fuel for intestinal cells and the immune system [17, 65].

Glutamine supplementation has been shown to have multiple benefits, including increasing nitrogen retention and reducing muscle mass loss, maintaining the permeability and structure of the gastrointestinal mucosa, enhancing immune function thereby reducing the risk of infection and maintaining organ glutamine [66, 67].

Sepsis is accompanied by increased consumption, impaired synthesis, and decreased supply of the semi-essential amino acid arginine. This state of arginine deficiency impairs immune homeostasis and increases the risk of nosocomial infections. L-arginine supplementation is thought to contribute to restoring physiological processes such as its role for protein synthesis, organ perfusion, and wound healing in septic patients [68].

Meanwhile, arginine is an essential amino acid which during pathophysiological stress such as sepsis and trauma, its synthesis decreases. The immunomodulatory effect of arginine lies in increasing the function of B and T lymphocytes and their macrophages. Arginine is also involved in many anabolic processes involved in wound growth and healing, as it participates in connective tissue synthesis, changes in blood flow, and angiogenesis [16, 65].

Arginine can stimulate the release of growth hormone, prolactin, and insulin, as well as increase the number of T cells and improve T cell function. During catabolic disease serum arginine levels decrease due to reduced food intake, increased uptake in the endothelium, liver, and intestines and increased metabolism [69]. In addition, increased arginase expression leads to arginine depletion and decreased T cell activation and immunocompetence, and an increased risk of infection. So it is hypothesized that arginine supplementation can inhibit arginase and prevent these negative symptoms [70].

6.2 Fatty acids related to immune function contained in coconut fruit for the treatment of infectious diseases and sepsis

Clinical trials have shown that unsaturated fatty acids can be considered as powerful disease-modifying nutrients in patients with acute lung injury and sepsis [71, 72]. In particular, feeding with polyunsaturated fatty acids (PUFA), eicosapentaenoic acid (EPA), and docasahexaenoic acid (DHA) has been found to attenuate the production of various cytokines, chemokines, and other effectors [73]. Moreover, the recent discovery of resolvin produced by EPA and DHA has shed more light on the resolution of inflammation, as a possible mechanism of the anti-inflammatory action of the 3 PUFAs during systemic inflammation [74].

To determine the fat quality of young coconut flesh, Rindengan *et al.* [75] have analyzed the fatty acid and amino acid composition of young coconut flesh. In addition, young coconut flesh contains carbohydrates, crude fiber, galactomannan, phospholipids and a number of macro and micro minerals. Coconut fruit contains unsaturated fatty acids (ALT) oleic or omega 9 and essential ALTJ linoleic or omega

6. In general, products on the market such as formula milk include the weight of the two types of fatty acids. Omega 9 and omega 6 fatty acids occur naturally in several types of plant foods [75]. Omega 6 is one type of essential fatty acid that must be obtained from food because it cannot be metabolized in the body. In the body, omega 6 will be metabolized into arachidonic acid (AA). AA and linoleic (omega 6) ranks 2nd and 3rd of the four types of fatty acids that support brain intelligence. Docosahexanoic acid (Docosahexaenoic acid, DHA) is in first place and linolenic acid (omega 3) is fourth. Linolenic acid is an essential that must be obtained from food and in the body will be metabolized into DHA [76].

Given the high content of omega 9 and omega 6 fatty acids in young coconut meat, young coconuts can be an alternative to meet the needs of these two types of fatty acids. Seeing the nutritional potential that is also contained in the flesh of young coconuts, it is better not only to consume coconut water but together with coconut meat. Omega 6 essential unsaturated fatty acids (ALTJ) (linoleic) are classified as double ALTJ (Polyunsaturated fatty acids, PUFAs) [33].

6.3 Vitamins, Carotenoids and Flavonoids related to immune function contained in coconuts for the treatment of infectious diseases and sepsis

6.3.1 Vitamin B

Vitamin B12, vitamin B6, folic acid and niacin are B vitamins that are beneficial for the immune system. Vitamin B6 contributes in the proliferation of lymphocytes, the formation of lymphoid tissue and in the antibody response. Vitamin B12 plays a role in augmenting the performance of phagocytes and T cell proliferation. Folic acid together with vitamin B12 can affect Natural Killer cells [24, 77, 78].

6.3.2 Vitamin C

Vitamin C is an enzyme catalyst and antioxidant. In addition, vitamin C is a regulator of immune cell activation to maintain the viability of immune cells. Vitamin C functions in the synthesis of nitric oxide produced by macrophages, regulates phagocytosis by reducing free radical production and increasing the activity of immune cells (natural killer) [79].

Vitamin C has important vascular protective effects by inhibiting oxidative stress, modulating intracellular signaling pathways, and maintaining homeostatic nitricoxide levels [80]. Vitamin C is also an important cofactor for the production of endogenous norepinephrine, epinephrine, and vasopressin [81]. Septic patients usually have very low or undetectable serum vitamin C levels [82].

Vitamin C can reduce the expression of iNOS ascorbate and can overcome radicals produced by the immune system. Ascorbate also reduces or prevents endotoxin translocation from the gut and is directly bactericidal, and can increase circulating GSH concentrations in the liver. Ascorbate also prevents the reduction of enzymes in the liver and is responsible for endotoxin clearance [26]. In a study conducted by Crimi *et al.*, administration of high doses of vitamin C and vitamin E can reduce mortality by 67.5% to 45.7% [83].

6.3.3 Vitamin E

Vitamin E (tocotrienol or -tocopherol) is a powerful antioxidant that can assist monocyte/macrophage-mediated immune responses and IL-2 [79]. Vitamin E and other antioxidants increase CD4 cells. Vitamin E inhibits the synthesis of prostaglandins produced in cells after membrane oxidation, prevents fatty acid peroxidation and is an immunoregulator of arachidonic acid metabolism through the synthesis of prostaglandins and leukotrienes. Vitamin E also affects T cells, B cells and monocytes and regulates the response of the cyclic element AMP that binds to protein [84].

6.3.4 Carotenoids and flavonoids

Supplementation of carotenoids and flavonoids causes an immunostimulator effect in the form of an increase in Th cells and NK cells, IL-2 receptors. Research has shown the ability of carotenoids to influence the production of cytokines, namely TNF alpha and IL-1, and T cell proliferation, as well as flavonoids to influence inflammation, cytokine production, lymphocyte and granuloside production through mechanisms of protection against free radicals, regulation of NO and arachidonic acid metabolism [85].

6.4 Minerals related to immune function contained in coconut fruit for the treatment of infectious diseases and sepsis

6.4.1 Zinc (Zn)

Zinc is an important component in the regulation of gene expression through its role in gene transcription, division, differentiation, and cell apoptosis [86]. Zinc in the immune system plays a role in mechanical barriers (the structure and function of the gastrointestinal epithelium), as an antioxidant, in thymid kinase activity (plays a role in the proliferation of lymphoid cells), thiomulin and increases IgAs [87, 88].

Zinc is a co-factor of more than 200 enzymes that play a role in the immune system. It is very important for the wound healing process, regenerate new cells and balance acid base. Zinc has a very important role for the immune system, oxidative stress response, wound healing process and protective homeostasis. Symptoms of zinc deficiency and sepsis are difficult to distinguish. Several enzymes that play a role in regulating oxidant defense, including SOD, catalase, and glutathione reductase, depend on normal zinc conditions. It is suitable because in sepsis there is a decrease in the detoxification capacity of ROS [88].

6.4.2 Selenium (Se)

Selenium is a component of selenoproteins with antioxidant, anti-inflammatory and immunomodulatory properties. Low selenium concentrations in patients with systemic inflammation or sepsis are associated with impaired neutrophil and macrophage function and decreased antioxidant defenses. The effect of selenium treatment may depend on dose, route of administration, combination with other nutrients, and the patient population studied [89].

Selenium has an antioxidant function through the activity of the enzyme glutathione peroxidase which protects cell membranes and organelles from peroxide damage and has a synergistic effect with vitamins C and E. In addition, selenoproteins (selenium derivatives) are components of the body's defenses that affect the function of neutrophils, macrophages, NK cells and lymphocytes T [79].

6.4.3 Copper (Cu)

Sepsis is often accompanied by acidosis and the release of cupric ions from ceruloplasmin and other proteins. With increased oxygen demand that is not accompanied by oxygen availability causes ischemia and acidosis in early sepsis and the release of cupric ions [90].

Copper is an essential trace mineral necessary for survival. It is found in all body tissues and plays a role in making red blood cells and maintaining nerve cells and the immune system. Copper may also have an antioxidant function. It may help reduce the production of free radicals [91].

Copper is an important component of several enzymes such as superoxide dismutase (SOD), cytochrome oxidase and several coenzymes. Necessary for hemoglobin formation, antioxidant effect, immune function and collagen synthesis. Copper consumption is limited for patients with liver failure and cholestasis because it is excreted through the gallbladder and will cause poisoning if it accumulates [92].

6.4.4 Iron (Fe)

Iron affects the function of lymphocytes and macrophages, which is related to its role as a cofactor for enzymes in various processes. Lymphocyte activation requires iron because iron plays an important role in the work of several enzymes including nucleotide reductase which is involved in DNA synthesis. Iron uptake is regulated by transferrin mRNA receptors by binding to iron regulatory proteins (IRPs). In the state of iron deficiency, transferrin only binds a small amount of iron which will interfere with proliferation, on the contrary, in iron overload, transferrin saturation will increase and will inhibit lymphocyte proliferation [93].

In sepsis, the decrease in iron concentration occurs because of increased permeability so that transferrin moves from the intravascular to the interstitial fluid. The increase in ferritin production in the liver is caused by the induction of IL-6 so that more Fe is stored in the liver. In sepsis, hepcidin production is increased and will inhibit Fe transport [94]. Neutrophils and macrophages require Fe for phagocytosis and the formation of oxygen intermediates which are toxic in killing bacteria. The reduction of nitroblue tetrazolium and hydrogen peroxide to neutrophils and macrophages is decreased in the presence of iron deficiency. Iron also plays a role in the Crebs cycle as an essential source of energy. Several enzymes such as glutathione, peroxidase, catalase and dehydrogenase require iron as a free radical scavenger [95, 96]. Increased venous permeability causes leakage of transferrin into the interstitial fluid. Iron stimulates bacterial growth because of its role as an essential nutrient for bacterial growth [94]. Polymorphonuclear (PMN) releases lactoferrin through the inflammatory process and bends iron which is then processed by macrophages. Neutrophils and macrophages need iron for phagocytosis and killing bacteria. Otherwise, excessive iron can decrease the ability of macrophages to carry out phagocytosis. This happens because the production of free radicals is increasing and damaging the lipid peroxidase contained in the phagosome membrane. Iron is also a growth factor for some bacteria and promotes overall proliferation in vivo [96].

7. Conclusions

An immunonutrient test preparation containing 20% young coconut flesh in coconut water and added kaffir lime juice has a very strong antioxidant activity influenced by the components found in coconut fruit (*Cocos nucifera* L.,) namely a component of a mixture of phytonutrients that can be used as immunonutrient agents in sepsis caused by Lipopolysaccaride *Escherichia coli* through antioxidant activity. The addition of kaffir lime juice can inhibit rancidity or rancidity arising from the oxidation of unsaturated fatty acids contained in processed coconut meat so as to maintain the stability of the components of the active compounds contained in processed coconuts so that these preparations can provide good treatment results.

Author details

Rahmayati Rusnedy
Sekolah Tinggi Ilmu Farmasi (STIFAR) Riau, Tampan, Pekanbaru, Indonesia

*Address all correspondence to: rahmayatikenedy@gmail.com

References

[1] Joshi RK. Role of natural products against microorganisms. Am J Clin Microbiol Antimicrob. 2018;1:1-5.

[2] Southwick F S. Infectious diseases: A clinical short course. Mc Graw Hill; 2007. 57- 65 p.

[3] Kang-Birken, S. Lena. Sepsis and Septic Shock. In: Dipiro, J.T., Talbert R.L., Yee, G.C., Matzke, G.R., Wells, B.G., and Posey, L.M., Pharmacotherapy A Pathophysiology Approach Ninth Edition. United States of America: The McGraw-Hill Companies Inc.; 2014. 1897-1910p.

[4] Gantner, D., Mason, C. Management of severe sepsis. Anaesth. Intensive Care Med. 2015;16:593-597. https://doi.org/10.1016/j.mpaic.2015.09.012

[5] Guntur A.H. Sepsis: SIRS, Sepsis, dan Syok Sepsis (Imunologi, Diagnosis, Penatalaksanaan). Surakarta: Sebelas Maret University Press; 2008. 1-8 p.

[6] S.B. Levy, B. Marshall. Antibacterial resistance worldwide: Causes, challenges and responses. Nat. Med. 2004;10: 122-129, https://doi.org/10.1038/nm1145.

[7] Garrido A.G, Poli de Figueiredo L.F, Rocha e Silva M. experimental models of sepsis and septic shock : An overview. Acta Cirurgica Brasileira. 2004;19(2):82-88.

[8] De Waele E, Malbrain MLNG, Spapen H. Nutrition in sepsis: A bench-tobedside review. Nutrients. 2020;12:1-16.

[9] Paul Wischmeyer, M.D. Nutrition therapy In sepsis. Crit Care Clin. 2018; 34(1):107-125.

[10] Hotchkiss, R.S.; Monneret, G.; Payen, D. Sepsis-induced immunosuppression: From cellular dysfunctions to immunotherapy. Nat. Rev. Immunol. 2013;13:862-874. https://doi.org/10.103

[11] Tom van der Poll, Frank L. van de Veerdonk, Brendon P. Scicluna & Mihai G. Netea. The immunopathology of sepsis and potential therapeutic targets. Nature Reviews Immunology. 2017;17:407-420.

[12] Cecconi, M.; Evans, L.; Levy, M.; Rhodes, A. Sepsis and septic shock. Lancet. 2018;392:75-87.

[13] Akram M. Salam and Cassandra L. Quave. Opportunities for plant natural products in infection control. Curr Opin Microbiol. 2018;45:189-194. doi: 10.1016/j.mib.2018.08.004.

[14] Vetvicka, V, Vetvickova, J. Concept of Immuno-Nutrition. Journal of Nutrition & Food Sciences. 2016; 6(3).

[15] Grimble, R. F. Basics in clinical nutrition: Immunonutrition – Nutrients which influence immunity: Effect and mechanism of action. E-SPEN. The European E-Journal of Clinical Nutrition and Metabolism. 2008;4(1):10-13. doi:10.1016/j.eclnm.2008.07.015

[16] Roehl, K. Immunonutrition in 2016: Benefit, harm or neither? Practical Gastroenterology. 2016; 154: 27-40.

[17] Calder, P. C. Immunonutrition may have beneficial effects in surgical patients. The BMJ, 2003;327(117): 117-118.

[18] Grimble, R. F. Basics in clinical nutrition: Immunonutrition – Nutrients which influence immunity: Effect and mechanism of action. E-SPEN. The European E-Journal of Clinical Nutrition and Metabolism, 2008;4(1):10-13. doi:10.1016/j.eclnm.2008.07.015

[19] Pierre JF, Heneghan AF, Lawson CM, Wischmeyer PE, Kozar RA, Kudsk KA. Pharmaconutrition review: Physiological mechanisms. J Parenter Enter Nutr. 2013;37:51-65.

[20] McCarthy MS, Martindale RG. Immunonutrition in critical illness: What is the role? Nutr Clin Pract. 2018;33(3):348-358.

[21] Zong J, Martirosyan DM. Anticancer effects of garlic and garlic-derived bioactive compounds and its potential status as functional food. Bioactive Compounds in Health and Disease. 2018;1(2):16-35.

[22] Osland E, Memon B, Memon MA. Pharmaconutrition administration on outcomes of elective oncological surgery for gastrointestinal malignancies: Is timing everything? — A review of published meta-analyses until the end of 2016. Translational Gastroenterology and Hepatology. 2018;3(52):1-8.

[23] McCarthy MS, Martindale RG. Immunonutrition in critical illness: What is the role? Nutr Clin Pract. 2018;33(3):348-358.

[24] Mizock BA, Sriram K. Perioperative immunonutrition. Expert Rev Clin Immunol. 2011;7(1):1-3.

[25] Agung Prasetiyo, Nasronudin. Micronutrient therapy for sepsis. Indonesian Journal of Tropical and Infectious Disease. 2015;5(5):119-123.

[26] Shenkin A. The key role of micronutrients. Clinical Nutrition. 2005;25:1-13.

[27] Rahmayati Rusnedy. Uji antioksidan campuran buah kelapa muda dan air perasan jeruk purut sebagai imunonutrisi pada tikus terinduksi sepsis. Riset Informasi Kesehatan. 2020;9(2):37-45.

[28] Putra AP. Pengaruh penambahan minyak jeruk purut terhadap proses penghambatan ransiditas pada minyak kelapa. Universitas Brawijaya; 2016.

[29] Berger MM, Chiolero RL. Antioxidant supplementation in sepsis and systemic inflammatory response syndrome. Crit Care Med. 2007;35:584-590.

[30] Heyland DK, Dhaliwal R, Suchner U, Berger M. Antioxidant nutrients: A systematic review of trace elements and vitamins in the critically ill patient. Intensive Care Med. 2005;31:327-337.

[31] M. DebMandal and S. Mandal, Coconut (Cocos nucifera L.: Arecaceae): In health promotion and disease prevention. Asian Pacific Journal of Tropical Medicine. 2011;1:241-247. doi:10.1016/S1995-7645(11)60078-3.

[32] Duarte, A.C.P., Coelho, M.A.Z., Leite, S.G.F. Identification of peroxidase and Tyrosinase in green coconut water. Cienc. Tecnol. Aliment. 2002;3(5):266-270.

[33] Barlina R,. Potensi Buah Kelapa Muda Untuk Kesehatan dan Pengolahannya. Perspektif. 2004;3(2):46-60.

[34] Farapti dan Savitri Sayogo. Air Kelapa Muda–Pengaruhnya terhadap Tekanan Darah. Jurnal CDK-23. 2014;41(12):896-900.

[35] Pulung ML, Yogaswara R. Oil Dari Tanaman Kelapa Asal Papua. Chem Prog. 2016;9(2):63-69.

[36] Barlina R. Pengaruh Perbandingan Air Kelapa Dengan Penambahan Daging Kelapa Muda. J Littri. 2007;13(2):73– 82.

[37] United States Department of Agriculture (USDA). National nutrient database for standard reference, Nuts, coconut water, 2008. [Online]. Available

from: http://www.nal.usda.gov/fnic/foodcomp/ cgi-bin/list_nut_edit.pl/. [Accessed on December 8, 2009].

[38] Yong WJWH, Ge L, Ng YF, Tan SN. The chemical composition and biological properties of coconut (Cocos nucifera L.). Molecules. 2009;14:5144-5164.

[39] A. M. Fonseca, F. J. Q Monte, M. da Conceic and F. de Oliveiraa ão. Coconut Water (*Cocos nucifera* L.)—A New Biocatalyst System for Organic Synthesis. Journal of Molecular Catalysis B: Enzymatic. 2009;57:78-82. doi:10.1016/j.molcatb.2008.06.022

[40] E. H. M. Walter, D. Y. Kabuki, L. M. R. Esper, A. S. Sant'Ana and A. Y. Kuaye. Modelling the growth of listeria monocytogenes in fresh green coconut (Cocos nucifera L.) water. Food Microbiology. 2009;26:653-657. doi:10.1016/j.fm.2009.04.003

[41] Campbell-Falck D. Thomas T. Falck TM. Tutuo N. Clem K. The intravenous use of coconut water. American Journal of Emergency Medicine. 2000;18(1):108-111.

[42] U. Santoso, K. Kubo, T. Ota, T. Tadokoro and A. Maekawa. Nutrient composition of Kopyor coconuts (Cocos nucifera L.). Food Chemistry. 1996;57(2):299-304. doi:10.1016/0308-8146(95)00237-5

[43] A. G. Pue, W. Riva, K. Sundarao, C. Kaluarin and K. Singh. Preliminary studies on changes in the coconut water during maturation of the fruit. Science in New Guinea. 1992;18(2):81-84.

[44] A. Jayalakshmy, C. Arumughan, C. S. Narayanan and A. G. Mathew. Changes in the chemical composition of coconut water during maturation. Journal of Food Science and Technology. 1986;23(4):203-207.

[45] Loki AL, Rajamohan T. Hepatoprotective and antioxidant effect of tender coconut water on CCl4 induced liver injury in rats. Indian J Biochem Biophy 2003;40(5):354-357.

[46] Effiong GS, Ebong PE, Eyong EU, Uwah AJ, Ekong UE. Amelioration of chloramphenicol induced toxicity in rats by coconut water. J Appl Sc Res. 2010; 6(4):331-335.

[47] Bankar GR, Nayak PG, Bansal P, Paul P, Pai KSR, Singla RK, et al. Vasorelaxant and antihypertensive effect of Cocos nucifera Linn. Endocarp on isolated rat thoracic aorta and DOCA saltinduced hypertensive rats. J Ethnopharmacol. 2010;134(1):50-54. doi:10.1016/ j.jep.2010.11.047

[48] Thormar H, Hilmarsson H, Bergsson G. Stable concentrated emulsions of the 1-monoglyceride of capric acid (monocaprin) with microbicidal activities against the food-borne bacteria campylobacter jejuni, salmonella spp., and Escherichia coli. Appl Environ Microbiol. 2006;72(1):522-526.

[49] Thormar H, Hilmarsson H. The role of microbicidal lipids in host defense against pathogens and their potential as therapeutic agents. Chem Phy lipids. 2007;150(1):1-11.

[50] Mandal S, Mandal MD, Pal NK, Saha K. Synergistic antiStaphylococcus aureus activity of amoxicillin in combination with Emblica officinalis and Nymphae odorata extracts. Asian Pacific J Trop Med. 2010;3:711-714.

[51] Mandal S, Mandal M, Pal NK. Antibacterial potential of Azadirachta indica seed and Bacopa monniera leaf extracts against multidrug resistant salmonella enterica serovar Typhi isolates. Archives Med Sci. 2007;3:14-18.

[52] Obi RC, Oyi AR, Onaolapo JA. Formulation and antimicrobial activities of coconut (Cocos nucifera Linne) oil. Research Journal of Applied Sciences,

Engineering and Technology. 2010;2(2):133-137.

[53] Pouillot A, Luigi LP, Philippe T, Alice N, Ada P and Barbara P. Formulating, Packaging, and Marketing of Natural Cosmetic Products. New York: Wiley; 2011.

[54] Mahalwal VS and AliM.Volatile Constituents of the Fruit Peels of C. reticulate. Blanco J Essent Oil Bearing Plants. 2001;4:45-49.

[55] Rahmi U, Manjang Y, Santoni A. Profil Fitokimia Metabolit Sekunder Dan Uji Aktivitas Antioksidan Tanaman Jeruk Purut (Citrus histrix DC) dan jeruk bali (Citrus maxima (Burm.f.) Merr). J Kim Unand. 2013;2(2):109-114.

[56] Swallah MS, Sun H, Affoh R, Fu H, Yu H. Antioxidant Potential Overviews of Secondary Metabolites (Polyphenols) in Fruits. Int J Food Sci. 2020. doi.org/10.1155/2020/9081686

[57] Al-Juhaimi FY, Ghafoor K. Bioactive compounds, antioxidant and physicochemical properties of juice from lemon, mandarin and orange fruits cultivated in Saudi Arabia. Pakistan J Bot. 2013;45(4):1193-1196.

[58] Ching LS, Mohamed S. AlphaTocopherol content in 62 edible tropical plants. J Agric Food Chem. 2001;49(6):3101–3105.

[59] Ghasemi K, Ghasemi Y, Ebrahimzadeh MA. Antioxidant activity, phenol and flavonoid contents of 13 citrus species peels and tissues. Pak J Pharm Sci. 2009;22(3):277-281.

[60] Siripongvutikorn, S., P. Thummaratwasik and Y. Huang. Antimicrobial and antioxidation effects of Thai seasoning, Tom-Yum. Lebensm. Wiss. U. Technol. 2005;38:347-352.

[61] Bourgou S, Ksouri R, Bellila A, Skandrani I, Falleh H, Marzouk B. Phenolic composition and biological activities of Tunisian Nigella sativa L. shoots and roots. Comptes Rendus - Biol. 2008;331(1):48-55.

[62] Naczk M, Shahidi F. Extraction and analysis of phenolics in food. J Chromatogr A. 2004;1054(1-2):95-111.

[63] Wischmeyer P.E. Glutamine: Mode of action in critical illness. Crit. CareMed. 2007;35:541-544.

[64] Cruzat V, Macedo Rogero M, Noel Keane K, Curi R, Newsholme P. Glutamine: Metabolism and immune function, Supplementation and Clinical Translation. Nutrients. 2018;10(11):1564.

[65] Calder, P: Overview of nutrients with their functions and effects. The BMJ. 2003;327(7407):117-118.

[66] Bengmark S. Modulation by enteral nutrition of the acute phase response and immune functions. Nutr Hosp. 2003;18(1):1-5.

[67] Novak F, Heyland D, Avenell A, Drover J, Su X. Glutamine Supplementation in Serious Illness ; A Sytematic Review of the Evidence. Crit Care Med. 2002;30(9):2022-2029.

[68] Davis, J.S.; Anstey, N.M. Is plasma arginine concentration decreased in patients with sepsis? A systematic review and meta-analysis*. Crit. Care Med. 2011;39:380-385.

[69] Waitzberg DL, Saito H, Plank LD, et al. Postsurgical infections are reduced with specialized nutrition support. World J Surg. 2006;30:1592-1604.

[70] Pan M, Choudry HA, Epler MJ, et al. Arginine transport in catabolic disease states. J Nutr. 2004;134(10):2826-2829.

[71] Singer P, Theilla M, Fisher H, et al. Benefit of an enteral diet enriched with

eicosapentaenoic acid and gamma-linolenic acid in ventilated patients with acute lung injury. Crit Care Med. 2006;34(4):1033-1038.

[72] Pontes-Arruda A, Aragao AM, Albuquerque JD. Effects of enteral feeding with eicosapentaenoic acid, gamma-linolenic acid, and antioxidants in mechanically ventilated patients with severe sepsis and septic shock. Crit Care Med. 2006;34(9):2325-2333.

[73] Singer P, Shapiro H, Theilla M, et al. Anti-inflammatory properties of omega-3 fatty acids in critical illness: Novel mechanisms and an integrative perspective. Intensive Care Med. 2008;34(9):1580-1592.

[74] Serhan CN, Savill J. Resolution of inflammation: The beginning programs the end. Nat Immunol. 2005;6(12):1191-1197.

[75] Rindengan, B., A. Lay., H. Novarianto., H. Kembuan dan Z. Mahmud. Karakterisasi daging buah Kelapa Hirbida untuk bahan baku industri makanan. Laporan Hasil Penelitian. Kerjasama Proyek Pembinaan Kelembagaan Penelitian Pertanian Nasional, Badan Litbang; 1995;49.

[76] Clandinin and Jumpsen. Brain development: Relationship to Dietary lipid and Lipid Metabolism. AOCS Press: Champaign. Illinois; 1995.

[77] Heys S, Schofield A, Wahle W. Immunonutrition in clinical practice : What is the current evidence? Nutr Hosp. 2004;14(6):325-332.

[78] Duggan C, Gannon J, Walker WA. Protective nutrients and functional foods for the gastrointestinal tract. Am J Clin Nutr. 2002;75(5):789-808.

[79] Cunningham-Rundles S, Moon A, McNeeley DF. Malnutrition and host defense. Dalam: Duggan C, Watkins JB, Walker WA, penyunting. Nutrition in pediatrics. Edisi. Ontario: BC Decker Inc; 2008.261-271p.

[80] Wilson, J.X.; Wu, F. Vitamin C in Sepsis. Sub-cell. Biochem. 2012;56:67-83.

[81] May, J.M.; Harrison, F.E. Role of vitamin C in the function of the vascular endothelium. Antioxid. Redox Sign. 2013;19(17):2068-2083.

[82] Carr A.C, Rosengrave P.C, Bayer S, Chambers S, Mehrtens J, Shaw G.M. Hypovitaminosis C and vitamin C deficiency in critically ill patients despite recommended enteral and parenteral intakes. Crit Care. 2017;21(1):300.

[83] Kalokerinos A, Dettman I, Meakin C. Endotoxin and vitamin C part 1 – Sepsis, endotoxin and vitamin C. J. Aust. Coll. Nutr. & Env. Med, 2005;24(1):17-21.

[84] Fernandes G, Jolly CA, Lawrence RA. Nutrition and the immune system. In: Shils ME, Shike M, Ross AC, Caballero B, Cousins RJ, penyunting. Modern Nutrition In Health And Disease, 10 Edition Baltimore: Lippincot Williams; 2006.

[85] Gershwin ME, German JB, Keen CL. Nutrition and Immunology Principles and Practice: Human Press; 2000.

[86] Savino W, Dardenne M, Velloso LA, Silva-Barbosa SD. The thymus is a common target in malnutrition and infection. Br J Nutr. 2007;98(1):11-16.

[87] Bhaskaram P. Micronutrient malnutrition, infection and immunity: An overview. Nutr Rev. 2002;60(5):40-45.

[88] Cunningham-Rundles S, Moon A, McNeeley DF. Malnutrition and host defense. In: Duggan C, Watkins JB, Walker WA, penyunting. Nutrition in

pediatrics. Edisi. Ontario: BC Decker Inc; 2008. 261-271p.

[89] Forceville X, Vitoux D, Gauzit R, Combes A, Lahilaire P, Chappuis P. Selenium, systemic immune response syndrome, sepsis, and outcome in critically ill patients. Crit. Care Med. 1998;26(9):1536-1544.

[90] Roberts A, Bar-Oy D, Winkler J, Rael L. Copper-induced oxidation of epinephrine: Protective effect of D-DHAK, a synthetic analogue of the high affinity copper binding site of human albumin. Biochemichal and Biophysical Research Communication. 2003;304:755-757.

[91] Megan Ware, RDN, L.D. Free Radicals Can Damage Cells and DNA, Leading to cancer and Other Diseases; 2017.

[92] Braunschweig C, Sowers M, Kovacevich D. Parenteral zinc supplementation in adult humans during the acute phase response increases the febrile response. The Journal of Nutrition. 1997;127(1):70-74.

[93] Brock J, Mulero V. Cellular and molecular aspects of iron and immune function. Proceedings of Nutrition Society. 2000;59(4):537-540.

[94] Shenkin A. The key role of micronutrients. Clinical Nutrition. 2006;25(1):1-13.

[95] Agarwal A, Khana P, Baidya D, Arora met. Trace elements in Criticall illness. Journal of Endocrinology and Metabolism. 2011;2(1):57-63.

[96] Doherty P, Weaver L, Prentice A. Micronutrient supplementation and infection: A double-edge sword?. Journal of Pediatric Gastroenterology and Nutrition. 2002;34(4):346-352.

Chapter 4

Empiric Antimicrobial Therapy in Critically Ill Septic Patients

Ahlem Trifi, Sami Abdellatif, Sameh Trabelsi and Salah Ben Lakhal

Abstract

Sepsis is a medical emergency and life-threatening condition due to a dysregulated host response to infection, which is time-dependent and associated with unacceptably high mortality. At the bedside of a patient with sepsis or septic shock, clinician must make immediate life-saving decisions including empirical initiation of broad-spectrum antimicrobials; the most likely to be appropriate. The empiric regimen should be initiated within the first hour of diagnosis and determined by assessing patient and epidemiological risk factors, likely source of infection based on presenting signs and symptoms, and severity of illness. Optimizing antibiotic use is crucial to ensure successful outcomes and to reduce adverse antibiotic effects, as well as preventing drug resistance. All likely pathogens involved should be considered to provide an appropriate antibiotic coverage. Herein, we tried to make suggestions of empirical therapeutic regimens in sepsis/septic shock according to most likely pathogens in cause and sepsis source based on the recent recommendations of learned societies. Some suggestions were adapted to an environment of low-resource regions where the ecology of multi drug resistant organisms is of concern.

Keywords: empiric, antimicrobial, sepsis, septic shock, intensive care

1. Introduction

Sepsis is a clinical syndrome characterized by systemic inflammation due to infection (presumed or confirmed). There is a continuum of severity ranging from sepsis to septic shock. Diagnosing sepsis remains difficult because it is not a single disease but a syndrome with various pathogen and host factor-associated symptoms. Sepsis-3 was established to improve risk stratification among patients with a suspected infection focusing on organ failures [1]. Sepsis should be immediately recognized because it is the primary cause of death from infection, especially if not diagnosed and treated promptly. Mortality has been estimated to be ≥10 percent and ≥ 40 percent when shock is present [1, 2]. In the United States, it is estimated that there are 270 000 deaths a year due to sepsis and 35 000 deaths attributable to antibiotic resistance [3, 4]. Herein, we discussed the immediate management of sepsis and septic shock mainly the empiric antimicrobials in critically ill patients.

2. Immediate conditioning

Correcting hypoxemia and establishing venous access for the **early** administration of fluids and antibiotics are priorities in the management of patients with sepsis and septic shock [5, 6].

2.1 Oxygenation

Intubation and mechanical ventilation (MV) may be required to support the increased work of breathing that typically accompanies sepsis. Oxygenation should be monitored continuously with pulse oximetry. Once MV is indicated, rapid sequence intubation (RSI) should incorporates a rapidly acting sedative (ie, induction) agent, in addition to a neuromuscular blocking (ie, paralytic) agent, to create optimal intubating conditions. Then ensure analgesia sedation throughout the duration necessary for the sepsis/septic shock management while regularly monitoring the possibility of weaning from ventilator.

2.2 Venous access

Venous access is essential in the immediate management of sepsis/septic shock. The peripheral access has the advantage of the quickness of its putting in (at least 2 lanes of good caliber). But anyway, we are going to need central venous access. Preferably, it is advisable to set up a central venous catheter (CVC) but that should not delay the administration of resuscitative fluids and antibiotics. A CVC is useful to infuse intravenous fluids, medications (particularly vasopressors) and antibiotics. As well as, it can be used to monitor the central venous pressure (CVP) and the central venous saturation ($ScvO_2$).

2.3 Initial investigations

Concomitantly to the initial conditioning including oxygenation and venous access, must be carried out: a history with a physical examination of rapid orientation, biological, microbiological and imaging examinations. This may allows having an orientation towards the source and sometimes the pathogen in cause and thus guiding the empirical choice of antibiotics.

- Laboratory tests include complete blood counts, Arterial blood gas (ABG), analysis of renal and liver functions, D-dimer level, Procalcitonin and serum lactate.

- Microbiologic samples include peripheral blood cultures (aerobic and anaerobic cultures from at least two different sites), and other samples depending of suspect sites should be obtained (e.g., cyto-bacteriologic examination of sputum if pneumonia suspected or urine if urinary tract infection evoked, catheter tip if catheter-related infection (CRI) evoked, surgical site, etc.). Regarding the bloodstream cultures, it is unnecessary to draw blood through a catheter, given the risk of contamination by skin flora. The sample should be taken from a peripheral venipuncture site.

- Imaging target at the suspected infection site is warranted (eg, chest radiography, computed tomography of chest and/or abdomen).

2.4 Rapid restoration of perfusion (first three hours)

Aggressive administration of intravenous fluids, usually crystalloids given at 30 ml/kg, started by one hour and completed within the first 3 hours following presentation.

Some patients may require higher than recommended volumes, particularly those who demonstrate clinical and/or hemodynamic indicators of fluid-responsiveness. The clinical and hemodynamic response and the presence or absence of pulmonary edema must be assessed before and after each bolus using passive leg raising, CVP variation, $ScvO_2$, pulsed pression variation (PPV) or ultrasound indicators etc.... Intravenous fluid challenges can be repeated until blood pressure and tissue perfusion become acceptable.

2.5 Vasopressors

Vasopressors on CVC if the blood volume is optimized and persistent hypoperfusion or immediately if the diastolic blood pressure is less than 40 mmHg.

Based on the SSC (survival sepsis campaign) guidelines 2016 [5], the response should be assessed using the following targets within 6 hours: $ScvO_2 \geq 70\%$, CVP 8–12 mmHg, mean arterial pressure (MAP) ≥65 mmHg, and urine output ≥0.5 ml/kg/hour.

3. Empiric antimicrobial therapy (EAT)

Initial selection of particular antimicrobial agents is empiric and is based on an assessment of the patient's underlying host defenses, the potential sources of infection, and the most likely pathogens depending on the locally epidemiological data. EAT is preferably administered within the first hour.

3.1 Times to antibiotics

Once a presumed diagnosis of sepsis or septic shock has been made, optimal doses of appropriate intravenous antibiotic therapy should be initiated, preferably within one hour of presentation and after cultures have been obtained. The Infectious Diseases society of America (IDSA) opts to that prompt administration of antibiotics is recommended once a presumed diagnosis of sepsis or shock has been made by the treating clinician [7]. The Surviving Sepsis Campaign recommends immediate antibiotics for all patients with suspected sepsis and septic shock, ideally within 1 hour of recognition.

The literature review does not find a clinical trials evaluating specially the target time of one hour to start antimicrobials. That is understandable given the enormous ethical concern that results. But almost all observational studies agree that a delay exceeding one hour is related to poor outcomes; as well as inadequate doses and inappropriate antibiotic therapy [8–14]. Ferrer R, et al. in a large population of patients with severe sepsis and septic shock (17,990 patients) demonstrated a linear increase in the risk of mortality for each hour delay in antibiotic administration [9]. In a retrospective study of 35,000 patients treated in emergency department, the increase in absolute mortality associated with an hour's delay in antibiotic administration was 0.3% ($p = 0.04$) for sepsis, 0.4% ($p = 0.02$) for severe sepsis, and 1.8% ($p = 0.001$) for shock [11].

In a large database study comparing patients with sepsis and septic shock treated with various types of protocolized treatment bundles (that included fluids and antibiotics, blood cultures, and serum lactate) versus those in whom a three-hour bundle (blood cultures before broad spectrum antibiotics and serum lactate level) was completed within the three-hour time frame [12]. Each 3-hour bundle delay achievement increased in-hospital mortality by 1.04 per hour [12]. In addition, a delayed completion of a fluid bolus did not increase mortality significantly (OR = 1.04) as the delay of antimicrobials [12].

3.2 Identification of suspected source/responsible pathogens

Establishing an accurate diagnosis of the infection site is a priority objective that must be fulfilled as soon as possible.

Sometimes the patient arrives with a visible source of infection (e.g. infected wound, cellulitis etc). In the case where the source is unclear, the process of its identification is based on a good anamnesis for collecting the medical and surgical history and a careful and exhaustive physical examination looking for local inflammatory signs or function loss. If the source is identified, targeted imaging and microbiological sampling should be done and therefore empiric antibiotic therapy should be initiated.

In the case where the source remains unclear, it is necessary to complete by an exhaustive imaging or even a whole body CT scan and extensive sampling.

Table 1 summarizes the most common sources of infection with a potential risk of progress to a sepsis and septic shock and the additional tests to be performed.

Additional diagnostic testing or interventions may be required to identify the anatomic site(s) of infection. In particular, in addition to antibiotics, closed space infections should be promptly drained or debrided (eg, empyema, abscess) for effective source control.

Besides bacteriological examinations, imaging is often essential to recognize sites of infection (chest radiography, ultrasound, tomography and MRI).

Sometimes in structures with limited resources, imaging is not always available, as are interventional radiology techniques. In this case, blood cultures before the administration of antibiotics becomes an essential measure and ideally that should be obtained from two sites.

3.3 Regimen to choose

The choice of empirical antibiotic therapy is not a simple attitude and must be reasoned upon the presumed primary focus, the history of the patient ((eg, recent antibiotics received, previous organisms) and its co-morbidities (eg, diabetes, organ failures, immune defect..), invasive devices, nosology (eg, community- or hospital-acquired) and the bacterial ecology and resistance patterns of the unit where the patient is hospitalized [13, 14, 16–18]. It must be preceded by directed bacteriological samples.

Also, the choice of the molecule is made according to its spectrum of action and its pharmacodynamics/pharmacokinetics (PK/PD) properties and the spectrum of the selected combination must be efficient against gram-positive, gram-negative, and anaerobic bacteria because all of these classes of organisms produce similar clinical presentations.

Regarding the administration route and dosing, it is recommended that the intravenous is mandatory and at high doses to achieve bactericidal serum levels. This later correlated with clinical improvement rather than the number of antibiotics prescribed.

Suspected site	Symptoms/signs	Suggested initial tests
Upper respiratory tract	Pharyngeal inflammation plus exudates ± swelling and lymphadenopathy	Throat swab for aerobic culture Cyto-bacteriological exam of sputum PCR-SARS CoV2 if pandemic context
Lower respiratory tract	Productive cough, pleuritic chest pain, consolidative auscultatory findings	Sputum of good quality, rapid influenza testing, urinary antigen testing (eg, pneumococcus, legionella) PCR-SARS CoV2 if pandemic context
Urinary tract	Dysuria, urination scorch	Urine culture, renal ultrasound (obstructive calculus)
Vascular catheters: arterial, central venous	Redness or pus at insertion site	Culture of blood (from the catheter and a peripheral site), catheter tip bacterial exam after removal
Abrasion, wound, burn, diabetic foot lesion	Erythema, pus, lymphangitis	Local swabs gram stain and culture, sampling of pus or per cleaning
Skin/soft tissue	Lividities, cyanic spots, subcutaneous crepitation, local hypo- or anesthesia, induration exceeding erythema, local necrosis	Culture of flowing liquid or draining pus, preoperative tissue samples
Urinary system	May differ by gender low abdominal pain and vaginal discharge in women, Dysuria, incontinence, cloudy urine, prostatic tenderness in men	Vaginal and endocervical sampling in women and cytobacteriological examination plus culture in both sexes
Deep intra-abdominal focus	abdominal pain depending on the organ affected, vomiting	Aerobic and anaerobic culture of abdominal fluid collections drained percutaneously or surgically
Gastrointestinal	Diarrhea, vomiting and intestinal spasms	Coproculture, parasitological stool examination
Meninges and brain	Meningitis: stiff neck, sign of Kernig and Brudzinski, osteotendinous hyper-reflexia Encephalitis: Altered state of consciousness, motor deficit, seizures	Lumbar puncture for exhaustive examination of the CSF (cytological, chemical, bacteriological, search for soluble Ag, culture and PCR if indicated)
Peritoneal catheter	Cloudy fluid, local inflammatory signs	Direct examination and culture of the discharged fluid
Bones and joints	Pain, Inflammatory signs	MRI, peroperative cultures or by interventional radiology Arthrocentesis, blood cultures

PCR: polymerase chain reaction, SARS CoV2: severe acute respiratory syndrome coronavirus 2, CSF: cerebrospinal fluid; PD: peritoneal dialysis; MRI: magnetic resonance imaging.
Source: Reference [15]

Table 1.
Identification of sources of sepsis and additional tests.

The regimen to choose should consider antipseudomonal in patients with neutropenia or burns and anti-anaerobes in intra-abdominal/perineal infections.

Antimicrobial choice should be tailored to each individual. In any case, appropriate cultures should be obtained which include two sets of blood cultures obtained before antibiotics are started and cultures of other suspected sites of infection (sputum, urine, etc.) obtained as soon as possible.

For most patients with sepsis without shock, antimicrobials may be administered in monotherapy or in combination. Anyway, the empiric chosen regimen must cover all the maximum number of pathogens most likely involved (ie gram-positive and gram-negative bacteria, fungi if presence of invasive candidiasis factors or immune-compromised for aim *Pneumocystis jirovecii*, and rarely viruses (eg, influenza, Cytomégalovirus (CMV)). For SARS CoV2, all the therapeutic means tried so far (chloroquine, macrolides, tocilizumab, remdesivir, monoclonal antibody, colchicine ...) are designed for immunomodulatory purposes and no treatment is directed specifically against COVID-19.

Patients with septic shock, in whom gram negative bacilli are suspected, must be treated with at least two antimicrobials from two different classes according to the considered likely organisms and local antibiotic susceptibilities. That is commonly called combination therapy defined as more than one antimicrobial agent given in the aim to improve efficiency against a known or suspected pathogen.

Escherichia coli, *Staphylococcus aureus, Klebsiella pneumoniae,* and *Streptococcus pneumoniae,* are the most common isolated organisms from patients with sepsis. Thus, these organisms should be taken into account when choosing empiric regimen [19]. Betalactams such carbapenem, piperacillin-tazobactam, in combination or not with aminosides or quinolones are a good alternative to cover a large batch of gram negative and positive organisms.

When nosocomial nature of sepsis or septic shock is suspected, the multiresistant profile of microorganisms (mainly non fermenting gram negative bacilli including *Acinetobacter Baumannii*) should be covered [20, 21].

Otherwise, the following pathogens must be included in the spectrum of antibiotics to be chosen and this according to the risk factors for their presence:

- **Methicillin-resistant *S. aureus***: Today, methicillin-resistant *S. aureus* (MRSA) is no longer classified among the pathogens of healthcare-related infections since it is increasingly described in community infections [22, 23]. That is why empirical intravenous vancomycin (be careful with the doses if renal impairement) should be added in subjects with sepsis/septic shock at risk of MRSA. Linezolid if MRSA refractory (VISA or GISA of susceptibility profile) or a contraindication to vancomycin can also be suggested as an anti MRSA. Daptomycin may be prescribed in cases of extra-pulmonary MRSA infection. In skin and soft structures infections, IDSA update 2014 proposed vacomycin, linezolid, clindamycin, daptomycin and ceftaroline/fosamil may be proposed.

- ***Pseudomonas aeruginosa***: if *Pseudomonas* is a likely pathogen and depending on local antibiotic susceptibility patterns, antimicrobials proposed are:

  - Antipseudomonal cephalosporin (eg, ceftazidime, cefepime), or

  - Antipseudomonal carbapenem (eg, imipenem, meropenem), or

  - Antipseudomonal beta-lactam/beta-lactamase inhibitor (eg, piperacillin-tazobactam, or Fluoroquinolone with good anti-pseudomonal activity (eg, ciprofloxacin), or Aminoglycoside (eg, gentamicin, amikacin), or Monobactam (eg, aztreonam)

- **Enterobacteria** (eg, *E. coli*, *K. pneumonia, Proteus, Providencia, Serratia*): They are pathogens treated, for a long time, by a regimen which combines several antibiotics although this is not proven by studies. Indeed, in the old meta-analysis of Safdar N, et al. the summary odds ratio was 0·96 (95% CI

0,70–1,32), indicating no mortality benefit with combination therapy compared to monotherapy with a third generation cephalosporin or a carbapenem [24]. Furthermore, the combination to an amino-glycoside was related to an increase of nephrotoxicity [24].
Therefore, it is recommended to administer a single antimicrobial agent known to have proven efficacy and the least possible toxicity. Patients with neutropenia or in whom *Pseudomonas* is suspected are to exclude from this rule and combination therpay should be contemplated.

- **Carbapenemase-producing *Enterobacteriaceae* (CPE)** are becoming an emerging concern worldwide. Infections caused by these pathogens are associated with high morbidity, mortality and costs while they are difficult to treat since only a small number of therapeutic options are available. Only a few clinical studies, often size-limited and retrospective, have been conducted mainly on infections caused by KPC - producing *Klebsiella pneumoniae* whereas there are more in vitro and animal data. In some cases, β-lactams can be used, such as carbapenems (if MIC ≤8 mg/L), aztreonam or ceftazidime. A double-carbapenem regimen also seems to be promising, with ertapenem. Polymyxins and tigecyline (with a loading dose and high dosages) are possible alternatives in combination. Aminoglycosides (especially gentamicin) in monotherapy are choice options for the treatment of urinary tract infections. Fosfomycin may be used in combination but there is a risk of emergence of resistant mutants during therapy. For the treatment of severe infections (bacteremia and pneumonia), combination therapy should be used since risks of clinical failure and mortality are significantly lower than with monotherapies in the majority of studies. The most frequent combinations are polymyxins-carbapenems, tigecycline-carbapenems and polymyxins-tigecycline, knowing that carbapenem-based regimens (if MIC ≤8 mg/L) must be favored [25].

  Acinetobacter Baumannii: *Acinetobacter* are opportunistic and ubiquitous bacteria that occur in the form of Gram-negative coccobacilli. Among the species of this genus, *Acinetobacter baumannii* is the most implicated in nosocomial infections, especially in ICU [26]. This bacterium is involved in a wide range of infections such as VAP, bacteremia, CRI, urinary tract infections, secondary wound infections or postoperative meningitis.
  A.baumannii exhibits a remarkable ability to acquire mechanisms of resistance to antibiotics, rapidly leading to multi-resistance to almost all commercially available antibiotics and sometimes to therapeutic dead ends [27].
  Acinetobacter baumannii is one of the ESCAPE organisms (*Enterococcus faecium*, *Staphylococcus aureus*, *Clostridium difficile*, *Pseudomonas aeruginosa*, and Enterobacteriaceae), a group of clinically important, predominantly health care-associated organisms that have the potential for substantial antimicrobial resistance [28].

Independent risk factors for colonization or infection with resistant strains of *Acinetobacter* include the following [29–32]: prior colonization with MRSA, prior beta-lactam (particularly carbapenems) or fluoroquinolone use, bedridden status, current or prior ICU admission, presence of a CVC, recent surgery, Mechanical ventilation, Hemodialysis, malignancy, steroids therapy.

Empiric antibiotic therapy for *Acinetobacter*, before results of antimicrobial susceptibility testing are available, should be selected based on local susceptibility patterns. In general, it should consist of a broad spectrum cephalosporin, a combination beta-lactam/beta-lactamase inhibitor (eg, a combination including sulbactam), or a carbapenem. An additional agent may be warranted if local resistance rates to the chosen antibiotic class are high (eg, greater than 10 to 15%).

When rates of resistance to the selected antimicrobial agent are low (ie, below 10 to 15 percent), monotherapy is likely adequate as there are no data to clearly demonstrate that combination therapy improves outcomes through synergistic effect. However, when rates of resistance are higher, it is reasonable to use one of the agents above in combination with an antipseudomonal fluoroquinolone, an aminoglycoside, or colistin to improve the likelihood of administering an antibiotic agent that retains activity. While there are no clear clinical data to support this practice for *Acinetobacter* infections, many experts favor empiric combination therapy for serious infections with these and other potentially resistant gram-negative organisms because of the increased mortality associated with inappropriate empiric therapy.

A prospective cohort study was made in 70 ICU patients with nosocomial sepsis/septic shock in whom imipenem/colistin was prescribed as first line antibiotic therapy [33]. The main findings were: this regimen was only appropriate in 52% of cases and inappropriateness was associated with an increased ICU mortality risk (OR = 6.27, 95% CI [1.83–21], p = 0.003) [33].

- If isolates susceptible to first line agents: we favor choosing the agent with the narrowest spectrum of activity. Other considerations in selection of a regimen include patient drug allergies or intolerance; need to cover additional infections, and hospital formulary.

- If resistant isolates: in the setting of resistance to first line agents, therapeutic options are generally limited to polymyxins (colistin [polymyxin E] and polymyxin B), and tigecycline. We generally use polymyxins, for which there is the most clinical experience in treating extensively drug-resistant *Acinetobacter*.

Susceptibility testing for these agents should be performed as well prior to their use given the possibility of resistance.

We generally favor using a second agent, such as a carbapenem, tigecycline, or rifampin, in addition to polymyxins for serious infections (eg, bacteremia, pneumonia, critical illness) with resistant isolates.

There are no definitive clinical data that demonstrate improved outcomes with combination versus monotherapy, and some randomized trials have suggested that certain combinations (colistin and rifampin or colistin and meropenem or fosfomycin) resulted in comparable clinical outcomes as monotherapy with colistin [34, 35]. Nevertheless, infections with multidrug-resistant *Acinetobacter* are associated with high mortality rates, and we are concerned that the use of a single agent is not adequate, particularly since resistance can develop during therapy, leaving no therapeutic alternatives. The synergistic pharmacological tests are a great contribution to the choice of treatment and consultation with an expert in the management of such infections is advised.

In case of ventilator acquired pneumonia (VAP) caused by *Acinetobacter*, additional considerations include the possible use of adjunctive inhaled antibiotics. Inhaled colistin may be beneficial in select patients [36–38], although not all studies suggest a benefit [39]. We favor use of inhaled colistin among patients with severe pneumonia due to *Acinetobacter* only sensitive to colistin, since intravenous colistin yields low lung concentration. The optimal dose of inhaled colistin is uncertain and ranges from 75 to 150 mg colistin base activity (2.25 to 4.5 million international units CMS) twice daily. Higher doses, up to 5 million international units colistimethate sodium (approximately 167 mg colistin base) every eight hours, have also been used for VAP with *Acinetobacter* [40].

- **Invasive fungal infections:** Fungal infections are a feared complication in ICU patients. Their epidemiology has deeply changed linked to major changes in medical practices (induced immunosuppression, organ transplants, cytotoxic chemotherapy, ICU invasive procedures, parenteral nutrition, and prolonged antimicrobial). Moreover, several factors depend on patient's morbidities (chronic liver or renal failure, diabetes, surgery, septic shock or multisite *Candida* colonization).

  The Arsenal antifungal therapy has also broadened considerably with new molecules, such echinocandins, well tolerated than amphotericin B. The use of an empiric antifungal in patients exhibiting sepsis and septic shock has been widely debated with a rather converging towards the absence of a favorable effect on mortality [41–44]:

Cortegiani A, et al. in a meta-analysis including 22 studies (total of 2761 participants) concluded that the use of untargeted antifungal is not associated with a significant reduction in all-cause mortality and may be associated with a reduction of invasive fungal infection among ICU patients [41]. Empiric antifungal treatment (mostly fluconazole) not decreased risk of mortality or occurrence of invasive candidiasis in ICU patients receiving mechanical ventilation for at least five days [42]. In addition, the multicenter randomized trial conducted in ICU (known as EMPIRICUS, n = 260 patients colonized with *Candida* and having sepsis), micafungin administered for 14 days did not improve 28 day-survival without infection [43].

In a 8-years retrospective double cohort (empiric antifungal group, n = 125 versus no empiric antifungal group, n = 122), no improvement of 28-day survival was found. Moreover, no preventing effect on a new episode of candidemia. Nevertheless, a beneficial effect of empiric antifungal on survival was found in patients with an Acute Physiology and Chronic Health (APACHE) II score < 16: OR = 0.68; CI 95% [0.53–0.87]; p = 0.002 [44]. That means; it is the less severe patients who can benefit from an empiric fungal.

However, if *Candida* or *Aspergillus* is strongly suspected or if neutropenia is present, echinocandin (for *Candida*) or voriconazole (for *Aspergillus*) are often appropriate [45].

Even if our focus here is the empirical choice of antibiotic therapy in septic ICU patients, but it would be wise to suggest a list of the more common potential pathogens that would need to be treated. The main pathogens to be considered in **community infections** depending on the infected site are:

Community acquired pneumonia (CAP): *Streptococcus pneumoniae, Mycoplasma pneumoniae, Chlamydia pneumoniae, Legionella pneumophyla, Haemophilus influenzae, Enterobacteria, anaerobies, Staphylococcus aureus.*

Community meningitides: *Streptococcus pneumoniae, Nesseria meningitis, Listeria monocytogenes Haemophilus influenzae, Enterobacteria, Streptococcus sp.*

Urinary tract infections: *Escherichia coli, Proteus mirabilis, Klebsiella pneumoniae, Staphylococcus saprophyticus, Enterobacter sp, Enterococcus sp.*

Skin and soft tissues infections: *Streptococcus pyogenes, Staphylococcus aureus, anaerobies.*

Intrabdominal infections: *Escherichia coli, Klebsiella pneumonia, anaerobies (Bacteroides fragilis) Enterobacter sp, Enterococcus sp, Streptococcus pneumoniae, Pseudomonas sp.*

For nosocomial infections, Gram-negative bacilli are mostly involved followed by Gram-positive cocci. The main multidrug-resistant bacteria (MDRs) to be considered are: Methicillin-resistant *Staphylococcus aureus* (MRSA), *Enterobacteriaceae* producing Extended spectrum beta-lactamases (ESBL) or hyperproducing cephalosporinases (HPCase), *Pseudomonas æruginosa, Acinetobacter Baumannii* and *Enterococci* Vancomycin Resistant (EVR).

Suspected source of sepsis/ septic shock	
Unknown Source (includes catheter related blood stream infection)	Vancomycin* **PLUS** Cefepime 1 g/6H or Aztreonam 2 g/8H or imipenem 1 g/ 8H (if known high incidence of MDR GNB in the unit) +/- Tobramycin 7 mg/kg IV EIAD+ + Consider addition of antifungal in those at high risk for candidemia (caspofungine 70 mg followed by 50 mg daily or anidulafungine 200 mg the 1st day relayed by 100 mg daily or micafungin 100 mg daily).
Intra-abdominal Source	Piperacillin/tazobactam 4 g/6H **OR** Ertapenem 1 g/d **OR** Aztreonam 2 g/8 h **OR** Cefepime 1 g/6H (failing cefotaxime 1 g/4H) **PLUS** Metronidazole 500 mg/8H +/- Gentamicin 5–7 mg/kg IV (adjust the dosing with dosage of the max and residual concentration +)
Urinary Tract	Cefotaxime 1 g/6H or Ceftriaxone 2 g daily +/– Gentamicin 7 mg/kg If History ESBL colonization: Ertapenem 1 g/d **OR** Aztreonam 2 g/8 h **PLUS** Gentamicin 7 mg/kg If history of MDR pathogen or Pseudomonas: Imipenem 1 g/8H PLUS Amikacine 25 mg/Kg/d
Skin/Soft Tissue Infection: Necrotizing Skin/Soft Tissue: Gas Gangrene or Necrotizing Fasciitis	**If MRSA not suspected:** Piperacillin/tazobactam 4 g/ 6H PLUS gentamycin 5–7 mg/Kg EIAD +/– Clindamycin 900 mg/8H (**only** if toxic shock present) **If MRSA suspected:** Vancomycin 30 mg/kg/d in 2 divided doses* +/– Clindamycin 900 mg/8H OR Linezolid 600 mg/12H OR Ceftaroline 600 mg/12H
Severe CAP	Ceftriaxone 2 g/24 h **PLUS Levofloxacin 500 mg/ 12 h OR** Azithromycin 500 mg /24 h Severe beta-lactam allergy: only Levofloxacin 500 mg /24H and Consider addition of vancomycin OR Linezolid 600 mg/12H if MRSA is suspected (CT features+)
Severe CAP with the following Risk factors: □Hospitalized ≥5 d in the past 90 days □Broad spectrum or IV antimicrobial for ≥5 days in the past 90 days □Known respiratory tract colonization with an MDR organism □Residence in a long-term care facility	Imipenem 1 g/8H OR Piperacillin/tazobactam 4 g/6H OR Cefepime 1 g/6 h **PLUS** Azithromycin 500 mg/24 h +/- Vancomycin IV or Linezolide 600 mg/12H if MRSA suspected +/- Tobramycin 7 mg/kg IV (if *Pseudomonas* colonization *such* COPD, cystic fibrosis...)
HAP/VAP: Risk factors: □Hospitalized ≥5 days □Broad spectrum or IV antimicrobial for ≥5 days in the past 90 days □Known respiratory colonization with an MDR organism □Septic shock	Imipenem 1 g/8H OR Meropenem 1 g/8 h OR Aztreonam 2 g/ 6 h **PLUS** Colistin 9MU in loading dose relayed by 4,5 MU /12H +/– Vancomycin (if MRSA suspected) Consider adjunction of inhaled colistin if high incidence *Acinetobacter* only susceptible to colistin

**Vancomycin dosed per pharmacy consult. Typically with loaded with 20–25 mg/kg dose initially (max 2 g initial dose).*
MDR GNB: multi drug resistant gram negative bacilli, ESBL: Extended spectrum betalactamases, MRSA: Methicillin-resistant Staphylococcus aureus, CAP: Community Acquired Pneumonia, HCAP: healthcare acquired pneumonia, HAP: hospital acquired pneumonia, VAP: ventilator acquired pneumonia.

Table 2.
Suggested regimens for empiric antimicrobials in sepsis/septic shock.

Table 2 displays suggested regimens for empiric antimicrobials in sepsis and septic shock according to the suspected Source (all antibiotics are to be administered intravenously).

3.4 Dosing and modality of administration

Maximizing the dose in patients with sepsis and septic shock is a judicious attitude. This strategy is based upon the known increased volume of distribution that can occur in patients with sepsis due to the administration of fluid and the action of inflammatory cytokines [46, 47] and that higher clinical success rates have been reported in patients with higher peak concentrations of antimicrobials [48, 49]. Continuous infusions of antibiotics as compared with intermittent dosing regimens remain investigational at this time [50].

The meta-analysis of Chen CH, et al. [51] (9 RCTs plus 4 retrospective studies, 1957 participants) compared continuous and intermittent groups. A significant difference was showed with mortality which was higher in the subgroup of continuous infusion (OR 1.433, 95% CI: 1.139–1.801). In this same group, length of stay in ICU was shorter and antibiotic duration was longer but without significance [(OR 0.834, 95% CI: 0.542–1.282) and (OR 1.055, 95% CI: 0.659–1.689) respectively] [51].

However, authors were unable to recommend continuous infusion of intravenous antibiotics better than traditional intermittent infusions of antibiotics at routine clinical care.

In general, the choice of the administration modality depends above all on the PK/PD characteristics of the antibiotic. Time-dependent antibiotics (eg betalactamins, vancomycin) their bactericide are based on the time of contact with the

Antimicrobial	Dose
Imipenem-cilastatin	0.5 to 1 g intravenously every 6 hours to 1 g every 8 hours
Meropenem	1 to 2 g intravenously every 8 hours
Doripenem	0.5 g intravenously every 8 hours
Gentamicin¶	1 to 2.5 mg/kg intravenously every 8 to 12 hours or 7 mg/kg every 24 to 48 hours depending on creatinine clearance
Tobramycin¶	1 to 2.5 mg/kg intravenously every 8 to 12 hours or 7 mg/kg every 24 to 48 hours depending on creatinine clearance
Amikacin¶	5 to 7.5 mg/kg intravenously every 8 hours or 15 mg/kg every 24 to 48 hours depending on creatinine clearance
Ciprofloxacin¶	400 mg intravenously every 8 hours
Colistin$^{\Delta}$	2.5 to 5 mg/kg/day as **colistin base**$^{\Delta}$ intravenously in two to four divided doses
Polymyxin B	25,000 units/kg (2.5 mg/kg) loading dose followed by 12,500 units/kg (1.25 mg/kg) intravenously every 12 hours
Minocycline	200 mg single dose, followed by 100 mg intravenously every 12 hours
Tigecycline$^{\Diamond}$	100 mg single dose, followed by 50 mg intravenously every 12 hours; 100 mg every 12 hours in serious infections

¶Aminoglycosides and fluoroquinolones are generally used in combination with another agent.
Source: Reference [52, 53]
$^{\Delta}$means that the recommended dosage corresponds to that of colistin base, the conversion is: 1 mg colistin base = 2.67 mg colistimethate = 33.3 IU. Thus 2.5 to 5 mg / kg / day of colistin base correspondsabout 6 to 12 million IU of colistimethate.
$^{\Diamond}$For severe hepatic dysfunction: loading dose is the same (100 mg) followed by 25 mg IV every 12 hours.

Table 3.
Dosage of most common prescribed systemic antibiotics in ICU adults with normal renal function.

microorganism at doses above the MIC. Therefore the administration of this type of antibiotic in continuous infusion or in multiple doses is preferred. On the other hand, dose-dependent antibiotics (eg aminosia, colistin), whose effectiveness depends on the peak concentration reached, their administration at a single or twice dose is preferred.

Dosing of the most common prescribed antimicrobials in ICU patients with normal renal function is summarized in the **Table 3.** When renal function impair, antibiotic's doses should be adjusted according to the creatinine clearance.

The follow up of infection's indices is mandatory, including complete blood count and additional cultures. Results should prompt modification of antibiotic choice if a better and safer regimen can be substituted and/or investigations directed towards source control.

3.5 Eradication of septic focus

It should be undertaken in timely manner when they feasible since undrained foci of infection may not respond to antibiotics alone. Typical examples are: infected catheter which must be removed (obviously after the establishment of another vascular access), plumonary abscess and chest wall, obstructive pyelonephritis which indicates percutaneous nephrostomy, cholecystectomy, peritonitis to be cleaned in the operative room, dermo-hypoderma which require debridement or amputation of soft tissues, etc.

Expert opinions recommend not exceeding 6 to 12 hours since the identification of septic focus and its eradication in order to facilitate access to antibiotics and thus improve survival.

3.6 De-escalation and duration of antibiotics

Antibiotics started for sepsis should be reassessed daily for potential discontinuing if sepsis is ruled out or narrowing if more data becomes available [54]. While there is no consensus on de-escalation criteria, most experts use follow-up clinical (improved vital signs), laboratory and imaging data, and a fixed course of broad-spectrum therapy (eg, 3 to 5 days). After culture and susceptibility results return and/or after patients clinically improve, antimicrobial therapy may be narrowed to a few days. When possible, antimicrobial therapy should also be pathogen/susceptibility-directed. However, since no pathogen is identified (almost in 50% of patients), de-escalation of empiric therapy requires a component of clinical judgment. For example, vancomycin is typically discontinued, if no *Staphylococcus* is cultured.

Concerning the duration of antibiotic therapy, it must be reasoned and reassessed on a case-by-case basis. Often duration of 7 to 10 days is sufficient [55]. For certain cases, this duration must be prolonged up to even three weeks (mainly septicaemic presentations with metastatic locations (endocarditis, osteomyelitis, large abscess), a lack of clinical improvement within the usual timeframes, deep infections with *Candida* or *aspergillus,* some viral infections (Herpes or cytomegalovirus), isolation of extensively drug resistant (XDR) Gram-negative bacilli, immune disorders [56].

3.7 Role of procalcitonin

PCT appears to be a more relevant marker in diagnostic for bacterial infections. Its serum level increases in case of severe bacterial or parasitic infection with a sensitivity comparable to that of PCR but with better specificity. The importance of its serum level at the time of initial treatment would be also correlated with a subsequent poor prognosis of patients.

Although many institutions and guidelines support the use of procalcitonin to limit antibiotic (empiric or therapeutic) use in critically ill patients with suspected infection or documented infection, the evidence to support this practice is limited. Other studies suggest that procalcitonin may distinguish infectious from noninfectious conditions and may therefore facilitate the decision to de-escalate empiric therapy [57, 58].

In addition, studies of the kinetics of PCT were more interesting and useful than studies of a static value of unadjusted PCT. MDT is a favorable marker to assess changes in clinical symptoms and patient prognosis. MDT may improve the judgment of disease severity in patients with sepsis or septic shock, thereby improving the ability of clinicians to accurately assess disease prognosis [59]. Hence, we suggest that PCT be assessed daily or at default every 48 hours for critical septic patients.

4. Conclusions

For patients with sepsis, we opt to an optimal doses of empiric broad spectrum intravenous therapy with one or more antimicrobials be administered, in a prompt fashion (eg, within one hour) of clinical presentation. For patients with septic shock with likely gram negative sepsis we suggest combination therapy (at least two) from different classes given with the intent of covering a known or suspected pathogen with more than one antibiotic. It is the only guarantor for sufficient activity to cover a broad range of gram negative and positive organisms and, if suspected, against fungi and viruses. Agent selection depends upon patient's history, co morbidities, immune defects, clinical context, suspected site of infection, presence of invasive devices, and local prevalence and resistance patterns.

The advent of new technologies (multiplex-PCR) with the ability to type and characterize microorganisms without the need for conventional culture techniques may negate the requirement for highly specialized microbiology staff and facilities. These methods could eventually contribute significantly to improved management of patients with sepsis and septic shock as well as antibiotic stewardship programs.

Conflict of interest

The authors declare no conflict of interest.

Acronyms and abbreviations

APACHE	Acute Physiology and Chronic Health
ABG	Arterial blood gas
CVC	Central venous catheter
CVP	Central venous pressure
$ScvO_2$	Central venous saturation
CMS	Colimesthate sodium
CAP	Community Acquired Pneumonia
CSF	Cerebrospinal fluid
EAT	Empiric Antimicrobial Therapy
EIAD	Extended Interval Aminoglycoside Dosing

ESBL	Extended spectrum betalactamases
GNB	Gram negative bacilli
HCAP	Healthcare acquired pneumonia
HAP	Hospital acquired pneumonia
ICU	intensive care unit
IDSA	Infectious Diseases society of America
MAP	Mean arterial pressure
MV	Mechanical ventilation
MRSA	Methicillin-resistant *Staphylococcus aureus*
MIC	Minimum inhibitory concentration
MRI	magnetic resonance imaging
CPE	Carbapenemase-producing *Enterobacteriaceae*
MDR	Multi drug resistant
OR	Odds ratio
PCR	polymerase chain reaction
PD	peritoneal dialysis
PPV	Pulsed pression variation
RCT	Randomized controlled trial
SARS CoV2	severe acute respiratory syndrome coronavirus 2
VAP	Ventilator acquired pneumonia

Author details

Ahlem Trifi[1,2*], Sami Abdellatif[1,2], Sameh Trabelsi[2,3,4] and Salah Ben Lakhal[1,2]

1 Medical Intensive Care Unit, University Hospital Center La Rabta, Tunis, Tunisia

2 Faculty of Medicine, University Tunis El Manar, Tunis, Tunisia

3 Clinical Pharmacology Department at the National Chalbi Belkahia Center for Pharmacovigilance, Tunis, Tunisia

4 Research Laboratory on Clinical and Experimental Pharmacology (LR16SP02), Tunis, Tunisia

*Address all correspondence to: trifiahlem2@gmail.com

References

[1] Singer M, Deutschman CS, Seymour CW, Shankar-Hari M, Annane D, Bauer M, et al. The third international consensus definitions for sepsis and septic shock (Sepsis-3). JAMA. 2016;315(8):801-810. doi:10.1001/jama.2016.0287

[2] Elixhauser A, Friedman B, Stranges E. Septicemia in U.S. Hospitals, 2009. Agency for Healthcare Research and Quality, Rockville, MD. http://www.hcup-us.ahrq.gov/reports/statbriefs/sb122.pdf

[3] Rhee C, Dantes R, Epstein L, Murphy DJ, Seymour CW, Iwashyna TJ, et al. Incidence and Trends of Sepsis in US Hospitals Using Clinical vs Claims Data, 2009-2014. JAMA. 2017 ;3;318(13):1241-1249. doi: 10.1001/jama.2017.13836.

[4] Centers for Disease Control and Prevention. Antibiotic threats in the United States. 2019.

[5] Rhodes A, Evans LE, Alhazzani W, Levy MM, Antonelli M, Ferrer R, et al. Surviving Sepsis Campaign: International Guidelines for Management of Sepsis and Septic Shock: 2016. Intensive Care Med. 2017 Mar;43(3):304-377. doi: 10.1007/s00134-017-4683-6.

[6] Howell MD, Davis AM. Management of Sepsis and Septic Shock. JAMA 2017; 317:847.

[7] IDSA Sepsis Task Force. Infectious Diseases Society of America (IDSA) POSITION STATEMENT: Why IDSA Did Not Endorse the Surviving Sepsis Campaign Guidelines. Clin Infect Dis 2018;66:1631.

[8] Kumar A, Ellis P, Arabi Y, Roberts D, Light B, Parrillo JE, et al. Initiation of inappropriate antimicrobial therapy results in a fivefold reduction of survival in human septic shock. Chest 2009; 136:1237. doi: 10.1378/chest.09-0087.

[9] Ferrer R, Martin-Loeches I, Phillips G, Osborn TM, Townsend S, Dellinger RP, et al. Empiric antibiotic treatment reduces mortality in severe sepsis and septic shock from the first hour: Results from a guideline-based performance improvement program. Crit Care Med 2014; 42:1749. doi: 10.1097/CCM.0000000000000330.

[10] Whiles BB, Deis AS, Simpson SQ. Increased time to initial antimicrobial administration is associated with progression to septic shock in severe sepsis patients. Crit Care Med 2017; 45:623. doi: 10.1097/CCM.0000000000002262.

[11] Liu VX, Fielding-Singh V, Greene JD, Baker JM, Iwashyna TJ, Bhattacharya J, et al. The timing of early antibiotics and hospital mortality in sepsis. Am J Respir Crit Care Med 2017; 196:856. doi: 10.1164/rccm.201609-1848OC.

[12] Seymour CW, Gesten F, Prescott HC, Friedrich ME, Iwashyna TJ, Phillips GS,et al. Time to treatment and mortality during mandated emergency Care for Sepsis. N Engl J Med 2017; 376:2235. DOI: 10.1056/NEJMoa1703058

[13] Johnson MT, Reichley R, Hoppe-Bauer J, Dunne WM, Micek S, Kollef M.. Impact of previous antibiotic therapy on outcome of gram-negative severe sepsis. Crit Care Med 2011; 39:1859. doi: 10.1097/CCM.0b013e31821b85f4.

[14] Weinberger J, Rhee C, Klompas, M. Time-to-antibiotics in suspected sepsis. J Infect Dis **2020.** doi: 10.1093/infdis/jiaa146.

[15] Schmidt GA, Mandel J. Evaluation and management of suspected sepsis

and septic shock in adults. Updated: Mar, 2021

[16] Verhoef J, Hustinx WM, Frasa H, Hoepelman AI. Issues in the adjunct therapy of severe sepsis. J Antimicrob Chemother 1996; 38:167. doi: 10.1093/jac/38.2.167. PMID: 8877531.

[17] Septimus EJ, Coopersmith CM, Whittle J, Hale CP, Fishman NO, Kim TJ. Sepsis National Hospital Inpatient Quality Measure (SEP-1): Multistakeholder work group recommendations for appropriate antibiotics for the treatment of sepsis. Clin Infect Dis. 2017 ;16;65(9):1565-1569. doi: 10.1093/cid/cix603..

[18] De Waele JJ, Akova M, Antonelli M, Canton R, Carlet J, De Backer D, et al. Antimicrobial resistance and antibiotic stewardship programs in the ICU: Insistence and persistence in the fight against resistance. A position statement from ESICM/ESCMID/WAAAR round table on multi-drug resistance. Intensive Care Med 2018; 44:189. doi: 10.1007/s00134-017-5036-1.

[19] Savage RD, Fowler RA, Rishu AH, Bagshaw SM, Cook D, Dodek P, et al. Pathogens and antimicrobial susceptibility profiles in critically ill patients with bloodstream infections: a descriptive study. CMAJ Open 2016; 4:E569. doi: 10.9778/cmajo.20160074.

[20] WHO, **The burden of health care-associated infection worldwide** (2016) Available on line from: http://www.who.int/gpsc/country_work/burden_hcai/en/

[21] CDC. **Types of healthcare-associated infections. Healthcare-associated infections (HAIs)** (2016) Available online from: https://www.cdc.gov/HAI/infectionTypes.html

[22] Becker, K.; Heilmann, C.; Peters, G. Coagulase-negative staphylococci. Clin. Microbiol. Rev. 2014, 27, 870-926. doi: 10.1128/CMR.00109-13.

[23] Sakr A, Brégeon F, Mège JL, Rolain JM, Blin O. *Staphylococcus aureus* nasal colonization: An update on mechanisms, epidemiology, risk factors, and subsequent infections. Front Microbiol; 2018;9:2419. doi:10.3389/fmicb.2018.02419

[24] Safdar N, Handelsman J, Maki DG. Does combination antimicrobial therapy reduce mortality in gram-negative bacteraemia? A meta-analysis. Lancet Infect Dis 2004; 4:519. doi: 10.1016/S1473-3099(04)01108-9.

[25] V. Cattoir, Traitement des infections dues à entérobactéries productrices de carbapénèmases, Journal des Anti-infectieux, Volume 16, Issue 3, 2014, Pages 99-105, doi:10.1016/j.antinf.2014.07.002.

[26] Fournier PE, Richet H. The epidemiology and control of Acinetobacter baumannii in health care facilities. Clin Infect Dis 2006; 42:692. doi: 10.1086/500202.

[27] Lolans K, Rice TW, Munoz-Price LS, Quinn JP. Multicity outbreak of carbapenem-resistant Acinetobacter baumannii isolates producing the carbapenemase OXA-40. Antimicrob Agents Chemother. 2006;50(9):2941-2945. doi:10.1128/AAC.00116-06

[28] De Rosa FG, Corcione S, Pagani N, Di Perri G. From ESKAPE to ESCAPE, from KPC to CCC. Clin Infect Dis 2015; 60:1289. DOI: 10.1093/cid/ciu1170

[29] Teerawattanapong N, Panich P, Kulpokin D, Na Ranong S, Kongpakwattana K, Saksinanon A, et al. A systematic review of the burden of multidrug-resistant healthcare-associated infections among intensive care unit patients in Southeast Asia: The rise of multidrug-resistant Acinetobacter baumannii. Infect

Control Hosp Epidemiol 2018; 39:525. doi: 10.1017/ice.2018.58.

[30] Kanafani ZA, Zahreddine N, Tayyar R, Sfeir J, Araj GF, Matar GM, et al. Multi-drug resistant Acinetobacter species: A seven-year experience from a tertiary care center in Lebanon. Antimicrob Resist Infect Control 2018; 7:9. DOI: 10.1186/s13756-017-0297-6

[31] Vitkauskiene A, Dambrauskiene A, Cerniauskiene K, Rimdeika R, Sakalauskas R. Risk factors and outcomes in patients with carbapenem-resistant Acinetobacter infection. Scand J Infect Dis 2013; 45:213. doi: 10.3109/00365548.2012.724178.

[32] Karruli A, Boccia F, Gagliardi M, Patauner F, Ursi MP, Sommese P, et al. Multidrug-resistant infections and outcome of critically ill patients with coronavirus disease 2019: A single center experience. Microb Drug Resist 2021. doi: 10.1089/mdr.2020.0489.

[33] Trifi A, Abdellatif S, Abdennebi C Daly F, Nasri R, Touil Y, *et al.* Appropriateness of empiric antimicrobial therapy with imipenem/colistin in severe septic patients: Observational cohort study. Ann Clin Microbiol Antimicrob 17, 39 (2018). doi: 10.1186/s12941-018-0292-7.

[34] Durante-Mangoni E, Signoriello G, Andini R, Mattei A, De Cristoforo M, Murino P, et al. Colistin and rifampicin compared with colistin alone for the treatment of serious infections due to extensively drug-resistant Acinetobacter baumannii: A multicenter, randomized clinical trial. Clin Infect Dis 2013; 57:349. doi: 10.1093/cid/cit253

[35] Paul M, Daikos GL, Durante-Mangoni E, Yahav D, Carmeli Y, Benattar YD, et al. Colistin alone versus colistin plus meropenem for treatment of severe infections caused by carbapenem-resistant gram-negative bacteria: An open-label, randomised controlled trial. Lancet Infect Dis 2018; 18:391. doi: 10.1016/S1473-3099(18)30099-9.

[36] Kmeid JG, Youssef MM, Kanafani ZA, Kanj SS. Combination therapy for gram-negative bacteria: What is the evidence? Expert Rev Anti Infect Ther 2013; 11:1355. doi: 10.1586/14787210.2013.846215.

[37] Abdellatif S, Trifi A, Daly F, Mahjoub K, Nasri R, Ben Lakhal S. Efficacy and toxicity of aerosolised colistin in ventilator-associated pneumonia: A prospective, randomised trial. Ann Intensive Care 2016; 6:26. doi: 10.1186/s13613-016-0127-7.

[38] Zheng JY, Huang SS, Huang SH, Ye JJ. Colistin for pneumonia involving multidrug-resistant Acinetobacter calcoaceticus-Acinetobacter baumannii complex. J Microbiol Immunol Infect 2020; 53:854. doi: 10.1016/j.jmii.2019.08.007.

[39] Demirdal T, Sari US, Nemli SA. Is inhaled colistin beneficial in ventilator associated pneumonia or nosocomial pneumonia caused by Acinetobacter baumannii? Ann Clin Microbiol Antimicrob 2016; 15:11. doi: 10.1186/s12941-016-0123-7.

[40] Lu Q, Luo R, Bodin L, Yang J, Zahr N, Aubry A, et al. Efficacy of high-dose nebulized colistin in ventilator-associated pneumonia caused by multidrug-resistant Pseudomonas aeruginosa and Acinetobacter baumannii. Anesthesiology 2012; 117:1335. doi: 10.1097/ALN.0b013e31827515de.

[41] Cortegiani A, Russotto V, Maggiore A, Attanasio M, Naro AR, Raineri SM, et al. Antifungal agents for preventing fungal infections in non-neutropenic critically ill patients. Cochrane Database Syst Rev 2016;: CD004920. doi: 10.1002/14651858.CD004920.pub3.

[42] Bailly S, Bouadma L, Azoulay E, Orgeas MG, Adrie C, Souweine B, et al. Failure of empirical systemic antifungal therapy in mechanically ventilated critically ill patients. Am J Respir Crit Care Med 2015; 191:1139. doi: 10.1164/rccm.201409-1701OC.

[43] Timsit JF, Azoulay E, Schwebel C, Charles PE, Cornet M, Souweine B, et al. Empirical micafungin treatment and survival without invasive fungal infection in adults with ICU-acquired sepsis, Candida colonization, and multiple organ failure: The EMPIRICUS randomized Clinical trial. JAMA 2016; 316:1555. doi: 10.1001/jama.2016.14655.

[44] Trifi A, Abdellatif S, Daly F, Nasri R, Touil Y, Ben Lakhal S. Empiric antifungal and outcome in ICU patients. Tunis Med. 2019;97(4):579-587. PMID: 31729709.

[45] Donnelly JP, Chen CS, Kauffman CA, Steinbach WJ, Baddley JW, Verweij PE, et al. Revision and update of the consensus definitions of invasive fungal disease from the European Organization for Research and Treatment of cancer and the mycoses study group education and research consortium. Clinical Infectious Diseases. 2020;71(6):1367-1376, doi:10.1093/cid/ciz1008

[46] Pletz MW, Bloos F, Burkhardt O, Brunkhorst FM, Bode-Böger SM, Martens-Lobenhoffer J,et al. Pharmacokinetics of moxifloxacin in patients with severe sepsis or septic shock. Intensive Care Med 2010; 36:979. doi: 10.1007/s00134-010-1864-y.

[47] Blot S, Koulenti D, Akova M, Bassetti M, De Waele JJ, Dimopoulos G, et al. Does contemporary vancomycin dosing achieve therapeutic targets in a heterogeneous clinical cohort of critically ill patients? Data from the multinational DALI study. Crit Care 2014; 18:R99. doi: 10.1186/cc13874.

[48] Zelenitsky S, Rubinstein E, Ariano R, Iacovides H, Dodek P, Mirzanejad Y,et al. Vancomycin pharmacodynamics and survival in patients with methicillin-resistant Staphylococcus aureus-associated septic shock. Int J Antimicrob Agents 2013; 41:255. doi: 10.1016/j.ijantimicag.2012.10.015.

[49] Kashuba AD, Nafziger AN, Drusano GL, Bertino JS Jr. Optimizing aminoglycoside therapy for nosocomial pneumonia caused by gram-negative bacteria. Antimicrob Agents Chemother 1999; 43:623. DOI: 10.1128/AAC.43.3.623

[50] Roberts JA, Abdul-Aziz MH, Davis JS, Dulhunty JM, Cotta MO, Myburgh J, et al. Continuous versus intermittent β-lactam infusion in severe sepsis. A meta-analysis of individual patient data from randomized trials. Am J Respir Crit Care Med 2016; 194:681. doi: 10.1164/rccm.201601-0024OC.

[51] Chen CH, Chen YM, Chang YJ, Wang SH, Chang CY, Yen HC. Continuous versus intermittent infusions of antibiotics for the treatment of infectious diseases: Meta-analysis and systematic review. Medicine (Baltimore). 2019;98(10):e14632. doi:10.1097/MD.0000000000014632

[52] Plachouras D, Karvanen M, Friberg LE, et al. Population pharmacokinetic analysis of colistin methanesulfonate and colistin after intravenous administration in critically ill patients with infections caused by gram-negative bacteria. Antimicrob Agents Chemother 2009; 53:3430

[53] Dalfino L, Puntillo F, Mosca A, et al. High-dose, extended-interval colistin administration in critically ill patients: Is this the right dosing strategy? A preliminary study. Clin Inf Dis 2012; 54:1720

[54] Tabah A, Bassetti M, Kollef MH, Zahar JR, Paiva JA, Timsit JF, et al. Antimicrobial de-escalation in critically ill patients: A position statement from a task force of the European Society of Intensive Care Medicine (ESICM) and European Society of Clinical Microbiology and Infectious Diseases (ESCMID) critically ill patients study group (ESGCIP). Intensive Care Med 2020; 46:245. doi: 10.1007/s00134-019-05866-w.

[55] Kalil AC, Metersky ML, Klompas M, Muscedere J, Sweeney DA, Palmer LB, et al. Management of Adults with Hospital-acquired and Ventilator-associated Pneumonia: 2016 Clinical practice guidelines by the Infectious Diseases Society of America and the American Thoracic Society. Clin Infect Dis 2016; 63:e61. DOI: 10.1093/cid/ciw353

[56] Jack L, Bal AM, Harte S, Collier A. International guidelines: The need to standardize the management of candidaemia. Infect Dis (Lond) 2016; 48:779. doi: 10.1080/23744235.2016.1207251.

[57] Westwood M, Ramaekers B, Whiting P, Tomini F, Joore M, Armstrong N, et al. Procalcitonin testing to guide antibiotic therapy for the treatment of sepsis in intensive care settings and for suspected bacterial infection in emergency department settings: a systematic review and cost-effectiveness analysis. Health Technol Assess 2015; 19:v. doi: 10.3310/hta19960.

[58] Schuetz P, Kutz A, Grolimund E, Haubitz S, Demann D, Vögeli A, Hitz F, et al. Excluding infection through procalcitonin testing improves outcomes of congestive heart failure patients presenting with acute respiratory symptoms: Results from the randomized ProHOSP trial. Int J Cardiol 2014; 175:464. doi: 10.1016/j.ijcard.2014.06.022.

[59] Samsudin I, Vasikaran SD. Clinical Utility and Measurement of Procalcitonin. Clin Biochem Rev. 2017 Apr;38(2):59-68. PMID: 29332972; PMCID: PMC5759088.

Chapter 5

Specific Bacterial Immunotherapy in Treating Chronic Osteomyelitis

Ferdinando Da Rin de Lorenzo

Abstract

The immunological experience is treating osteomyelitis chronic forms at the Istituto Putti in Cortina starts in 1963 by introducing immunotherapy, applied by the progressive administration in growing doses of a staphylococci pool, that had been collected from some patients with bone infections by the same germ and then inactivated in an aqueous solution suspension. This therapy is coadjutant of antibiotics, surgical and hyperbaric therapy and not substitutive of these. This study ascertained indeed a reduction of the phagocytic activity as a whole, and especially the opsonisation activity It has been thought therefore that in immunotherapy more factors are involved; their principal property is to reduce the allergising effect and therefore to desensitise vs. the germ proteins and to increase the phagocytic activity. This condition, neither whose entity nor its lasting may be defined, does not appear to be unlimited. Obviously this desensitisation can be obtained also by the right antibiotic choice that, as already said mainly in acute forms, may develop their bactericidal properties and sterilise the focus. In the chronic forms it is possible to provoke this mechanism by carrying out a surgical toilette that restores the vascularization and stimulation conditions needed for a correct antibiotic action. Checks upon immuno-stimulation treatment termination clearly showed corresponding results between laboratory deficit corrected and clinical conditions bettering. The casuistry is based on 50 patients with hematogenic osteomyelitis, all under the age of 16, age at which the growth plate is still active, and 117 post-traumatic septic non-union, where this term was adopted for cases that showed a lack of non-solidification at 6 months after trauma. We have expressly made a distinction between hematogenic and post-traumatic forms, since the relationships between bacterial counts vs. host response do differ.

Keywords: immunotherapy, osteomyelitis, non union, psudoarthritis, vaccine

1. Introduction

The Codivilla-Putti Institutes has been a strong will of Prof. Vittorio Putti, especially for treating chronic infections; it started its activity in 1930 and had been located in a famous winter sport resort, as it was the case for almost all sanatoriums build in those years to treat septical diseases with "good air" and sun (UV rays), that were then the only therapeutic treatments available to the medical science.

We are now facing in modern therapeutic treatment of chronic osteomyelitis some growing obstacles in using antibiotics, as we find often resistance, principally concerning staphylococcus, which are the major responsible concerning bone infections. The clinician therefore has to dispose not only of surgical knowledge, but

1884	Leucotoxin	Van de Velde
1901	Anti-Staphylolysin	Neisser, Wechsberg
1925	Anti-Staphylococcus-Sera	Baker, Shands
1936	Anatoxin-Therapy	Ramon
1938	Exp. Allergic Osteomyelitis	Derizanov
1939	Autovaccination	Schoolfield
1953	Sensitisation and Osteomyelitis	Grundmann
1968	Opsonin Activity	Williams
1971	Prophylactic Immunisation	Weber
1972	Anti-Staphylolysin-titre	Queneau, Bertoye
1973	Anti-Nuclear Factors	Hierholzer
1973	Wound-Specific Antibodies	Ring, Seifert
1976	The Staphylococci	Cohen

Table 1.
Historical list of work on immunotherapy in osteomyelitis.

he has to be also acquainted with all most recent advances in the field of antibiotic therapies. Moreover, he has to be acquainted with the immunoresponses offered by the body in special circumstances. As a matter of fact the lack of success in such cases induced many scientists to re-evaluate the immunological system by considering its possible deficit.

An immunodeficiency may also show itself in the clinical picture as an increased tendency to chronicize, a reduced phlogistic reaction and an increased frequency of multifocal processes [1].

The use of the so-called "immunotherapy" started at the beginning of the 20th century and is still a field of investigation (**Table 1**) [1–3].

2. Definition of chronic

Chronic osteomyelitis as all forms of bone inflammatory lesions, sustained by pyogenic germs, who selectively involved from the start bone marrow and intra-trabecular spaces and therefore are not healing anyhow, as they brought about a suppuration process, but engender foci in the internal part of bones, who maintain themselves active or more or less weakened [4].

Chronicizing may be:

1. The consequence of initially acute osteomyelitis (hematogenous, post-traumatic, iatrogenous), that passes gradually into the chronic phase (reduced reaction by the patient owing to the symbiosis guest-host through a progressive reduction in acuteness;

2. Induced by rapid evolution from the acute form into the chronical form (it happens sometimes as an effect of the antibiotic's administration);

3. A chronic form "ab initio" without any initial acuteness or a generalisation of the process.

3. Characteristics of the Staphylococcus

Staphylococci are the most important micro-organisms in the Microccaceae family: they have been denominated by Ogston, as in microscopic slides their elements dispose themselves in clusters. They have a spherical form and are asporigenic and normally non-capsulated, gram-positive, aerobic and optionally anaerobic. It is easy to grow them on common culture media; optimal temperature is 37°C. They are among the most resistant germs to heating and disinfectants. With reference to the colony colours they are classed in aureus, albus, citreus and aurantiacus.

More recently they have been divided in aureus and epidermidis, as the former produces coagulasis and is able to ferment mannitol in anaerobic conditions. By phagic typisation 4 groups have been ascertained, whose major representatives in chronic bone pathologies are type 5 and type 8 [5].

Staphylococcus produces many extracellular substances that show almost all antigenic properties. The most interesting is coagulase that fosters a fibrin barrier around the staphylococcus that might oppose the action of phagocytes and opsonins [6].

It can also induce in the host a form of "allergy" that further reduces his defences [2–4]. It seems moreover that the bacterial resistance develops proportionally to its capacity to produce para-aminobenzoic acid, necessary to its metabolism, or producing its precursor folic acid. It is supposed that para-aminobenzensulfonamide displaces para-aminobenzoic acid from the bacterial body, i.e. owing to the antibiotic action the bacterial bodies may lose their strong cellular wall transforming themselves in sferoblasts with a weakened antigenic function or without any antigenic function, who are responsible for some infections with a chronic evolution.

4. Some immunological information

Before discussing this point some general knowledge concerning immunology is required. We do not refer to immunology as a whole (as the matter covers very wide aspects), but only to infection resistance.

The host defence to bacterial infections happens through two classical mechanisms, i.e.:

a. natural **non-specific** immunoresistance (humoral and cellular factors mainly related to phagocyte reactions) [7].

b. acquired **specific** immunity (specific antibodies production and Ag-Ab reaction).

We shall mainly focus on the **former** mechanism, as its deficiency is considered as the major cause of chronic septical forms; it is the fastest and it arises through humoral and cellular factors (in order to summarise we shall treat the matter in very schematic terms).

Humoral factors may be divided principally in three species.

- **The complement (C)** (a biological entity showing itself through the concomitant action of several constituents, some of which are thermolabile) comprehends a group of known substances, that are present in fresh serum and able to interact, in clearly defined sequence, with all possible kind of Ag-Ab combination.

The **C** does not show any antibody activity and there is no evidence that its blood levels increase as a consequence of immunisation processes. It has been however evidenced (Lopow, Beker) that at least some C components have enzymatic activity against the bacterial cellular walls, that therefore are opsonised and become weaker to the phagocyte action.

- **The bacteriocidines** are produced mainly by leukocytes and in their majority thermostable. They are principally active against Gram+.

- **Lysozime** is an enzyme discovered by Fleming in 1922 and it has been confirmed in many body fluids and tissues and in the internal parts of neutrophile granulocytes. It is constituted by a protein that should be able to depolymerise some polysaccharides contained in many bacterial species. Moreover it should stimulate: phagocytosis, bacterial suspensions agglutinations (Ferrina), phlogistic processes inhibition (Matracia).

- **Opsonins** [8] act on micro-organisms by making them easier to be phagocitated. Generally neutrophyles are able to phagocytate aggressive micro-organisms only after a specific Opsonin has covered (opsonisation) the micro-organisms. Their action fosters also the elimination of micro-organisms from blood by means of the reticuloendothelial system.
  As far as the non-specific cellular immunity is concerned, it is mainly related to phagocytosis, i.e. the capacity showed by some cells to take up corpuscular matter of different nature and origin; the cells are part of the so-called reticulohistocytic system (R.H.S).
  Metchnikoff considers that cells with the capability to phagocitate are essentially:

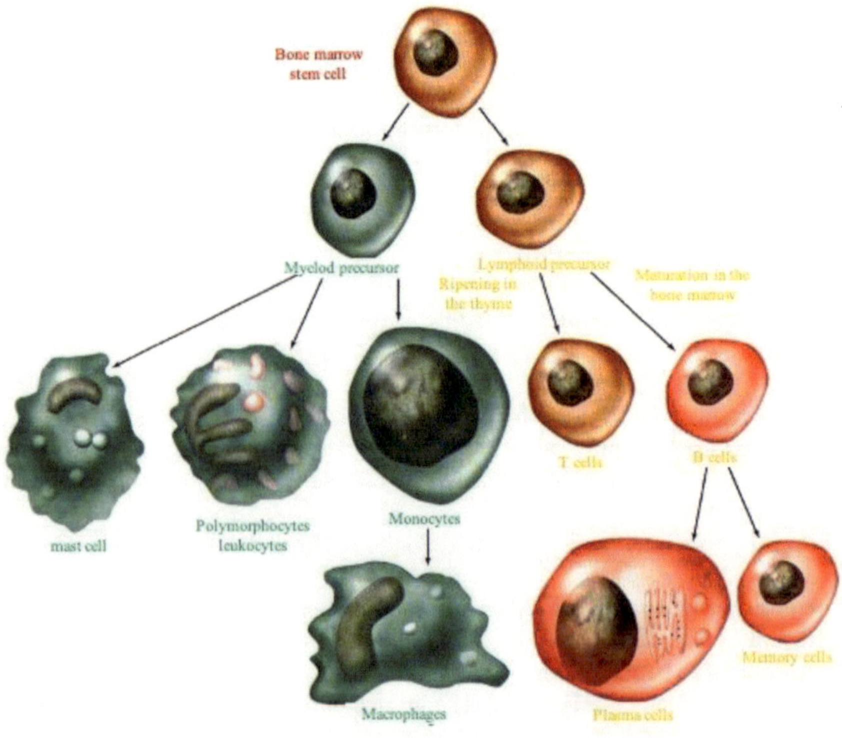

Figure 1.
Genesis of the immunolgical cells.

- **The macrophages** [9], classed in fixed and mobile, are the reticular cells in the spleen and in the lymphonodules and the Küpfer cells in the liver, the fixed osteoclasts and the histiocytes, which pass from the tissues into circulation (mobile) (see macrophages origin in **Figure 1**).

- **Microphages** are represented by the blood polymorphonucleic leukocytes, essentially by neutrophyles.

With reference to **specific activity** brought about by the production of most often Permanent Ab, it does not seem that staphylococci infections have such characteristics. A study by Ring shows indeed that only 26 cases on 112 have an increased antistaphylolysinic level.

It has been observed that the staphylococci pathogenicity appears on one side as an increased resistance to the defensive powers of the patient and on the other side as a capacity to establish a kind of allergy that further reduces body defences. The production of toxins might have only a minor role in the pathogenicity (Zironi) [2]; as a matter of fact there is no parallelism between germ virulence and the seriousness of the illness. It has been observed that the two factors provoking allergy (hypersensitivity against the germ or its products and increased reaction capacity) do not always evolve in parallel but may show different evolution.

Sensitivity to the micro-organism and its antigens, without variation of the host reactivity may beobserved and such a mechanism induces a very dangerous condition, called by immunologists "specific hyperreceptivity". Such a mechanism could account as an explication how this state may grow by inappropriate use of antibiotics.

Insufficient immunitary system predisposition to the entrance of the germ inadequate microbial sterilisation (inappropriate antibiotics – dosage – choice) bacterial persistence, even only latent stimulation repeated in the time hyper-receptivity (**Figure 2**).

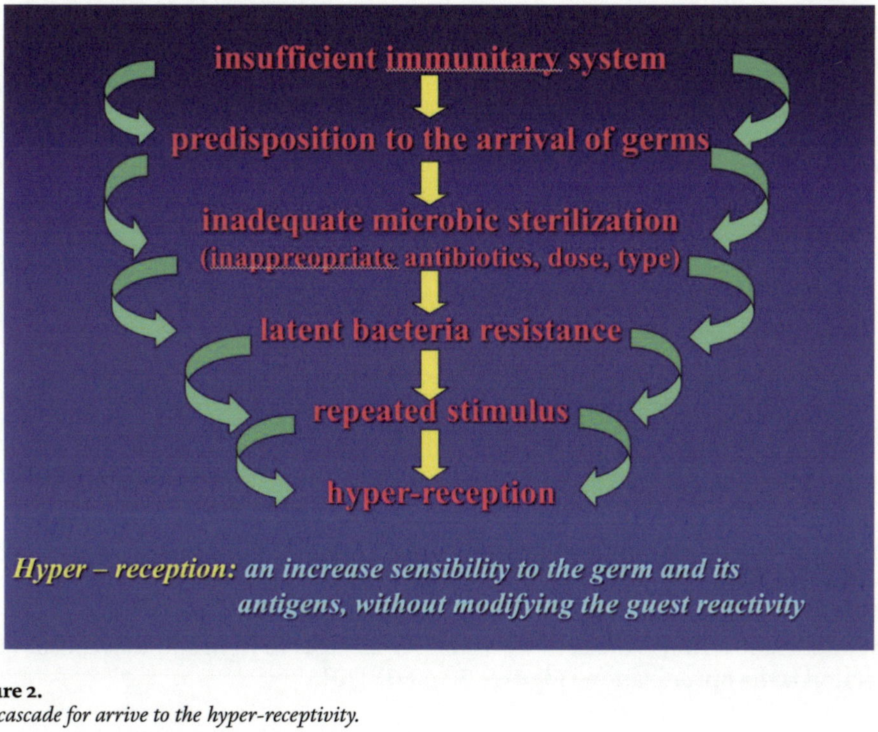

Figure 2.
The cascade for arrive to the hyper-receptivity.

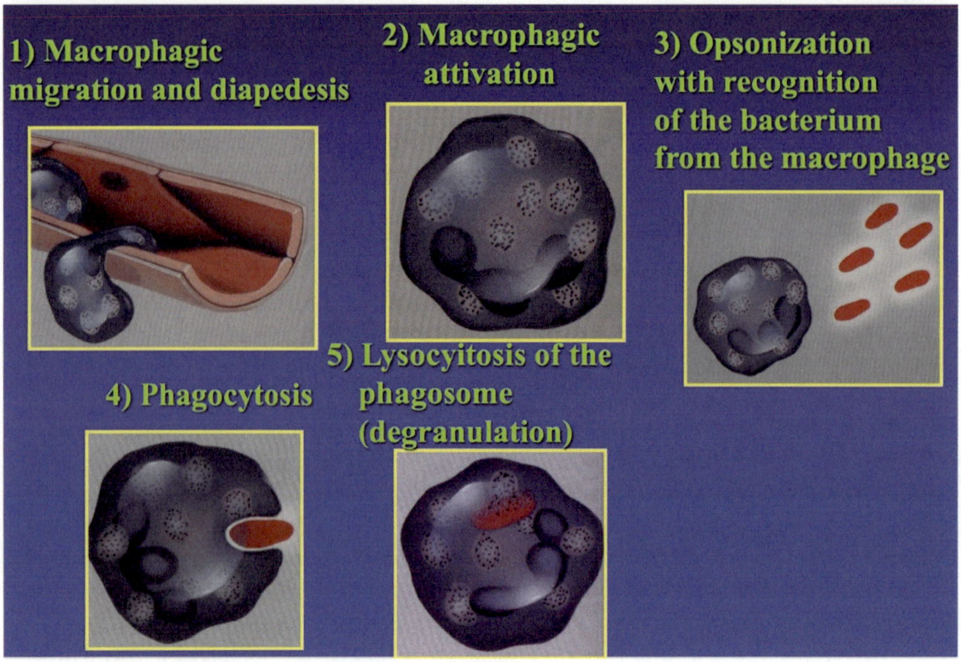

Figure 3.
Summary opsonization-phagocytosis of the "macrophages".

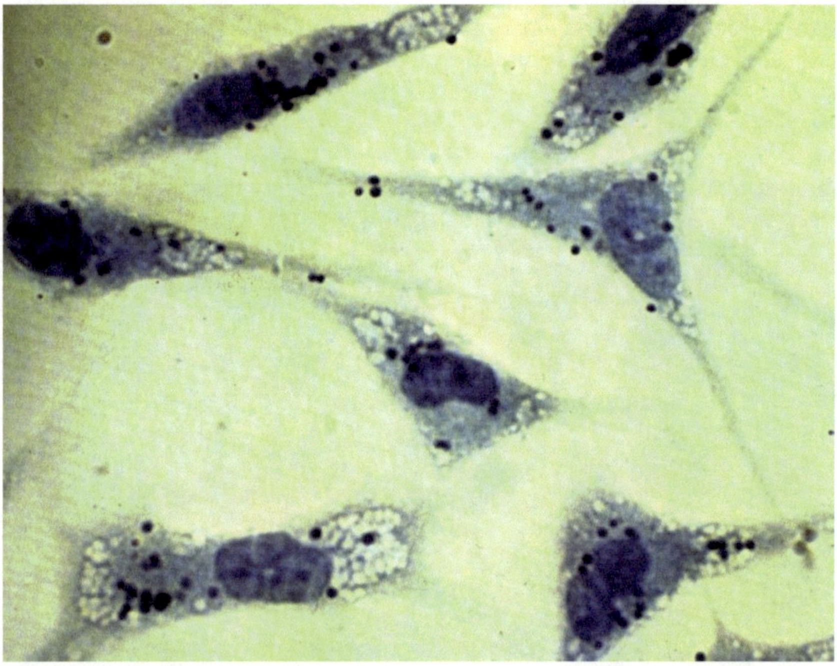

Figure 4.
Phagocytosis of the staphylococci from "macrophagis".

We have many actions in the aspecific immunological activity but one of the most important action is the activity of the Macrofages to fight staphylococcus and the action is the opsonization (**Figures 3** and **4**) [10].

5. Specific bacterial immunotherapy (S.B.I.T)

The immunological experience is treating osteomyelitis chronic forms at the Istituto Putti in Cortina starts in 1963 [11–13] by introducing immunotherapy, applied by the progressive administration in growing doses of a staphylococci pool, that had been collected from some patients with bone infections by the same germ and then inactivated in an aqueous solution suspension. At that time also autologous immunostimulation was carried out, i.e. a therapy prepared by isolating the responsible bacterial agent directly in the patient's exudate.

Also experiences with a *Pseudomonas aeruginosa* autologous immunotherapy have been carried out, but we abandoned it, as we saw that this bacterium wasn't the principal pathogenic agent, which provoked bone infections.

Nowadays only the isolation of Staphylococcus strains 5 and 8 is carried out, as only these strains are responsible for 98% of the bone infections. This aspect has been showed by a joint research with Institut Pasteur in Paris. We are working now only with these kinds of staphylococci and were able to better the general characteristics.

As already mentioned, administration is performed at growing dosages according to patterns adopted since long avoiding that too approached stimulation may exhaust the capacity responses as a consequence of a too prolonged stress.

The preparation is inoculated subcutaneously, and the therapy lasts about three months. After at least one month stop treatment may be repeated (**Figure 5**).

With reference to the above said we tried, together with "Immuno" in Vienna, to find out whether among chronic osteomyelitis patients there was some immunological deficit. We did not consider this evaluation had to be made on acute forms, as they show different characteristics while the host reactivity is still within the norm.

We evaluated therefore about 150 cases, with different ages and causes (hematogenic, post-traumatical and iatrogenous) and referred to following parameters:

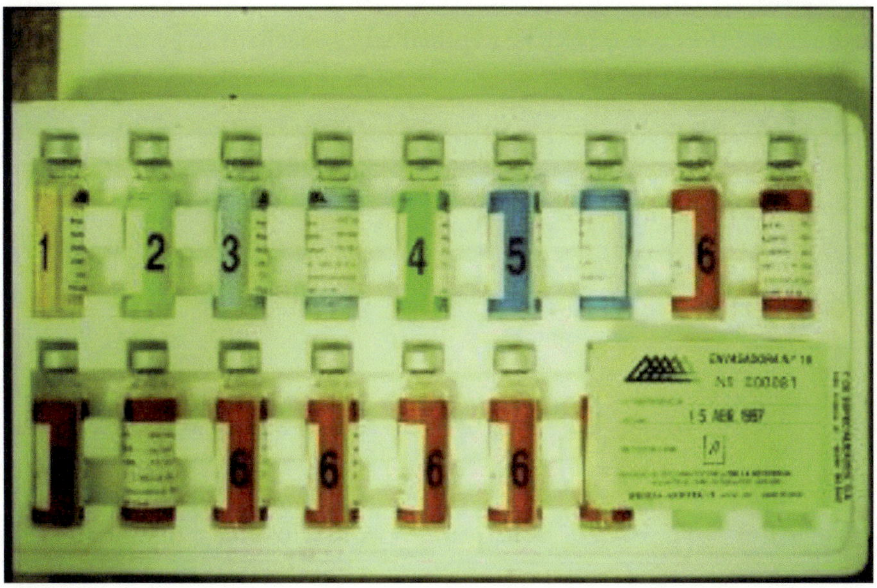

Figure 5.
Increasing subcutaneous injections of doses, according to a widely scheme (since 1963) of an inactivated staphylococci pool of type 5 and 8.

- Antibody titre
- Complement (fraction 3)
- Phagocytic activity
- Opsonisation capacity
- Bactericidal reaction
- Bacterial agglutinins
- "T" lymphocyte count

This study ascertained indeed a reduction of the phagocytic activity as a whole, and especially the opsonisation activity.

• Opsonisation capacity deficit	62%
• Antibody activity deficit	34%
• "T" lymphocytes decrease	4%

It has been thought therefore that in immunotherapy more factors are involved; their principal property is to reduce the allergising effect and therefore to desensitise vs. the germ proteins and to increase the phagocytic activity.

This condition, neither whose entity nor its lasting may be defined, does not appear to be unlimited.

Obviously, this desensitisation can be obtained also by the right antibiotic choice that, as already said mainly in acute forms, may develop their bactericidal properties and sterilise the focus.

In the chronic forms it is possible to provoke this mechanism by carrying out a surgical toilette that restores the vascularization and stimulation conditions needed for a correct antibiotic action.

Checks upon immuno-stimulation treatment termination clearly showed corresponding results between laboratory deficit clinical conditions bettering laboratory bettering.

6. Laboratory

Parameters normalisation	35%
Minor increases	34%
No variations	25%

7. Clinical

Good	50%
Reduced	28%
Bad	22%

Patients	Phagocytosis*		LIF**
	PMN	Monocyte	
19 Non-responders	60.6 ± 19.1^	52.6 ± 11.7^	30.5 ± 9.3^
3 responders	87.0 ± 3.2	87.6 ± 5.3	54.3 ± 12.4
40 (controllo)	86.9 ± 4.45	87.1 ± 4.2	48.3 ± 6.9

Table 2.
*The phagocytosis: Is valued as percentage of cells that englobe the specific Bacterias. *Description of the study.*

Patients	Phagocytosis*					
	PMN		Monocyte		LIF**	
	Before	After	Before	After	Before	After
19 Non-responders	65.7 ± 19.1	72.4 ± 12.4	30.6 ± 8.9	70.4 ± 8.9	25.8 ± 8.1	30.6 ± 8.9
3 Responders	87.0 ± 3.1	85.3 ± 6.1	87.3 ± 5.3	85.2 ± 4.7	54.3 ± 12.4	60.3 ± 11.2

Table 3.
*The valuation was repeated after the sominiстration of S.B.I.T and the results were significant, as you can see on the table, between the beginning and the end of treatment. *The results.*

8. Another immunological evaluation in the use of S.B.I.T

Dr. G. Mastrorillo Work Bari's School (**Tables 2** and **3**) [14].

- LIF: inhibition of the leucocytic migration in percentage
- ^: Relevant statistic values

This work considers the immunological effects of S.B.I.T.

In 22 patients with chronic osteomyelitis with a follow up of 20 months the Authors valued:

- The phagocytosis of polymorphonucleate and monocytes versus some bacteria that were identified in at least two samples on three.
- The dosage of LIF (inhibition of the leukocytes migration in percentage).

The patients were divided in two categories and compared with 40 volunteers.

The responders (3) who had almost normal parameters.

The non responders (19) who were immuno-compromised.

From this valuation, we understand that in chronic osteomyelitis there is unimportant immunological compromise.

9. Clinical effect with the S.B.I.T. treatment

We clinically evaluated the results obtained by using immunotherapy and we observed different facts recorded on about 7,500 cases treated since 1963 till 2016.

- Spontaneous elimination of sequestra,
- Demarcation or resorption,
- Output colour change,
- Trend to fistula healing,
- Reduction of congestive facts,
- Less frequent reacutisation,
- Reduced articular rigidity,
- Stimulation of bone reparation,
- Reduction of soft tissues calcification.

Some of these effects (sequestrum resorption or demarcation, reduced articular rigidity, increased repairing capacity) may be explained only by hypothesising a stimulating action on the reticuloendothelial cells that are able to differentiate themselves in different tissues [9].

We studied also possible differences between children, known for their evolutive receptive potentiality, and adults leaving the kind pf suffered infection out of consideration.

10. Result

The results on 100 adults and 100 children have been compared by referring to following parameters:

100 adults	♂:90	♀:10
100 children	♂:80	♀:20

11. Form

	Children	Adults
Hematogen	66	19
Post-traumatic	30	40
Iatrogenic	4	4

12. Stabilisation

Time	Children	Adults
1–6 months	36	15
6–12 months	30	26

Time	Children	Adults
> 1 year	31	37
Non attained	3	22

13. Healing

	Children	Adults
Obtained	90	73
Not obtained	10	27

Whereas healed are the patients who do not show any restart at least after 1 year from stabilisation, stabilised are those, who do not show any clinical, radiographic or bio-humoral sign of inflammation. As however chronic infections may show restarts, even after more than 1 year from stabilisation, the word "healing" has been adopted by us only to quantitize the research results and we have to evidence that it is more a language term than a truth, as it is well known to our colleagues who deal with these pathologies [15].

Another study has been made by us in order to define the Immunotherapy potentiality concerning both hematogenic and post-traumatic forms.

14. The casuistry

The casuistic is based on 50 patients with hematogenous osteomyelitis, all less than 16 years old, age at which the growth cartilage knit, and 117 post-traumatic infective pseudoarthroses, where this term has been adopted for cases who showed a lack of non-solidification at 6 months after trauma.

We expressly made a distinction between hematogenic and post-traumatic forms, as the relations bacterial count vs. host response do differ. Let us first consider the hematogenic form with all patients infected by coagulase positive *Staphylococcus aureus*.

Males were infected most often (78%); the prevailing age were between 10 and 16 years old.

Lower limbs were involved three times more than arms, while there was no difference between proximal diaphyseal and distal diaphyseal localisation. In 30% of cases the lesion involved the whole bone segment (panostytis), while the remaining 70% showed a localisation at the diaphysis half (42%) or at the diaphysis (28%).

In males diffused forms are more frequent, while in females the same applies to localised forms.

Patients have been checked with a following-up lasting from 1 till 10 years after healing (where healing has already been defined).

With the depicted criteria we obtained 86% of healing (88.5% when considering localisation), of which 74% already from the first treatment, and only 12% after possible recurrences. Of these relapses only the half involved a bone, while in the other cases they were the periodical opening of abscesses and fistulae, without any bone involvement. 50% of the patients healed by adopting only immunotherapy; in 38% immunotherapy complemented a surgical intervention, and remaining 11.5% did not heal.

As far as time elapsed from treatment beginning till healing is concerned, we observed 46% healing within 6 months, 30% between 6 months and 1 year, and 24% between 1 and 5 years with an average duration of 9.6 months.

With reference to radiographic belated evidences 20 patients showed the damaged bone segments fully leaked, whereas in later checks 33 patients showed a bone rearrangement (residual osteosclerosis without periostal reaction or osteolytic area).

In 7 cases there were still traces of active infection.

In 3 cases the later checks showed growth disturbs higher than 2.5 cm (in 2 cases there had been a contraction owing to growth cartilage lesions and in 1 case there was a lengthening). In 5 further cases, that initially showed limb lengthening, such dysmetrias disappeared afterwards.

In 5 cases the later checks showed a limitation in movements concerning the articulation near the focus; in 4 cases such limitation was already ascertained at the first control and imputable to the treatment with plaster. The joint limitation has never been imputable to joint involvement by the inflammation process (osteoarthritis).

In 3 cases there were deformities of the bone segments (coxa varia, femur procurvation).

We discuss now the data concerning the 147 cases of post-traumatic infective pseudoarthrosis.

The higher percentage of 75.5% concerns pseudoarthrosis subsequent to osteosynthesis.

In this percentage there were 118 males (83.3%) and 29 female patients (19.7%). Mean age has been 32 years and 5 months; the youngest patient was 18 years old, whereas the oldest was 68 years old. The most frequently interested bone has been the shinbone with 99 cases and secondarily the femur with 35 cases.

25 cases were a two bone fractures and there were exactly 19 tibia and fibula and 6 radius and ulna fractures.

We had 7 cases concerning radius and ulna, 3 cases collar bone, 1 case humerus and 1 case hand. The time elapsed between trauma and infection beginning has been in the male 30 days with 7 days in the shortest case and 5 months in the most belated.

The tome between infection initial and our therapy start has been on an average 8 months, varying from minimal 6 months till maximal 4 years. Our treatment allowed almost always precocious weight bearing; as a matter of fact only the most serious cases had to wait 6 months before being in condition to use the sick limb.

At first hospitalisation already 89.1% of the patients showed a fistula.

In all cases therapy has been immunotherapy+antibioticotherapy. In 11 cases immunotherapy has been repeated and in 5 cases it has been administered 3 times.

We carried out 98 surgical toilets and sequestrectomies, of which 22 cases were more than once. In 4 cases we carried out Paltrinieri parafocal osteotomy (all tibial). In 45 cases the Ilizarof system has been adopted with resection of the focus and compactotomy. We had to amputate only in 1 case. Solidification rimes vary according to the involved bone. On the tibiae they vary from at least 3 till maximal 36 months, on average 9.9 months.

More frequently (76.8% of cases) healing was attained within 1 year from therapy start, 26 cases (equalling 26%) did not attain solidification, of which 18 cases are still under treatment.

Very similar times have been observed on femurs, from 3 till 35 months with 9.2 months average duration.

Also for the femur the 84% of cases heals after 12 months therapy, whereas the non consolidated cases are 10 equalling 28.6%, of which 6 cases are still under treatment.

The forearm does not show substantial differences concerning ulna and radius; the same results indeed have been obtained for both bone segments; in 2 cases on 7 we observed a lack of solidification with bone material loss/this happened in the pre-microsurgical period of our experience).

Fistulae closed fairly fast 6 months in 53.48 of cases. The main check control has been 15 months, varying from 4 months at least up to 7 years.

Belated consequences have been:

Articular rigidity. Patients who have been treated with immunotherapy and submitted to plaster casts, both cylinder or valve casts, and precocious walking showed significant articular functional limitations only in 26 cases, equalling 17.6%. 14 cases concerned the talocrural articulation, 8 cases the knee and 4 cases on 7 concerned the elbow.

Shortenings have been significant (more than 4 cm) only in 2% of cases, whereas there have been 30.5% with less than 4 cm. In the whole 102 cases showed shortenings, that were compatible with a good functionality of the sick limb with good walking.

Axial deviations appeared in 18.3% of cases: 15 cases in varus dislocation, 12 in valgus dislocation, 17 in recordation and 10 in procurvation. Calcification of soft parts have been only 3.4%, whereas they were very frequent before systematically introducing immunotherapy.

Relapses concern 26.5% of our patients, i.e. about 39 cases. In 15 cases (10.2%) it was a simple reopening of the fistula that healed soon, in 13 cases the restart of the infective focus was associated with a new relaxation of the fracture. Afterwards 9 cases healed and these have been the precocious relapses (within 1 year from healing), the belated ones have been 11 cases (7.5%) with 10 healings.

15. Final considerations of the results

The efficacy of immunotherapy is certainly higher in children, as it is confirmed by a lower number of surgical interventions and by the stabilisation and healing results. *We analysed 50 cases of hematogenous osteomyelitis in order to consider which factors might have influenced the prognoses.*

1. No negative influences have been brought about by age.

2. The same applied to sex, though males showed major lesions. Daoud and Martin consider the female sex a favourable prognostic factor.

3. Prognoses are more difficult in cases with lesions, that are localised on the femur (21% without healing, whereas these reduce themselves to 5–6% in other localisation).

4. Also the extension (pandiaphysis) and the deep localisation (diaphysis) of the infection adversely influence the illness evolution.

5. Finally the prognoses is very sensible to the lesion chronicity. As a matter of fact the healing frequency is adversely proportional to the lesion duration (94%, 77%, 36%, 5%). The failures have been observed only with symptoms

that has been lasted more than 1 year. Immunotherapy has to be started as soon as possible.

Another analysis with similar considerations has been made by us on 147 cases of infected pseudoarthrose:

1. Healing is significantly influenced by the fistula healing. As a matter of fact we found 86% healing when fistula closes within 6 months. Healing frequency is lower when fistula has staid open for longer times.

2. the contrary recovery is not influenced by time elapsed from trauma till infection beginning.

3. Presence of a fistula upon hospitalisation did not affect healing.

4. Very important has been time elapsed from infection beginning and immunological treatment. With times less than 6 months recoveries show satisfactory percentages that reduce themselves to 50.6% when elapsed times are more than 1 year.

5. Localisation influences results. Whereas hands recover soon, times are on an average when tibiae are involved to become long lasting on femurs.

6. Male patients are more frequent than women (118 cases vs. 29 cases).

16. Conclusions

By comparing the results obtained in chronic osteomyelitis (both hematogenous and post-traumatic) before introducing immunotherapy and reconsidered afterwards, after having acquired a long experience in its administration, we feel following conclusions have to be drawn.

1. Immunotherapy (eventually associated to surgical therapy) ensures high recovery percentages (among the lightest mentioned in the scientific literature) [16–22].

2. Such therapy notably reduces recurrences (12% instead of 40% mentioned in the literature), as it fosters natural defences.

3. Immunological therapy is somewhat more efficacious (and certainly less toxic) than antibioticotherapy. The two approaches have to be associated, as immunotherapy does not substitute antibioticotherapy (only 15% of patients affected by chronic osteomyelitis fully recover by administering only antibiotics).

4. Immunotherapy remarkably reduced surgical interventions.

We may conclude that Specific Bacterial Immunotherapy (S.B.I.T.) has to be considered an important defence, that does not exclude, but has to be associated to antibiotico therapy and even more to surgery. The obtained positive results shall be studied with complex research methods, as the concept “immunity messenger” opens therapeutical approaches, still difficult to evaluate.

17. Some cases

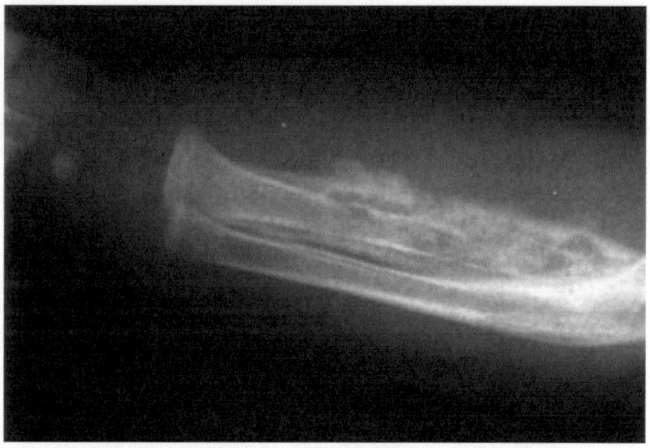

A case of hemathogenous osteomyelitis of radio in the young patient, 3 year old treated with only S.B.I.T (doses reduction) and antibiotics of course.

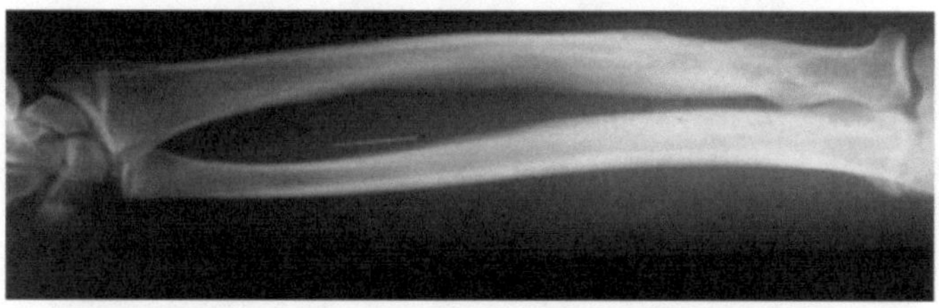

X-ray control after 13 years. Completed reconstruction of the bone. The infection health after 6 months of treatement with immunotherapy and antibiotics.

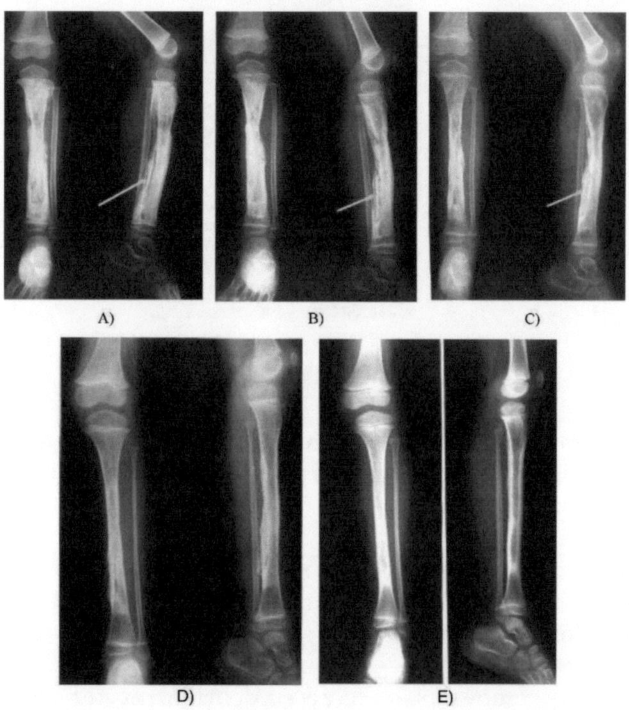

a. Heavy hematogenic pandiaphysitis in a 10 years old child, who has been treated only with S.B.I.T. according to a reduced therapeutical scheme.

b. After 2 months of treatment the whole diaphysis partially recovers there are still sequestrum of wich one is postero cortical. Fistulae closed.

c. After 2 months reabitation of big sequestrum. (The arrow indicates bone sequestrum and its revitalization)

d. Rx control after 15 months after the beginning of the treatment

e. Rx control one year after the previous one, please note the complete reconstruction of the bones of the leg, absence of flogosi markers (clinical and laboratory)

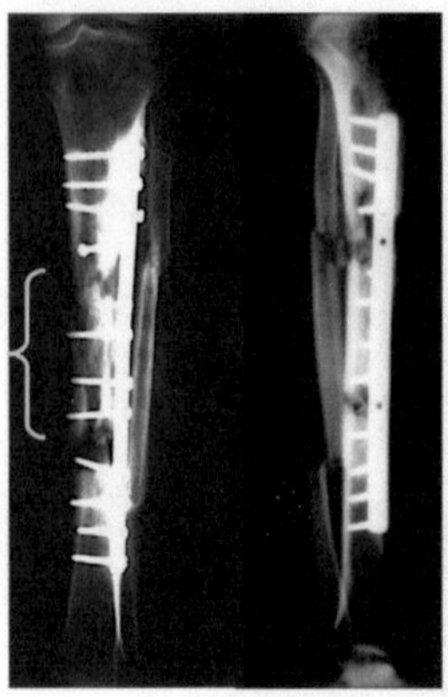

A)

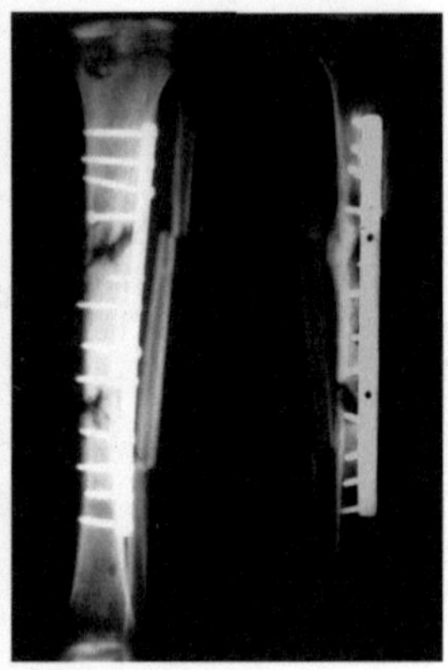

B)

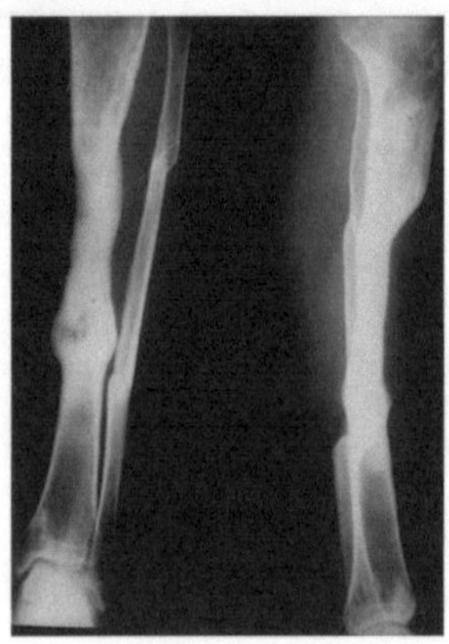

C)

a. 45 years old man after an open fracture of the leg. Arrived to our hospital after 12 months; he had two fistulae and two focuses of non union and a wide sequestrum was presented.

b. Rx control after 3 months of treatment with S.B.I.T. and you can see the reabitation of the central sequestrum and the beginning of callification on the two focuses (of non union

c. Rx control after removal plate, screw e a debridment and 3 months in plaster.

Author details

Ferdinando Da Rin de Lorenzo
National Center of Reference for the Bone Infections, Codivilla-Putti Institutes, Cortina d'Ampezzo, Italy

*Address all correspondence to: darin.ferdinando@iol.it

References

[1] Eisen H. Immunologia. Piccin Editore, Padova 1977 Stookey P.F., Scarpellino L.a., Weavar J.B.: Immunology of osteomyelitis. Arch. Surg., 32, 494-505, 1935.

[2] Zironi A.: L'allergia nelle malattie infettive – Es. Ist. Sier. Milanese – Milano – 1951.)

[3] Meloni C. A.: Nozioni di Microbiologia. Libreria Cortina Ed., Padova, 1970.

[4] Sorice F., Ortona L.: L'infezione Stafilococcica. – Ed. Scient. It. – Napoli – 1955.

[5] Fournier J.M., K. Hannon, M. Moreau, W. W. Karakawa, and W. F. Vann. 1987. Isolation of type 5 capsular polysaccharide from Staphylococcus aureus. Ann. Inst. Pasteur Microbiol. 138:561-567.

[6] Tager M., Drumond M. C. Staphylocoagulase; Ann. N. Y. Acad. Sci.; 1965, 128, 92.

[7] Savoini E., Capanna R., Gherlinzoni F.: Immunità umorale ed osteomielite cronica. COM, 66 (4), 511-515, 1980.

[8] Pozzi C, Wilk K, Lee JC, Gening M, Nifantiev N, Pier GB. Source Channing Laboratory, Department of Medicine, Brigham and Women's Hospital, Harvard Medical School, Boston, Massachusetts, USA. Opsonic and protective properties of antibodies raised to conjugate vaccines targeting six Staphylococcus aureus antigens. PLoS One. 2012;7(10):e46648. doi:10.1371/journal.pone.0046648. Epub 2012 Oct 15.

[9] Snyderman R., Mergenhagen S.: Chemotaxis of macrofages – in Nelson DS (Ed) – Immunobiology of the Macrofage – New York Accademic press p. 323 – 1976.

[10] S. Giedrys-Galant; J. Halasa Phagocytosis and Intracellular Killing of Various Strains of *Staphylococcus aureus* in Rabbits Immunized by aureus Smith Dep of Microbiology and Immunology Pomeranian Medical Academy, Szczecin, Poland. Janusz Jeljaszewicz (Ed.). The Staphylococci, Zbl. Bakt. Suppl. 14 Gustav Fischer Verlag * Stuttgart * New York * 1985

[11] Savoini E., L'autovaccino Antistafilococcico Nella Cura Della Osteomielite Ematogena Cronica, Clin. Ortop. Vol. XVII magg.-giu, 1965 Fasc. III.

[12] Savoini E., Capanna R., Mercuri M., Stilli S.: Risultati nel trattamento immunoterapico e chirurgico nelle osteomieliti croniche dell'infanzia. COM, 67 (4), 397-404, 1981.

[13] Ciotti M., Argazzi M., Bergami P.L.: La vaccinoterapia nell'osteomelite cronica. Atti S.E.R.T.O.T., Vol. XXXIV – Fasc. 2, 1992.

[14] Mastrorillo G., Minoia L., Jirillo E., De Vito D.: "Il vaccino autogeno antistafilococcico, trattamento delle osteomieliti croniche: basi scientifiche". Quad. Inf. Osteoart. Apr. 2001, 23-30 Ed. Masson

[15] Morrey B.F.: Hematogenus osteomyelitis at uncommon sites in children. Mayo Clin. Proc. 53: 707, 1978.

[16] Halasa J., Giedrys-Galant S., Podkowinska I., Braun J., Strzelecka G. and Dabrowski W.: Evaluation of certain immunological parameters in the course of autovaccine treatement in patients with chronic ostitis and carbunculosis. Arch. Immunol. Ter. Exp. 26: 589-593, 1978.

[17] Fattom A., Schneerson R., C. Szu S., F. Vann W. Shiloach J., W. Karakawa W. and Robbins J.B.: Synthesis and

Immunologic properties in mice of vaccines composed of *Staphylococcus aureus* type 5 and type 8 capsular polysaccharides conjugated to *Pseudomonas aeruginosa* exotoxin A. Infection and Immunity July 1990, p. 2367-2374.

[18] Ing-Marie Nilsson,* Joseph M. Patti,‡ Tomas Bremell,* Magnus Höök,‡ and Andrzej Tarkowski* Department of Rheumatology, University of Göteborg, Sweden; Center for Extracellular Matrix Biology, Institute of Biosciences and Technology, Texas a&M University, Houston, Texas 77030 vaccination with a recombinant fragment of collagen Adhesin provides protection against Staphylococcus aureus-mediated septic death. The American society for clinical investigation, Inc. Volume 101, Number 12, June 1998, 2640-2649

[19] Foster TJ. Potential for vaccination against infections caused by Staphylococcus aureus. Vaccine. 1991 Apr;9(4):221-227.

[20] Nilsson IM, Verdrengh M, Ulrich RG, Bavari S, Tarkowski A. Source Department of Rheumatology, S-41346 Göteborg, Sweden. Ing-Marie. Nilsson@immuno.gu.se protection against Staphylococcus aureus sepsis by vaccination with recombinant staphylococcal enterotoxin a devoid of superantigenicity. Department of Rheumatology, S-41346 Göteborg, Sweden. Ing-Marie. J Infect Dis. 1999 Oct;180(4):1370-1373.

[21] Bagnoli, F., Bertholet, S., and Grandi, G. (2012). Inferring reasons for the failure of Staphylococcus aureus vac-cines in clinical trials. Front. Cell. Infect. Microbiol. 2:16. doi:10.3389/fcimb.2012.00016

[22] R.A. Proctor.: Recent developments for *Staphylococcus aureus* vaccines: clinical and basic science challenges. European Cells and Materials Vol. 30 2015 (pages 315-326) DOI: 10.22203/eCM. V030a22 ISSN 1473-2262. University of Wisconsin – Medical Microbiology/Immunology 835 Asa Gray, Ann Arbor, Michigan 48105, USA

Chapter 6

Prevalence, Antimicrobial Resistance and Pathogenicity of Non-O1 *Vibrio cholerae* in Suburban and Rural Groundwater Supplies of Marrakesh Area (Morocco)

Hafsa Lamrani Alaoui, Khalid Oufdou and Nour-Eddine Mezrioui

Abstract

This synthesis of research work considers the dynamic, antibiotic resistance, hemolytic, and hemagglutination activities of non-O1 *Vibrio cholerae* in comparison with those of fecal coliforms, fecal streptococci, and *Pseudomonas aeruginosa* isolated from suburban and rural groundwater supplies in a Marrakesh area (Morocco). In addition, it assesses the influence of some chemical factors on the distribution of all these bacterial groups. The obtained results showed that the prospected well waters contain them at varying abundance degrees while undergoing generally spatial and temporal fluctuations. The total occurrence of these bacteria during the period of study was 94%. Detectable non-O1 *V. cholerae* was present in 81% of the samples and the mean abundances ranged from 0 to 11100 MPN/100 ml. According to WHO standards for drinking water, they were heavily contaminated and could have significant health risks for the local population consuming them. Non-O1 *V. cholerae* and the other studied bacteria are virulent since most of them were found to be adhesive, producers of hemolysins and multi-resistant to antibiotics. Pollution activities around the wells lead to an increase of virulence and antimicrobial resistance in groundwater. This shows the role of these bacteria in several cases of gastro-enteric and systemic pathologies noted in Marrakech local population.

Keywords: non-O1 *Vibrio cholerae*, antibiotic resistance, groundwater, hemagglutination, hemolysin, chemical factors

1. Introduction

Currently, pollution, water scarcity and seasonal droughts are emerging as major development challenges for many developing countries. According to data for the world's most water-stressed countries [1], Morocco is among the most vulnerable and will become a water-stressed country by 2040 [2, 3]. Thus, the preservation and management of its aquifers against various forms of pollution is a major national and regional concern. In Marrakesh area, groundwater supplies are a valuable resource for wide suburban and rural populations. However, their consumers' growth and anthropogenic activities heavily influence these wells water. In fact, due to the lack of sewerage networks and the absence of household waste collection, these people are directly discharging wastewater and solid waste onto the ground. Then, the chemical and microbial quality of well water under such environments is seriously threatened. Also, these communities rely only on these untreated wells' water as a source of human and animal drinking, domestic activities, and cultural irrigation. The use of these well waters without any previous treatment involves serious health problems due to the potential presence of pollutants and pathogenic bacteria. Water pollution has a direct impact on human health so that about 884 million people are living without access to clean drinking water in 2019 [4, 5]. According to WHO, about 1.8 million people die every year because of cholera and diarrhea, and 3900 children die every day as a result of contaminated water consumption and sanitation conditions inadequacy [6, 7]. Indeed, emergences of some aquatic diseases and sporadic outbreaks of acute diarrhea were reported on several occasions in Marrakesh area especially in the hot period [8, 9]. Even so, etiological information related to such outbreaks in this region is very limited. The occurrence of antibiotic-resistant bacteria in these wells' water could worsen more than in this previous situation. Many research studies have noted the important public health implications of the presence of antibiotic-resistant bacteria and especially multiple antibiotic-resistant bacteria, in suburban and rural groundwater [10, 11]. The horizontal gene transfer and clonal spread of resistant bacteria can mediate the transfer of not only antibiotic resistance genes but also virulence factors [12, 13].

There is a growing trend toward infection due to *Vibrio* spp., their capacity to persist in the aquatic environment and their association with abiotic and biotic factors [14, 15]. Non-O1 *Vibrio cholerae* is ubiquitously distributed in diverse aquatic environments where water acts as a reservoir and source of its transmission [16]. They are an essential and potentially life-threatening cause of infections that are primarily related to the consumption of feces-contaminated water and person-to-person transmission [17–19]. This pathogen leads to self-limiting gastroenteritis, septicemia, bacteremia, meningoencephalitis, oral infection, wound or ear infections, and non-epidemic diarrhea with a fatal outcome in immunocompromised hosts with predisposing medical conditions [19–23]. Different virulence factors have been suggested to be involved in these diseases such as a heat-stable toxin, hemolysin and other cell-associated hemagglutinins [24–26]. Few studies have been conducted in Morocco on the occurrence of antibiotic resistance and virulence factors of non-O1 *V. cholerae* in groundwater supplies in Morocco and particularly in the Marrakesh area. Accordingly, this study presents a synthesis of our research works on the dynamics, occurrence of antibiotic resistance, and potential virulence of non-O1 *V. cholerae* in supplying well water in comparison with other bacteria. The incidence of hemolytic and hemagglutination activities and the importance of some chemical parameters on the distribution of non-O1 *V. cholerae*, *Pseudomonas aeruginosa*, fecal coliforms (FC), and fecal streptococci (FS) is discussed.

2. Dynamics, pathogenicity of non-O1 *V. cholerae* in suburban and rural groundwater supplies in Marrakesh area (Morocco)

2.1 Dynamics and ecology of non-O1 *V. cholerae*

Diarrheic diseases caused by contaminated water continue to be a serious problem in developing countries and a lesser, but chronic problem in developed countries [4, 5]. More than half of the reported waterborne disease outbreaks have been linked to contaminated groundwater [27]. The importance of the ecology, distribution, and pathogenicity of non-O1 *V. cholerae* in water ecosystems is underestimated in the Mediterranean region [28] and particularly in Morocco. In preliminary research, the bacteriological and physicochemical quality was studied in sixteen well waters [29]. The prospected wells were located in two regions (Tensift and Jbilet aquifers) with environments representing different vulnerability to contamination. Sampling stations are situated at the north of Marrakesh city. The hydrology of these regions was relatively similar but they were geologically different. In the Jbilet region where the 10 studied wells (W1, W2, W3, W4, W5, W6, W7, W8, W9, and W10) are situated, the geological formations are almost all represented by Schist [30]. They are altered on the surface and give a stony soil with a few centimeters of clay soil. However, runoff waters seep partly into cracked and altered areas and fault zones [30, 31]. In the Tensift region where the other 6 monitored wells are sited, there is a predominance of superficial limestone formations and very permeable alluvial deposits [32]. In these two areas, the groundwater contained in these permeable formations was relatively slightly deep (6–30 m). To study the dynamic of non-O1 *V. cholerae*, we have targeted essentially six wells depending on their level of fecal contamination, proximity to pollution sources. The other reasons were their relative importance for local populations, and given that the research methodology of this pathogen is arduous and pricey. We have also selected wells that are highly susceptible to degradation by anthropogenic activities. W11 was the control well as it's not damaged by any pollutant source categories. Taking into account all these factors and risks, we opt for the following wells to identify non-O1 *V. cholerae*: W2, W3, W5, W9, W11, and W14. Spatial and temporal distributions of non-O1 *V. cholerae*, *P. aeruginosa*, and fecal indicators abundances were conducted over a year. Sampling was done each month from April 2004 to April 2005.

For non-O1 *V. cholerae* enumeration, the three tubes MPN technique was accomplished to search this bacterium according to the methodology described by Mezrioui et al. [33], Mezrioui and Oufdou [12] and Lamrani Alaoui et al. [34]. Concentration by the membrane filtration technique (Millipore size, pore: 0.45 μm) of volumes of 100, 10, and 1 ml or their dilutions was the perfect way to inoculate non-O1 *V. cholerae* into three tubes using the MPN technique. It consists of three steps: alkaline peptone water enrichment step (1% peptone, 1% NaCl, pH 8.6) for 18 hours of incubation at 37 °C. Seeding stage on thiosulfate-citrate-bile-sucrose selective media (TCBS) with incubation at 37 °C for 24 h. Identification of colonies presumed to be non-O1 *V. cholerae* through screening tests cited previously.

The standard bacterial indicators of fecal pollution in waters are FC. They are the most used to know the bacterial load of groundwater and testify the potential presence of enteric pathogens in water. But, to differentiate the fecal contamination of human and animal origin, it is proposed to use FS [35–37]. *P. aeruginosa* is an environmental microorganism that has become a major cause of opportunistic infections. It is regarded as complicated and can be life-threatening, especially respiratory tract infection in patients with cystic fibrosis and corneal infection or septicemias and diarrhea [38]. The counts of FC, FS, and *P. aeruginosa* were carried out on filtered volumes by 100, 10, and 1 ml of water samples by the membrane filtration technique (Φ = 0.45 μm). The appropriate selective media to each bacterial group was used like the following: lactose 2, 3, 5-Triphenyl Tetrazolium Chloride (TTC) agar with tergitol 7 (Biokar Diagnostics) for FC, Slanetz agar with TTC (Pasteur Diagnostics) for FS, and Cetrimid agar medium (Merck Diagnostics) for *P. aeruginosa*. For FC, the yellow colonies were enumerated after incubation at 44.5 °C for 24 h. For FS, the pink colonies were enumerated after incubation at 37 °C for 24 h. For *P. aeruginosa*, the fluorescent colonies were enumerated after incubation at 42 °C for 24 h to 48 h. The densities of these bacteria were expressed by the indirect count of colonies forming units (cfu). For the physicochemical analyses, water temperature, pH, salinity, conductivity, and dissolved oxygen were measured *in situ* by the multiline engine parameters P4 SET. The other measured parameters (nitrate, nitrite, ammonium, organic matter, sodium, chloride, calcium, potassium, and sulphates) were determined at the laboratory according to the methods described by Lamrani Alaoui et al. [29].

The dynamics of non-O1 *V. cholerae*, *P. aeruginosa*, FC, and FS were statistically analyzed using SPSS 10.0 for windows. The two factor analysis of variance (ANOVA) was used for seasonal variation and the difference between the stations' comparison of bacterial abundances. Bacterial densities were transformed into a log10 unit to realize data analysis. Significant differences between each pair of average were established when $p \leq 0.05$. While being based on the Spearman correlation test, the nature of relationships between bacterial abundances and physicochemical factors was performed. Densities variation of non-O1 *V. cholerae*, *P. aeruginosa*, FC, and FS underwent high spatial and temporal fluctuations. The degree of pollution in these wells was different. Detectable non-O1 *V. cholerae* was present in 81% of samples and the average abundances ranged from 0 to 11100 MPN/100 ml. The annual average abundances of non-O1 *V. cholerae* were 4903 MPN/100 ml in all samples. Detectable *P. aeruginosa* was present in 88% of samples and its abundances ranged from 0 to 1670 cfu/100 ml with annual average densities of 206 cfu/100 ml. Throughout the year of study, the total incidence of FC and FS was 94%. The considerable variations of their densities were respectively recorded from a minimum of 0 cfu/100 ml to a maximum of 10200 cfu/100 ml for FC and 6700 cfu/100 ml for FS. Nevertheless, the annual mean abundances of FC and FS were respectively 1891 cfu/100 ml and 1246 cfu/100 ml. Among the studied physical parameters, the water temperature was important to define cold and hot periods. The average water temperature during the whole period of our study was 22 °C. Temperature values varied between 15 °C and 30 °C. Based on the average water temperature, two periods were defined: October to March (cold period: $T < 22$ °C) and April to September (hot period: $T \geq 22$ °C). This has served to scrutiny the temporal evolutions of non-O1 *V. cholerae*, FC, FS, and *P. aeruginosa* which generally appeared to be similar. Relatively, their highest densities were noted during the hot period, while their low levels were noted during the cold period. The average abundances of non-O1 *V. cholerae* were 7696 MPN/100 ml in the hot period and 2109 MPN/100 ml in the cold period. The hot period was characterized by average abundances of FC of 3083 cfu/100 ml and 699 cfu/100 ml in the cold period. FS registered 1821 cfu/100 ml in the warm season and 671 cfu/100 ml in the cool season. But, *P. aeruginosa* was distinguished by mean densities of 308 cfu/100 ml in the warm period and 104 cfu/100 ml in the cold period.

For non-O1 *V. cholerae* and FC, W9 was the most contaminated. This well is located near a municipal landfill and sewage effluent. The bacterial abundances were compared in the studied wells. The average densities of FC, FS, *P. aeruginosa*, and non-O1 *V. cholerae* were very significantly ($p < 0.05$, ANOVA test) higher in the whole wells compared to the control well (W11). On the other hand, indicators of fecal contamination showed significantly higher abundances than those of *P. aeruginosa* ($p < 0.05$, ANOVA test). *P. aeruginosa* is requiring more interest as an indicator in the assessment of swimming pool water quality, drinking water, recreational and wastewater [39, 40]. This opportunistic pathogen provides differentiation of the human origin feces most likely rather than animal origin feces in waters [41]. All of these results demonstrated that the studied well waters were heavily contaminated with non-O1 *V. cholerae*, indicators of fecal contamination, and *P. aeruginosa*. The prospected wells play a crucial role in the supply of rural and suburban populations in the Marrakesh area to meet their needs for drinking water, domestic water supply, and recreation activities. This fact points out potential health effects on populations using them directly without any previous treatment.

The comparison of these bacterial abundances in the different sampling locations has shown that the most loaded wells were surrounded by several sources of pollution such as septic pit, manure, wastes, spreading wastewater, animal stools and detergents. Based on the results of our study, it is possible to conclude that groundwater can play an important role as a transmission vehicle of non-O1 *V. cholerae* and the other studied bacteria. Our findings are in agreement with those reported by Nogueira et al. [42] and Isaac-Marquez [17]. These authors investigated water quality at sources and points of consumption of urban and rural communities. According to them, the water distribution system, spring water and private wells samples had high coliforms positive and high percentages of non-O1 *V. cholerae*. Several reports have demonstrated that gastrointestinal and extraintestinal infections caused by non-O1 *V. cholerae* are linked with contaminated water and other activities in aquatic environments, and this bacterium could therefore pose a problem for public health [43, 44]. In this study, it appears that the contamination of the two prospected aquifers was not only due to a simple process of diffusion but also to the various sources of pollution around the wells. The wells situated close to many sources of pollution showed the greatest densities of the studied bacteria. These sources of contamination include faulty septic systems, landfill leachates, and infiltration of untreated sewage. Also, septic tanks seepage or runoffs of human and animal activities nearby the studied wells have an impact on their safety. All of these factors led to the contamination of the groundwater. The majority of the studied wells are situated 20 to 400 m from pollution sources. Furthermore, Tensift and Jbilet aquifers are found under the highly porous texture of the ground, allowing rapid infiltration of contaminants into groundwater. Next to that the extreme permeability subsurface formations generate hydraulic fracturing made up through cracks, root channels, and fissures in these sloping areas. The nature of these subsurface formations produces an accelerated flow of pollutants derived from the surface build-up of solid waste and sewage. The shallowness of the monitored wells is also involved in the contamination of Tensift and Jbilet groundwaters. In addition, these unprotected dug wells facilitate the introduction of polluting substances. These combined factors revealed the vulnerability of Tensift and Jbilet groundwater. Besides, the obtained results indicated that the distributions of FC, FS, *P. aeruginosa*, and non-O1 *V. cholerae* undergo spatio-temporal fluctuations. Their abundances increased in the hot season and were lower in the cold season. The effects of the temperature on the microbial growth rate, lag phase, and cell yield have been defined in previous studies [45]. Indeed, *Pseudomonas putida* presented a shorter growth phase lag of only 10 h at 17.5 °C but was longer within 3 days at 7.5 °C [45].

To evaluate the impact of some chemical factors on the evolutions of the studied bacterial groups, the evolutions of physicochemical parameters were followed. According to the survey, the water pH of these two studied aquifers remained neutral or slightly basic and varied from 6.8 to 8.1. Total mineralization of the studied water wells was expressed by electrical conductivity. Its values average showed that the prospected wells were fair to greatly mineralized. Moreover, the wells situated downstream are the most loaded. When conductivity values exceed 2000 μS/cm, water presents laxative effects for the consumers [46]. The water of the two-studied groundwater presented strong concentrations of major elements (Ca^{2+}, Na^{+}, Cl^{-}, SO_4^{2-} and K^{+}) with high concentrations of nitrogenous ions. They were particularly very hard, very salt, very chlorinated, and present high concentrations of sulphate. According to the international standard limits, the gauged concentrations of nitrites, calcium, sodium, and chloride overtake these requirements [47]. Seasonal impacts are expressed by ammonium, nitrites, calcium, and organic matter. Their fluctuations were similar to those of the counted bacterial groups, but there was no temporal pattern for the other chemical parameters. These influences result from rainwater runoff and temperature variation that upload greatly calcium, ammonium, nitrites, and organic matter from soil to groundwater during the wet season compared to the dry season.

Based on the above results, the relationship between bacteriological and physicochemical parameters was determined using the Spearman correlation test. The studied wells are a dynamic system where bacteriological and chemical components might interact in a complex synergistic or antagonistic manner. Analysis of potential correlations between the different abundances of non-O1 *V. cholerae* and FC reflected that there is a stronger linkage among them in the studied wells. FC can testify to the existence of non-O1 *V. cholerae* in Marrakesh groundwater. However, no significant statistical correlation could be shown between the concentrations of non-O1 *V. cholerae* and *P. aeruginosa*. Several studies were conducted for the purpose of correlating the densities of fecal indicators with the presence of pathogens. Gallacher and Spino [48] emphasized that a correlation between the levels of total and fecal coliforms and the possibility of isolating pathogens would be valuable in setting reliable bacteriological standards, particularly for recreation and fishing uses. Hoi et al. [49] also demonstrated significant correlations between the occurrence of coliform bacteria and that of FS and also between coliform bacteria and *Vibrio vulnificus*. However, Mezrioui et al. [33] and Mezrioui and Oufdou [12] have shown that the spatial–temporal dynamic of non-O1 *V. cholerae* abundances was reverse to that of FC in other ecosystems such as sewage waters or water purified by the stabilization pond system.

The simulation of the sixteen well water points to a single ecosystem indicates a strong and positive relationship between calcium and FC and FS abundances. It was also indicated that a synergistic relationship exists between non-O1 *V. cholerae*, salinity, chlorides, calcium, sulphates, and nitrates ($p < 0.05$) especially after the mock of the six wells water like a single ecosystem. However, there is a significant negative correlation between calcium and *P. aeruginosa* abundances. These same correlations between nitrites and FC, FS, and *P. aeruginosa* abundances were recorded. Sjogren and Gibson [50] have revealed an important effect of acidic pH linked with the concentrations of calcium, magnesium, and other ions commonly present in hard-water, on the survival of enteric bacteria in the environment. These elements contributed to the adsorption of Fe^{3+} and Al^{3+} in the environment [51]. Ca^{2+} or Mg^{2+} are necessary for the physical integrity of many microbial components and intervene in some *Bacillus* species metabolism in the organic molecules transportation through the cell wall [52].

2.2 Pathogenesis of non-O1 *V. cholerae*

Infections caused by pathogenic *Vibrios* remain a severe threat to the public. Most of these infections result from the consumption of contaminated water or undercooked seafood products [53]. Non-O1 *V. cholerae* can also cause infections to range from self-limiting gastroenteritis to severe life-threatening septicemia and necrotizing fasciitis [53]. However, their infections are under-detected and under-reported because clinicians and microbiologist underestimate their abilities to induce diarrhea, and given that searching non-O1 *V. cholerae* is not subjected to routine testing [54]. Between 1 and 3.4% of cases of acute diarrhea are believed to be due to non-O1 *V. cholerae*, in developing and developed countries alike [55]. Up to now, there are few reports of the frequency of isolation of non-O1 *V. cholerae* and there is an under-diagnosis of their infections, especially for those taken as milder cases, from the consumption of contaminated groundwater supplies in Morocco. The significant abundances of non-O1 *V. cholerae*, FC, FS, and *P. aeruginosa* recorded in this work confirm the presence of pathogenic microorganisms in groundwater consumed by the suburban and rural population in Marrakesh area. So that also informed the need to conduct the study about their virulence factors.

The enteropathogenicity of non-O1 *V. cholerae* is multifactorial [56]. The various putative virulence determinants identified in non-O1 *V. cholerae* include the production of cholera toxin CT [57, 58], enterotoxin LT or ST [59, 60], *V. cholerae* cytolysin (VCC) referred to a hemolysin and cytolysin with activity against a range of eukaryotic cells [61], shiga-like toxin [62] and cell-associated hemagglutinins [63]. It has been demonstrated that non-O1 *V. cholerae* adheres and invades the epithelial cells of gut mucosa and starts its multiplication [64]. It includes mild watery diarrhea of 1 or 2 days duration, a severe dehydrating disease resembling cholera, and dysentery [65]. This situation occurs only with the expression of certain virulence factors as previously cited [60–62, 64]. Alternatively, *V. cholerae* virulence factors encoded on a mobile genetic element, can spread through horizontal transfer. This underscores the importance of the environmental strains of non-O1 *V. choleare* as a reservoir of virulence genes that generate the dissemination of new variants [66].

In this work to characterize the virulence factors of the bacterial isolates recovered during our study, hemolysis and hemagglutination with human erythrocytes were realized. The potential virulence of non-O1 *V. cholerae* in supplying well waters in comparison with *P. aeruginosa*, FC, and FS. To our knowledge, this is the first report on the incidence of hemolytic and hemagglutination activities and antibiotic resistance of bacteria isolated from rural and suburban well waters from Morocco and particularly in Marrakesh groundwater. For hemolytic activity and hemagglutination assays 317 strains of non-O1 *V. cholerae*, 208 strains of *P. aeruginosa*, 320 strains of FC, and 338 strains of FS were collected from the prospected wells over the year. After bacterial strains, isolation was streaked onto Trypticase Soy Agar (TSA) for purification. The ability of all these isolates to adhere and destroy host cells was verified with human O erythrocytes. Quantification of hemolytic activity of bacterial cells was performed according to the procedure described by Rahim et al. [67] and Lamrani Alaoui et al. [34]. The hemagglutination test was realized according to the methodology described by Pal et al. [68] and Lamrani Alaoui et al. [34]. To statistically analyze the percentage of hemolytic and hemagglutination activities, the test of two proportions or frequencies was carried out as referred by Schwartz [69].

This test enables comparisons and identification of significant differences between two frequencies: f_1 noted on n_1 samples and f_2 noted on n_2 samples as shown below:

$$t = \frac{f1 - f2}{\sqrt{f(1-f)\left(\frac{1}{n1} + \frac{1}{n2}\right)}} \quad \text{With} \quad \frac{n1f1 + n2f2}{n1 + n2} \tag{1}$$

If $|t| < 1.96$: the difference between f1 and f2 was not significant ($p > 0.05$).

If $|t| \geq 1.96$: the difference was significant ($p \leq 0.05$).

Non-O1 *V cholerae*, *P. aeruginosa*, FC, and FS strains have distinct hemolysin production. Complete and partial hemolytic activities of non-O1 *V. cholerae* isolates indicate major percentages of 71.29%. Hemolysin productions, among FS and FC strains have reached respectively considerable levels of 20.71% and 16.88%

compared to *P. aeruginosa* isolates (9.13%). Non-O1 *V. cholerae* expressed significantly the greatest β hemolytic activity of 33.12%, while only 3.44% of FC and 4.44% of FS strains were β hemolytic ($p \leq 0.05$, the test of two proportions). The lowest β hemolytic activities were recorded among *P. aeruginosa* strains (1.44%). Hemolysin of *V. cholerae* is suggested to be a virulence factor contributing to pathogenesis [70]. Guhathakurta et al. [71] Purified a bifunctional hemolysin-phospholipase C molecule from non-O1 *V. cholerae* (O139) showing enterotoxic activity, as shown by fluid accumulation in the ligated rabbit ileal loop and in the intestine of suckling mice [68]. In this work, obtained hemolytic activity percentages were comparable to those registered by Begum et al. [72]. They noted that 80% of non-O1 and non-O139 *V. cholerae* strains were hemolysin producers. Nevertheless, our findings were inferior in number to those given by Amaro et al. [73]. They demonstrated that hemolytic activity within environmental non-O1 *V. cholerae* strains achieved a percentage of 97%. Adhesion to the intestinal mucosa represents the first step in the infectivity of bacterial pathogens such as *V. cholerae* [74].

The extent of the results of hemagglutination activities of the adhesive bacterial strains isolated from Marrakesh groundwater was fluctuating from 63.09% for non-O1 *V. cholerae* to 65.09% for FS, 84.06% for FC, and 87.98% for *P. aeruginosa*. From a total of 317 strains of non-O1 *V. cholerae*, 18.93% were highly adhesive and 44.16% did not agglutinate completely to the erythrocytes. Besides, 69.06% of FC strains and 62.02% of *P. aeruginosa* possessed a complete agglutination ability, and respectively 15% and 25.96% of them agglutinated partially. Our results are consistent with prior research related to the distribution of hemagglutination in environmental non-Ol *V. cholerae* [73]. They noted that 78% of the tested strains presented agglutinating ability. Baffone et al. [75] study on the identification of virulence factors among *V. fluvialis*, *V. alginolyticus*, non-O1 *V. cholerae*, and *V. parahaemolyticus* showed that their adhesive capability was respectively expressed with varying percentages of 40% to 55–80%.

2.3 Antimicrobial susceptibility of non-O1 *V. cholerae*

Antibiotics and other antimicrobial agents have been used, since their discovery, for the treatment and management of bacterial infections in humans and animals [76]. Waterborne bacterial pathogens such as *Vibrio* spp., *Escherichia coli*, *Pseudomonas*, fecal coliforms and *enterococci*, and other enteric pathogens cause diseases around the world and still with their increasing antibiotic resistance the major drinking water health threats in developing countries [35–37]. Disappointingly, the rapid overuse of recommended antimicrobials drives mainly to the development of drug-resistant pathogens. So, antibiotic resistance is a global health threat that requires more expensive medication and can compromise therapeutic success leading to morbidity and mortality [77, 78]. On the other side, many people, especially in rural areas, rely on untreated groundwater for their water supplies. Consumption of contaminated water is one of the sources of *Vibrio* infections. Among the other virulence factors, resistance to antibiotics is more important. Several authors have noted that *V. cholerae* species are rapidly adapting to new drugs commonly used in medicine [79, 80], becoming a potential risk to public health. In addition, molecular analyses demonstrated that resistance to antibiotics and the other virulence factors are chromosomally mediated [81, 82]. Few studies have been done to determine the antibiotic resistance of isolates from groundwater. Non-O1 *V. cholerae* and *Pseudomonas* were resistant to ampicillin, chloramphenicol, and streptomycin have been isolated [35, 83]. According to our knowledge, no study has been developed on the occurrence of antibiotic resistance of non-O1 *V. cholerae* in groundwater supplies in Morocco and particularly in Marrakesh area. For this reason, the other objective was focused on the study of the antibiotic resistance of non-O1 *V. cholerae* in untreated suburban and rural well water of Marrakesh region. A comparison was made between the dynamics and antibiotic resistance of non-O1 *V. cholerae* and those of fecal coliforms (FC).

In order to estimate the sanitary risk associated with antibiotic resistant bacteria, a total of 317 strains of non-O1 *V. cholerae*, 320 strains of FC, 338 strains of FS, and 204 strains of *P. aeruginosa* were collected from the prospected wells over the year and were tested for their antibiotic susceptibility. The strain antibiotic resistance study was carried out using the multipoint inoculation method reported by Oufdou et al. [84] and Lamrani Alaoui et al. [34]. The antibiotic was incorporated into molten Muller-Hinton agar in order to prepare the plates. After their inoculation, they were incubated at 37 °C for 24 h.

The control plate was elaborated without antibiotic and was inoculated in the same way. In comparison with the control plate and if no growth of the strain is observed in the medium containing the concentration of antibiotic tested the bacterium is considered resistant. The concentrations (given in $\mu g\ ml^{-1}$) of the antibiotics tested have been cited in the above studies. These antibiotics were chosen for two reasons: (i) they have been used in the treatment of human and/or livestock illnesses; and (ii) they have been used in previous surveys of antibiotic resistance in aquatic environments [12, 84–86]. Similarly, the test of two proportions or frequencies described by Schwartz [69] was used to compare percentages of antibiotic resistance between non-O1 *V. cholerae*, FC, FS, and *P. aeruginosa*. Obtained results showed that the overall resistance (resistance to at least one antibiotic) of non-O1 *V. cholerae* strains was 79%, while it was 100% for *P. aeruginosa*, FC, and FS strains. The mono-resistance (resistance to one antibiotic) of non-O1 *V. cholerae* was 10% while it was 5% for FC and FS strains. The multi-resistance of non-O1 *V. cholerae* strains remain at a degree (69%) significantly below those of FC and FS strains (95%) ($p < 0.05$, the test of two proportions), while all *P. aeruginosa* strains were multi-resistant. On the other hand, the multi-resistance of non-O1 *V. cholerae* and FC strains was significantly higher ($p < 0.05$, the test of two proportions) than that of their monoresistance. The susceptibility of non-O1 *V. cholerae* to all antibiotics tested is estimated at 21%, while none of the isolates *P. aeruginosa*, FC and FS was susceptible to all antibiotics tested. Our findings highlighted the most common antibiotics for which non-O1 *V. cholerae* strains resistance is recorded are in ascending order: trimethoprim (49%), cephalothin (60%), streptomycin (62%) and sulfamethoxazole (75%). The lowest proportions of resistance were toward erythromycin (18%), kanamycin and polymyxin B (12%), cephotaxim (8%), gentamycin (7%), and tetracycline (2%). It's important to perceive that all the 317 non-O1 *V. cholerae* isolates were susceptible to chloramphenicol, nalidixic acid, and novobiocin. Amaro et al. [73] have demonstrated that non-O1 *V. cholerae* environmental isolates were resistant to sulfanilamide (80%), to ampicillin (63%) and to amoxicillin (61%) and were susceptible to chloramphenicol, nalidixic acid, tetracycline, novobiocin and trimethoprim. Radu et al. [87] showed that all *V. cholerae* isolates were susceptible to chloramphenicol and exhibited high rates of resistance to cephalothin (90.9%), streptomycin (87.9%), and tetracycline (77.79%). Isolates of non-O1 *V. cholerae* from the aquatic environment in India were found to have multiple antibiotic resistance. Thirty-nine percent of *V. cholerae* isolates were resistant to two drugs [88]. Furthermore, several cases of antimicrobial resistance have been described in environmental as well as in clinical strains, involving cefotaxime, nalidixic acid, tetracyclines, cotrimoxazole, ciprofloxacin, and depending on location, certain multidrug resistant strains having been reported [55, 89]. Nevertheless, FC results are in perfect agreement with the findings of McKeon et al. [10] indicating that the overall resistance of the coliforms is around 87%. This one comprises respectively 14, 64, and 94% of *E. coli*, *Citrobacter freundii* and *Enterobacter cloacae* isolates. The multi-resistance was registered by all bacterial strains isolated from groundwater and fluctuated as great as 100% for *Enterobacter cloacae*, *Klebsiella pneumoniae*, and *Klebsiella ozonae*. These authors have also demonstrated that 100% of the non-coliforms isolated from groundwater were multiple antibiotics resistant. El-Zanfaly et al. [90] observed a high multiple antibiotic resistance (63%) for gram-negative bacteria isolated from rural waters. Amundsen et al. [91] noted that 45% of total coliforms isolated from untreated well water were multidrug-resistant.

Antimicrobial resistance of FC strains was most widely manifested against sulfamethoxazole (91%), followed by cephalothin (88%) and ampicillin (84%). More than 30% of the FC isolates were resistant to kanamycin, gentamycin, streptomycin, trimethoprim, and tetracycline. However, the smaller susceptibility proportion was noted to chloramphenicol (13%) and nalidixic acid (28%). FS isolates were resistant to polymyxin (87%), sulfamethoxazole (86%), and nalidixic acid (85%), cephalothin (82%), and to streptomycin (74%), while they were less resistant to ampicillin (28%) and amoxicillin-clavulanic acid (34%). 28%, 34%, and 40% of FS isolates were resistant respectively to ampicillin, amoxicillin-clavulanic acid, and cephotaxim. The highest prevalence of resistance was observed among *P. aeruginosa* strains. More than 90% of these isolates were resistant to cephalothin (95%), cephotaxim (93%), polymyxin (92%), and cephamandole (90%). Also, 86% of *P. aeruginosa* isolates were resistant to tetracycline and nalidixic acid, 83% to ampicillin and kanamycin, 81% to streptomycin and 80% to trimethoprim, respectively. *P. aeruginosa* strains were generally resistant to the antibiotics tested, whereas they were less resistant only to imipenem (12%). The predominant resistance property observed was to β-lactam antibiotics, either alone or in combination with resistance to other antibiotics. Bell et al. [92] have also noted ampicillin and cephalothin resistance exhibited by most fecal coliform strains isolated from both rural and urban environments. McKeon et al. [10] analyzed antimicrobial susceptibility toward sixteen antibiotics of 265 coliform and non-coliform strains isolated from rural groundwater. They established that the overall resistance was approximately 70% and frequently indicated against novobiocin, cephalothin, and ampicillin. They have found that resistance toward tetracycline and nitrofurantoin was more than 30%.

The main multi-resistant patterns identified for non-O1 *V. cholerae* were to seven antibiotics with a percentage of around 24.09%. These strains were characterized with six profiles to seven antibiotics while the maximal multidrug resistance was to ten antibiotics with two profiles: "Gm, Str, Km, Tpm, Smx, Amp, Amx, Cfl, Cfm, Ery", and "Gm, Str, Km, Tpm, Smx, Tc, Amp, Amx, Cfl, Cfm". For the isolated FC, antimicrobial susceptibility toward five or more antibiotics was registered by 80% of them. The prevalent multi-resistant profile recorded for FC was to eight antibiotics (11.6%). The maximal multidrug resistance was to fourteen antibiotics with two patterns: "Amp, Amx, Amx-clav, Cfl, Cfm, Cft, Gm, Km, Na, PB, Smx, Str, Tc, Tpm" and "Amp, Amx, Amx-clav, Cfl, Cfm, Cft, Chl, Gm, Na, PB, Smx, Str, Tc, Tpm".

3. Conclusion

Groundwater is the primary drinking water source for a large suburban and rural population in Morocco. Hence, it is critical to ensure that groundwater resources are protected and of acceptable drinking quality. To the best of our knowledge, this study presents the most comprehensive monitoring of non-O1 *V. cholerae*, *P. aeruginosa*, and fecal indicator bacteria from Marrakech wells waters. Our findings show that microbial presence within Marrakech groundwater supplies is a persistent issue, with a total occurrence of 81% for non-O1 *V. cholerae* and 94% for FC, FS, and *P. aeruginosa*. Another ecological challenge was elucidated since these bacteria with other physicochemical parameters underwent generally spatial and temporal fluctuations that structure bacterial variability. The temporal evolutions of non-O1 *V. cholerae* and FC appeared to be similar. Relatively, the highest densities were noted during the hot period, while the low levels were noted during the cold period. This heavy colonization of the prospected wells, with potentially pathogenic bacteria, implies that they are unsuitable for drinking and other domestic activities according to the international norms. Also, a highly significant relationship was observed between non-O1 *V. cholerae* and FC abundances in the studied wells. FC can be used to detect the presence of non-O1 *V. cholerae* in Marrakesh groundwater. Generally, no significant correlation was detected between these fecal indicator bacteria and *P. aeruginosa*. This opportunistic pathogenic bacterium is acquiring greater importance and may be useful in evaluating groundwater quality. The degrees of antibiotic resistance and particularly of multi-resistance of non-O1 *V. cholerae*, FC, FS, and *P. aeruginosa* strains are high. The multi-resistance of non-O1 *V. cholerae* strains (69%) was significantly lower than that of FC strains (94%). Non-O1 *V. cholerae*, FC, FS, and *P. aeruginosa* strains resistant to antibiotics occurred during the whole study period. The multiple antibiotic resistant bacteria once introduced into the studied groundwater supplies are capable of long-term survival in this ecosystem. In addition, non-O1 *V. cholerae* and the other studied bacteria isolated from Marrakesh groundwater are virulent since most of them are producers of hemolysins, hemagglutinins. These wells are used directly without any previous treatment for drinking water supply and domestic and recreation activities of these rural and suburban populations. This fact could be at the origin of the emergence of diarrheal diseases noted among them. It is well known that the incidence of multiple antibiotic resistant bacteria is a cause for concern because of possible colonization of the gastrointestinal tract and conjugal transfer of antibiotic resistance to the normal flora, serving to further amplify the number introduced into aquatic environments such as groundwater reservoirs. The ability of non-O1 *V. cholerae* and the other bacteria to survive in groundwater throughout the period of the study indicated a continuing trend of human and animal fecal contamination. The leachates from the reservoir of animal fertilizer which contaminate the groundwater might be a source of antibiotics in this water ecosystem. The manure runoff, leakage from septic tanks or broken sewage channels, led to the input of antibiotic resistant bacteria into groundwater. Given that the groundwater may play an important role in the spread of resistant and virulent bacteria, further study using molecular tools is warranted to properly evaluate the public health and ecological significance of these antibiotic and virulent bacteria in rural drinking water supplies. Non-O1 *V. cholerae* and the other bacteria could act as a reservoir of resistance and virulence genes in the groundwater environment.

Ultimately, the study highlights the need to remain highly suspicious of non-O1 *V. cholerae* infections related to consumption of contaminated wells water with known risk factors. Adaptation of special strategies should be taken to avoid poor maintenance, inappropriate well location and a historical lack of regulation that has led to many instances of groundwater contamination and associated public health issues. Consumption of these wells water requires an urgent reaction to apply adequate solutions. The protection of these wells waters, implementation and management of sanitation systems and sewerage network, the disinfection of groundwater should be adopted to cope with unforeseen situations and to decrease the water-related disease burden. As shown in reported results, this approach is still valuable in indicating potential avenues for future research. It's vital to link education and social awareness with these measurements which play a major role in confronting and controlling groundwater pollution, water-related diseases, and subsequently in improving the human health of these suburban and rural populations.

Acknowledgements

This work was supported by the International Foundation for Science (i.f.s.) (Project No. F/2826-2 and F/2826-3). We also thank Dr. Zioua Tawfik for the supply of human blood from the bank of Avicennes Military hospital of Marrakesh (Morocco).

Author details

Hafsa Lamrani Alaoui[1]*, Khalid Oufdou[2] and Nour-Eddine Mezrioui[2]

1 Laboratory of Microbiology, Faculty of Medicine and Pharmacy, Mohammed V University in Rabat, Rabat, Morocco

2 Laboratory of Microbial Biotechnologies, Agrosciences, and Environment, Faculty of Sciences, Semlalia, Cadi Ayyad University, Marrakesh, Morocco

*Address all correspondence to: h.alaoui@um5s.net.ma

References

[1] Reig, P., Maddocks, A., Gassert, F. (2013). World's 36 most Water Stressed Countries Data. World Resources Institute, Available online: http://www.wri.org/blog/2013/12/world%E2%80%99s-36-most-waterstressed-countries (accessed on 12 January 2021).

[2] Rijsberman, F.R. (2006). Water scarcity: Fact or fiction? Agricultural Water Management, 80: 5-22.

[3] Maddocks, A., Young, R.S., Reig, P. (2015). Ranking the World's most Water-Stressed Countries in 2040. World Resources Institute: Washington, DC, USA, Available online:http://www.wri.org/blog/2015/08/ranking-world%E2%80%99s-most-water-stressed-countries-2040 (accessed on 12 January 2021).

[4] Vineis, P., Chan, Q., Khan, A. (2011). Climate change impacts on water salinity and health. Journal of Epidemiology and Global Health, 1: 5-10.

[5] Abedin, M.A., Collins, A.E., Habiba, U., Shaw, R. (2019). Climate change, water scarcity, and health adaptation in southwestern coastal Bangladesh. International Journal of Disaster Risk Science, 10: 28-42.

[6] World Health Organization. Drinking Water. Fact Sheet. (2016). Available online: http://www.who.int/ mediacentre/factsheets/fs391/en/ (accessed on 12 January 2021).

[7] Ashbolt, N.J. 2004. Microbial contamination of drinking water and disease outcomes in developing regions. Toxicology, 198: 229-238.

[8] Bouhoum K., Habbari Kh., Jana M. (1997). Etude épidémiologique des helminthiases intestinales chez l'enfant de la zone d'épandage des eaux usées de la ville de Marrakech. In "Conception, naissance et petite enfance au Maghreb". Cahier de l'IREMAN, Institut de recherche et d'étude sur le monde arabe et musulman, CNRS-Univ. Aix-Marseille, 9/10: 275-291.

[9] Ait Melloul, A., Hassani, L. (1999). Antibiotic resistance of Salmonella strains isolated from children living in the wastewater spreading area of Marrakesh city (Morocco). World Journal of Microbiology and Biotechnology, 15: 91-96.

[10] McKeon, M.D., Calabrese, J.P., Bissonnette G.K. (1995). Antibiotic resistant gram-negative bacteria in rural groundwater supplies. Water Research, 29: 1902-1908.

[11] Arvanitidou M., Katsouyan nopoulos V., Tsakris A. (2001). Antibiotic resistance patterns of enterococci isolated from coastal bathing waters. Journal of Medical Microbiology, 50: 1001-1005.

[12] Mezrioui, N., Oufdou K. (1996). Abundance and antibiotic resistance of non-O1 *Vibrio cholerae* strains in domestic wastewater before and after treatment in stabilization ponds in an arid region (Marrakesh, Morocco). FEMS Microbiology Ecology, 21: 277-284.

[13] Wellington, E. M., Boxall, A. B., Cross, P., Feil, E. J., Gaze, W. H., Hawkey, P. M., Johnson-Rollings, A. S., Jones, D. L., Lee, N. M., Otten, W., Thomas, C. M., A. P. Williams. (2013). The role of the natural environment in the emergence of antibiotic resistance in gram-negative bacteria. The Lancet Infectious Diseases, 13(2):155-65.

[14] Grimes, D. J., Johnson, C. N., Dillon, K. S., Flowers, A. R., Noriea III, N. F., Berutti, T. (2009). What genomic sequence information has revealed

about *Vibrio* ecology in the ocean-a review. Microbial Ecology, 58: 447-460. doi:10.1007/s00248-009-9578-9.

[15] Johnson, C.N. (2013). Fitness factors in *Vibrios*: a mini-review. Microbial Ecology, 65: 826-851. doi:10.1007/s00248-012-0168.

[16] Colwell, R.R. (2004). Infectious disease and environment: cholera as a paradigm for waterborne disease. International Microbiology, 7: 285-289.

[17] Isaac-Marquez, A. P., Lezama-Davila, C. M., Eslava-Campos, C., Navarro-Ocana, A., Cravioto-quintana, A. (1998). Serotype of *Vibrio cholerae* non-O1 isolated from water supplies for human consumption in Campeche, Mexico and their antibiotic resistance susceptibility pattern. Memorias do Instituto Oswaldo Cruz, Rio de Janeiro, 93: 17-21.

[18] Haley, B.J. , Choi, S. Y., Grim, C. J., Onifade, T. J., Cinar, H. N., Tall, B. D., Taviani, E., Hasan N. A., Abdullah, AS. H., Carter, L., Sahu, S. N., Kothary, M. H., Chen, A., Baker, R., Hutchinson, R., Blackmore, C., Cebula, T. A., Huq, A., Colwell, R. R. (2014) Genomic and phenotypic characterization of *Vibrio cholerae* non-O1 isolates from a US Gulf Coast cholera outbreak. PLoS ONE 9: (4) e86264

[19] Deshayes, S., Daurel, C., Cattoir, V., Parienti, J. J., Quilici, M-L., de La Blanchardière A. 2015. Non-O1, non-O139 *Vibrio cholerae* bacteraemia: case report and literature review. Springer Plus, 4(575): 1-9. DOI 10.1186/s40064-015-1346-3.

[20] Kueh, C.S.W., Kutarski, P., Brunton, M. (1992). Contaminated marine wounds: the risk of acquiring acute bacterial infection from marine recreational beaches. Journal of Applied Bacteriology, 73: 412-420.

[21] Petsaris, O., Nousbaum, J.B., Quilici, M.L., Le Coadou, G., Payan, C., Abalain, M.L. (2010). Non-O1, non-O139 *Vibrio cholerae* bacteraemia in a cirrhotic patient. Journal of Medical Microbiology, 59:1260-1262.

[22] Kaki, R., El-Hossary, D., Jiman-Fatani, A., Al-Ghamdi, R. (2017). Non-O1/non-O139 *Vibrio cholerae* septicaemia in a Saudi man: a case report. JMM Case Reports, 4: 1-6 DOI 10.1099/jmmcr.0.005077

[23] Xie, H., Wu, Y., Liu, C., Guo, J., Ma, J., Li, X., Sun X. (2020). Oral infection caused by non-O1/non-O139 *Vibrio cholerae* in a patient with esophageal cancer undergoing esophagectomy and chemoradiotherapy: A case report. Infection and Drug Resistance, 13: 3923-3927.

[24] Banerjee, K. K., Ghosh, A. N., Dutta-Roy, K., Pal, S. C., Ghose, A. C. (1990). Purification and characterization of a novel hemagglutinin from *Vibrio cholerae*. Infection and Immunity, 58: 3698-3705.

[25] Dalsgaard, A., Albert, M.J., Taylor, D.N., Shimada, T., Meza, R., Serichantalergs, O. Echeverria, P. (1995). Characterization of *Vibrio cholerae* non-O1 serogroups obtained from an outbreak of diarrhoea in Lima, Peru. Journal of Clinical Microbiology, 33: 2715-2722.

[26] Sharma, C., Thungapathra, M., Ghosh, A., Mukhopadhyay, A.K., Basu, A., Mitra, R., Basu, I., Bhattacharya, S.K., et al. (1998). Molecular analysis of non-O1, non-O139 *Vibrio cholerae* associated with an unusual upsurge in the incidence of cholera-like disease in Calcutta, India. Journal of Clinical Microbiology, 36: 756-763.

[27] Craun, G. F., Berger, P. S., Calderon, R. L. (1997). Coliform bacteria and water borne disease outbreaks. *Journal (American Water Works Association)*, 89: 96-104.

[28] Dumontet, S., Krovacek, K., Svenson, S. B., Pasquale, V., Baloda, S. B, Figliuolod, G. (2000). Prevalence and diversity of *Aeromonas* and *Vibrio* spp. in coastal waters of Southern Italy. Comparative Immunology, Microbiology and Infectious Diseases, 23: 53-72.

[29] Lamrani Alaoui, H., Oufdou, K., Mezrioui, N. (2008). Environmental pollutions impacts on the bacteriological and physicochemical quality of suburban and rural groundwater supplies in Marrakesh area (Morocco). Environmental Monitoring and assessment, 145: 195-207.

[30] Boulanouar M., Yacoubi-khebiza M., Messouli M., Coineau N. (1995). Un nouveau Microcharbon (Isopoda, Janiroidea) du Maroc-Origine et biogéographie historique. Contribution to Zoology, 65: 53-64.

[31] Hakkou R., Wahbi M., Bachnou A., Elamari K., Hanich L., Hibti M. (2001). Impact de la décharge publique de Marrakech (Maroc) sur les ressources en eau. Bulletin of Engineering Geology and Environment, 60: 325-336.

[32] El Omari L. (1975). Note géothermique concernant le périmètre urbain de Marrakech et ses environs. Rap. SRG/ MAR / N° 36 Ministère du Commerce de l'industrie des Mines et de la marchandise.

[33] Mezrioui N., Oufdou K., Baleux B. (1995). Dynamics of non-O1 *Vibrio cholerae* and fecal coliforms in experimental stabilization ponds in the arid region of Marrakesh, Morocco, and the effect of pH, temperature and sunlight on their experimental survival. Canadian Journal of Microbiology, 41: 489-498.

[34] Lamrani Alaoui, H., Oufdou, K., Mezrioui, N. (2010). Determination of several potential virulence factors in non-o1 *Vibrio cholerae*, *Pseudomonas aeruginosa*, fecal coliforms and streptococci isolated from Marrakesh groundwater. Water Science and Technology, 61 (7): 1895-1905.

[35] Gangle, J.B. (2005). Sources and occurrence of antibiotic resistance in the environment. Thesis submitted to the Faculty of the Graduate School of the University of Maryland, College Park in partial fulfillment of the requirements for the degree of Master of Science, 125p

[36] Hynds, P. D., Thomas, M. K., Pintar K. (2014). Contamination of Groundwater Systems in the US and Canada by Enteric Pathogens, 1990-2013: A Review and Pooled-Analysis. PLoS ONE, 9 (5): e93301.

[37] Pons, W., Young, I., Truong, J., Jones-Bitton A., McEwen, S., Pintar, K., Papadopoulos A. (2015). A systematic review of waterborne disease outbreaks associated with small non-community drinking water systems in Canada and the United States. PLoS ONE, 10(10): e0141646.

[38] Costerton, J.W., Stewart, P.S., Greenberg, E.P. (1999). Bacterial biofilms: a common cause of persistent infections. Science, 284: 1318-22.

[39] Bahlaoui , M.A., Baleux, B., Troussellier, M. (1997). Dynamics of pollution-indicator and pathogenic bacteria in high-rate oxidation wastewater treatment ponds. Water Research, 31: 630-638.

[40] De Victorica, J., Galvan, M. (2001). *Pseudomonas aeruginosa* as an indicator of health risk in water for human consumption. Water Science Technology, 43, 49-52.

[41] Olivieri, V. P. (1982). Bacterial indicators of pollution. In: Pipes W.O. (ed.) Bacterial indicators of pollution. CRC Press, Boca Raton, FL, p. 21-41.

[42] Nogueira, G., Nakamura, C. V., Tognim, M. C. B., Abreu Filho, B. A., Dias Filho, B. P. (2003). Microbiological quality of drinking water of urban and rural communities. Review Saùde Pùblica, 37: 232-236.

[43] WHO (World Health Organization). (1993). Epidemic diarrhea due to *Vibrio cholerae* non-O1. Weekly Epidemiological Record, 68: 141-142.

[44] Chakraborty, S., Nair, G. B., Shinoda, S. (1997). Pathogenic *Vibrio*s in the natural aquatic environment. Reviews on Environmental Health, 12: 63-80.

[45] Fransolet, G., Delavalentina, D. J., Masschelein, W. J. (1985). Influence of temperature on bacterial development in water. Ozone Science, 7: 205-227.

[46] WHO (World Health Organization) (1986). Directives de la qualité pour l'eau de boisson. Vol. 2. Critères d'hygiène et documentation à l'appui. Genève: OMS, 341 p.

[47] Diop, E. S., Tandia, A. A. (1997). Qualité de l'eau de la nappe phréatique à Yeumbeul, Sénégal. Etude sur le terrain, CSI info N° 3 UNESCO, Paris, 27 pp.

[48] Gallacher, T., Spino, D. (1968). The significance of numbers of coliform bacteria as an indicator of enteric pathogens. Water Research, 2: 169-175.

[49] Hoi, L., Larsen, J., Dalsgaard, I., Dalsgaard, A. (1998). Occurrence of *Vibrio vulnificus* biotypes in Dannish marine environments. Applied and Environmental Microbiology, 64: 7-13.

[50] Sjogren, R. E., Gibson, M. J. (1981). Bacterial survival in a dilute environment. Applied and Environmental Microbiology, 41: 1331-1336.

[51] Dommergues, Y., Mangenot, F. (1970). In: Masson et Cie, editor. Soil microbial ecology. Paris, 796 pp.

[52] Pelmont, J. (1993). Bacterium and environment. Physiological adaptation. Presse universitaire de Grenoble ed., Grenoble, 899 p.

[53] Centers for Disease Control and Prevention (CDC). (2014). "National enteric disease surveillance: covis annual summary," Summary of Human *Vibrio* Cases Reported to CDC, Centers for Disease Control and Prevention, Atlanta, GA.

[54] Pierce, A. B., Broughton, S. J., Johnson, P.D., Grayson, M. L. (2000) *Vibrio cholerae* in Victoria. Medical Journal of Australia, 172:44-46

[55] Luo, Y., Ye, J., Jin, D., Ding, G., Zhang, Z., Mei, L., Octavia, S., Lan, R. (2013). Molecular analysis of non-O1/ non-O139 *Vibrio cholerae* isolated from hospitalized patients in China. BMC Microbiology, 13:52.

[56] Ramamurthy, T., Bag, P. K., Pal, A., Bhattacharya, S. K., Bhattacharya, M. K., Shimada, T., Takeda T., Karasawa, T., Kurazono H., Takeda Y., Nair G. B. (1993). Virulence patterns of *Vibrio cholerae* non-O1 strains isolated from hospitalized patients with acute diarrhoea in Calcutta, India. Journal of Medical Microbiology, 39:310-317.

[57] Spira, W. M., Fedorka-Cray, P. J. (1983). Production of cholera toxin-like toxin by *Vibrio mimicus* and non-O1 *Vibrio cholerae*. Infection and Immunity, 42: 501-509.

[58] Yamamoto, K., Takeda, Y., Miwatani, T. Craig, J. P. (1983). Purification and some properties of a non-O1 *Vibrio cholerae* enterotoxin that is identical to cholera enterotoxin. Infection and Immunity, 39: 1128-1135.

[59] Arita, M., Takeda, T., Honda, T. Miwatani, T. (1986). Purification and

characterization of *Vibrio cholerae* non-Ol heat-stable enterotoxin. Infection and Immunity, 52: 45-49.

[60] Ichinose, Y., Yamamoto, K., Nakasone, N. (1987). Enterotoxicity of El Tor-like hemolysin of non-O1 *Vibrio cholerae*. Infection and Immunity, 55: 1090-1093.

[61] Ruenchit, P., Reamtong, O., Siripanichgon, K., Chaicumpa, W., Diraphat, P. (2018). New facet of non-O1/non-O139 *Vibrio cholerae* hemolysin A: a competitive factor in the ecological niche. FEMS Microbiology Ecology, 94: (1).

[62] O'Brien, A. D., Chen, M. E., Holmes, R. K., Kaper, J., Levine, M. M. (1984). Environmental and human isolates of *Vibrio cholerae* and *Vibrio parahaemlovticus* produce a *Shigella dysenteriae* 1 (Shiga)-like cytotoxin. The Lancet, 323(8368): 77-78.

[63] Yamamoto, T., T. Yokota. (1988). *Vibrio cholerae* non-O1: production of cell-associated hemagglutinins and *in vitro* adherence to mucus coat and epithelial surfaces of the villi and lymphoid follicles of human small intestines treated with formalin. Journal of Clinical Microbiology, 26:2018-2024.

[64] Nishibuchi, M., Seidler, R. J., Rollins, D. M., Joseph, S. W. (1983). *Vibrio* factors cause rapid fluid accumulation in suckling mice. Infection and Immunity. 40: 1083-1091.

[65] Spira, W. M., Daniel R. R. (1979). Biotype cluster on the basis of virulence characteristics in non-O group 1 *Vibrio cholerae*, p. 440-457. In N. Pierce and K. Takeya (ed.), Symposium on cholera: Bethesda 1979. Proceedings of the 15th Joint Conference U.S.-Japan Cooperative Medical Science Program, Cholera Panel. NIH publication no. 80-2003. National Institutes of Health, Bethesda, Md.

[66] Chakraborty, S., Mukhopadhyay, A. K., Bhadra R. K., Ghosh A. N., Mitra R., Shimada, T., Yamasaki, S., S. M. Faruque, Y. Takeda, Colwell R., Nair G. B. (2000). Virulence Genes in Environmental Strains of *Vibrio cholerae*. Applied and Environmental Microbiology, 66(9): 4022-4028.

[67] Rahim, Z., Sultan Aziz, K. M. (1994). Enterotoxigenicity, hemolytic activity and antibiotic resistance of *Aeromonas* spp. Isolated from freshwater prawn marketed in Dhaka, Bangladesh. Microbiology and Immunology, 38: 773-778.

[68] Pal, S., Datta, A., Nair, G. B., Guhathakurta, B. (1998). Use of monoclonal antibodies to identify phospholipase C as the enterotoxic factor of the bifunctional hemolysin phospholipase C molecule of *Vibrio cholerae* O139. Infection and Immunity. 66, 3974-3977.

[69] Schwartz, D. (1963). Méthodes statistiques à l'usage des Médecins et des Biologistes (Statistical methods used for the medicine and the biology), 3rd edition, Paris, Medecine Flammarion Sciences ISBN 2-257-10326-2.

[70] Nagamune, K., Yamamoto, K., Honda, T. (1995). Cloning and sequencing of a novel hemolysin gene of *Vibrio cholerae*. FEMS Microbiology Letters, 128: 265-269.

[71] Guhathakurta, B., Sasmal, D., Pal, S., Chakraborty, S., Nair, G. B. Datta, A. (1999). Comparative analysis of cytotoxin, hemolysin, hemagglutinin and exocellular enzymes among clinical and environmental isolates of *Vibrio cholerae* O139 and non-O1, non-O139. FEMS Microbiology Letters, 179: 401-407.

[72] Begum, K., Ahsan, C. R., Ansaruzzaman, M., Dutta, D. K., Ahmad, Q. S. Talukder, K. A. (2006). Toxin(s), other than cholera toxin,

produced by environmental non O1 non O139 *Vibrio cholerae*. Cellular and Molecular Immunology. 3: 115-121.

[73] Amaro, C., Toranzo, A. E., Gonzalez, E. A., Blanco, J., Pujalte, M. J., Aznar, R. & Garay, E. (1990). Surface and virulence properties of environmental *Vibrio cholerae* non-O1 from Albufera Lake (Valencia, Spain). Applied and Environmental Microbiology, 56: 1140-1147.

[74] Booth, B. A., Finkelstein, R. A. (1986). Presence of hemagglutinin/protease and other potential virulence factors in O1 and non-O1 *Vibrio cholerae*. Journal of the Infectious Diseases, 154: 183-186.

[75] Baffone, W., Citterio, B., Vittoria, E., Casaroli, A., Pianetti, A., Campana, R., Bruscolini, F. 2001 Determination of several potential virulence factors in *Vibrio* spp. isolated from seawater. Food Microbiology, 18: 479-488.

[76] Saga T., Yamaguchi K., "History of antimicrobial agents and resistant bacteria," Japan Medical Association Journal, vol. 52, pp. 103-108, 2009.

[77] Carlet, J. P., Collignon, D., Goldmann D., Goossens, H., Gyssens I. C., Harbarth, S., Jarlier, V., Levy, S. B., N'Doye B., Pittet, D., Richtmann, R., Seto, W. H., Van der Meer J. WM., Voss, A. (2011). "Society's failure to protect a precious resource: antibiotics" Lancet, 378(9788): 369-371,

[78] Finley, R. L., Collignon, P., Larsson, D. G. J. McEwen, S. A., Li, X-Z., Gaze, W. H., Reid-Smith, R., Timinouni, M., Graham, D. W., Topp, E. (2013). "The scourge of antibiotic resistance: the important role of the environment". Clinical Infectious Diseases, 57(5): 704-710.

[79] Garg, P., Chakraborty, S., Basu, I., Datta, S., Rajendran, K., Bhattacharya, T., Yamasaki, S., Bhattacharya, S. K., Takeda, Y., Nair, G. B., Ramamurthy, T. (2000). Expanding multiple antibiotic resistance among clinical strains of *Vibrio cholerae* isolated from 1992-7 in Calcutta. India. Epidemiology and Infection, 124: 393-399.

[80] Thiagarajah, J. R., Verkman, A. S. (2005). New drug targets for cholera therapy. Trends in Pharmacological Sciences, 26: 172-176.

[81] Yamamoto, T., Nair, G. B., Takeda, Y. (1995). Emergence of tetracycline resistance due to a multiple drug resistance plasmid in *Vibrio cholerae* O139. FEMS Immunology and Medical Microbiology, 11: 131-136.

[82] Trucksis, M., Michalski, J., Deng, Y. K., Kaper, J. B. (1998). The *Vibrio cholerae* genome contains two unique circular chromosomes. Proceeding of the National Academy of sciences of the United States of America. 95: 14464-14469.

[83] Louis, V.R., Russek-Cohen, E., Choopun, N., Rivera, I.N., Gangle, B., Jiang, S.C., Rubin, A., Patz, J.A., Huq, A., Colwell R. R. (2003). Predictability of *Vibrio cholerae* in Chesapeake Bay. Applied Environmental Microbiology, 69: 2773-2785.

[84] Oufdou, K., Mezrioui, N., Ait Melloul, A., Barakate, M. Ait alla, A. (1999). Effects of sunlight and *Synechocystis* sp. (picocyanobacterium) on the incidence of antibiotic resistance in waste water enteric bacteria. World Journal of Microbiology and Biotechnology. 15: 553-559.

[85] Kelch, W. J., Lee, J. S. (1978). Antibiotic resistance patterns of gram-negative bacteria isolated from environmental sources. Applied Environmental Microbiology, 36: 450-456.

[86] Hassani, L., Imziln, B., Boussaid, A., Gauthier, M. J. (1992).

Antibiotic-resistant *Escherichia coli* from wastewater before and after treatment in stabilization ponds in the arid region of Marrakesh, Morocco. Letters in Applied Microbiology, 15: 228-231.

[87] Radu, S., Vincent, M., Apum, K., Abdul Rahim, R., Benjamin, P. G., Yuherman Rusul, G. (2002). Molecular characterization of *Vibrio cholerae* O1 outbreak strains in Miri, Srawak (Malaysia). Acta Tropica, 83: 169-176.

[88] Pathak, S. P., Bhattacherjee J. W., Ray P. K. (1993). Seasonal variation in survival and antibiotic resistance among various bacterial populations in a tropical river. Journal of General and Applied Microbiology, 39: 47-56.

[89] Lu, B., Zhou, H., Li, D., Li, F., Zhu, F., Cui, Y., Huang, L., Wang, D. (2014). The first case of bacteraemia due to non-O1/non-O139 *Vibrio cholerae* from type 2 diabetes mellitus in mainland China. International Journal of Infectious Diseases, 25:116-118

[90] El-Zanfaly, H. T., Hosny, I., Fayez, M., Shaban, A. M. (1988). Incidence of antibiotic resistant bacteria in undergroundwater. Environment International, 14: 391-394.

[91] Amundsen, D., Lindholm, C., Goyal, S. M., Robinson, R. A. (1988). Microbial pollution of well water in south-eastern Minnesota. Journal of Environmental Science and Health, 23: 453-468.

[92] Bell, J. B., Elliott, G. E., Smith, D. W. (1983). Influence of sewage treatment and urbanization on selection of multiple resistance in faecal coliform populations. Applied Environmental Microbiology, 46: 227-232.

Chapter 7

Community Change and Pathogenicity of *Vibrio*

Lixing Huang, Qiancheng Gao, Youyu Zhang, Wei Xu and Qingpi Yan

Abstract

Vibrio is a rod-shaped Gram-negative bacteria, which is widely distributed in marine and estuarine environments worldwide. It is an important component of the aquatic ecosystem and plays an important role in biogeochemical cycle. Its population dynamics are usually affected by climate and seasonal factors. Most of the *Vibrios* in the environment are not pathogenic, but some of them are pathogenic bacteria for human and animal, such as *Vibrio* cholerae, *Vibrio* vulnificus, *Vibrio parahaemolyticus*, and *Vibrio* anguillarum, etc., which are generally reported to be related to aquatic animal diseases and human food-borne diseases. Over the last couple of years, due to the influence of the rising seawater temperature and climate change, the incidence of diseases caused by *Vibrio* infection has increased significantly, which poses a great threat to human health and aquaculture. The research on pathogenic *Vibrio* has attracted more and more attention. The abundance and community changes of *Vibrio* in the environment are usually controlled by many biological and abiotic factors. The *Vibrio* pathogenicity is related to the virulence factors encoded by virulence genes. The process of *Vibrio* infecting the host and causing host disease is determined by multiple virulence factors acting together, instead of being determined by a single virulence factor. In this chapter, community changes of *Vibrio*, as well as the virulence factors of *Vibrio* and the related virulence genes of Vibiro are summarized, and their important roles in *Vibrio* infection are also discussed.

Keywords: *Vibrio*, community change, foodborne diseases, pathogenicity, virulence factors

1. Introduction

The *Vibrio* belongs to the *Vibrionaceae* family of the *Gammaproteobacteria*, is a thermophilic, rod-shaped, heterotrophic Gram-negative bacterium [1]. *Vibrio* has genetic and metabolic diversity, and there are great phenotypic and genotypic differences among different species. It widely exists in estuaries and marine habitats all over the world and is an important part of aquatic ecosystems [2].

Vibrio usually has chemotaxis and motility, which can quickly respond to fluctuations of nutrient concentration and make use of nutrients in the environment to grow rapidly [3, 4]. In addition, *Vibrio* has the ability to degrade the common carbon substrates. It can decompose and utilize a variety of substrates by producing chitinase, protease, lipase and other extracellular proteases. The production and secretion of these enzymes can provide *Vibrio* rich nutrients unavailable for other organisms, enabling *Vibrio* to quickly transform from a relatively small part to a dominant bacteria in response to environmental and climate changes [5]. *Vibrio* plays an important role in the biogeochemical cycle, which regulates inorganic nutrients and carbon flux by fixing and re-mineralize nutrients [6].

Most *Vibrio* are not pathogenic, but there are several *Vibrio* that are pathogens of humans, fish, shellfish, or other species and can cause a range of clinical manifestations including gastroenteritis, acute diarrhea, sepsis, narcotizing soft tissue infection, high mortality in cultured aquatic animals, and, in some reported cases, human death [7–10]. Vibriosis usually occurs by eating raw or under cooked seafood products, drinking contaminated water, or by direct contact with the contaminated environment through wounds [11, 12]. In the United States, the most common cause of gastroenteritis is the consumption of oysters infected or under cooked with *V. parahaemolyticus* [13]. According to the report of the Centers for Disease Control and Prevention (CDC) in 2006, *V. parahaemolyticus* is a major food-borne pathogen in the United States, and there are about 34,664 food-borne cases every year [14]. In another report, 80,000 people were infected with food-borne *Vibrio* annually in the United States in 2016, resulting in more than 500 hospitalizations and 100 deaths, the vast majority of which were *V. vulnificus* and *V. parahaemolyticus* [15]. Moreover, *V.parahaemolyticus* is a common source of food borne disease in Asian countries such as China, Japan and South Koala [7].

Aquaculture is a fast growing sector and continues to grow to meet the increasing global demand for seafood. From 2000 to 2017, aquaculture business grew by approximately 150%. China is the world's largest aquaculture producer (accounting for 58% of global production) producing 46.8 million tons of aquaculture animals per year [9]. In order to further meet the needs of the national economy and food security, the mariculture industry in southern China has gradually developed into intensive and industrialized [16]. However, high-density farming, severe human activities and global climate change have led to frequent Vibriosis, which has posed a huge threat to human health and social and economic development [17]. Vibriosis is one of the most common bacterial diseases affecting a variety of marine fish and shellfish [18, 19]. Studies have demonstrated that the content of *Vibrio* in aquaculture facilities is very high, especially during the outbreak of disease. The culturable *Vibrio* community in the affected facilities is composed of single or few *Vibrio* species, including *V. alginolyticus*, *V. parahaemolyticus*, *V. vulnificus* and *Vibrio harveyi*. These species include human and animal pathogens, which can lead to high mortality of aquatic animals [20]. For example, from May 2000 to November 2003, the mortality rate of large yellow croakers reared in marine cages due to infection with *V. alginolyticus* and *V. harveyi* ranged from 30% to 40% and even as high as 80% in Zhejiang province, China [21]. In addition, wastewater from aquaculture farms is often released to the environment without treatment, potentially causing large quantities of pathogenic *Vibrio* to enter the environment, posing a potential threat to human health. Therefore, understanding the dynamic changes of *Vibrio* community and the pathogenicity of *Vibrio* is of great significance for the healthy development of aquaculture and reducing the impact on human public health [22, 23].

2. Dynamic changes of *Vibrio* community

2.1 Abundance of *Vibrio*

Vibrio are widely distributed in estuaries and marine environments, and mainly in nearshore areas. *Vibrio* generally exhibit two different growth strategies, either as a free-living form or attached to biological or non-biological surfaces, where they can co-exist with the host or cause host disease [24]. For example, some *Vibrio* living in squid or other organisms can be used as the source of luminescence of light-emitting organs and also an important part of the combination of biofilm and macroalgae [25].

Vibrio easily grow on conventional medium (such as seawater 2216E agar medium) and selective medium (such as thiosulfate citrate bile salt sucrose agar medium, TCBS) and can carry out a variety of metabolic activities [26]. In some studies based on culture, *Vibrio* can account for 10% of culturable marine bacteria [27], and the average abundance in estuaries and nearshore waters is 103 ~ 106 CFU L−1. However, in studies using non-culture methods, *Vibrio* population only accounts for about 1% of the total plankton bacteria in nearshore waters, and the average abundance in estuaries and nearshore waters is $10^4 \sim 10^8$ 16 s rRNA copies L^{-1} [28]. Their *Vibrio* abundance was found to be between 15 and 2395 CFU mL^{-1} in a study of tropical estuaries and coastal water in Malaysia [29]. In addition, studies have shown a high density of *Vibrio* on the surface and in the body of marine animals such as fish, shrimp, mollusks, corals, sponges, zooplankton, algae and seaweed [30]. For example, in a study examining the effects of aquaculture on *Vibrio* communities, the relative abundance of the 16SrRNA gene sequence reads 16 from seaweed samples were the highest by sequencing water, sediment, seaweed and tissue samples obtained in the aquaculture area of Hainan [9]. This is also consistent with studies describing *Vibrio* communities as important components of seagrass bacterial communities. These bacteria account for 25% of the culturable bacteria in seaweed off the coast of Hainan province [31].

2.2 Diversity of *Vibrio*

At least 110 *Vibrios* have been found and reported, and more may be found in the future. Among the *Vibrios* that have been described, several are commonly associated with human diseases, among which *V. cholerae*, *V. parahaemolyticus*, and *V. vulnificus* are recognized as human pathogenic bacteria, while *Vibrio alginolyticus*, *V. anguillarum*, *V. harveyi*, *Vibrio* fluvialis, *Vibrio* furniss, *Vibrio* metschnikovii, and *Vibrio* mimicus are primarily marine animal pathogenic bacteria but occasionally associated with human infections [32–36].

Vibrio usually has species-specific salinity and temperature preferences, and different kinds of *Vibrio* may exist in different environments. They exit from deep-sea hydrothermal vents and sediment are more than 6, 000 meters deep to seawater 10, 500 meters deep in the mariana trench [37, 38]. For example, the optimal growth temperature and salinity for *Vibrio devil*, first isolated from deep-sea hydrothermal vents, is 30 ~ 45 °C and 20 ~ 50 ppt, respectively [39]. The salinity-dependent *Vibrio* carinii is mainly present in seawater in the range of salinity from the Baltic Sea to the Mediterranean Sea [40]. *Vibrio pacinii*, *Vibrio cyclotrophicus*, *Vibrio lentus*, and some unnamed *Vibrio* have also been found at low temperatures [32].

At present, studies on the diversity of *Vibrio* communities in marine environments are mainly based on *Vibrio* isolated and cultured [41]. However, due to the low interspecific resolution of the 16S rRNA gene, the use of 16S rRNA gene similarity as a major interspecific marker for the phylogenetic relationships of *Vibrios* appears to have lost its effect. Multiple-locus sequence analysis (MLSA) and other novel phylogenetic markers such as the iron absorption regulatory gene *fur* have been used as alternative approaches [42, 43]. In order to study the diversity of environmental *Vibrio*, Siboni et al. first extracted DNA from seawater, and then used 16S rRNA gene primers specific to *Vibrio* to conduct high-throughput sequencing, thus making it possible to more intuitively and effectively explore the diversity of *Vibrio* communities [44]. In another study by Bei et al., the abundance and community structure of *Vibrio* species at different depths was studied using *Vibrio-specific* 16S rRNA gene high-throughput sequencing and quantitative PCR (qPCR) techniques as well as traditional culture methods [5].

2.3 The influence of environmental factors on *Vibrio* community

In a marine environment, abundance and community composition of *Vibrio* is affected by many factors, including temperature, salinity, pH, water depth, dissolved oxygen and transparency [45, 46]. Chemical factors are mainly the concentrations of inorganic and organic nutrients. In addition, biological factors such as protozoa, viruses, marine animals and algae also affect the change of *Vibrio* community. Therefore, under the interaction between biological and non-biological factors, the *Vibrio* community in the environment shows complex dynamic changes.

The abundance and community structure of *Vibrio* in seawater is generally considered to be related to temperature and salinity. Temperature is the most important factor affecting the change of *Vibrio* community. Under general conditions, the relationship between *Vibrio* and water temperature shows a positive correlation. Growth of *Vibrio* population can be observed in short-term temperature rise and long-term temperature change related to climate change [47–49]. At present, many coastal areas around the world have been reported an increase in the number of *Vibrio*. For example, some researchers have used continuous plankton recording equipment to show that the increase in sea temperature has caused an increase in the number of *Vibrio* in parts of the North Atlantic and North Sea [50]. In Peru, Alaska and the gulf of Mexico and other regions also reported that due to the increase in water temperature, some pathogenic *Vibrio* species began to increase [51]. Moreover, some cases of infection caused by *Vibrio* have also been reported to be associated with abnormally high water temperatures [52].

Salinity was the second largest factor affecting the abundance of *Vibrio*, and *Vibrio* had a positive correlation with salinity, but the relationship might also be covered by increases in temperature and nutrient concentration [53, 54]. Not only that, some studies found that short-term salinity changes do increase the concentration of *Vibrio*, but long-term salinity changes have no significant effect on the overall trend of *Vibrio*, for example, there are studies found that abundance of *Vibrio* is affected by salinity and chlorophyll A concentration, but only when the salinity is less than 20 ppt, the effect of salinity is significant [29]. In another study on the abundance of microbial communities in Guanabara Bay, the researchers constructed an artificial neural network that could simulate the response of environmental microbial communities to environmental parameters. The results showed that temperature had a positive correlation with the abundance of *Vibrio*, and salinity had a negative correlation with the abundance of *Vibrio*. Transparency had a positive correlation with chlorophyll concentration but had little to do with the number of *Vibrio*. Moreover, these physical parameters were more related to the abundance of *Vibrio* than in total phosphorus and total nitrogen [55]. The authors deduced that due to the high degree of eutrophication in the bay, the microbial community had reached its maximum capacity to absorb and utilize nutrients, and the growth of the microflora was no longer restricted by nutrients. On the contrary, salinity, temperature and transparency jointly determined the number of *Vibrio*.

Although the composition and abundance of *Vibrio* communities are closely related to temperature and salinity, in temperate regions, concentrations of organic and inorganic nutrients and phytoplankton communities appear to be more important drivers of seasonal changes in *Vibrio* communities because annual changes in temperature are not significant.

In a study of wetlands in Macchiatonda Regional Nature Reserve, it was found that the CFU abundance of TCBS depended on temperature and salinity, and the effect of temperature was greater than that of salinity (27% and 20%, respectively), but since temperature and salinity accounted for only 40% of the total CFU abundance, other environmental and biological factors had to play a role in driving *Vibrio* abundance in the system of the region [32]. In another ten-year study of the mouth of the Newz River in North Carolina, the United States, it seems that similar views have been confirmed. During the study, the temperature of the estuary did not change significantly, but the number of some *Vibrios* closely related to the temperature increased. The salinity of the estuary showed a trend of increasing to the highest and decreasing during the study. The increase of the number of *Vibrio* in the estuary had to be in conformity with the decrease in salinity. When the salinity increased, the number of *Vibrios* in the mouth of the river increased. Some specific *Vibrio*, such as *V. vulnificus*, had almost declined to undetectable levels, and the final conclusion was that the concentration of *Vibrio* in the area appeared to be independent of changes in the three factors commonly used to predict *Vibrio* abundance, including salinity, temperature, and dissolved oxygen. Although the overall abundance of *Vibrio* was on the rise, the number of some potential pathogenic species was decreasing, and the concentration of *Vibrio* in the estuaries was predicted to be related to nitrogen and carbon in the environment [2]. In addition, studies have shown that ammonium radical promotes the growth of *Vibrio*, while silicic acid and phosphate have opposite effects on *Vibrio* population [56]. Dissolved organic carbon (DOC) has a strong impact on the ecology of *Vibrio.* DOC provides a large amount of nutrients needed for *Vibrio* living in estuarine and marine habitats. *Vibrio* can absorb, metabolize and produce organic matter, thus changing its chemical properties and bioavailability [57]. Therefore, in temperate regions where the temperature is relatively stable, factors other than physical parameters such as temperature and salinity may play a more important role. However, when the degree of nutrition is high and the microbial community has reached the maximum capacity to absorb and utilize nutrition, physical factors are more relevant to the abundance of *Vibrio*.

Dissolved oxygen is an important hydrological parameter, which affects the number of *Vibrio* bacteria by affecting their metabolism. Due to hypoxia, the *Vibrio* population will switch from breathing mode to fermentation mode [58]. The abundance of free-living and particulate-related fractions of *Vibrio* was negatively correlated with dissolved oxygen (48.7% ~ 105.8% saturation) in the coastal area of georgia, USA [59]. A negative correlation between *Vibrio* abundance and dissolved oxygen (5 ~ 11 mg L^{-1}) was found in the North Carolina estuary [60]. In addition, a study on Yongle Blue Cave in Sansha, Hainan, China found that in the deepest Blue Cave in the world, due to the strong stratification limiting the vertical exchange of oxygen, the water body was divided into an upper aerobic zone and a lower anoxic zone. The strong DO gradient resulted in no significant correlation between *Vibrio* abundance and temperature, but *Vibrio* abundance was very high at a depth of 100 m (the interface between aerobic and anoxic) [5].

In addition to physical factors, biological factors also play an important role in affecting changes in the *Vibrio* community. The virus has a strong lethal effect on *Vibrio* and can greatly affect the change of *Vibrio* community. Some researchers have identified a virus with a wide host range from infected *Vibrio*, which can kill 34 *Vibrio* strains of four species [61]. For some special species, changes in biological factors may have a stronger effect on their abundance than non-biological parameters [62, 63]. Recently, it has been proved that there is a significant correlation between the abundance of particle-associated *Vibrio* and the community composition of phytoplankton, and it is speculated that this may be related to the bioavailability of dissolved organic matter released from phytoplankton [64].

Finally, *Vibrio* can enter a viable but non-culturable state (VBNC) under adverse environmental conditions (such as oligotrophic, excessively high or low temperature, high salt, extreme pH, and sunlight radiation). This physiological state is reversible, and when the conditions become favorable again, the pathogen will recover [65]. The cells could still survive in this dormant state, but it could not be detected by the traditional culture method, which might show a higher resistance to exogenous stress and maintain the active virulence factors [66]. However, conditions for *Vibrio* to enter "recovery" from "dormancy" are not completely clear.

3. Pathogenicity of *Vibrio*

Vibrio is usually reported being related to food-borne diseases and aquaculture diseases. Diseases or even death of aquatic animals caused by *Vibrio* infection have been reported worldwide and are showing an increasing trend [7, 11, 18, 67]. Therefore, Vibriosis has caused significant impacts on human health and the development of aquaculture [68–70]. The pathogenicity of *Vibrio* is determined by multiple virulence factors encoded by its virulence genes [71–74]. *Vibrio* infects and destroys the host through a series of processes, including adhesion, invasion, immune escape, in vivo proliferation and production of toxins [46]. *Vibrio* mainly includes adhesion factor, the capsule and polysaccharide, cytotoxin and other virulence factors [75]. Therefore, infection and pathogenesis of *Vibrio* are not completed by a single virulence factor, but the result of the combined action of multiple virulence factors.

3.1 Adhesion factor

Adhesion is the prerequisite for pathogenic bacteria to cause disease to the body infection, and it is of great significance in invading the host and effectively exerting the virulence [76]. Adhesion is mainly achieved by adhesion factors that specifically recognize and bind to host cells, the ability of *Vibrio* to adhere to and form biofilm on the surfaces of organisms and non-organisms can enhance the virulence and pathogenicity of *Vibrio* [77]. Moreover, adhesion is strongly related to the biofilm formation ability, movement ability and quorum sensing of bacterial [78].

Adhesion factor is a kind of macromolecular substance that can make pathogenic bacteria adhere to the surface of eukaryotic cells, and it plays an important role in the host infection process of *Vibrio*. *Vibrio* has a variety of adhesin, such as fimbriae, cilia, outer membrane protein (OMP), lipopolysaccharide (LPS), extracellular polysaccharide, etc. Among them, fimbriae and cilia belong to fimbriae adhesin, while OMP, LPS, and extracellular polysaccharides belong to non-pilin adhesin [79]. The exposure of OMP to the bacterial surface is a unique and important component of the outer membrane of Gram-negative bacteria, which plays an important role in maintaining the outer membrane structure, ensuring the transport of substances, and stimulating the body to produce antibodies and cytokines. It has been found that the outer membrane protein is an important pathogenic factor closely related to the process of bacterial adhesion and iron uptake [80]. LPS is a lipopolysaccharide substance located in the outermost layer of the cell wall of Gram-negative bacteria. It is not only the main component of the cell wall of Gram-negative bacteria, but also the material basis for the endotoxin of the virulence factor of Gram-negative pathogens [81]. In *Vibrio* pathogens (such as *V. anguillarum*, *V.*

vulnificus, V. cholerae, V. mimicus, V. parahaemolyticus, etc.), LPS has been proven to be an important pathogenic factor [82].

Although *Vibrio* has a variety of adhesion factors, previous studies on the adhesion of *Vibrio* generally focused on flagellum, and some researchers proposed that flagellum plays an irreplaceable role in the adhesion process of bacteria-infected host [83]. According to the location of the flagellum, the flagellum can be divided into two types: terminal flagellum and peri-flagellum. Belas investigated the differences in the adsorption characteristics of *Vibrio* with different types of flagellum on chitin, and found that peri-flagellum had a stronger affinity for chitin than terminal flagellum [84]. The adhesion of *V. alginolyticus* to the epidermal mucus of *Sparus macrocephalus* was studied by Bordas, which also proved this viewpoint [85]. In addition, studies have found that pili seems to have a strong correlation with the pathogenicity of *Vibrio*. Wright first found in 1989, most clinical isolates of *V. vulnificus* have pili, while environmental isolates lack pili [86]. Analysis of pili protein gene expression during infection indicated that the pili protein expression of the strong strain was higher than that of the weak strain [87]. Moreover, the mobility of the strain was also one of the main factors affecting the adhesion. Kogure found that under the condition of having flagella at the same time, strains with mobility showed faster and stronger adhesion than the strains without mobility [88].

3.2 Capsular and polysaccharide

After entering the host, bacteria usually activate the host immune system to cause a series of immune responses to eliminate pathogens [89]. In order to survive and reproduce in the host, bacteria must adopt a series of strategies to improve their viability and virulence in the host as well as their resistance to phagocytosis and antibiotics.

The correlation between the capsular and polysaccharide and virulence has been confirmed [90]. The capsule encapsulated on the surface of bacteria is a dense, high molecular weight capsule that plays a major role in evading the host's immune defense. The encapsulated pathogen shows strong resistance to phagocytosis and complement-mediated lethality. Studies have shown that organisms with capsular polysaccharides are more likely to survive in serum, that isolates expressing opaque colonies are more resistant to serum than translucent isolates, and there are differences in colony characteristics between seafood isolates and clinical isolates. Clinical isolates were more resistant to serum complement proteins than environmental isolates, and the clinical genotype had a consistent survival advantage when exposed to serum [91–93]. In addition, the formation of biofilm will also promote the adhesion of pathogens to the host, coordinate the quorum sensing between bacteria, and improve the resistance of pathogens to antibiotics, playing a major role in the escape of pathogens from host immunity.

3.3 Cytotoxins

Cytotoxic is the main killer factor of pathogens in the process of attacking the host. Toxins secreted by *Vibrio* can be divided into endotoxin and exotoxin. Endotoxin is the lipid part of lipopolysaccharide released after cell death, and the exotoxin is secreted out of cells to cause damage to the host. At present, the toxins produced by *Vibrio* have been studied in depth, and the expression of many virulence factors is related to the pathogenicity of *Vibrio*, including: Thermostable direct hemolysin (TDH), TDH-related hemolysin (TRH), *V. vulnificus* cytolytic toxin (VVC), cholera toxin (CT), and zonulaoccludens toxin (Zot).

V. parahaemolyticus is one of the main bacterial isolates of food poisoning caused by seafood contamination and is usually associated with outbreaks of foodborne diseases [11]. The thermostable direct hemolysin (TDH) and TDH-related hemolysin (TRH) encoded by the *tdh* and *trh* genes are considered to be the main virulence factors of *V. parahaemolyticus*. TDH has a variety of biological activities, such as hemolytic activity, cytotoxicity, cardiotoxicity and enterictoxicity. TDH is a perforated toxin, and its toxic mechanism is to create pores with a diameter of 0 ~ 2 nm on the erythrocyte membrane, among which the larger pores can make the water and ions in the cells flow out of the cell membrane, and changes in these ion fluxes in the intestine are also the main cause of diarrhea [94, 95]. TRH is a thermolabile toxin, which is similar to TDH in immunology, and can also activate chloride channels and cause changes in ion flux [96]. TDH and TRH share approximately 70% homology [97], and these two genes are considered to be the most important virulence markers of *V. parahaemolyticus* and are commonly used for virulence testing of *V. parahaemolyticus* [98].

V. vulnificus is a conditionally pathogenic human pathogen, which can cause severe wound infection, acute gastroenteritis and life-threatening septicemia. In susceptible or immunocompromised individuals, the mortality rate exceeds 50% [99]. VVC encoded by *VvhA* gene of *V. vulnificus* is the key virulence factor of *V. vulnificus,* which mainly plays a role through two mechanisms: cytolysis and apoptosis induction [100]. VVC has species specificity in *V. vulnificus*, which is the only exotoxin that can be secreted out of cells, and belongs to cholesterol-dependent cytolysin of pore-forming protein family [101]. The cytotoxic mechanism of cytotoxin is that it combines with non-esterified cholesterol on cell membrane and aggregates on the cell surface, which makes the cell membrane form a channel and leads to the outflow of intracellular potassium ions, which leads to the rupture of colloid permeable cells. The main mechanism of apoptosis induced by cytotoxin is related to mitochondria. Cytotoxin can lead to the production of mitochondrial reactive oxygen species (ROS) in intestinal epithelial cells, and then lead to cell necrosis and apoptosis [102].

V. cholerae has caused several epidemics in history. Cholera toxin (CT) is the main pathogenic factor of O1/O139 *V. cholerae*, which can cause serious damage to intestinal cell function and lead to cholera watery secretory diarrhea [103]. CT is encoded by *ctxA* and *ctxB*. These genes are encoded by CTXΦ of lysogenic filamentous phage and can be transferred between virulent and non-virulent strains [104]. *zot* is also encoded by lysogenic filamentous bacteriophage CTXΦ [105], and its encoded zona-linked toxin (ZOT) is the second virulence index of *V. cholerae*, which can make mucosal cells adhere together, maintain the tight connection structure of mucosal integrity and increase the permeability of intestinal mucosa [106]. Except as a cytotoxin, Zot seems to be related to the assembly of CTX phage in structure and function. *Zot* gene has sequence homology with the coat protein gene, which is probably the coat protein of CTX Φ. This indicates that it may have dual functions [107].

3.4 Other virulence factors

In addition to secreting toxins, some pathogenic bacteria can secrete a variety of extracellular products, which are also the main factors causing host diseases. For example, Balebona and Morinigo discovered in 1995 that the extracellular products of *V. alginolyticus* have various enzyme activities such as caseinase, gelatinase, amylase, phospholipase, collagenase, etc., and these extracellular products have strong toxicity to fish cells, which can dissolve fish cells and cause fish death [108]. Balebona et al. infected fish by intramuscular injection with extracellular protease.

After 6 h, it was observed that the injected extracellular products were lysed, which could lead to fish death in 24 ~ 72 h [109]. Lee et al. found that alkaline serine protease produced by *V.* alginolyticus can reduce thrombin in prawn plasma and prevent hemolymph from agglutinating, which is one of the main lethal factors secreted by *V. alginolyticus. V. vulnificus* metalloproteinases (VVP) is a kind of zinc ion-dependent protease with hemolysis. Miyoshi et al. studies have proved that VVP can enhance vascular permeability, destroy the basement membrane, cause bleeding reaction, cause cell and tissue damage, and eventually develop into sepsis [110].

Iron, as an indispensable trace element, is also an important component of various cellular enzymes, and plays an important role in the growth, reproduction, pathogenicity and cellular metabolism of pathogenic bacteria [111]. The iron carrier of *Vibrio* is an important pathogenic factor, and the iron uptake system mediated by it plays a very important role in bacterial growth and host colonization. Under the condition of lack of iron, the strain will produce a chelation agent iron carrier with high affinity for heme iron ions and low molecular weight, and the iron absorbed from transferrin and lactoferrin will be transported to bacterial cells for its own use through the receptor [112].

4. Conclusion

Vibrio, as a kind of human and animal pathogen, exists widely in the world, and its increasing number and pathogenicity are great challenges to human public health and healthy aquaculture. The changes of *Vibrio* community in the environment are related to abiotic factors (temperature, salinity, pH, water depth, dissolved oxygen, transparency, nutrient concentration, etc.) and biological factors (protozoa, viruses, marine animals and algae, etc.), among which temperature and salinity are considered to be the most important factors affecting the changes of *Vibrio* community, but in temperate regions where salinity and temperature are relatively stable, nutrient concentration and phytoplankton community contribute more to the changes of *Vibrio* community. In recent years, with the outbreak of *Vibrio* in some areas caused by climate change and rising seawater temperature, the number of some pathogenic *Vibrio* began to increase. The pathogenicity of *Vibrio* is related to virulence factors encoded by virulence genes (adhesion factors, cytotoxins, extracellular enzymes, capsular polysaccharides, iron uptake system, etc.), and different virulence factors play different roles in the infection process. In this chapter, the influencing factors of *Vibrio* community change and various virulence factors of *Vibrio* in the process of infecting the host were summarized, in order to provide reference and help for human public health and aquaculture industry.

Author details

Lixing Huang[1*], Qiancheng Gao[1], Youyu Zhang[2], Wei Xu[3] and Qingpi Yan[1]

1 Fisheries College, Key Laboratory of Healthy Mariculture for the East China Sea, Ministry of Agriculture, Jimei University, Xiamen, Fujian, PR China

2 Institute of Electromagnetics and Acoustics, School of Electronic Science and Engineering, Xiamen University, Xiamen, Fujian, PR China

3 Third Institute of Oceanography, Ministry of Natural Resources, Xiamen, PR China

*Address all correspondence to: lixinghuang@outlook.com

References

[1] Thompson FL, Iida T, Swings J. Biodiversity of vibrios. Microbiol Mol Biol Rev, 2004,68(3): 403-431.

[2] Froelich B, Gonzalez R, Blackwood D, et al. Decadal monitoring reveals an increase in Vibrio spp. concentrations in the Neuse River Estuary, North Carolina, USA. PLoS One, 2019,14(4): e215254.

[3] Westrich JR, Griffin DW, Westphal DL, et al. Vibrio Population Dynamics in Mid-Atlantic Surface Waters during Saharan Dust Events. Frontiers in Marine Science, 2018,5.

[4] Huang L, Huang L, Zhao L, et al. The regulation of oxidative phosphorylation pathway on Vibrio alginolyticus adhesion under adversities. MicrobiologyOpen, 2019.

[5] Bei L, Jiwen L, Shun Z, et al. Vertical variation in Vibrio community composition in Sansha Yongle Blue Hole and its ability to degrade macromolecules. Marine Life Science & Technology, 2020,2(1).

[6] Zeng J, Lin Y, Zhao D, et al. Seasonality overwhelms aquacultural activity in determining the composition and assembly of the bacterial community in Lake Taihu, China. Sci Total Environ, 2019,683: 427-435.

[7] Dahanayake PS, Silva BCJD, Hossain S, et al. Occurrence, virulence factors, and antimicrobial susceptibility patterns of Vibrio spp. isolated from live oyster (*Crassostrea gigas*) in Korea. Journal of food safety, 2018,38(5): e12490.

[8] Ford CL, Powell A, Lau D, et al. Isolation and characterization of potentially pathogenic Vibrio species in a temperate, higher latitude hotspot. Environ Microbiol Rep, 2020,12(4): 424-434.

[9] Möller L, Kreikemeyer B, Luo Z, et al. Impact of coastal aquaculture operation systems in Hainan island (China) on the relative abundance and community structure of Vibrio in adjacent coastal systems. Estuarine, coastal and shelf science, 2020,233: 106542.

[10] Huang L, Guo L, Xu X, et al. The role of rpoS in the regulation of Vibrio alginolyticus virulence and the response to diverse stresses. J Fish Dis, 2019,42(5): 703-712.

[11] Jeamsripong S, Khant W, Chuanchuen R. Distribution of phenotypic and genotypic antimicrobial resistance and virulence genes in *Vibrio parahaemolyticus* isolated from cultivated oysters and estuarine water. FEMS Microbiol Ecol, 2020,96(8).

[12] Zuo Y, Zhao L, Xu X, et al. Mechanisms underlying the virulence regulation of new Vibrio alginolyticus ncRNA Vvrr1 with a comparative proteomic analysis. Emerg Microbes Infect, 2019,8(1): 1604-1618.

[13] Daniels NA, Mackinnon L, Bishop R, et al. *Vibrio parahaemolyticus* Infections in the United States, 1973-1998. The Journal of infectious diseases, 2000,181(5): 1661-1666.

[14] Scallan E, Hoekstra RM, Angulo FJ, et al. Foodborne illness acquired in the United States--major pathogens. Emerg Infect Dis, 2011,17(1): 7-15.

[15] FoodNet 2015 Annual Foodborne Illness Surveillance Report[R].

[16] Hong W, Zhang Q. Review of captive bred species and fry production of marine fish in China. Aquaculture, 2003,227(1): 305-318.

[17] Xu X, Huang L, Su Y, et al. The complete genome sequence of Vibrio aestuarianus W-40 reveals virulence

factor genes. Microbiologyopen, 2018,7(3): e568.

[18] Deng Y, Xu L, Chen H, et al. Prevalence, virulence genes, and antimicrobial resistance of Vibrio species isolated from diseased marine fish in South China. Sci Rep, 2020,10(1): 14329.

[19] Guo L, Huang L, Su Y, et al. secA, secD, secF, yajC, and yidC contribute to the adhesion regulation of Vibrio alginolyticus. Microbiologyopen, 2018,7(2): e551.

[20] Huang L, Wang L, Lin X, et al. mcp, aer, cheB, and cheV contribute to the regulation of Vibrio alginolyticus (ND-01) adhesion under gradients of environmental factors. Microbiologyopen, 2017,6(6).

[21] Jin S, Wang G, Zhao Q, et al. Epidemiology of vibriosis in large yellow croaker *Pseudosciaena crocea* (richardson) in marine cage culture[Z]. 2005: 24, 17-19.

[22] Sung HH, Hsu SF, Chen CK, et al. Relationships between disease outbreak in cultured tiger shrimp (*Penaeus monodon*) and the composition of Vibrio communities in pond water and shrimp hepatopancreas during cultivation. Aquaculture, 2001,192(2-4): 101-110.

[23] Al-Harbi AH, Uddin N. Bacterial diversity of tilapia (*Oreochromis niloticus*) cultured in brackish water in Saudi Arabia. Aquaculture, 2005,250 (3-4): 566-572.

[24] Reen FJ, Almagro-Moreno S, Ussery D, et al. The genomic code: inferring Vibrionaceae niche specialization. Nat Rev Microbiol, 2006,4(9): 697-704.

[25] Fidopiastis PM, Boletzky SV, Ruby EG. A new niche for Vibrio logei, the predominant light organ symbiont of squids in the genus Sepiola. J Bacteriol, 1998,180(1): 59-64.

[26] Thompson FL, Brian A, Jean S. The Biology of Vibrios[M]. ASM Press, 2006.

[27] Eilers H, Pernthaler J, Glockner FO, et al. Culturability and In situ abundance of pelagic bacteria from the North Sea. Appl Environ Microbiol, 2000,66(7): 3044-3051.

[28] Thompson JR, Polz MF. Dynamics of Vibrio Populations and Their Role in Environmental Nutrient Cycling[M]. John Wiley & Sons, Ltd, 2014.

[29] Wong YY, Lee CW, Bong CW, et al. Environmental control of Vibrio spp. abundance and community structure in tropical waters. FEMS Microbiol Ecol, 2019,95(11).

[30] Liu W, Huang L, Su Y, et al. Contributions of the oligopeptide permeases in multistep of Vibrio alginolyticus pathogenesis. Microbiologyopen, 2017,6(1).

[31] Jiang YF, Ling J, Wang YS, et al. Cultivation-dependent analysis of the microbial diversity associated with the seagrass meadows in Xincun Bay, South China Sea. Ecotoxicology, 2015,24(7-8): 1540-1547.

[32] Matteucci G, Schippa S, Di Lallo G, et al. Species diversity, spatial distribution, and virulence associated genes of culturable vibrios in a brackish coastal Mediterranean environment. Annals of microbiology, 2015,65(4): 2311-2321.

[33] Huang L, Huang L, Yan Q, et al. The TCA Pathway is an Important Player in the Regulatory Network Governing Vibrio alginolyticus Adhesion Under Adversity. Front Microbiol, 2016,7: 40.

[34] Wang L, Huang L, Su Y, et al. Involvement of the flagellar assembly

pathway in Vibrio alginolyticus adhesion under environmental stresses. Front Cell Infect Microbiol, 2015,5: 59.

[35] Huang L, Hu J, Su Y, et al. Genome-Wide Detection of Predicted Non-coding RNAs Related to the Adhesion Process in Vibrio alginolyticus Using High-Throughput Sequencing. Front Microbiol, 2016,7: 619.

[36] Luo G, Huang LX, Su YQ, et al. flrA, flrB and flrC regulate adhesion by controlling the expression of critical virulence genes in Vibrio alginolyticus. Emerging Microbes & Infections, 2016.

[37] Liu J, Zheng Y, Lin H, et al. Proliferation of hydrocarbon-degrading microbes at the bottom of the Mariana Trench. Microbiome, 2019,7(1): 47.

[38] Hasan NA, Grim CJ, Lipp EK, et al. Deep-sea hydrothermal vent bacteria related to human pathogenic Vibrio species. Proc Natl Acad Sci U S A, 2015,112(21): E2813-E2819.

[39] Raguenes G, Christen R, Guezennec J, et al. Vibrio diabolicus sp. nov., a new polysaccharide-secreting organism isolated from a deep-sea hydrothermal vent polychaete annelid, Alvinella pompejana. Int J Syst Bacteriol, 1997,47(4): 989-995.

[40] Thompson, FL. Vibrio kanaloae sp. nov., Vibrio pomeroyi sp. nov. and Vibrio chagasii sp. nov., from sea water and marine animals. INTERNATIONAL JOURNAL OF SYSTEMATIC AND EVOLUTIONARY MICROBIOLOGY, 2003,53(3).

[41] Amin AK, Feng G, Al-Saari N, et al. The First Temporal and Spatial Assessment of Vibrio Diversity of the Surrounding Seawater of Coral Reefs in Ishigaki, Japan. Front Microbiol, 2016,7: 1185.

[42] Machado H, Gram L. The fur gene as a new phylogenetic marker for Vibrionaceae species identification. Appl Environ Microbiol, 2015,81(8): 2745-2752.

[43] Pascual J, Macian MC, Arahal DR, et al. Multilocus sequence analysis of the central clade of the genus Vibrio by using the 16S rRNA, recA, pyrH, rpoD, gyrB, rctB and toxR genes. Int J Syst Evol Microbiol, 2010,60(Pt 1): 154-165.

[44] Siboni N, Balaraju V, Carney R, et al. Spatiotemporal Dynamics of Vibrio spp. within the Sydney Harbour Estuary. Front Microbiol, 2016,7: 460.

[45] Kong W, Huang L, Su Y, et al. Investigation of possible molecular mechanisms underlying the regulation of adhesion in Vibrio alginolyticus with comparative transcriptome analysis. Antonie Van Leeuwenhoek, 2015,107(5): 1197-1206.

[46] Huang L, Hu J, Su Y, et al. Identification and characterization of three Vibrio alginolyticus non-coding RNAs involved in adhesion, chemotaxis, and motility processes. Front Cell Infect Microbiol, 2015,5: 56.

[47] Baker-Austin C, Trinanes JA, Salmenlinna S, et al. Heat Wave–Associated Vibriosis, Sweden and Finland, 2014. Emerging infectious diseases, 2016,22(7): 1216-1220.

[48] Baker-Austin C, Trinanes JA, Taylor NGH, et al. Emerging Vibrio risk at high latitudes in response to ocean warming. Nature Climate Change, 2013,3(1): 73-77.

[49] Sterk A, Schets FM, Husman AMDR, et al. Effect of Climate Change on the Concentration and Associated Risks of Vibrio Spp. in Dutch Recreational Waters. Risk Analysis, 2015,35(9): 1717-1729.

[50] Vezzulli L, Grande C, Reid PC, et al. Climate influence on Vibrio and associated human diseases during the

past half-century in the coastal North Atlantic. Proc Natl Acad Sci U S A, 2016,113(34): E5062-E5071.

[51] Martinez-Urtaza J, Bowers JC, Trinanes J, et al. Climate anomalies and the increasing risk of *Vibrio parahaemolyticus* and Vibrio vulnificus illnesses. Food Research International, 2010,43(7): 1780-1790.

[52] Baker-Austin C, Trinanes JA, Salmenlinna S, et al. Heat Wave-Associated Vibriosis, Sweden and Finland, 2014. Emerg Infect Dis, 2016,22(7): 1216-1220.

[53] Oberbeckmann S, Fuchs BM, Meiners M, et al. Seasonal dynamics and modeling of a Vibrio community in coastal waters of the North Sea. Microb Ecol, 2012,63(3): 543-551.

[54] Hsieh JL, Fries JS, Noble RT. Dynamics and predictive modelling of Vibrio spp. in the Neuse River Estuary, North Carolina, USA. Environ Microbiol, 2008,10(1): 57-64.

[55] Coutinho FH, Thompson CC, Cabral S, et al. Modelling the influence of environmental parameters over marine planktonic microbial communities using artificial neural networks. Sci Total Environ, 2019,677: 205-214.

[56] Asplund ME, Rehnstam-Holm AS, Atnur V, et al. Water column dynamics of Vibrio in relation to phytoplankton community composition and environmental conditions in a tropical coastal area. Environ Microbiol, 2011,13(10): 2738-2751.

[57] Takemura AF, Chien DM, Polz MF. Associations and dynamics of Vibrionaceae in the environment, from the genus to the population level. Front Microbiol, 2014,5: 38.

[58] Garcia-Amado MA, Bozo-Hurtado L, ASTOR Y, et al. Denaturing gradient gel electrophoresis analyses of the vertical distribution and diversity of Vibrio spp. populations in the Cariaco Basin. FEMS Microbiol Ecol, 2011,77(2): 347-356.

[59] Turner JW, Good B, Cole D, et al. Plankton composition and environmental factors contribute to Vibrio seasonality. ISME J, 2009,3(9): 1082-1092.

[60] Blackwell KD, Oliver JD. The ecology of Vibrio vulnificus, Vibrio cholerae, and *Vibrio parahaemolyticus* in North Carolina estuaries. J Microbiol, 2008,46(2): 146-153.

[61] Kauffman KM, Hussain FA, Yang J, et al. A major lineage of non-tailed dsDNA viruses as unrecognized killers of marine bacteria. Nature, 2018,554(7690): 118-122.

[62] Davis B, Jacobs JM, Davis MF, et al. Environmental Determinants of *Vibrio parahaemolyticus* in the Chesapeake Bay. Appl Environ Microbiol, 2017,83(21).

[63] Kopprio GA, Streitenberger ME, Okuno K, et al. Biogeochemical and hydrological drivers of the dynamics of Vibrio species in two Patagonian estuaries. Sci Total Environ, 2017,579: 646-656.

[64] Main CR, Salvitti LR, Whereat EB, et al. Community-Level and Species-Specific Associations between Phytoplankton and Particle-Associated Vibrio Species in Delaware's Inland Bays. Appl Environ Microbiol, 2015,81(17): 5703-5713.

[65] Colwell RR. Viable but Not Cultivable Bacteria[M]. 2009.

[66] Li L, Mendis N, Trigui H, et al. The importance of the viable but non-culturable state in human bacterial pathogens. Front Microbiol, 2014,5: 258.

[67] Yang L, Wang Y, Yu P, et al. Prophage-Related Gene VpaChn25_0724 Contributes to Cell Membrane Integrity and Growth of *Vibrio parahaemolyticus* CHN25. Frontiers in cellular and infection microbiology, 2020,10: 595709.

[68] Biswas S, Chouhan OP, Bandekar D. Diguanylate Cyclases in Vibrio cholerae: Essential Regulators of Lifestyle Switching. Front Cell Infect Microbiol, 2020,10: 582947.

[69] Qin Z, Yang X, Chen G, et al. Crosstalks Between Gut Microbiota and Vibrio Cholerae. Front Cell Infect Microbiol, 2020,10: 582554.

[70] Perez-Reytor D, Pavon A, Lopez-Joven C, et al. Analysis of the Zonula occludens Toxin Found in the Genome of the Chilean Non-toxigenic *Vibrio parahaemolyticus* Strain PMC53.7. Front Cell Infect Microbiol, 2020,10: 482.

[71] Schroeder M, brooks BD, Brooks AE. The Complex Relationship between Virulence and Antibiotic Resistance. Genes (Basel), 2017,8(1).

[72] Ramamurthy T, Nandy RK, Mukhopadhyay AK, et al. Virulence Regulation and Innate Host Response in the Pathogenicity of Vibrio cholerae. Front Cell Infect Microbiol, 2020,10: 572096.

[73] Kumar A, Das B, Kumar N. Vibrio Pathogenicity Island-1: The Master Determinant of Cholera Pathogenesis. Front Cell Infect Microbiol, 2020,10: 561296.

[74] Wu C, Zhao Z, Liu Y, et al. Type III Secretion 1 Effector Gene Diversity Among Vibrio Isolates From Coastal Areas in China. Front Cell Infect Microbiol, 2020,10: 301.

[75] Wu HJ, Wang AH, Jennings MP. Discovery of virulence factors of pathogenic bacteria. Curr Opin Chem Biol, 2008,12(1): 93-101.

[76] Wilson. Bacterial adhesion to host tissues. 2002.

[77] Efstathios G, Even H, Micka LD, et al. Intra- and inter-species interactions within biofilms of important foodborne bacterial pathogens. Frontiers in Microbiology, 2015,6(841): 841.

[78] Thakur P, Chawla R, Tanwar A, et al. Attenuation of adhesion, quorum sensing and biofilm mediated virulence of carbapenem resistant *Escherichia coli* by selected natural plant products. Microb Pathog, 2016,92: 76-85.

[79] Wang XH, Leung KY. Biochemical characterization of different types of adherence of Vibrio species to fish epithelial cells. Microbiology (Reading), 2000,146 (Pt 4): 989-998.

[80] Bricknell IR, King JA, Bowden TJ, et al. Duration of protective antibodies, and the correlation with protection in Atlantic salmon (*Salmo salar* L.), following vaccination with an *Aeromonas salmonicida* vaccine containing iron-regulated outer membrane proteins and secretory polysaccharide. Fish & Shellfish Immunology, 1999,9(2): 139-151.

[81] Hisatsune K, Kiuye A, Kondo S. A comparative study of the sugar composition of O-antigenic lipopolysaccharides isolated from Vibrio alginolyticus and *Vibrio parahaemolyticus*. Microbiol Immunol, 1981,25(2): 127-136.

[82] Milton DL, Norqvist A, Wolf-Watz H. Sequence of a novel virulence-mediating gene, virC, from Vibrio anguillarum. Gene, 1995,164(1): 95-100.

[83] Meadows PS. The attachment of bacteria to solid surfaces. Archiv Für Mikrobiologie, 1971,75(4): 374-381.

[84] Belas MR, Colwell RR. Adsorption kinetics of laterally and polarly flagellated Vibrio. J Bacteriol, 1982,151(3): 1568-1580.

[85] Bordas MA, Balebona MC, Zorrilla I, et al. Kinetics of adhesion of selected fish-pathogenic Vibrio strains of skin mucus of gilt-head sea bream (*Sparus aurata* L.). Appl Environ Microbiol, 1996,62(10): 3650-3654.

[86] Wright AC, Simpson LM, Oliver JD, et al. Phenotypic evaluation of acapsular transposon mutants of Vibrio vulnificus. Infect Immun, 1990,58(6): 1769-1773.

[87] Kim IH, Kim BS, Lee KS, et al. Identification of virulence factors in vibrio vulnificus by comparative transcriptomic analyses between clinical and environmental isolates using cDNA microarray. J Microbiol Biotechnol, 2011,21(12): 1228-1235.

[88] Kogure K, Ikemoto E, Morisaki H. Attachment of Vibrio alginolyticus to glass surfaces is dependent on swimming speed. J Bacteriol, 1998,180(4): 932-937.

[89] Sperandio B, Fischer N, Sansonetti P J. Mucosal physical and chemical innate barriers: Lessons from microbial evasion strategies. Semin Immunol, 2015,27(2): 111-118.

[90] Wright AC, Simpson L M, Oliver JD, et al. Phenotypic evaluation of acapsular transposon mutants of Vibrio vulnificus. Infect Immun, 1990,58(6): 1769-1773.

[91] Williams TC, Ayrapetyan M, Ryan H, et al. Serum Survival of Vibrio vulnificus: Role of Genotype, Capsule, Complement, Clinical Origin, and in Situ Incubation. Pathogens, 2014,3(4): 822-832.

[92] Johnson DE, Calia FM, Musher DM, et al. Resistance of Vibrio vulnificus to serum bactericidal and opsonizing factors: relation to virulence in suckling mice and humans. J Infect Dis, 1984,150(3): 413-418.

[93] Garrett SB, Garrison-schilling KL, Cooke JT, et al. Capsular polysaccharide production and serum survival of Vibrio vulnificus are dependent on antitermination control by RfaH. FEBS Lett, 2016,590(24): 4564-4572.

[94] Matsumoto C, Okuda J, Ishibashi M, et al. Pandemic spread of an O3:K6 clone of *Vibrio parahaemolyticus* and emergence of related strains evidenced by arbitrarily primed PCR and toxRS sequence analyses. J Clin Microbiol, 2000,38(2): 578-585.

[95] Honda T, Ni Y, Miwatani T, et al. The thermostable direct hemolysin of *Vibrio parahaemolyticus* is a pore-forming toxin. Can J Microbiol, 1992,38(11): 1175-1180.

[96] Takahashi A, Kenjyo N, Imura K, et al. Cl(−) secretion in colonic epithelial cells induced by the *Vibrio parahaemolyticus* hemolytic toxin related to thermostable direct hemolysin. Infect Immun, 2000,68(9): 5435-5438.

[97] Honda T, Ni YX, Miwatani T. Purification and characterization of a hemolysin produced by a clinical isolate of Kanagawa phenomenon-negative *Vibrio parahaemolyticus* and related to the thermostable direct hemolysin. Infect Immun, 1988,56(4): 961-965.

[98] Letchumanan V, Pusparajah P, Tan LT, et al. Occurrence and Antibiotic Resistance of *Vibrio parahaemolyticus* from Shellfish in Selangor, Malaysia. Front Microbiol, 2015,6: 1417.

[99] Jones MK, Oliver JD. Vibrio vulnificus: disease and pathogenesis. Infect Immun, 2009,77(5): 1723-1733.

[100] Gavin HE, Beubier NT, Satchell KJ. The Effector Domain Region of the Vibrio vulnificus MARTX Toxin Confers Biphasic Epithelial Barrier Disruption

and Is Essential for Systemic Spread from the Intestine. PLoS Pathog, 2017,13(1): e1006119.

[101] Jeong HG, Satchell KJ. Additive function of Vibrio vulnificus MARTX(Vv) and VvhA cytolysins promotes rapid growth and epithelial tissue necrosis during intestinal infection. PLoS Pathog, 2012,8(3): e1002581.

[102] Lee SJ, Jung YH, Oh SY, et al. Vibrio vulnificus VvhA induces NF-kappaB-dependent mitochondrial cell death via lipid raft-mediated ROS production in intestinal epithelial cells. Cell Death Dis, 2015,6: 1655.

[103] Vezzulli L, Colwell RR, Pruzzo C. Ocean warming and spread of pathogenic vibrios in the aquatic environment. Microb Ecol, 2013,65(4): 817-825.

[104] Waldor MK, Mekalanos JJ. Lysogenic conversion by a filamentous phage encoding cholera toxin. Science, 1996,272(5270): 1910-1914.

[105] Castillo D, Kauffman K, Hussain F, et al. Widespread distribution of prophage-encoded virulence factors in marine Vibrio communities. Sci Rep, 2018,8(1): 9973.

[106] Fasano A, Baudry B, Pumplin DW, et al. Vibrio cholerae produces a second enterotoxin, which affects intestinal tight junctions. Proc Natl Acad Sci U S A, 1991,88(12): 5242-5246.

[107] Di-Pierro M, Lu R, Uzzau S, et al. Zonula occludens toxin structure-function analysis. Identification of the fragment biologically active on tight junctions and of the zonulin receptor binding domain. J Biol Chem, 2001,276(22): 19160-19165.

[108] Balebona MC, Morinigo MA, Borrego JJ. Role of extracellular products in the pathogenicity of Vibrio strains on cultured gilt-head seabream (*Sparus aurata*). Microbiologia, 1995,11(4): 439-446.

[109] Balebona MC, Andreu MJ, Bordas MA, et al. Pathogenicity of Vibrio alginolyticus for cultured gilt-head sea bream (*Sparus aurata* L.). Appl Environ Microbiol, 1998,64(11): 4269-4275.

[110] Miyoshi SI, Narukawa H, Tomochika KI, et al. Actions of Vibrio vulnificus metalloprotease on human plasma proteinase-proteinase inhibitor systems: a comparative study of native protease with its derivative modified by polyethylene glycol. Microbiol Immunol, 1995,39(12): 959-966.

[111] Bagg A, Neilands J B. Molecular mechanism of regulation of siderophore-mediated iron assimilation. Microbiol Rev, 1987,51(4): 509-518.

[112] Braun V, Hantke K, Koster W. Bacterial iron transport: mechanisms, genetics, and regulation. Met Ions Biol Syst, 1998,35: 67-145.

Chapter 8

The Secretome of *Vibrio cholerae*

Annabelle Mathieu-Denoncourt, Sean Giacomucci and Marylise Duperthuy

Abstract

Vibrio cholerae is a facultative human pathogen responsible for the cholera disease which infects millions of people worldwide each year. *V. cholerae* is a natural inhabitant of aquatic environments and the infection usually occurs after ingestion of contaminated water or food. The virulence factors of *V. cholerae* have been extensively studied in the last decades and include the cholera toxin and the coregulated pilus. Most of the virulence factors of *V. cholerae* belong to the secretome, which corresponds to all the molecules secreted in the extracellular environment such as proteins, exopolysaccharides, extracellular DNA or membrane vesicles. In this chapter, we review the current knowledge of the secretome of *V. cholerae* and its role in virulence, colonization and resistance. In the first section, we focus on the proteins secreted through conventional secretion systems. The second and third sections emphasize on the membrane vesicles and on the secretome associated with biofilms.

Keywords: *Vibrio cholerae*, secretome, secretion system, membrane vesicles, biofilm

1. Introduction

Vibrio cholerae is a Gram-negative bacterium responsible for the cholera disease, which infects millions of people per year worldwide. In the environment, *V. cholerae* is a common inhabitant of aquatic ecosystems. Over more than 200 serotypes of *V. cholerae* have been described, but only two are responsible of the pandemics, *i.e.* O1 and O139 serotypes. The O1 serotype is divided in two biotypes, classical and El Tor. The *V. cholerae* O1 El Tor is responsible for the ongoing 7th pandemic [1]. The infection usually begins with the ingestion of contaminated water or food. Once inside the human host, *V. cholerae* colonizes the small intestine where biofilm-like structures have been observed [2]. The colonization and virulence inside the host are highly correlated with the secretion of a panel of proteins, including the cholera toxin (CT). The toxin is responsible for the misfunction of the calcium channel of the host epithelial cells, leading to the cholera characteristic massive loss of water and the diarrhea [3]. This review aims to focus on the secretome of *V. cholerae* and the secretion systems used by this bacterium to colonize the human host, compete with other bacteria, and survive in the environment.

2. Secretion systems

V. cholerae possesses as many as five multicomponent secretion systems, allowing secretion or translocation of a broad range of molecules into the extracellular milieu

IntechOpen

or directly into the neighbouring cells. These molecules are essential for niche competition in the environment and for persistence in the host.

2.1 Type II secretion system for virulence and environmental fitness

The type II secretion system (T2SS) shares many structural characteristics with the type IV pilus (T4P) and is conserved among Gram-negative bacteria for delivery of colonization and virulence factors in the extracellular milieu [4, 5]. In *V. cholerae*, it is used in the aquatic environment and in the human host to secrete exoproteins from the periplasm to the extracellular milieu or to anchor the bacteria to the host cells [4, 6]. The loss of T2SS altered growth, biofilm formation, antimicrobial resistance, and cell envelope integrity, suggesting that the T2SS has an essential role in this bacterium, which makes it a suitable target for therapeutic development [7–9]. The T2SS genes are referred to as extracellular protein secretion (*eps*) [7]. Hydrolyzation of ATP is required to provide energy for secretion [5]. The T2SS is anchored in both bacterial membranes and is distributed all over the bacterial surface [10, 11].

The growth defect of mutants lacking essential components or regulators of the T2SS shows that it is a vital component for *V. cholerae*, mostly since all the proteins secreted by the T2SS seem to act together to facilitate *V. cholerae* colonization and survival in ecological niches or in the human host. Majority of experiments occur in controlled laboratory conditions which do not represent the complexity of the intestinal nor the marine niches. These conditions might influence the type of proteins that are secreted by the bacteria, as seen in the Sikora et al. study where the CT has not been detected in the supernatant while it is a known T2SS secreted protein [6].

2.1.1 Structure and secretion through the T2SS

The structural components [5] and secreted proteins [4] of the T2SS have recently been the object for reviews. Briefly, the T2SS assembles in 4 complexes; (i) the secretin, a pore located in the outer membrane, (ii) the inner membrane anchoring platform, (iii) the intracytoplasmic ATPase complex and (iv) the pseudopilus. Even though the exact sequence of biogenesis is still unknown, a general pathway of assembly has been suggested.

The targeted proteins with signal peptides are firstly translocated to the periplasm by Sec or Tat, where they are assembled to acquire a secretion competent conformation [12, 13]. Then, it has been proposed that they bind to the pseudopilin trimeric tip and to the inner membrane platform. This interaction activates the ATPase hydrolysis activity, thus the pseudopilus elongation by addition of pseudopilin subunits and leads to the thrust of the secreted protein through the secretin channel as a piston [5]. It has been proposed that the signals for T2SS transportation are dependent on the protein conformation on the N-terminal signal peptides, but they have not been clearly identified yet [14].

2.1.2 Genes and regulation

The T2SS apparatus is composed of a dozen types of proteins, which are encoded on the *eps* operon (*epsC* to *epsN*), plus *epsAB* and the *vcpD* (*pilD*) genes in *V. cholerae* [7, 10]. Few studies have concentrated on the regulation of the T2SS in *V. cholerae*. Under laboratory conditions, the T2SS is constitutively expressed in *V. cholerae* following the growth rate of the bacteria with a higher expression at 25°C than at 37°C [15]. In addition, studies on the T2SS regulation suggest that several major regulatory pathways, including the quorum sensing, the c-di-GMP, the σE envelope stress response, might be involved [15, 16]. Finally, as more than 20 extracellular proteins with important activities throughout the infection are secreted through the T2SS [6], this system must be tightly controlled over time to allow their synchronized secretion. Therefore, the expression of the cargo proteins is regulated by a panoply of regulators.

2.1.3 Secreted proteins

In *V. cholerae*, the T2SS ensures the transportation of more than 20 proteins with extracellular activities such as enzymes, toxins, virulence and colonization effectors [6]. The T2SS is essential for survival in the aquatic environment and to infect the human gut. An essential process to colonize both environments is the ability to adhere to abiotic and biotic surfaces such as copepods and zooplankton exoskeletons and epithelial cells, respectively [17–19]. The surface-exposed GlcNAc binding protein (GbpA - VCA0811) is secreted by the T2SS and is an adhesion factor used by *V. cholerae* to bind chitinous surfaces, intestinal epithelial cells and mucin [18–21]. Chitin is the second most abundant polymer in nature and consists on N-acetyl-D-glucosamine (GlcNAc) monomers linked in β-1,4 and the main component of copepods and zooplankton exoskeleton [22]. Attachment to marine crustacea and zooplankton is an advantage for nutrients acquisition, survival and dispersion in aquatic environment. GlcNAc-containing glycoconjugates are often beared by some glycoproteins at the surface of the intestinal epithelial cells and might insure adhesion to the epithelial cells [17, 23, 24]. GbpA possesses 4 domains, the 1 and 4 being the most important for chitin binding, while only the 1 is needed for mucin binding [18]. As a secreted protein, GbpA must be able to interact with *V. cholerae* to allow its adhesion to the substrate. This function is assumed by the domains 3 and 4 of GbpA, that bind to the bacterial surface [18]. GbpA is regulated by the quorum sensing and produced at low cell density [25]. At high cell density, HA/P and PrtV digest GbpA to allow cell detachment and propagation [25, 26]. Also, higher temperatures increase the production of GbpA, promoting cell adhesion [27]. GbpA induces mucin secretion by intestinal epithelium, and mucin increases expression of GbpA [21]. Studies also determined that GbpA can induce necrosis of intestinal cells by increasing their membrane permeability [28]. Recently, a chitin cleavage activity under copper saturation has been described for GbpA and would therefore make it a lytic polysaccharide monooxygenase, a metalloenzyme copper-dependant capable of polysaccharide cleavage by oxidation [29]. Taken together, these findings suggest that GbpA is not only an early adhesion factor but might also have a more important role in pathogenesis.

In the aquatic environment, after binding to zooplankton, copepods and insect egg masses, *V. cholerae* can use chitin as source of carbon and nitrogen [14, 30]. To do so, *V. cholerae* secretes at least 2 chitinases: ChiA-1 and ChiA-2. The chitinase-1 (ChiA-1 - VC1952) and 2 (ChiA-2 – VC0027) are secreted by the T2SS and synergistically hydrolyzes the β1,4 bond between the GlcNAc monomers in the extracellular milieu [6, 14, 31]. The expression and activity of *V. cholerae* chitinases are influenced by environmental factors such as pH, salinity or temperature [32]. In the extracellular milieu, ChiA-1 expression is induced by chitin via the sensor kinase of the orphan two-component system ChiS [31]. In the intestine, the expression of the chitinases is constitutive and a role for ChiA-2 in mucin degradation and in virulence has been reported [33]. Besides ChiA-1 and ChiA-2, other proteins might have a role in chitin utilization including the VCA0140 gene that encodes for the spindolin-related protein, the VC0769 gene product and the chitin oligosaccharide deacetylase (COD - VC1280) [6, 31, 34]. All of them are secreted by the T2SS [6]. Regarding COD, Xibing Li *and coll.* demonstrated that it removes the GlcNAc from chitin oligosaccharides [34].

Besides chitin, collagen can also be used as carbon source by *V. cholerae*. Collagen is one of the most abundant components of host tissues and aquatic animals, and can therefore be found in aquatic environments in association with marine life and sedimentation of decomposing animals [35]. Its degradation provides a nitrogen source, giving a growth advantage to collagenases producing bacteria [35]. The collagenase (VchC - VC1650) is a metalloprotease that degrades type I collagen, providing another carbon source for *V. cholerae* [36]. VchC has been recognized as a T2SS dependant extracellular protein [36]. In other *Vibrio* species, collagenases are recognized as virulence factors as it facilitates their dispersion by degradation of the cellular basal lamina, but this role has not been attributed to VchC yet [36].

After the ingestion, *V. cholerae* navigates through the digestive tract, where it survives many physical and chemical barriers such as gastric acid, peristaltic movement, bile, mucin and microbiota. In the small intestine, it crosses mucin using its flagellum and the mucinase complex, that includes the vibriolysin, a zinc dependant metalloprotease hemagglutinin/protease (HA/P - VCA0865) secreted *via* the T2SS as a free protease or in a cell associated form [26, 37]. The structure, regulation, secretion mechanism and functions of HA/P have been reviewed recently [37]. Briefly, HA/P is expressed when cell density is high or when there is nutrient limitation through the HapR and RpoS regulators [38, 39]. It is translated as an inactive protein and chaperones ensure its inactive state inside the cytoplasm, then the secretion occurs in 2 steps; (i) HA/P is translocated *via* Sec into the periplasm, (ii) the T2SS exports the protease in the extracellular space where an autocatalytic event activates HA/P [37]. HA/P has multiple targets to facilitate spreading of *Vibrio* and increases its virulence [37]. *V. cholerae* gains access to the intestinal epithelial cells by degradation of the mucus layer, lactoferrin and fibronectin by HA/P in order to release toxic effectors into the epithelial cells [26]. In addition, HA/P can cleave toxins such as CT and lactoferrin to activate or increase their activity [26, 40, 41] and disrupts tight junctions between intestinal epithelial cells by occludin cleavage [42]. HA/P participates in *V. cholerae*'s release into the stool by degradation of mucin to detach bacteria from epithelial cells [43].

A second important component of the mucinase complex is the neuramidase (VCNA - VC1784). The sialidase, or neuraminidase, is encoded on the pathogenicity island of every toxigenic *V. cholerae* strains and is secreted by the T2SS [44]. VCNA removes the sialic acid that hides the ganglioside GM1, which is the receptor of the CT, on the surface of epithelial cells [45]. It binds to sialic acid to modify it by its N-terminal lectin domain [46]. Multiple enzymes (VesA, HA/P, and VCNA) appear to work synergistically and with redundancy, ensuring access to the receptor and the activation of the toxin immediately after its secretion [6].

The CT (VC1456-57) is an AB5 toxin secreted by the T2SS in the intestinal lumen, which represents the main virulence factor of *V. cholerae* found in O1 and O139 strains [3, 47]. The subunits are individually translocated by Sec into the periplasm, and the assembled toxin is translocated to the extracellular milieu by the T2SS [7]. The toxin is secreted in an inactive form and must be cleaved by human or bacterial protease to be activated [40]. CT is composed of five B subunits linked in a ring shape that bind to the ganglioside membrane receptor GM1 on the apical surface of intestinal epithelial cells [3]. CT is internalised and transits to the endoplasmic reticulum. The A subunit is heterodimeric with the A2 as the linker between B and A1 subunits, and A1 as a mono-ADP-rybosyltransferase [3]. A1 is released in the endoplasmic reticulum by disulfide isomerase and translocated to the cytosol where it activates the adenylate cyclase G protein by addition of an ADP. Thereby, the activated adenylate cyclase increases the intracellular levels of cyclic AMP, which in turn, activates the protein kinase A (PKA). Finally, PKA activates the chloride anion (Cl^-) excretion by phosphorylation of the chloride channel, that leads to major water secretion by osmose [3]. *ctxA* and *ctxB* genes are organized as an operon on the integrated CTXφ lysogenic phage [48]. The secretin complex of the T2SS is required by CTXφ to exit the bacteria, which makes the T2SS essential for virulence and horizontal transfer of CT [49]. CT is expressed when the cell density is low, inversely to HA/P, which is why it has been suggested that HA/P could cleave the remaining non-activated CT when the cell density rises [50].

Prior to GM1 binding, the CT must be processed by extracellular proteases to be activated. These proteases are therefore important for virulence and colonization. Besides their capacity to activate the toxin, they have a role in finding a substrate (modification of integrin) and nutrients, and in deactivating host defense mechanisms. Among the T2SS secreted proteins, 3 serine proteases with 30% homology between them have been identified, the *Vibrio* extracellular serine proteases (VesA - VCA0803; VesB - VC1200; VesC - VC1649) [6]. All three proteins have a N-terminal protease domain [6, 51]. VesB has a similar structure and specificity to trypsin [51]. Mutation of *vesABC* allowed to identify that VesB is the main responsible of the proteolytic activity, while VesA and VesC are responsible of 20% of the total proteolytic activity [6]. VesABC do not require bivalent ions for their enzymatic activity [6]. Under laboratory growth conditions, VesA, and in a lesser extend VesB and HA/P, activate the CT in the extracellular milieu [6, 40]. VesC induces a hemorrhagic response in rabbit ileal loop model, which might also reflect a role in virulence [52]. VesB and VesC are expressed at low cell density while VesA is expressed at high cell density [4].

Other virulence factors secreted by the T2SS have been identified in *V. cholerae*. The extracellular metalloprotease (PrtV) is a Zn-dependant metalloprotease [53, 54]. Its activity depends on several autocatalytic events occurring inside and outside the cell for activation [55]. PrtV uses two mechanisms of secretion, in association with membrane vesicles (MV) and *via* the T2SS [6, 56]. PrtV cleaves host proteins such as extracellular matrix and substrate proteins, inducing a change in host cell conformation leading to cell death [53]. In addition, PrtV is necessary for killing of *Caenorhabditis elegans* and protection against predators [57]. To do so, PrtV has many substrates such as, but not limited to, fibronectin, fibrinogen and plasminogen [53]. PrtV is composed of two domains usually known to allow protein-protein or protein-carbohydrates interactions [55, 58]. Thus, PrtV is important for the colonization of ecological niches and in pathogenesis.

The cytolytic toxin cytolysin/hemolysin A (VCC or HlyA - VCA0219), is secreted by the T2SS [6]. All *V. cholerae* strains produce VCC, an iron-dependant secondary toxin activated by cleavage [59]. VCC leads to cell death by vacuolization of the target cell, after production of anions channels in the membrane [60]. Since VCC leads to chloride efflux in intestinal cells, and subsequently to sodium and water by osmosis, it has been suggested that VCC is the major factor responsible of diarrhea in non-producing CT strains.

Leucine aminopeptidase (Lap - VCA0812) and aminopeptidase (LapX - VCA0813) are other secreted proteases using T2SS [6]. Lap is a zinc dependant metallo-exopeptidase that cleaves leucin in N-terminal position, while the role of LapX remains unknown [61]. Both Lap and LapX have no role in virulence in a *C. elegans* model [57]. While the TagA-related protein (Tarp - VCA0148), the unidentified VCA0583 and VCA0738 proteins, as well as the putative lipoprotein VC2298, have been recognized as T2SS secreted proteins, their role in *V. cholerae* is still unknown [6].

Finally, several proteins involved in biofilm formation and dissemination are also secreted by the T2SS in *V. cholerae*. Biofilm protects bacteria from antibiotics, immune system and poor environmental conditions, thus allows their survival in diversified range of ecological niches. Many components are secreted into the extracellular milieu to form the matrix. Among them, Biofilm associated protein 1 (Bap1 - VC1888) and rugosity and biofilm structure modulator A (RbmA - VC0928) and C (RbmC - VC0930) are the matrix proteins and are secreted by the T2SS [9]. In addition, the DNase Xds, an exonuclease would also be secreted by the T2SS [62].

Xds is expressed at the late stage of infection, can contribute to survival against neutrophiles NET traps, to acquisition of new DNA and dispersion of the biofilm [62, 63]. More details about the roles of the matrix proteins and nucleases in biofilm formation are presented in the Biofilms and Flagella section.

2.2 Type VI secretion system for competition and DNA acquisition

The type VI secretion system (T6SS) is a versatile syringe-like apparatus with homology to the phage T4 and produced by more than 25% Gram-negative bacteria that, upon contact with a target cell, punctures its cell wall, allowing translocation of toxic effectors directly into the neighboring cells [64, 65]. The cellular targets of these effectors are multiple; peptidoglycan, actin, cellular membrane, nucleic acids and immune system components, for instance [66]. As the target cells release their DNA into the extracellular milieu upon lysis, another function of the T6SS is to capture the extracellular DNA (eDNA) in order to acquire new features such as antibiotic resistance factors and new effectors or immunity proteins [67]. Bacteria use this device as a competition effector to take over the environmental niche and a single bacterium can possess as much as 6 different types of T6SS [65]. In *V. cholerae*, the T6SS is as efficient at killing bacterial competitors as it is at delivering toxic effectors to eukaryotic host cells, making it an important colonization and virulence factor [68].

2.2.1 Structure and secretion through the T6SS

The T6SS is anchored in the cell membrane and contains 4 distinct domains; (i) the membrane complex, (ii) the baseplate, (iii) the contractile sheath and (iv) the syringe. The current knowledge on the structure of the T6SS have been reviewed elsewhere [64].

Valine glycine rich proteins G 1, 2 and 3 (VgrG1-3) and a single proline-alanine-alanine-arginine repeated motif protein (PAAR) form the tip of the syringe [69]. There are multiple PAAR proteins in *V. cholerae*'s genome but only one binds and folds in order to form a sharpened tip and it has been shown to be essential for an efficient secretion by the T6SS [69]. The PAAR proteins also have toxic effector functions. The syringe is a tube composed of multiple hexameric rings of hemolysin-coregulated protein (Hcp) [70]. Almost simultaneously, the syringe is wrapped by the helical contractile sheath made of VipA and VipB [71] which polymerizes in an extended conformation. This high-energy conformation provides enough energy, upon contraction signal, to propel the Hcp syringe, the VgrG-PAAR tip and the associated effectors into the extracellular milieu or directly into a near target cell by contraction and rotation of VipB [71]. VipA would function as a chaperone for the VipB subunits [71]. The contracted arrangement of VipB would expose the ClpV binding sites on VipB, which are hidden in the extended conformation. ClpV is the ATPase responsible for recycling the sheath components that can be reused for further effectors translocation [72, 73]. Adaptor proteins are required to load the effectors on the tip of the syringe; however, they are not secreted by the T6SS [74].

2.2.2 Genes and regulation

In *V. cholerae*, the core genes are organized in a main cluster operon that includes *vipAB*, *hsiF*, *vasA* to *vasM* and *clpV*, on the small chromosome [68]. It contains most of the structural components of the T6SS, except for Hcp, in addition to the regulator VasH and recycling protease ClpV. At least 2 auxiliary clusters (Hcp –1 and –2), harbouring Hcp, VgrGs, adaptor and effector/immunity proteins, are distributed in the genome [75]. Some strains, including pandemic strains, have an additional auxiliary cluster (Aux –3) coding for a second PAAR protein and extra effector/immunity module set [75]. Recently, two other auxiliary clusters, Aux –4, coding for the predicted Tse4, and Aux –5, coding for Hcp, a VgrG protein, an adaptor protein and effector/immunity module set, have been identified [75, 76]. While the genes from the main cluster are highly conserved, the auxiliary clusters, even from the pandemic strains harbouring the same effectors/immunity module sets, only share about 30 % homology between them [77].

The complexity of the apparatus and its organization require a fine regulation to insure its efficiency and recycling. The transcriptional regulation of the T6SS in *V. cholerae* is strain dependant [78, 79], complex and not entirely understood yet. As the environmental strains constitutively express the T6SS to control the surrounding bacterial populations and survive predators of the ecological niche, the pathogenic strains tightly regulate their T6SS [79, 80]. Quorum sensing, the chitin and bacterial competence pathways, osmolarity and other environmental conditions are involved in the regulation of the T6SS (for a more detailed review of the T6SS see: [64]).

2.2.3 Secreted proteins

As mentioned before, the T6SS apparatus carries toxic effectors directly into the target bacterial or eukaryotic cells. A single contraction event allows the translocation of many of these effectors at the same time into the target cell [69]. The cellular targets for these effectors are multiple; they go from peptidoglycan to cellular membrane, actin and nucleic acids [64]. To protect themselves against the toxic effectors they produce, bacterial cells express immunity proteins, which brings the notion of strains compatibility (for more information see: [81]). The secreted effectors and structure components can be reused by recipient cells to form a new T6SS [82].

Hcp is one of the proteins transported by the T6SS into the target cell, in addition to be part of its structure by forming the inner tube and serving as a chaperone to the effector molecules [83]. Hcp is encoded by two different yet functional genes (VC1415; VCA0017) producing the same protein [68, 84]. Both genes must be knocked out to suppress the T6SS activity [68]. Hcp is co-expressed with HlyA, and its secretion was observed before the discovery of the T6SS [84].

Similarly to Hcp, the VgrG proteins (VC1416; VCA0018; VCA0123) are part of the T6SS structure and are secreted into the target cell upon contraction of the T6SS [68, 85]. VgrG-1 has an actin cross-linking activity in eukaryotic cells, thus preventing cytoskeleton reorganization and phagocytosis [86]. VgrG-2 is homologous to VgrG-1, but without a functional C-terminal effector domain [85]. Both appear to be essential for secretion of other T6SS components as a mutational inactivation of one of these gene makes the mutant unable to secrete any T6SS-dependant effectors [85]. Since its toxicity is exclusive to eukaryotic cells, no immunity coupled protein is required against VgrG-1. The VgrG-3 protein is known to be active against other bacteria by hydrolyzing peptidoglycan with its lysozyme-like domain, after a translocation to the periplasm [85, 87]. It might also have a muramidase activity, which could be useful in its aquatic niche to gain access to chitin or in infection to cross mucin [88]. TsiV3 (VCA0124) acts as the antitoxin for VgrG-3 by biding to it and prevents the degradation of the cell wall in the predator bacteria [87]. Thus, VgrG-3 might be important for infection by killing gut microbiota and by hydrolysing mucin.

The PAAR proteins (VCA0284; VCA0105), along with VgrGs, form the tip of the syringe of T6SS, bind the effectors and are therefore essential for T6SS effectors' secretion. There are two proteins with a PAAR domain in *V. cholerae*'s genome with enzymatic activities that could be toxic for eukaryotic or prokaryotic cells, thus acting as effectors [69]. PAAR proteins are secreted by the T6SS by caping the tip of the syringe, the PAAR domain allowing the bond with the VgrG trimeric tip. As Hcp, VgrG and PAAR proteins can bind and load effectors, the multiple effector translocation VgrGs (MERV) model has been proposed, suggesting that the T6SS spike (Hcp-VgrG-PAAR) can deliver different cargo effectors at the same time into the targeted cell [69].

The cargo effector VasX (VCA0020) acts as a colicin and targets the inner bacterial membrane or eukaryotic membrane in which it is believed to form pores, increase permeability and lead to its disruption [89]. It is encoded downstream of Hcp-2 and VgrG-2 and is regulated by VasH [89]. Its immunity coupled protein is TsiV2 (VCA0021) [88]. The VasW (VCA0019) protein encoded right upstream VasX is an adaptor protein that plays a role in secretion of VasX and an accessory role to VasX bactericidal activity [90].

The type six effector Lipase (TseL - VC1418) is another cargo effector and its secretion depends on the presence of VgrG-3. It carries a phospholipase domain that is believed to cause damage to cell membranes in both eukaryotic and prokaryotic cells [88, 91]. Its immunity coupled protein is TsiV1 (VC1419).

The type six effector Hydrolase (TseH - VCA0285) is encoded next to the PAAR protein and its secretion is dependant of the T6SS [92]. It has been shown that TseH is able to degrade peptidoglycan, a main component of the bacterial cell wall, by hydrolysis and would therefore make it an important effector as for interbacterial competition. Its immunity coupled protein is the type six immunity hydrolase (TsiH - VCA0286), which prevents cell wall degradation.

Recently, another lipase, the Type VI lipase effector *Vibrio* (TleV1) has been discovered in environmental *V. cholerae*'s genome [75]. TleV1 has a toxic activity in bacteria, mainly in periplasm, by targeting phospholipids and destabilizing the cellular membrane. Two immunity coupled proteins are associated with TleV1, TliV1a and TliV1b (type VI lipase immunity Vibrio 1a and 1b), but only TliV1a has an effective neutralizing effect against TleV1.

It is most likely that, as genome analysis of more *V. cholerae* strains will occur, new effector/immunity modules will be identified as they can be transferred between strains by genetic transfer or acquisition of eDNA upon target cell lysis [67, 75, 76, 93]. All the pandemic strains encode the same effector/immunity module sets (TseL/TsiV1, VasX/TsiV2 and VgrG3/TsiV3, called AAA), as a result of intraspecific competition [93]. Some strains harbour immunity genes without the coupled effector that they acquired from gene transfer, named orphan immunity proteins, allowing their survival from multiple toxic effectors [80]. The modules found within strains may differ from each other, however, their diversity and their omnipresence testify of their value for virulence and competition of the niche.

2.3 Type I secretion system, a tool for auxiliary toxins secretion

The type I secretion system (T1SS) is used by Gram-negative bacteria to secrete, in a one-step process using ATP, proteins directly into the extracellular milieu.

2.3.1 Structure and secretion through the T1SS

The most studied T1SS is the hemolysin A associated T1SS (HlyA-T1SS) from *E. coli* and its general structure has been reviewed elsewhere [94]. Briefly, the T1SS are composed of 3 proteins encoded on the same operon, next to their associated secreted protein and activator; (i) an outer membrane protein (TolC), (ii) an ATP binding cassette (ABC) transporter in the inner membrane (HlyB), and (iii) a linker protein (HlyD) anchored in the inner membrane, linking the two other components.

The secreted proteins carry a C-terminal secretion signal sensed by the inner membrane proteins upon binding [95]. The porin TolC is then recruited to the complex, and the proteins pass through the HlyB and HlyD channel. The binding of TolC to the inner membrane complex allows its opening and the secretion of the protein to the extracellular milieu, whereafter TolC leaves the complex [94]. As the inner membrane proteins bind to specific substrates, the TolC can be used by multiple T1SS within a cell [96]. The secreted proteins have a functional domain in N-terminal and are secreted shortly after their translation in their unfolded state. In *V. cholerae*, the T1SS structure is atypical and is composed of 4 components: the periplasmic linker RtxD, the outer membrane protein TolC, and 2 ATPases RtxB and RtxE, which most probably form heterodimers in the inner membrane instead of the conventional homodimer ATPase [97].

2.3.2 Genes and regulation

The *rtx* gene cluster is encoded near the CTXφ phage, but their regulation is not linked [98]. RtxA is secreted by its own unorthodox T1SS that requires two ABC transporters for the secretion [97]. The *rtx* locus is composed of 2 operons, the first one is left oriented and contains a conserved hypothetical gene VC1449, the activator (*rtxC*) and the toxin (*rtxA*). The second, right oriented, contains the ABC transporter (*rtxB*) and the fusion protein (*rtxD*) genes, plus the extra ABC transporter *rtxE*. The *tolC* is encoded further. The RtxA toxin secretion is optimal during the exponential phase of growth but is inhibited in stationary phase [98].

2.3.3 Secreted proteins

The repeat in toxin (RTX) proteins are a class of proteins exclusively secreted by the T1SS [99]. They include the HlyA of *E. coli* (but not of *V. cholerae* – see T2SS) and RtxA and FrhA of *V. cholerae*. Briefly, these proteins contain glycine and aspartate-rich sequence in C-terminal, before their T1SS secretion signal, and a functional domain originally associated with toxin activities. They require activation by the acetyl transferase activator encoded within the operon. The RTX region offers many Ca^{2+} binding sites. Once bound to the sites, the Ca^{2+} generates a sudden conformation change and formation of the secondary structure of the RTX protein. As the Ca^{2+} concentrations are low inside the cells, the RTX proteins keep their unfolded state until they reach the extracellular milieu, where the Ca^{2+} concentrations are higher.

One T1SS has been described in *V. cholerae.* It is associated to the RTX toxin (RtxA), a large toxin found in many *V. cholerae* strains, including O1 El tor, O139 and non-O1/O139 strains, but not in the O1 classical strains that contain a deletion into the gene cluster [98, 100]. The omnipresence of RtxA toxin among currently circulating strains lets us think that it is an important virulence factor that could be responsible for the non-O1/O139 strains' emergence [100]. RtxA leads to the depolarization of actin, by cross-linking the actin monomers into dimers, trimers or multimers, which causes rapid rounding of host cells [101–104].

Three other T1SS could be found in *V. cholerae*'s genome. The first one is associated to two putative RTX toxins with hemolytic activity (RtxL1 and RtxL2) that have been discovered in the genome of many *V. cholerae* strains [105]. They induce cell rounding and cytotoxicity and, unlike RtxA, also have a hemolytic activity. The locus has been identified but the secretion pathway has not, although all RTX proteins are secreted through a T1SS, the RtxL associated T1SS is yet to be described. Another of the putative T1SS of *V. cholerae* is associated to another RTX-like toxin, the Flagellum-regulated hemagglutinin A (FrhA - VC1620) [106]. The decreased hemagglutination in non-motile *V. cholerae* mutant has led to the discovery of FrhA. FrhA contains a RTX-like domain and a T1SS signal and has a role in hemagglutination, adhesion to human host cells and chitin, thus in colonization and biofilm formation [107]. Its regulation is comprised in the four-step hierarchy regulation of motility, which includes the regulation of several virulence factors. FrhA is encoded in a gene cluster harbouring components with homology to TolC (FrhC - VC1621) and HlyB (VC1628). However, no HlyD homolog has been found in the surrounding genes and the homology of VC1618 to HlyB is poor, as the ATP binding site, essential to the translocation process through the T1SS, is missing [106]. This secretion system is yet to be described. The retention module-containing protein (CraA - VCA0849) also contains a glycine rich module used as T1SS secretion signal, but its secretion system remains to be described [108]. CraA is an adhesin that has a role in early stage of biofilm formation by binding chitin. It has some homology to RtxA. In other Gram-negative bacteria, it serves as an adhesin on the bacterial surface.

2.4 Type III secretion system for colonization and injection of effectors into eukaryotic host cells

The Type III secretion system (T3SS) is a multicomponent device translocating various effectors directly into the neighbouring eukaryotic host cells and is found in many *Vibrio* species, including *V. cholerae* [109]. Many non O1/O139 strains, which can lead to severe diarrhea even though they do not produce the CT and toxin coregulated pilus (TCP), possess a T3SS [110, 111]. Unlike the pandemic strains, the diarrhea induced by non O1/O139 strains shows damages to the intestinal epithelium [112]. The T3SS would in fact be essential for intestinal colonization and invasive diarrhea in those strains. The T3SS is composed of a basal structure that shares similarities with the flagella, and a needle, connecting the bacterial cytoplasm to the eukaryotic cell using a pore at its end [113]. While the structure of the T3SS is conserved among Gram-negative bacteria, the effectors encoded differ from one another, subsequently to the intended host. In *V. cholerae*, the translocated effectors are multiple, and their accumulation disrupts host cellular processes with a key role in the early stages of infection, such as cytoskeletal rearrangement and cytotoxicity, resulting in intestinal epithelial damages and colonization of the gut [109, 114].

2.4.1 Structure and secretion through the T3SS

The T3SS is a multicomponent apparatus spawning both bacterial membranes. While the effectors' secretion through T3SS is Sec independent, the translocation of the membrane components of the injectosome requires it [113]. The T3SS uses ATP for the active translocation of the effectors through both bacterial membranes directly into host cell cytoplasm. The T3SS consists of an injectosome with structural and genetic homology to the flagellum and a molecular syringe, the structure has been reviewed elsewhere [113]. In brief, the syringe connects the membrane complex to the host cell cytoplasm. It is composed of (i) a basal needle, (ii) a tip and, at its end, (iii) a translocation pore. The membrane complex is composed of an assembly of concentric rings creating a channel through both bacterial membranes. It includes an outer membrane ring connected, in the periplasm, to the inner membrane ring, in addition to a cytoplasmic portion, made of a cytoplasmic ring and an ATPase complex. The exact T3SS assembly in *V. cholerae* has not been studied yet, and some components remain to be identified [109].

2.4.2 Genes and regulation

While some *Vibrio* species (*V. parahaemolyticus*) possess two T3SS (T3SS1 and T3SS2), only one, with similarities to the T3SS2 of *V. parahaemolyticus*, has been found in *V. cholerae*'s genome [111]. The T3SS genes are located on a genomic island of approximatively 49kb, which includes an integrase, structural components, effectors and regulators (*vttR*$_A$, *vttR*$_B$) [114]. The T3SS genomic island is acquired by horizontal transfer [115]. The core region contains most of the structural components and some effectors, while the upstream and downstream regions, more affected by the gene transfer, harbor a variety of effectors [109]. The *Vibrio* type three regulators VttR$_A$ and VttR$_B$ share similarities with ToxR, an important virulence regulator in *V. cholerae* [116]. The regulators VttR$_A$ and ToxR control the expression of VttR$_B$, which, afterwards, controls the expression of the T3SS structural genes in presence of bile [117]. The deletion of either of these regulators leads to a decreased T3SS-dependant cytotoxicity. VttR$_A$ and VttR$_B$ might also regulate genes outside the T3SS island [110].

2.4.3 Secreted proteins

The presence of T3SS in non O1/O139 strains leads to intestinal epithelium damages, such as alteration of the brush border and disruption, as seen in the infant rabbit model of infection [112]. It is the result of the translocation of many effectors into the eukaryotic host cytoplasm by the T3SS. In *V. cholerae*, there are 7 effectors encoded within the T3SS core genomic island and at least 5 others have been identified in the up and downstream regions [109]. The first effector to be identify is *Vibrio* outer protein F (VopF - NT01VC2350) [118, 119]. VopF possesses 2 actin binding domains, the formin homology-1 like and WASP homology 2 domains, that intervene in actin polymerization of the host intestinal epithelial cells. It has been shown to be essential for virulence in infant mouse model of infection [119]. VopF has a homolog in other non O1/O139 strains, VopN, that shares 55% similarity [119]. Just like VopF, VopN disturbs actin polymerization by nucleation, but unlike VopF, locates in the stress fibers by binding filamin. Both would also have an anti-apoptotic effect.

A total of 11 proteins that use the T3SS for their secretion have been identified by using a FRET technique to visualize the translocation of proteins in HeLa cells, including an effector specific to *V. cholerae,* VopX (A33_1663) [114]. VopX has been found to be essential for colonization in infant mouse model of infection and to induce an important growth defect in *S. cerevisiae* by destabilization of the cell wall through Cell Wall Integrity MAP kinase pathway activation [114, 120].

Another of the secreted effectors is VopE (A33_1662) [121]. VopE is translocated to the mitochondria after its secretion by the T3SS, where it acts as a GTPase-activating protein. Its presence in the mitochondria intervenes with the normal process of Rho GTPases Miro1 and 2, thus with the immune response using mitochondrial signalisation pathways [121, 122]. Along with VopF, VopE would lead to the loosening of the tight junctions, a primordial structure of the intestinal epithelium [119]. VopM (A33_1684) is another effector secreted by the T3SS that leads to actin stress fibers formation and brush border effacement [110].

Other effectors have been identified, but their function remains unclear, such as VopZ (A33_1704), VopW (A33_1690), VopA (A33_1680), VopG (A33_1697), VopI (A33_1687), VopY (A33_1700), VopH (A33_1678) and VopK (A33_1699) [110, 114]. VopW is known as a hydrophilic translocator that would both have structural and effector roles [114]. Despite the lack of information, a study on multiple effectors brought some light on their potential role in infection [110]. It stated that VopA, VopM, VopW and VopH seemed to be required for intestinal colonization in infant mouse model of infection, as mutants of these effectors where not recovered from infected animals. VopA could also have a role in adhesion to the intestinal cells in the early stages of infection. Along with VopH, VopI and VopW, VopA could be part of the structural apparatus as it is essential for other effectors secretion.

2.5 Type IV secretion system, a crucial virulence factor

Three T4Ps can be found at the surface of *V. cholerae*, TCP, the chitin regulated pilus (ChiRP) and the mannose sensitive hemagglutinin pilus (MSHA). T4P have structural similarities with the T2SS, and their structure has been reviewed elsewhere [123]. An inner membrane complex, docking an ATPase cytoplasmic complex, recruits a secretion pore in the outer membrane. The pilin subunits are then assembled and secreted to form a strong but malleable filament. They have a role in many biological processes leading to virulence such as, in *V. cholerae*, acquisition of mobile genetic elements (MGE), micro-colonies formation in the intestinal lumen, adhesion to abiotic surfaces or chitin and biofilm formation [123]. The bacterial aggregation by pilus-pilus interaction with TCP, in form of micro-colonies, allows concentration of the toxin at the site of colonization and protection of the immune system (as would a biofilm) [124]. Most T4Ps have cytoplasmic ATPases that allow their elongation and retraction, which can lead to eDNA capture and motility. The main secreted components of the T4P are the pilin subunits.

2.5.1 The toxin coregulated pilus

The pandemic virulence potential of *V. cholerae* resides in its MGE, harbouring both the CT and TCP apparel on the integrated CTXφ phage and *Vibrio* Pathogenic Island 1 (VPI-1), respectively [125]. TCP is essential for effective colonization of the intestinal epithelium in pandemic O1/O139 strains [126]. The VPI-1 harbours the receptor for the CTXφ phage, the major pilin of TCP (TcpA), allowing its entry into *V. cholerae*. It also regulates the CT production with ToxT, which also regulates TCP expression [48, 125]. It is believed that acquisition of both these MGE is enough to convert environmental strains into pathogenic strains [125]. Considering this information, it is clear that the gene acquisition by horizontal transfer is important for the toxigenic potential of *V. cholerae*. Obviously, TcpA, being the major component of the filament, is responsible for the pilus:pilus interaction that leads to the formation of the micro-colonies [124]. TCP also has a minor pilin, TcpB, which is also secreted and initiates pilus polymerization and retraction, despite the lack of a retraction ATPase in TCP [127]. TcpB would also bind to CTXφ minor coat protein and then leads to its internalization into *V. cholerae* by initializing the retraction of the T4P [127].

2.5.2 The mannose sensitive hemagglutinin pilus

MSHA is produced by O1 El Tor and O139 strains, but not by the O1 classical strains, and is important for adhesion to chitinous surface and biofilm formation, although it does not seem to play a role in virulence nor colonization in humans [27, 31, 126, 128]. Its filament is composed of the single major pilin MshA [129]. The dynamic of retraction/polymerization of the MSHA is controlled by c-di-GMP [129].

2.5.3 The chitin regulated pilus

The third T4P identified in *V. cholerae* is ChiRP [31]. Because, in its marine life, *V. cholerae* can use chitin as a carbon source, the capacity to colonize shellfish is then primordial to acquire this element. The expression of PilA, the major pilin of ChiRP, is induced when the bacteria are grown in presence of chitin [31]. The absence of PilA, thus of ChiRP, decreases, but does not suppress, the ability of *V. cholerae* to colonize crab shell, even though it has no effect in infant mouse model nor on adhesion to human cells [130]. It suggests that ChiRP has a role in adhesion to chitin in collaboration with other chitin binding structures and proteins (MSHA, GbpA). The colocalization of ChiRP at the pole of *V. cholerae* along with the T2SS, secreting chitinases required for chitin acquisition, would increase the effectiveness of chitin uptake by limiting the secretion to an adhesion site [31]. In other *Vibrio*, ChiRP could also have a role in biofilm formation by mediating bacterium:bacterium interactions, a phenomenon that has also been observed in *V. cholerae* and that could further increase chitin uptake [131, 132]. It is important to note that the chitin utilization pathway is linked with natural competence pathway and that ChiRP is implied in eDNA uptake [131]. eDNA uptake is used by bacteria to gain new functions, such as virulence and resistance factors, and to increase their fitness and survival in environment.

2.6 Other secreted molecules

The cholix toxin (ChxA) is a eukaryotic elongation factor-2 specific ADP-rybosyl transferase that induces cell death [133]. ChxA is produced by many *V. cholerae* strains [134, 135].

Accessory cholera enterotoxin (Ace - VC1459) and zonula occludens toxin (Zot - VC1458) are accessory toxins that are both encoded near the CT genes on the CTXφ phage [136, 137]. Zot leads to the disruption of the tight junctions between intestinal epithelial cells, an important structure in the intestinal permeability [138, 139]. It is translocated and anchored in the outer membrane and has two functional domains. The N-terminal domain is important for CTXφ phage's morphogenesis and the C-terminal domain is cleaved by proteases. Once released into the intestinal lumen, the C-terminal domain acts as a toxin [139, 140]. Thus, Zot does not employ a conventional secretion system for its release into the extracellular milieu. Regarding Ace, it leads to fluid secretion in rabbit ileal loop model by unbalancing calcium secretion and the secretion mechanism has not been determined yet [138].

3. Membrane vesicles, the type 0 secretion system

Most bacteria, including Gram-negative and Gram-positive bacteria, release MV, also known as the type 0 secretion system [141]. Different types of MV can be produced including the outer membrane vesicles (OMV), the outer-inner membrane vesicles (OIMV), the cytoplasmic membrane vesicles (CMV) and the tube-shaped membranous structures (TSMS). The different types of MV differ in their composition and their biogenesis mechanisms, which will not be presented here since they have already been reviewed elsewhere [142]. *V. cholerae* can secrete OMV and OIMV, which contain lipopolysaccharides, phospholipids, proteins [143], DNA and RNA [144, 145]. An hypervesiculation has been reported in *V. cholerae* at the early stages of intestine colonization by silencing the phospholipid transporter VacJ/Yrb involved in the maintenance of the outer membrane lipid asymmetry. This hypervesiculation is characterized by a drastic modification of the membrane composition and a better colonization of the host intestine [146].

In vitro, the protein cargo of MV is highly dependent on the bacterial growth conditions [147]. The protein cargo of the MV secreted by *V. cholerae* El Tor O1 has been determined under virulence activating conditions. A total of 90 proteins associated to MV have been identified, 50 % being outer membrane or periplasmic proteins [143]. Among these proteins, some are secreted in association with the vesicles, such as the membrane and periplasmic proteins, while others are secreted independently and associated with the vesicles in the extracellular compartment, such as Bap1 [148]. The proteins associated with the vesicles can have a role in resistance (antimicrobials, plasma and bacteriophages), in biofilm formation or in virulence.

3.1 Membrane vesicles and resistance

A role for the MV in antimicrobial peptides (AMP) resistance has been reported in several Gram-negative bacteria including *V. cholerae*. Our previous studies demonstrated that PrtV-associated MV can protect *V. cholerae* from the lysis by LL-37, a cathelicidin secreted by the epithelial cells in response to *V. cholerae* infection [56]. In addition, the matrix protein Bap1 can bind to OmpT, a porin located in the outer membrane, on the surface of the MV of *V. cholerae* in presence of polymyxin B and confer cross-resistance to LL-37 [148]. Interestingly, the hypervesiculation observed during the early stages of infection leads to a decrease of OmpT in the outer membrane correlated with an increase in OmpT abundance in the MV [146]. The authors suggest that the hypervesiculation is a process used by *V. cholerae* to quickly modify the outer membrane protein content in order to increase the intestinal colonization fitness. Therefore, the hypervesiculation *in vivo* may contribute to the Bap1 mediated AMP resistance in the intestine where analogues of polymyxin B are secreted by the microbiota. In *V. cholerae*, the expression of *ompT* is negatively correlated with the expression of *ompU* through the ToxR switch [149, 150]. During the hypervesiculation process, *ompU* expression increases, leading to an accumulation of OmpU in the membrane [148]. A role of OmpU in AMP and bile resistance has been reported in *V. cholerae* [151]. Therefore, the hypervesiculation in *V. cholerae* might represent a double advantage in terms of AMP resistance through vesicles associated OmpT-Bap1 and membrane bounded OmpU.

Besides AMP, MV are also involved in serum resistance in *V. cholerae*. Septicemia caused by *V. cholerae* has been reported, especially in patients suffering liver disorders, which can lead to a 50% mortality rates [152]. In an elegant study, Aung *et al.* demonstrated that IgG present in the serum of healthy people can recognize OmpU of *V. cholerae*, which leads to the recruitment of the complement through C1q binding and to the clearance of *V. cholerae* [153]. However, the presence of OmpU in the MV can sequester the anti-OmpU IgG before they reach the bacterial cells, leading to an increased resistance of the bacteria to serum [153].

A role of the MV in resistance to bacteriophages has also been demonstrated in *V. cholerae* [154]. The authors proposed that, similarly to Bap1 and AMP and to OmpU and IgG, the presence of MV is used as bacterial decoy to lure the phages before they can reach the bacterial cell. In this case, it is the presence of phage receptors on the surface of the MV that is responsible for the sequestration of the phages [154].

3.2 Membrane vesicles and biofilm

A significant part of antimicrobial resistance is associated with the biofilm lifestyle of bacteria. The bacteria growing in a biofilm are up to 1000 times more resistant to antimicrobials and disinfectants than their planktonic counterparts [155]. It has been demonstrated that MV are involved in the formation of biofilms in several Gram-negative bacteria [156]. In *V. cholerae*, the association of Bap1, PrtV and eDNA with the MV might have a role in biofilm formation by strengthening the structure and by recruiting planktonic bacteria. More information on the role of MV in biofilm is provided in the Biofilms and Flagella section.

3.3 Membrane vesicles and virulence

The MV can also carry virulence factors including the CT, the major virulence factor of *V. cholerae* [157]. After secretion, The B subunits interact with the GM1 receptor at the surface of the epithelial cells and the toxin is endocytosed. The A subunit dissociates from the rest of the toxin in the endoplasmic reticulum and spontaneously unfold. The unfolded form of the A subunit is responsible for the toxic activity of the CT. The vesicle-associated toxin is biologically active although only A subunits are encapsulated [158]. It has been demonstrated that the MV can enter inside the host cells using different mechanisms involving clathrin coated pits, formation of caveolae, use of lipid rafts and direct fusion with host cell membrane [159]. Therefore, it is likely that the lack of B subunits is not an issue for the delivery of active A subunits of the CT while encapsulated inside the MV.

Besides the CT, other biologically active virulence factors can also be transported to the host cells through MV. It is the case for HA/P and VesC [160], PrtV metalloprotease [56] and the VCC [161]. Therefore, the MV of *V. cholerae* can carry a concentrated arsenal of virulence factors that can be efficiently delivered to the host cells and have a role in *V. cholerae* pathogenesis.

4. Biofilms and flagella

Most of the bacteria, including pathogens, form biofilm to survive and persist in different environments. Biofilms are organized bacterial communities attached to a surface and producing a matrix. *V. cholerae* form biofilms at different stages of its life cycle. An increasing number of evidences suggest that *V. cholerae* forms biofilm during the gut infection and biofilm-like aggregates display a hyper-infective phenotype [162]. To persist in the environment, *V. cholerae* forms biofilm on different biotic and abiotic substrates such as floating aggregates, ship hulls, microalgae and copepods [163]. The transition between planktonic motile and non-motile biofilm states is highly regulated [162, 164]. The composition and abundance of the secreted factors involved in biofilm formation, maturation and dispersion largely depend on environmental conditions and on surface composition. In this section, we will review the current knowledge about the biofilm secretome in *V. cholerae* at different stages of the biofilm formation and the interplay between biofilm and motility.

4.1 From motility to initial adhesion

Planktonic *V. cholerae* are motile cells and their motility is ensured by a single polar flagellum. The flagellum is composed of three major structural components: i) the basal body, ii) the hook and iii) the filament (for detailed structure: [165]). Structurally, the flagellum is closely related to the T3SS and therefore has been referred as fT3SS (flagellum Type-3 Secretion System) [166]. The main proteins secreted through the fT3SS are the flagellins. In *V. cholerae*, five different flagellins (FlaA-E) encoded on two chromosomally distinct loci (*flaAC and flaEDB)* have been described. From these 5 flagellins, only FlaA is essential for the motility [167]. Recently, an elegant study from Dongre *and coll*. demonstrated that the cytotoxin MakA is also secreted through the fT3SS [168]. This toxin is involved in colonization and virulence in zebrafish and *C. elegans* infection models and represents the first characterization of a toxin secreted through the fT3SS in *V. cholerae* [168].

V. cholerae motility and chemotaxis are important for the virulence in the human gut [169]. They are necessary for the bacteria to travel from the lumen to the epithelial cells, where the virulence factors are secreted after attachment of the bacteria. Motility also plays a key role in biofilm formation on surfaces as an essential element of the initial adhesion of the bacteria. On abiotic surfaces, *V. cholerae*'s adhesion involves MSHA to "scan the surface" [170]. The flagellum is responsible for the bacterial rotation on the surface of the support, which allows MSHA to reach a spot of high affinity. This adhesion is signaled through the flagellum rotor and results in an inhibition of motility pathways and the secretion of the *Vibrio* polysaccharides (VPS) [171]. Two other T4Ps are implicated in bacterial adhesion; ChiRP and TCP (see T4SS section). Initial adhesion to biotic surface is promoted by GbpA, which is secreted through the T2SS and induces mucin secretion [21].

Additionally, FrhA (hemagglutinin) and CraA (adhesin) secreted through the T1SS are involved in adhesion and biofilm formation (see T1SS section). The expression of both *frhA* and *craA* is controlled by a c-di-GMP-dependent regulatory system [108]. In addition, *frhA* is regulated by the flagella regulation pathways, reinforcing the role of flagella in the initial stages of biofilm formation [106].

4.2 Biofilm maturation

Once attached, *Vibrio* starts secreting VPS, which represent more than 50% of matrix composition. VPS polymers are secreted throughout the biofilm production and are mostly composed of [→4)-α-L-Gul*p*NAcAGly3OAc-(1→4)-β-D-Glc*p*-(1→4)-α-d-Glc*p*-(1→4)-α-D-Gal*p*-(1→] subunits. A variant representing around 20% of VPS consists on the same pattern except for the α-D-Glc*p* moiety that is replaced by α-D-Glc*p*NAc [172]. The VPS biogenesis and export systems are encoded on two clusters: VpsI and VpsII, encoding VpsA-K and VpsL-Q, respectively [173, 174]. Among the 18 *vps* genes, 15 of them induced highly impaired biofilm formation in *V. cholerae* when suppressed [174]. Recently, a model has been proposed for the production and secretion of VPS. In this model, the VPS are synthesized by formation and polymerization of individual subunits. The polymers are then transferred across the outer membrane through VpsM/N [175]. This system is tightly controlled by the tyrosine phosphoregulatory system VpsO/VpsU, which controls the level of phosphorylation of the C-terminal tyrosine-cluster of VpsO. High level of phosphorylation results in VpsO oligomer dissociation and VPS production reduction, whereas low level of VpsO phosphorylation results in high oligomerization and increased VPS production [175].

Shortly after VPS secretion has been initiated, the sequential secretion of the 3 major biofilm matrix proteins through the T2SS occurs. The first matrix protein to be secreted is RbmA, followed by Bap1 and RbmC [176]. More specifically, RmbC has a role in maintaining and stabilizing the biofilm [177]. A study using mutants lacking RbmC and its homolog Bap1 showed a change of colonial morphology and the loss of biofilm formation capacity [177, 178]. On the other hand, RbmA controls the structure of the biofilm [9, 179].

Growth of the biofilm is ensured by two different processes: (i) the bacteria inside the matrix are dividing inside an envelope formed by the VPS, RbmC and Bap1 [176] and (ii) new bacteria are recruited inside the biofilm. This recruitment requires the cleavage of the N-terminal domain of RbmA by PrtV. Once cleaved, RbmA can bind bacterial cells that are not producing VPS (planktonic) and recruits them into the biofilm [180]. Since MV have been observed in the biofilm matrix and PrtV can be associated to the surface of the MV, it is possible that MV play an important role in biofilm maturation in *V. cholerae* [181]. In addition, the association of Bap1 to the MV in specific conditions is likely to lead to the adhesion of the MV to the surface and to the exopolysaccharides [181]. Three other proteins with no role in biofilm formation and adhesion have been identified in biofilm preparation, *i.e.* the hemolysin HylA, HA/P and ChiA-2 [182].

Besides VPS, proteins and MV, a significant amount of eDNA is entrapped in the biofilm matrix. The roles of eDNA in bacterial physiology have been reviewed elsewhere and include nutrient source, horizontal gene transfer and adherence [183]. Recently, a role in the tridimensional matrix structure of the biofilm in *V. cholerae* has been reported [184]. The eDNA inside the biofilm most probably results from cell autolysis and MV secretion [185].

4.3 Biofilm dispersion and detachment

Biofilm dispersal is a complex process by which bacteria actively succeed to evade biofilm matrix [186]. Conversely to adhesion and biofilm maturation, little is known about the dispersion process of *V. cholerae* biofilms. It requires specific environmental signals, which trigger the quorum sensing and the general stress response pathways [187], matrix degradation and motility resumption [188]. The matrix degradation requires RbmB, an extracellular polysaccharide lyase that digests the VPS, and LapG, a periplasmic protease that cleaves the adhesins FrhA and CraA located at the outer membrane [188]. Under substrate specific conditions, the extracellular protease HA/P also participates in biofilm dispersion by degrading the mucin [189]. Finally, secreted nucleases such as Dns and Xds have a role in biofilm dispersion by cleaving the eDNA present in the matrix [185]. The motility resumption requires the ability to switch the flagella rotation from counterclockwise to clockwise direction mediated by CheY3 independently of chemotaxis [188].

5. Conclusion

Over the last decades, numerous studies have focused on the secreted molecules and secretion systems used by *V. cholerae* to deliver extracellular effectors. Various roles have been assigned to the secreted molecules especially regarding the host colonization and virulence, and the environmental survival and persistence, denoting their importance in *V. cholerae*'s pathogenesis and life cycle. Additionally, the redundancy of some functions carried by multiple secreted effectors testifies of their importance. With gene acquisition, MGE, strain sequencing and the emergence of more efficient technologies, it is most likely that additional secreted effectors and secretion systems will be identified and characterized.

The recent characterization of the MakA toxin secretion through the fT3SS [168] and the numerous studies on the T6SS since its discovery 15 years ago [68] clearly demonstrate that there is still work to do on the secretome and secretion systems in *V. cholerae*. The secretion mechanism of some extracellular proteins - with characterized functions - remains to be determined. It is the case of ChxA, Ace, RbmB and the DNAse Dns.

The regulation of the secretion systems and their cargo molecules is a complex process. It involves numerous regulators that can be activated or repressed depending on the detection of specific intracellular and extracellular signals. So far, most of the studies aiming to decipher the regulation pathways have been performed under laboratory conditions. The featuring of conditions that characterize the intestinal environment before and during diarrhea, including the peristaltic movement, anaerobia, the presence of the microbiota, water efflux and high osmolarity, is likely to modify *V. cholerae* secretion in terms of regulation and nature, abundance and activity of the secreted molecules. Therefore, it would be highly beneficial to study the secretion mechanisms, the secreted molecules and their regulation in models that are closer to the physiological conditions encountered in the host, such as *ex vivo* devices. Understanding the regulation and the mechanisms of colonization, virulence and resistance in these physiological conditions is crucial for the development of treatments and vaccines against *V. cholerae*.

Acknowledgements

This work was supported by the Natural Sciences and Engineering Research Council of Canada (NSERC http://www.nserc-crsng.gc.ca/index_eng.asp) Discovery grant number RGPIN-2017-05322. AMD received financial support from the Fonds de recherche du Québec en Santé, doctoral training scholarship #290352.

Author details

Annabelle Mathieu-Denoncourt, Sean Giacomucci and Marylise Duperthuy*
Département de Microbiologie, Infectiologie et Immunologie, Université de Montréal, Montreal, Canada

*Address all correspondence to: marylise.duperthuy@umontreal.ca

References

[1] Zuckerman JN, Rombo L, Fisch A. The true burden and risk of cholera: implications for prevention and control. Lancet Infect Dis. 2007;7(8):521-530.

[2] Sengupta C, Mukherjee O, Chowdhury R. Adherence to Intestinal Cells Promotes Biofilm Formation in *Vibrio cholerae*. J Infect Dis. 2016; 214(10):1571-1578.

[3] Vanden Broeck D, Horvath C, De Wolf MJ. *Vibrio cholerae*: cholera toxin. Int J Biochem Cell Biol. 2007;39(10): 1771-1775.

[4] Sikora AE. Proteins secreted via the type II secretion system: smart strategies of *Vibrio cholerae* to maintain fitness in different ecological niches. PLoS Pathog. 2013;9(2):e1003126.

[5] Korotkov KV, Sandkvist M, Hol WG. The type II secretion system: biogenesis, molecular architecture and mechanism. Nat Rev Microbiol. 2012;10(5):336-351.

[6] Sikora AE, Zielke RA, Lawrence DA, Andrews PC, Sandkvist M. Proteomic analysis of the *Vibrio cholerae* type II secretome reveals new proteins, including three related serine proteases. J Biol Chem. 2011;286(19):16555-16566.

[7] Sandkvist M, Michel LO, Hough LP, Morales VM, Bagdasarian M, Koomey M, et al. General secretion pathway (eps) genes required for toxin secretion and outer membrane biogenesis in *Vibrio cholerae*. J Bacteriol. 1997;179(22): 6994-7003.

[8] Sikora AE, Lybarger SR, Sandkvist M. Compromised outer membrane integrity in *Vibrio cholerae* Type II secretion mutants. J Bacteriol. 2007;189(23):8484-8495.

[9] Johnson TL, Fong JC, Rule C, Rogers A, Yildiz FH, Sandkvist M. The Type II secretion system delivers matrix proteins for biofilm formation by *Vibrio cholerae*. J Bacteriol. 2014;196(24):4245-4252.

[10] Lybarger SR, Johnson TL, Gray MD, Sikora AE, Sandkvist M. Docking and assembly of the type II secretion complex of *Vibrio cholerae*. J Bacteriol. 2009;191(9):3149-3161.

[11] Johnson TL, Abendroth J, Hol WG, Sandkvist M. Type II secretion: from structure to function. FEMS Microbiol Lett. 2006;255(2):175-186.

[12] Voulhoux R, Ball G, Ize B, Vasil ML, Lazdunski A, Wu LF, et al. Involvement of the twin-arginine translocation system in protein secretion via the type II pathway. EMBO J. 2001;20(23):6735-6741.

[13] Hofstra H, Witholt B. Kinetics of synthesis, processing, and membrane transport of heat-labile enterotoxin, a periplasmic protein in Escherichia coli. J Biol Chem. 1984;259(24):15182-15187.

[14] Connell TD, Metzger DJ, Lynch J, Folster JP. Endochitinase is transported to the extracellular milieu by the eps-encoded general secretory pathway of *Vibrio cholerae*. J Bacteriol. 1998;180(21):5591-5600.

[15] Zielke RA, Simmons RS, Park BR, Nonogaki M, Emerson S, Sikora AE. The type II secretion pathway in *Vibrio cholerae* is characterized by growth phase-dependent expression of exoprotein genes and is positively regulated by sigmaE. Infect Immun. 2014;82(7):2788-2801.

[16] Sloup RE, Konal AE, Severin GB, Korir ML, Bagdasarian MM, Bagdasarian M, et al. Cyclic Di-GMP and VpsR Induce the Expression of Type II Secretion in *Vibrio cholerae*. J Bacteriol. 2017;199(19).

[17] Benktander J, Angstrom J, Karlsson H, Teymournejad O, Linden S, Lebens M, et al. The repertoire of glycosphingolipids

recognized by *Vibrio cholerae*. PLoS One. 2013;8(1):e53999.

[18] Wong E, Vaaje-Kolstad G, Ghosh A, Hurtado-Guerrero R, Konarev PV, Ibrahim AF, et al. The *Vibrio cholerae* colonization factor GbpA possesses a modular structure that governs binding to different host surfaces. PLoS Pathog. 2012;8(1):e1002373.

[19] Stauder M, Huq A, Pezzati E, Grim CJ, Ramoino P, Pane L, et al. Role of GbpA protein, an important virulence-related colonization factor, for *Vibrio cholerae's* survival in the aquatic environment. Environ Microbiol Rep. 2012;4(4):439-445.

[20] Kirn TJ, Jude BA, Taylor RK. A colonization factor links *Vibrio cholerae* environmental survival and human infection. Nature. 2005;438(7069):863-866.

[21] Bhowmick R, Ghosal A, Das B, Koley H, Saha DR, Ganguly S, et al. Intestinal adherence of *Vibrio cholerae* involves a coordinated interaction between colonization factor GbpA and mucin. Infect Immun. 2008;76(11): 4968-4977.

[22] Keyhani NO, Roseman S. Physiological aspects of chitin catabolism in marine bacteria. Biochim Biophys Acta. 1999;1473(1):108-122.

[23] Finne J, Breimer ME, Hansson GC, Karlsson KA, Leffler H, Vliegenthart JF, et al. Novel polyfucosylated N-linked glycopeptides with blood group A, H, X, and Y determinants from human small intestinal epithelial cells. J Biol Chem. 1989;264(10):5720-5735.

[24] Zampini M, Pruzzo C, Bondre VP, Tarsi R, Cosmo M, Bacciaglia A, et al. *Vibrio cholerae* persistence in aquatic environments and colonization of intestinal cells: involvement of a common adhesion mechanism. FEMS Microbiol Lett. 2005;244(2):267-273.

[25] Jude BA, Martinez RM, Skorupski K, Taylor RK. Levels of the secreted *Vibrio cholerae* attachment factor GbpA are modulated by quorum-sensing-induced proteolysis. J Bacteriol. 2009;191(22): 6911-6917.

[26] Finkelstein RA, Boesman-Finkelstein M, Holt P. *Vibrio cholerae* hemagglutinin/lectin/protease hydrolyzes fibronectin and ovomucin: F.M. Burnet revisited. Proc Natl Acad Sci U S A. 1983;80(4):1092-1095.

[27] Stauder M, Vezzulli L, Pezzati E, Repetto B, Pruzzo C. Temperature affects *Vibrio cholerae* O1 El Tor persistence in the aquatic environment via an enhanced expression of GbpA and MSHA adhesins. Environ Microbiol Rep. 2010;2(1):140-144.

[28] Mandal S, Chatterjee NS. *Vibrio cholerae* GbpA elicits necrotic cell death in intestinal cells. J Med Microbiol. 2016;65(8):837-847.

[29] Loose JS, Forsberg Z, Fraaije MW, Eijsink VG, Vaaje-Kolstad G. A rapid quantitative activity assay shows that the *Vibrio cholerae* colonization factor GbpA is an active lytic polysaccharide monooxygenase. FEBS Lett. 2014; 588(18):3435-3440.

[30] Garay E, Arnau A, Amaro C. Incidence of *Vibrio cholerae* and related vibrios in a coastal lagoon and seawater influenced by lake discharges along an annual cycle. Appl Environ Microbiol. 1985;50(2):426-430.

[31] Meibom KL, Li XB, Nielsen AT, Wu CY, Roseman S, Schoolnik GK. The *Vibrio cholerae* chitin utilization program. Proc Natl Acad Sci U S A. 2004;101(8):2524-2529.

[32] Bhowmick R, Ghosal A, Chatterjee NS. Effect of environmental factors on expression and activity of chitinase genes of vibrios with special reference to *Vibrio cholerae*. J Appl Microbiol. 2007;103(1):97-108.

[33] Mondal M, Nag D, Koley H, Saha DR, Chatterjee NS. The *Vibrio cholerae* extracellular chitinase ChiA2 is important for survival and pathogenesis in the host intestine. PLoS One. 2014;9(9):e103119.

[34] Li X, Wang LX, Wang X, Roseman S. The chitin catabolic cascade in the marine bacterium *Vibrio cholerae*: characterization of a unique chitin oligosaccharide deacetylase. Glycobiology. 2007;17(12):1377-1387.

[35] Zhang YZ, Ran LY, Li CY, Chen XL. Diversity, Structures, and Collagen-Degrading Mechanisms of Bacterial Collagenolytic Proteases. Appl Environ Microbiol. 2015;81(18):6098-6107.

[36] Park BR, Zielke RA, Wierzbicki IH, Mitchell KC, Withey JH, Sikora AE. A metalloprotease secreted by the type II secretion system links *Vibrio cholerae* with collagen. J Bacteriol. 2015;197(6): 1051-1064.

[37] Benitez JA, Silva AJ. *Vibrio cholerae* hemagglutinin(HA)/protease: An extracellular metalloprotease with multiple pathogenic activities. Toxicon. 2016;115:55-62.

[38] Zhu J, Miller MB, Vance RE, Dziejman M, Bassler BL, Mekalanos JJ. Quorum-sensing regulators control virulence gene expression in *Vibrio cholerae*. Proc Natl Acad Sci U S A. 2002;99(5):3129-3134.

[39] Vance RE, Zhu J, Mekalanos JJ. A constitutively active variant of the quorum-sensing regulator LuxO affects protease production and biofilm formation in *Vibrio cholerae*. Infect Immun. 2003;71(5):2571-2576.

[40] Booth BA, Boesman-Finkelstein M, Finkelstein RA. *Vibrio cholerae* hemagglutinin/protease nicks cholera enterotoxin. Infect Immun. 1984;45(3): 558-560.

[41] Silva AJ, Leitch GJ, Camilli A, Benitez JA. Contribution of hemagglutinin/protease and motility to the pathogenesis of El Tor biotype cholera. Infect Immun. 2006;74(4):2072-2079.

[42] Wu Z, Nybom P, Magnusson KE. Distinct effects of *Vibrio cholerae* haemagglutinin/protease on the structure and localization of the tight junction-associated proteins occludin and ZO-1. Cell Microbiol. 2000;2(1):11-17.

[43] Finkelstein RA, Boesman-Finkelstein M, Chang Y, Hase CC. *Vibrio cholerae* hemagglutinin/protease, colonial variation, virulence, and detachment. Infect Immun. 1992; 60(2):472-478.

[44] Moustafa I, Connaris H, Taylor M, Zaitsev V, Wilson JC, Kiefel MJ, et al. Sialic acid recognition by *Vibrio cholerae* neuraminidase. J Biol Chem. 2004;279(39):40819-40826.

[45] Galen JE, Ketley JM, Fasano A, Richardson SH, Wasserman SS, Kaper JB. Role of *Vibrio cholerae* neuraminidase in the function of cholera toxin. Infect Immun. 1992;60(2):406-415.

[46] Crennell S, Garman E, Laver G, Vimr E, Taylor G. Crystal structure of *Vibrio cholerae* neuraminidase reveals dual lectin-like domains in addition to the catalytic domain. Structure. 1994; 2(6):535-544.

[47] Finkelstein RA, Mukerjee S, Rudra BC. Demonstration and Quantitation of Antigen in Cholera Stool Filtrates. J Infect Dis. 1963;113:99-104.

[48] Waldor MK, Mekalanos JJ. Lysogenic conversion by a filamentous phage encoding cholera toxin. Science. 1996;272(5270):1910-1914.

[49] Davis BM, Lawson EH, Sandkvist M, Ali A, Sozhamannan S, Waldor MK. Convergence of the secretory pathways for cholera toxin and the filamentous phage, CTXphi. Science. 2000;288(5464):333-335.

[50] Chaudhuri K. Structure, Genetics, and Mode of Disease of Cholera Toxin. In: Gopalakrishnakone P. B-MM, Llewellyn L., Singh B., editor. Biological Toxins and Bioterrorism. Toxinology. 1. Dordrecht: Springer; 2014. p. 3-27.

[51] Gadwal S, Korotkov KV, Delarosa JR, Hol WG, Sandkvist M. Functional and structural characterization of *Vibrio cholerae* extracellular serine protease B, VesB. J Biol Chem. 2014;289(12):8288-8298.

[52] Syngkon A, Elluri S, Koley H, Rompikuntal PK, Saha DR, Chakrabarti MK, et al. Studies on a novel serine protease of a DeltahapADeltaprtV *Vibrio cholerae* O1 strain and its role in hemorrhagic response in the rabbit ileal loop model. PLoS One. 2010;5(9).

[53] Vaitkevicius K, Rompikuntal PK, Lindmark B, Vaitkevicius R, Song T, Wai SN. The metalloprotease PrtV from *Vibrio cholerae*. FEBS J. 2008;275(12):3167-3177.

[54] Ogierman MA, Fallarino A, Riess T, Williams SG, Attridge SR, Manning PA. Characterization of the *Vibrio cholerae* El Tor lipase operon lipAB and a protease gene downstream of the hly region. J Bacteriol. 1997;179(22):7072-7080.

[55] Edwin A, Grundstrom C, Wai SN, Ohman A, Stier G, Sauer-Eriksson AE. Domain isolation, expression, purification and proteolytic activity of the metalloprotease PrtV from *Vibrio cholerae*. Protein Expr Purif. 2014;96:39-47.

[56] Rompikuntal PK, Vdovikova S, Duperthuy M, Johnson TL, Ahlund M, Lundmark R, et al. Outer Membrane Vesicle-Mediated Export of Processed PrtV Protease from *Vibrio cholerae*. PLoS One. 2015;10(7):e0134098.

[57] Vaitkevicius K, Lindmark B, Ou G, Song T, Toma C, Iwanaga M, et al. A *Vibrio cholerae* protease needed for killing of Caenorhabditis elegans has a role in protection from natural predator grazing. Proc Natl Acad Sci U S A. 2006;103(24):9280-9285.

[58] Edwin A, Persson C, Mayzel M, Wai SN, Ohman A, Karlsson BG, et al. Structure of the N-terminal domain of the metalloprotease PrtV from *Vibrio cholerae*. Protein Sci. 2015;24(12): 2076-2080.

[59] Stoebner JA, Payne SM. Iron-regulated hemolysin production and utilization of heme and hemoglobin by *Vibrio cholerae*. Infect Immun. 1988;56(11):2891-2895.

[60] Debellis L, Diana A, Arcidiacono D, Fiorotto R, Portincasa P, Altomare DF, et al. The *Vibrio cholerae* cytolysin promotes chloride secretion from intact human intestinal mucosa. PLoS One. 2009;4(3):e5074.

[61] Toma C, Honma Y. Cloning and genetic analysis of the *Vibrio cholerae* aminopeptidase gene. Infect Immun. 1996;64(11):4495-4500.

[62] Seper A, Hosseinzadeh A, Gorkiewicz G, Lichtenegger S, Roier S, Leitner DR, et al. *Vibrio cholerae* evades neutrophil extracellular traps by the activity of two extracellular nucleases. PLoS Pathog. 2013;9(9):e1003614.

[63] Blokesch M, Schoolnik GK. The extracellular nuclease Dns and its role in natural transformation of *Vibrio cholerae*. J Bacteriol. 2008;190(21):7232-7240.

[64] Joshi A, Kostiuk B, Rogers A, Teschler J, Pukatzki S, Yildiz FH. Rules of Engagement: The Type VI Secretion System in *Vibrio cholerae*. Trends Microbiol. 2017;25(4):267-279.

[65] Coulthurst S. The Type VI secretion system: a versatile bacterial weapon. Microbiology (Reading). 2019;165(5):503-515.

[66] Cherrak Y, Flaugnatti N, Durand E, Journet L, Cascales E. Structure and Activity of the Type VI Secretion System. Microbiol Spectr. 2019;7(4).

[67] Borgeaud S, Metzger LC, Scrignari T, Blokesch M. The type VI secretion system of *Vibrio cholerae* fosters horizontal gene transfer. Science. 2015;347(6217):63-67.

[68] Pukatzki S, Ma AT, Sturtevant D, Krastins B, Sarracino D, Nelson WC, et al. Identification of a conserved bacterial protein secretion system in *Vibrio cholerae* using the Dictyostelium host model system. Proc Natl Acad Sci U S A. 2006;103(5):1528-1533.

[69] Shneider MM, Buth SA, Ho BT, Basler M, Mekalanos JJ, Leiman PG. PAAR-repeat proteins sharpen and diversify the type VI secretion system spike. Nature. 2013;500(7462):350-353.

[70] Brunet YR, Henin J, Celia H, Cascales E. Type VI secretion and bacteriophage tail tubes share a common assembly pathway. EMBO Rep. 2014;15(3):315-321.

[71] Kube S, Kapitein N, Zimniak T, Herzog F, Mogk A, Wendler P. Structure of the VipA/B type VI secretion complex suggests a contraction-state-specific recycling mechanism. Cell Rep. 2014;8(1):20-30.

[72] Bonemann G, Pietrosiuk A, Diemand A, Zentgraf H, Mogk A. Remodelling of VipA/VipB tubules by ClpV-mediated threading is crucial for type VI protein secretion. EMBO J. 2009;28(4):315-325.

[73] Pietrosiuk A, Lenherr ED, Falk S, Bonemann G, Kopp J, Zentgraf H, et al. Molecular basis for the unique role of the AAA+ chaperone ClpV in type VI protein secretion. J Biol Chem. 2011;286(34):30010-30021.

[74] Unterweger D, Kostiuk B, Pukatzki S. Adaptor Proteins of Type VI Secretion System Effectors. Trends Microbiol. 2017;25(1):8-10.

[75] Crisan CV, Chande AT, Williams K, Raghuram V, Rishishwar L, Steinbach G, et al. Analysis of *Vibrio cholerae* genomes identifies new type VI secretion system gene clusters. Genome Biol. 2019;20(1):163.

[76] Labbate M, Orata FD, Petty NK, Jayatilleke ND, King WL, Kirchberger PC, et al. A genomic island in *Vibrio cholerae* with VPI-1 site-specific recombination characteristics contains CRISPR-Cas and type VI secretion modules. Sci Rep. 2016;6:36891.

[77] Unterweger D, Miyata ST, Bachmann V, Brooks TM, Mullins T, Kostiuk B, et al. The *Vibrio cholerae* type VI secretion system employs diverse effector modules for intraspecific competition. Nat Commun. 2014;5:3549.

[78] Dong TG, Mekalanos JJ. Characterization of the RpoN regulon reveals differential regulation of T6SS and new flagellar operons in *Vibrio cholerae* O37 strain V52. Nucleic Acids Res. 2012;40(16):7766-7775.

[79] Ishikawa T, Sabharwal D, Broms J, Milton DL, Sjostedt A, Uhlin BE, et al. Pathoadaptive conditional regulation of the type VI secretion system in *Vibrio cholerae* O1 strains. Infect Immun. 2012;80(2):575-584.

[80] Drebes Dorr NC, Blokesch M. Interbacterial competition and anti-predatory behaviour of environmental *Vibrio cholerae* strains. Environ Microbiol. 2020;22(10):4485-4504.

[81] Yang X, Long M, Shen X. Effector(-) Immunity Pairs Provide the T6SS Nanomachine its Offensive and Defensive Capabilities. Molecules. 2018;23(5).

[82] Vettiger A, Basler M. Type VI Secretion System Substrates Are Transferred and Reused among Sister Cells. Cell. 2016;167(1):99-110 e12.

[83] Silverman JM, Agnello DM, Zheng H, Andrews BT, Li M, Catalano CE, et al. Haemolysin coregulated protein is an exported receptor and chaperone of type VI secretion substrates. Mol Cell. 2013;51(5):584-593.

[84] Williams SG, Varcoe LT, Attridge SR, Manning PA. *Vibrio cholerae* Hcp, a secreted protein coregulated with HlyA. Infect Immun. 1996;64(1):283-289.

[85] Pukatzki S, Ma AT, Revel AT, Sturtevant D, Mekalanos JJ. Type VI secretion system translocates a phage tail spike-like protein into target cells where it cross-links actin. Proc Natl Acad Sci U S A. 2007;104(39):15508-15513.

[86] Ma AT, Mekalanos JJ. In vivo actin cross-linking induced by *Vibrio cholerae* type VI secretion system is associated with intestinal inflammation. Proc Natl Acad Sci U S A. 2010;107(9):4365-4370.

[87] Brooks TM, Unterweger D, Bachmann V, Kostiuk B, Pukatzki S. Lytic activity of the *Vibrio cholerae* type VI secretion toxin VgrG-3 is inhibited by the antitoxin TsaB. J Biol Chem. 2013;288(11):7618-7625.

[88] Dong TG, Ho BT, Yoder-Himes DR, Mekalanos JJ. Identification of T6SS-dependent effector and immunity proteins by Tn-seq in *Vibrio cholerae*. Proc Natl Acad Sci U S A. 2013;110(7): 2623-2628.

[89] Miyata ST, Kitaoka M, Brooks TM, McAuley SB, Pukatzki S. *Vibrio cholerae* requires the type VI secretion system virulence factor VasX to kill Dictyostelium discoideum. Infect Immun. 2011;79(7):2941-2949.

[90] Miyata ST, Unterweger D, Rudko SP, Pukatzki S. Dual expression profile of type VI secretion system immunity genes protects pandemic *Vibrio cholerae*. PLoS Pathog. 2013;9(12):e1003752.

[91] Kamal F, Liang X, Manera K, Pei TT, Kim H, Lam LG, et al. Differential Cellular Response to Translocated Toxic Effectors and Physical Penetration by the Type VI Secretion System. Cell Rep. 2020;31(11):107766.

[92] Altindis E, Dong T, Catalano C, Mekalanos J. Secretome analysis of *Vibrio cholerae* type VI secretion system reveals a new effector-immunity pair. mBio. 2015;6(2):e00075.

[93] Kostiuk B, Unterweger D, Provenzano D, Pukatzki S. T6SS intraspecific competition orchestrates *Vibrio cholerae* genotypic diversity. Int Microbiol. 2017;20(3):130-137.

[94] Kanonenberg K, Spitz O, Erenburg IN, Beer T, Schmitt L. Type I secretion system-it takes three and a substrate. FEMS Microbiol Lett. 2018;365(11).

[95] Gray L, Mackman N, Nicaud JM, Holland IB. The carboxy-terminal region of haemolysin 2001 is required for secretion of the toxin from Escherichia coli. Mol Gen Genet. 1986;205(1):127-133.

[96] Costa TR, Felisberto-Rodrigues C, Meir A, Prevost MS, Redzej A, Trokter M, et al. Secretion systems in Gram-negative bacteria: structural and mechanistic insights. Nat Rev Microbiol. 2015;13(6):343-359.

[97] Boardman BK, Satchell KJ. *Vibrio cholerae* strains with mutations in an atypical type I secretion system accumulate RTX toxin intracellularly. J Bacteriol. 2004;186(23):8137-8143.

[98] Boardman BK, Meehan BM, Fullner Satchell KJ. Growth phase regulation of *Vibrio cholerae* RTX toxin export. J Bacteriol. 2007;189(5):1827-1835.

[99] Linhartova I, Bumba L, Masin J, Basler M, Osicka R, Kamanova J, et al. RTX proteins: a highly diverse family secreted by a common

mechanism. FEMS Microbiol Rev. 2010;34(6):1076-1112.

[100] Lin W, Fullner KJ, Clayton R, Sexton JA, Rogers MB, Calia KE, et al. Identification of a *Vibrio cholerae* RTX toxin gene cluster that is tightly linked to the cholera toxin prophage. Proc Natl Acad Sci U S A. 1999;96(3):1071-1076.

[101] Cordero CL, Kudryashov DS, Reisler E, Satchell KJ. The Actin cross-linking domain of the *Vibrio cholerae* RTX toxin directly catalyzes the covalent cross-linking of actin. J Biol Chem. 2006;281(43):32366-32374.

[102] Cordero CL, Sozhamannan S, Satchell KJ. RTX toxin actin cross-linking activity in clinical and environmental isolates of *Vibrio cholerae*. J Clin Microbiol. 2007;45(7):2289-2292.

[103] Fullner KJ, Mekalanos JJ. In vivo covalent cross-linking of cellular actin by the *Vibrio cholerae* RTX toxin. EMBO J. 2000;19(20):5315-5323.

[104] Sheahan KL, Cordero CL, Satchell KJ. Identification of a domain within the multifunctional *Vibrio cholerae* RTX toxin that covalently cross-links actin. Proc Natl Acad Sci U S A. 2004;101(26):9798-9803.

[105] Chatterjee R, Nag S, Chaudhuri K. Identification of a new RTX-like gene cluster in *Vibrio cholerae*. FEMS Microbiol Lett. 2008;284(2):165-171.

[106] Syed KA, Beyhan S, Correa N, Queen J, Liu J, Peng F, et al. The *Vibrio cholerae* flagellar regulatory hierarchy controls expression of virulence factors. J Bacteriol. 2009;191(21):6555-6570.

[107] Syed KA. Regulation of hemagglutinin by flagellar hierarchy in *Vibrio cholerae*. Ann Arbor: University of Texas; 2010.

[108] Kitts G, Giglio KM, Zamorano-Sanchez D, Park JH, Townsley L, Cooley RB, et al. A Conserved Regulatory Circuit Controls Large Adhesins in *Vibrio cholerae*. mBio. 2019;10(6).

[109] Miller KA, Tomberlin KF, Dziejman M. Vibrio variations on a type three theme. Curr Opin Microbiol. 2019;47:66-73.

[110] Chaand M, Miller KA, Sofia MK, Schlesener C, Weaver JW, Sood V, et al. Type 3 Secretion System Island Encoded Proteins Required for Colonization by Non-O1/non-O139 Serogroup *Vibrio cholerae*. Infect Immun. 2015;83(7): 2862-2869.

[111] Dziejman M, Serruto D, Tam VC, Sturtevant D, Diraphat P, Faruque SM, et al. Genomic characterization of non-O1, non-O139 *Vibrio cholerae* reveals genes for a type III secretion system. Proc Natl Acad Sci U S A. 2005;102(9):3465-3470.

[112] Shin OS, Tam VC, Suzuki M, Ritchie JM, Bronson RT, Waldor MK, et al. Type III secretion is essential for the rapidly fatal diarrheal disease caused by non-O1, non-O139 *Vibrio cholerae*. mBio. 2011;2(3):e00106-11.

[113] Portaliou AG, Tsolis KC, Loos MS, Zorzini V, Economou A. Type III Secretion: Building and Operating a Remarkable Nanomachine. Trends Biochem Sci. 2016;41(2):175-189.

[114] Alam A, Miller KA, Chaand M, Butler JS, Dziejman M. Identification of *Vibrio cholerae* type III secretion system effector proteins. Infect Immun. 2011;79(4):1728-1740.

[115] Morita M, Yamamoto S, Hiyoshi H, Kodama T, Okura M, Arakawa E, et al. Horizontal gene transfer of a genetic island encoding a type III secretion system distributed in *Vibrio cholerae*. Microbiol Immunol. 2013;57(5):334-339.

[116] Alam A, Tam V, Hamilton E, Dziejman M. vttRA and vttRB Encode

ToxR family proteins that mediate bile-induced expression of type three secretion system genes in a non-O1/non-O139 *Vibrio cholerae* strain. Infect Immun. 2010;78(6):2554-2570.

[117] Miller KA, Sofia MK, Weaver JWA, Seward CH, Dziejman M. Regulation by ToxR-Like Proteins Converges on vttRB Expression To Control Type 3 Secretion System-Dependent Caco2-BBE Cytotoxicity in *Vibrio cholerae*. J Bacteriol. 2016;198(11):1675-1682.

[118] Tam VC, Serruto D, Dziejman M, Brieher W, Mekalanos JJ. A type III secretion system in *Vibrio cholerae* translocates a formin/spire hybrid-like actin nucleator to promote intestinal colonization. Cell Host Microbe. 2007;1(2):95-107.

[119] Tam VC, Suzuki M, Coughlin M, Saslowsky D, Biswas K, Lencer WI, et al. Functional analysis of VopF activity required for colonization in *Vibrio cholerae*. mBio. 2010;1(5).

[120] Seward CH, Manzella A, Alam A, Butler JS, Dziejman M. Using S. cerevisiae as a Model System to Investigate V. cholerae VopX-Host Cell Protein Interactions and Phenotypes. Toxins (Basel). 2015;7(10):4099-4110.

[121] Suzuki M, Danilchanka O, Mekalanos JJ. *Vibrio cholerae* T3SS effector VopE modulates mitochondrial dynamics and innate immune signaling by targeting Miro GTPases. Cell Host Microbe. 2014;16(5):581-591.

[122] Kay LJ, Sangal V, Black GW, Soundararajan M. Proteomics and bioinformatics analyses identify novel cellular roles outside mitochondrial function for human miro GTPases. Mol Cell Biochem. 2019;451(1-2):21-35.

[123] Hospenthal MK, Costa TRD, Waksman G. A comprehensive guide to pilus biogenesis in Gram-negative bacteria. Nat Rev Microbiol. 2017;15(6):365-379.

[124] Lim MS, Ng D, Zong Z, Arvai AS, Taylor RK, Tainer JA, et al. *Vibrio cholerae* El Tor TcpA crystal structure and mechanism for pilus-mediated microcolony formation. Mol Microbiol. 2010;77(3):755-770.

[125] Kumar A, Das B, Kumar N. Vibrio Pathogenicity Island-1: The Master Determinant of Cholera Pathogenesis. Front Cell Infect Microbiol. 2020;10:561296.

[126] Tacket CO, Taylor RK, Losonsky G, Lim Y, Nataro JP, Kaper JB, et al. Investigation of the roles of toxin-coregulated pili and mannose-sensitive hemagglutinin pili in the pathogenesis of *Vibrio cholerae* O139 infection. Infect Immun. 1998;66(2):692-695.

[127] Gutierrez-Rodarte M, Kolappan S, Burrell BA, Craig L. The *Vibrio cholerae* minor pilin TcpB mediates uptake of the cholera toxin phage CTXphi. J Biol Chem. 2019;294(43):15698-15710.

[128] Watnick PI, Fullner KJ, Kolter R. A role for the mannose-sensitive hemagglutinin in biofilm formation by *Vibrio cholerae* El Tor. J Bacteriol. 1999;181(11):3606-3609.

[129] Floyd KA, Lee CK, Xian W, Nametalla M, Valentine A, Crair B, et al. c-di-GMP modulates type IV MSHA pilus retraction and surface attachment in *Vibrio cholerae*. Nat Commun. 2020;11(1):1549.

[130] Fullner KJ, Mekalanos JJ. Genetic characterization of a new type IV-A pilus gene cluster found in both classical and El Tor biotypes of *Vibrio cholerae*. Infect Immun. 1999;67(3):1393-1404.

[131] Adams DW, Stutzmann S, Stoudmann C, Blokesch M. DNA-uptake pili of *Vibrio cholerae* are required for chitin colonization and capable of kin recognition via sequence-specific self-interaction. Nat Microbiol. 2019;4(9):1545-1557.

[132] Shime-Hattori A, Iida T, Arita M, Park KS, Kodama T, Honda T. Two type IV pili of Vibrio parahaemolyticus play different roles in biofilm formation. FEMS Microbiol Lett. 2006;264(1):89-97.

[133] Ogura K, Yahiro K, Moss J. Cell Death Signaling Pathway Induced by Cholix Toxin, a Cytotoxin and eEF2 ADP-Ribosyltransferase Produced by *Vibrio cholerae*. Toxins (Basel). 2020;13(1).

[134] Jorgensen R, Purdy AE, Fieldhouse RJ, Kimber MS, Bartlett DH, Merrill AR. Cholix toxin, a novel ADP-ribosylating factor from *Vibrio cholerae*. J Biol Chem. 2008;283(16):10671-10678.

[135] Taverner A, MacKay J, Laurent F, Hunter T, Liu K, Mangat K, et al. Cholix protein domain I functions as a carrier element for efficient apical to basal epithelial transcytosis. Tissue Barriers. 2020;8(1):1710429.

[136] Trucksis M, Galen JE, Michalski J, Fasano A, Kaper JB. Accessory cholera enterotoxin (Ace), the third toxin of a *Vibrio cholerae* virulence cassette. Proc Natl Acad Sci U S A. 1993;90(11):5267-5271.

[137] Fasano A, Baudry B, Pumplin DW, Wasserman SS, Tall BD, Ketley JM, et al. *Vibrio cholerae* produces a second enterotoxin, which affects intestinal tight junctions. Proc Natl Acad Sci U S A. 1991;88(12):5242-5246.

[138] Perez-Reytor D, Pavon A, Lopez-Joven C, Ramirez-Araya S, Pena-Varas C, Plaza N, et al. Analysis of the Zonula occludens Toxin Found in the Genome of the Chilean Non-toxigenic Vibrio parahaemolyticus Strain PMC53.7. Front Cell Infect Microbiol. 2020;10:482.

[139] Uzzau S, Cappuccinelli P, Fasano A. Expression of *Vibrio cholerae* zonula occludens toxin and analysis of its subcellular localization. Microb Pathog. 1999;27(6):377-385.

[140] Goldblum SE, Rai U, Tripathi A, Thakar M, De Leo L, Di Toro N, et al. The active Zot domain (aa 288-293) increases ZO-1 and myosin 1C serine/threonine phosphorylation, alters interaction between ZO-1 and its binding partners, and induces tight junction disassembly through proteinase activated receptor 2 activation. FASEB J. 2011;25(1):144-158.

[141] Guerrero-Mandujano A, Hernandez-Cortez C, Ibarra JA, Castro-Escarpulli G. The outer membrane vesicles: Secretion system type zero. Traffic. 2017;18(7):425-432.

[142] Toyofuku M, Nomura N, Eberl L. Types and origins of bacterial membrane vesicles. Nat Rev Microbiol. 2019;17(1):13-24.

[143] Altindis E, Fu Y, Mekalanos JJ. Proteomic analysis of *Vibrio cholerae* outer membrane vesicles. Proc Natl Acad Sci U S A. 2014;111(15):E1548-E1556.

[144] Langlete P, Krabberod AK, Winther-Larsen HC. Vesicles From *Vibrio cholerae* Contain AT-Rich DNA and Shorter mRNAs That Do Not Correlate With Their Protein Products. Front Microbiol. 2019;10:2708.

[145] Sjostrom AE, Sandblad L, Uhlin BE, Wai SN. Membrane vesicle-mediated release of bacterial RNA. Sci Rep. 2015;5:15329.

[146] Zingl FG, Kohl P, Cakar F, Leitner DR, Mitterer F, Bonnington KE, et al. Outer Membrane Vesiculation Facilitates Surface Exchange and In Vivo Adaptation of *Vibrio cholerae*. Cell Host Microbe. 2020;27(2):225-237 e8.

[147] Orench-Rivera N, Kuehn MJ. Environmentally controlled bacterial vesicle-mediated export. Cell Microbiol. 2016;18(11):1525-1536.

[148] Duperthuy M, Sjostrom AE, Sabharwal D, Damghani F, Uhlin BE, Wai SN. Role of the *Vibrio cholerae*

matrix protein Bap1 in cross-resistance to antimicrobial peptides. PLoS Pathog. 2013;9(10):e1003620.

[149] Miller VL, Mekalanos JJ. A novel suicide vector and its use in construction of insertion mutations: osmoregulation of outer membrane proteins and virulence determinants in *Vibrio cholerae* requires toxR. J Bacteriol. 1988;170(6):2575-2583.

[150] Champion GA, Neely MN, Brennan MA, DiRita VJ. A branch in the ToxR regulatory cascade of *Vibrio cholerae* revealed by characterization of toxT mutant strains. Mol Microbiol. 1997;23(2):323-331.

[151] Mathur J, Waldor MK. The *Vibrio cholerae* ToxR-regulated porin OmpU confers resistance to antimicrobial peptides. Infect Immun. 2004;72(6):3577-3583.

[152] Blake PA, Weaver RE, Hollis DG. Diseases of humans (other than cholera) caused by vibrios. Annu Rev Microbiol. 1980;34:341-367.

[153] Aung KM, Sjostrom AE, von Pawel-Rammingen U, Riesbeck K, Uhlin BE, Wai SN. Naturally Occurring IgG Antibodies Provide Innate Protection against *Vibrio cholerae* Bacteremia by Recognition of the Outer Membrane Protein U. J Innate Immun. 2016;8(3):269-283.

[154] Reyes-RoblesT, DillardRS, CairnsLS, Silva-Valenzuela CA, Housman M, Ali A, et al. *Vibrio cholerae* Outer Membrane Vesicles Inhibit Bacteriophage Infection. J Bacteriol. 2018;200(15).

[155] Mah TF. Biofilm-specific antibiotic resistance. Future Microbiol. 2012;7(9): 1061-1072.

[156] Fong JNC, Yildiz FH. Biofilm Matrix Proteins. Microbiol Spectr. 2015;3(2).

[157] Chatterjee D, Chaudhuri K. Association of cholera toxin with *Vibrio cholerae* outer membrane vesicles which are internalized by human intestinal epithelial cells. FEBS Lett. 2011;585(9):1357-1362.

[158] Rasti ES, Brown AC. Cholera Toxin Encapsulated within Several *Vibrio cholerae* O1 Serotype Inaba Outer Membrane Vesicles Lacks a Functional B-Subunit. Toxins (Basel). 2019;11(4).

[159] O'Donoghue EJ, Krachler AM. Mechanisms of outer membrane vesicle entry into host cells. Cell Microbiol. 2016;18(11):1508-1517.

[160] Mondal A, Tapader R, Chatterjee NS, Ghosh A, Sinha R, Koley H, et al. Cytotoxic and Inflammatory Responses Induced by Outer Membrane Vesicle-Associated Biologically Active Proteases from *Vibrio cholerae*. Infect Immun. 2016;84(5):1478-1490.

[161] Elluri S, Enow C, Vdovikova S, Rompikuntal PK, Dongre M, Carlsson S, et al. Outer membrane vesicles mediate transport of biologically active *Vibrio cholerae* cytolysin (VCC) from V. cholerae strains. PLoS One. 2014;9(9):e106731.

[162] Silva AJ, Benitez JA. *Vibrio cholerae* Biofilms and Cholera Pathogenesis. PLoS Negl Trop Dis. 2016;10(2):e0004330.

[163] Lutz C, Erken M, Noorian P, Sun S, McDougald D. Environmental reservoirs and mechanisms of persistence of *Vibrio cholerae*. Front Microbiol. 2013;4:375.

[164] Conner JG, Teschler JK, Jones CJ, Yildiz FH. Staying Alive: *Vibrio cholerae's* Cycle of Environmental Survival, Transmission, and Dissemination. Microbiol Spectr. 2016;4(2).

[165] Echazarreta MA, Klose KE. Vibrio Flagellar Synthesis. Front Cell Infect Microbiol. 2019;9:131.

[166] Galan JE, Collmer A. Type III secretion machines: bacterial devices for

protein delivery into host cells. Science. 1999;284(5418):1322-1328.

[167] Klose KE, Mekalanos JJ. Differential regulation of multiple flagellins in *Vibrio cholerae*. J Bacteriol. 1998;180(2):303-316.

[168] Dongre M, Singh B, Aung KM, Larsson P, Miftakhova R, Persson K, et al. Flagella-mediated secretion of a novel *Vibrio cholerae* cytotoxin affecting both vertebrate and invertebrate hosts. Commun Biol. 2018;1:59.

[169] Butler SM, Camilli A. Both chemotaxis and net motility greatly influence the infectivity of *Vibrio cholerae*. Proc Natl Acad Sci U S A. 2004;101(14):5018-5023.

[170] Utada AS, Bennett RR, Fong JCN, Gibiansky ML, Yildiz FH, Golestanian R, et al. *Vibrio cholerae* use pili and flagella synergistically to effect motility switching and conditional surface attachment. Nat Commun. 2014;5:4913.

[171] Lauriano CM, Ghosh C, Correa NE, Klose KE. The sodium-driven flagellar motor controls exopolysaccharide expression in *Vibrio cholerae*. J Bacteriol. 2004;186(15):4864-4874.

[172] Yildiz F, Fong J, Sadovskaya I, Grard T, Vinogradov E. Structural characterization of the extracellular polysaccharide from *Vibrio cholerae* O1 El-Tor. PLoS One. 2014;9(1):e86751.

[173] Yildiz FH, Schoolnik GK. *Vibrio cholerae* O1 El Tor: identification of a gene cluster required for the rugose colony type, exopolysaccharide production, chlorine resistance, and biofilm formation. Proc Natl Acad Sci U S A. 1999;96(7):4028-4033.

[174] Fong JCN, Syed KA, Klose KE, Yildiz FH. Role of Vibrio polysaccharide (vps) genes in VPS production, biofilm formation and *Vibrio cholerae* pathogenesis. Microbiology (Reading). 2010;156(Pt 9):2757-2769.

[175] Schwechheimer C, Hebert K, Tripathi S, Singh PK, Floyd KA, Brown ER, et al. A tyrosine phospho-regulatory system controls exopolysaccharide biosynthesis and biofilm formation in *Vibrio cholerae*. PLoS Pathog. 2020;16(8):e1008745.

[176] Teschler JK, Zamorano-Sanchez D, Utada AS, Warner CJ, Wong GC, Linington RG, et al. Living in the matrix: assembly and control of *Vibrio cholerae* biofilms. Nat Rev Microbiol. 2015;13(5):255-268.

[177] Fong JC, Yildiz FH. The rbmBCDEF gene cluster modulates development of rugose colony morphology and biofilm formation in *Vibrio cholerae*. J Bacteriol. 2007;189(6):2319-2330.

[178] Kaus K, Biester A, Chupp E, Lu J, Visudharomn C, Olson R. The 1.9 A crystal structure of the extracellular matrix protein Bap1 from *Vibrio cholerae* provides insights into bacterial biofilm adhesion. J Biol Chem. 2019;294(40):14499-14511.

[179] Fong JC, Karplus K, Schoolnik GK, Yildiz FH. Identification and characterization of RbmA, a novel protein required for the development of rugose colony morphology and biofilm structure in *Vibrio cholerae*. J Bacteriol. 2006;188(3):1049-1059.

[180] Smith DR, Maestre-Reyna M, Lee G, Gerard H, Wang AH, Watnick PI. In situ proteolysis of the *Vibrio cholerae* matrix protein RbmA promotes biofilm recruitment. Proc Natl Acad Sci U S A. 2015;112(33):10491-10496.

[181] Duperthuy M, Uhlin BE, Wai SN. Biofilm recruitment of *Vibrio cholerae* by matrix proteolysis. Trends Microbiol. 2015;23(11):667-668.

[182] Absalon C, Van Dellen K, Watnick PI. A communal bacterial adhesin anchors biofilm and bystander cells to surfaces. PLoS Pathog. 2011;7(8): e1002210.

[183] Vorkapic D, Pressler K, Schild S. Multifaceted roles of extracellular DNA in bacterial physiology. Curr Genet. 2016;62(1):71-79.

[184] Kanampalliwar A, Singh DV. Extracellular DNA builds and interacts with vibrio polysaccharide in the biofilm matrix formed by *Vibrio cholerae*. Environ Microbiol Rep. 2020;12(5):594-606.

[185] Seper A, Fengler VH, Roier S, Wolinski H, Kohlwein SD, Bishop AL, et al. Extracellular nucleases and extracellular DNA play important roles in *Vibrio cholerae* biofilm formation. Mol Microbiol. 2011;82(4):1015-1037.

[186] Kaplan JB. Biofilm dispersal: mechanisms, clinical implications, and potential therapeutic uses. J Dent Res. 2010;89(3):205-218.

[187] Singh PK, Bartalomej S, Hartmann R, Jeckel H, Vidakovic L, Nadell CD, et al. *Vibrio cholerae* Combines Individual and Collective Sensing to Trigger Biofilm Dispersal. Curr Biol. 2017;27(21):3359-3366 e7.

[188] Bridges AA, Fei C, Bassler BL. Identification of signaling pathways, matrix-digestion enzymes, and motility components controlling *Vibrio cholerae* biofilm dispersal. Proc Natl Acad Sci U S A. 2020;117(51):32639-32647.

[189] Mewborn L, Benitez JA, Silva AJ. Flagellar motility, extracellular proteases and *Vibrio cholerae* detachment from abiotic and biotic surfaces. Microb Pathog. 2017;113:17-24.

Chapter 9

Challenges in Controlling Vibriosis in Shrimp Farms

Hethesh Chellapandian, Jeyachandran Sivakamavalli, A. Vijay Anand and Balamuralikrishnan Balasubramanian

Abstract

Recently the shrimp farming has blooming as a crucial counterpart in the aquaculture industry which contribute the remarkable role in sea food production as well economy of the country. However, this could be fluctuated every year through several circumstances such as unfavorable (Poor water and soil quality) environmental factors. The environmental factors includes disease causing bacterial pathogens in the soil and water which causes the bacterial diseases in the aquatic animals, like this hectic problems are prevented through bioaugmentation strategies. The pond environment plays a vital role in determining the healthy culture system, but there is high risk for manipulation by bacterial community which takes care of waste generated in the system through *in situ* bioremediation. Due to the impact of rapidly growing bacterial diseases of shrimps throughout the world, numerous studies have been carried out to find immunostimulants, immunomodulators and biotic component that can be used against vibrio causing pathogens, and can also be used as an alternative for antibiotics. Recent research focus towards the marine resources such as microalgae, seaweed, live feeds (like artemia, copepods, rotifers), bacteriophage, and probiotics have been found to have higher potential in reducing vibriosis. Eco-based shrimp farming includes green water technology, phage therapy bio-floc technology (BFT) and integrated multi-trophic aquaculture (IMTA), these methods hold a promising alternative to antibiotics in the near future. Bacterial diseases caused by vibrios have been reported in penaeid shrimp culture systems implicating at least 14 species and they are *Vibrio harveyi, V. splendidus, V. parahaemolyticus, V. alginolyticus, V. anguillarum, V. vulnificuslogei* etc.

Keywords: Immunity, Hypoxia, Salinity, pH, Vibriosis, Probiotics

1. Introduction

Vibriosis is a bacterial disease caused by *Vibrio* which is Gram-negative, motile, facultative anaerobe bacteria of the family Vibrionaceae. It is ubiquitous throughout the world and in all marine crustaceans, including shrimp. Vibriosis is one of the major disease problems in shellfish and finfish aquaculture, especially in shrimp farming. Vibriosis is a bacterial disease responsible for mortality of cultured shrimp worldwide. Various studies has been done to find a remedy for vibriosis in rearing as well as shrimp culture ponds. Certain studies show that usage of microalgae, bacteriophage, and probiotic bacteria have been found to have higher potential in reducing vibriosis. Vibriosis is a series of bacterial infections caused by a bacterium belongs to the genus *Vibrio*. Black shell disease, bacterial septicemia, hepatopancreatic necrosis, brown gill disease, swollen hindgut syndrome and luminous bacterial disease [1]. High density of the bacterial species in culture pond increases the probability of getting viral diseases, especially white spot syndrome

The pacific white shrimp (*Litopenaeus vannamei*), Indian white shrimp (*Fenneropenaeus indicus*), Black tiger shrimp (*Penaeus monodon)* are important commercial species of the penaeid family. *Fenneropenaeus indicus* supports commercial fisheries in both marine and brackish water environments on the east and west coasts of India. India is one of the major suppliers of shrimp to Japan, Europe, Thailand and USA [2]. The secondary infection of vibrios in *P. monodon* occurs due to poor water quality, stress, high stocking density, unstable environmental conditions, toxins and virion particles. Vibriosis is caused by a number of bacteria belongs to *vibrio* species which includes; *Vibrio harveyi, V. splendidus, V. parahaemolyticus, V. alginolyticus*. There have been occasional reports of vibriosis caused *by V. damsella, V. fluvalis* and other undefined *vibrio* species [3].

2. Vibrio diseases

2.1 Bacterial septicemia

This is one of the severe systemic diseases caused by bacteria, which affects shrimps and exhibits the symptoms such as lethargic, show abnormal swimming behavior, expansion of chromatophores, followed by reddish color change in the pleopods which can be seen in the abdominal musculature. In chronic cases, the gill covers appear flared up and eroded along with the melanized black blisters on the carapace and abdomen. The disease caused by *Vibrio alginolyticus, V. anguillarium or V. parahaemolyticus* and diagnosed based on gross signs like its swimming patterns, Food consumption ratio (FCR) and confirmed by analyzing the isolated pathogen from haemolymph or muscle sample by standard microbiological methods and histopathology. Bacterial septicemia can be prevented by maintaining good water quality and by reducing the organic load by increased water exchange. This can be prevented by giving high protein feed with antibiotics, repeated water exchange might help to decrease the density of disease causing pathogens [4].

2.2 Necrosis (Hepatopancreas, muscle and appendages)

Inflammation in the cells explores the proteins release from tissues and cells, which reflects on the color change of the animals as like milky white. This disease could be caused due to several unfavorable environmental conditions such as water quality, organic load, malnutrition and wastes producecd from the animals, in chronic cases, melanization of setae, antennae, appendages and muscle can be witnessed. Necrosis is usually caused by *Vibrio spp, Pseudomonas spp, Aeromonas spp* and *Flavobacterium spp* and can be diagnosed based on swimming patterns and other symptoms like white patches in cephalothorax and can be prevented by repeated water exchange and feeding nutrient rich feed. Necrosis is controlled by induced molting by applying 5–10 ppm fermented rice cake (**Figure 1**) [5].

3. Brown spot diseases: (Shell disease or rust disease)

This kind of disease in shrimps showed brown to black enodsed areas on the body surface and appendages, *Aeromonas spp*, and *Flavobacterium spp*., are the crucial causative agents involved in the pathogenisis through chitinolytic activity.

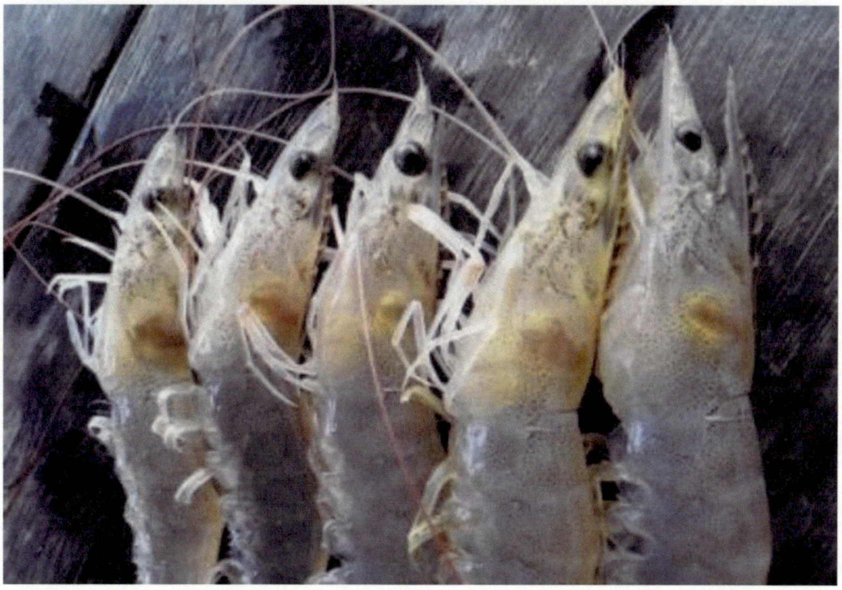

Figure 1.
Shrimps affected by Necrosis 1.

Major symptoms are stooped posture and brown to back spots on the exoskeleton, in extreme conditions it might even lead to necrosis [6]. Brown spot disease can be prevented by reducing organic load in water, with repeated water exchange and by feeding the shrimps with nutritional supplement.

3.1 Vibriosis in shrimp

Members of the microorganism genus *Vibrio* have become a major constraint on production and trading in shrimp industry. *Vibrio* is responsible for several diseases and causing mortalities up to 100 percent and global losses of around 4.5 billion USD. *Vibrio spp.* is a natural micro flora of wild and cultured shrimps, and become opportunistic pathogens when natural defense mechanisms are suppressed. In intensive

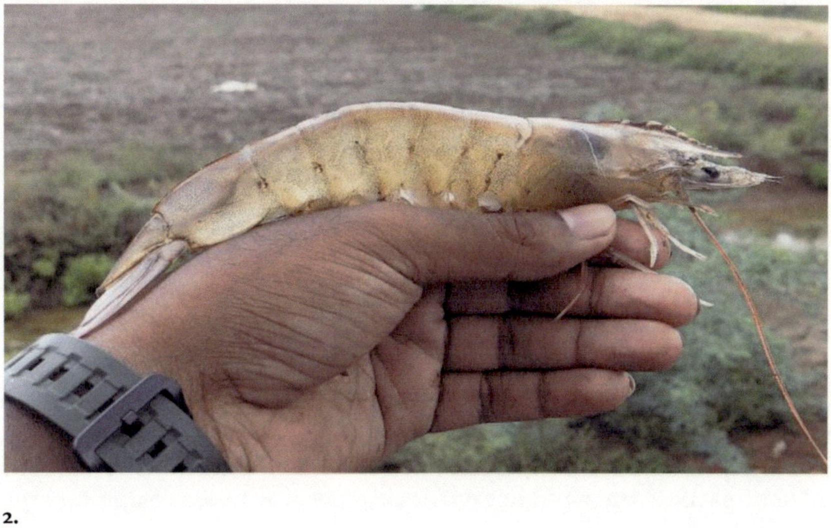

Figure 2.
Vibriosis in shrimp 1.

systems, crustaceans especially shrimps are often exposed to stressful conditions due to the high stocking density, leading to vibriosis [7]. *Vibrio* usually associated with etiological agents, however some vibrio species have been identified as primary pathogen. Several species of *vibrio* including *V. parahaemolyticus* and *V. harveyi* have been described as the main pathogenic species in shrimps (**Figure 2**) [8].

3.2 Filamentous bacterial disease

The disease was characterized by fouling of gills, setae, appendages and body surface. Molting is impaired and the larval shrimp may die due to stress and hypoxia, which is caused by filamentous bacteria such as *Leucothrix mucor*, which is diagnosed microscopically. This can be prevented by maintaining good water quality with optimal physical – chemical conditions controlled by 0.25–1 ppm copper sulphate bath treatment for 4–6 hours [9].

3.3 Factors responsible for disease outbreaks

- Unfavorable environment such as poor soil and water quality.
- Poor water exchange facilities with high stock density.
- Usage of poor quality feeds with low protein content.
- Accumulation of sludge in the pond bottom due to the presence of unutilized feed.
- Presence of gut micro flora and numerous virulent pathogens in the pond.

3.4 Disease controlling methods

3.4.1 Bacteriophage therapy

Bacteriophage therapy acts as a prophylactic alternative instead of antibiotics usage in shrimp industry. These are viruses that kill only specific disease causing pathogens and acts as therapeutic agents in pathogenic infections. Unlike antibiotics, bacteriophage therapy has no residual issues and has advantages of being specific to their host bacteria, without harming other micro-organisms [10]. In aquaculture hatcheries, bacterial diseases often cause considerable economic loss across globe for hatchery operators. Bacteriophages and their lytic enzymes are in use for therapy of bacterial infections in human and animals, as biocontrol agents for food protection also as tools in molecular biology, the penentration of phage DNA inside a bacteria is promoted by lysossome produced by the phage. In yellow tail fish, a pathogen named *Lactococcus garveyi* is inhibited by bacteriophage therapy in the early 1990s (**Figure 3**) [11].

3.4.2 Herbs as antibiotics

Herbs act as antibiotic for controlling or reduce the infection of pathogen in aquaculture sector and also increases the survival rate of organisms, during outbreak of disease managements. In *Fenneropeneaus indicus,* the *vibrio* disease controlled by garlic extract and hot water extracts of seaweeds *Sargassum sp* acts

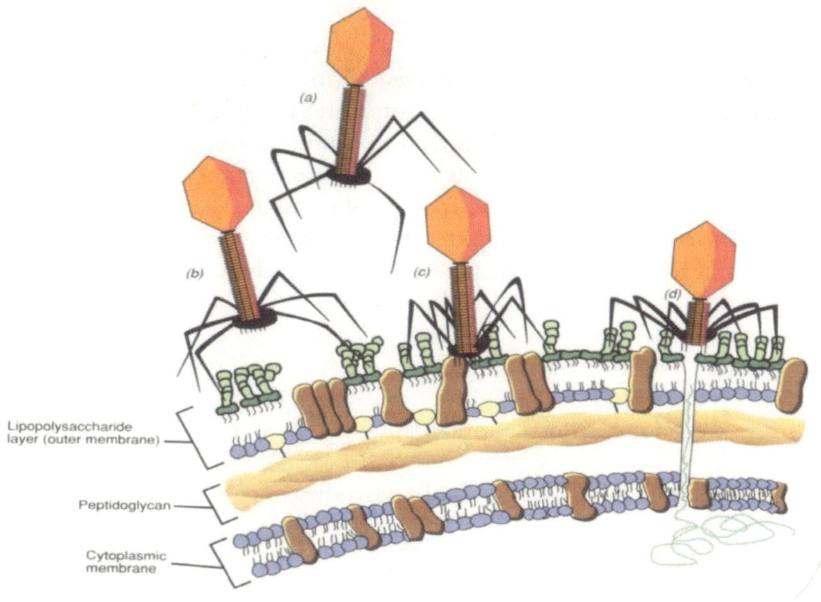

Figure 3.
Bacteriophage attached to bacterial cell 1.

as immunomodulator for white spot syndrome virus (WSSV) in shrimp *P. monodon.* Similarly, *Azardiracta indica* plant extract used as an ailment for *Citrobactor freundii* bacterial infection in *Oreochromis mosambicus* [12]. The majority of herbs act as anti-pathogenic agent, acts as antibiotic to strengthen the immune system of organisms prevent from disease or forming disease resistance variety in aquaculture sector.

3.4.3 Probiotics

Probiotics gaining more attention in recent scenario in all sectors including aquaculture, agriculture and animal husbandry when considering other remedies probiotics acts as a better option rather than incorporating antibiotics to control pathogens in aquaculture. The term probiotic has been defined as a mono or mixed culture of live microorganisms which can be applied to animal or human to enhance the immune system. The animal health is then improved by the removal or decrease in population density of pathogens and by improving water quality through more rapid degradation of waste organic matter (sludge). Environmental microbiology and biotechnology have advanced in the past decade, to the point that commercial products and technologies are available for treating large areas of water and land to enhance population densities of desired microbial species or biochemical activities. The practice of bioremediation is applied in many areas of interest, but success rate varies in different areas, depending on the environmental conditions, nature of products and the method of usage by the consumer, the probiotic that are added must be selected for specific functions. Bioaugmentation and the use of probiotics are significant tools for aquaculture but their efficiency depends on understanding the nature of competition between disease causing pathogens and desired strains of bacteria. *Bacillius* spp., *Lactobacillius* spp., *Pseudomonas* spp., nitrifying and denitrifying bacteria are some of the commonly used probiotic in shrimp culture.

3.4.4 Disease control

The disease control programmers in aquaculture must include examination of diseases and mortalities in a holistic manner and consider various factors such as stocking densities, environment (turbidity, temperature, pH, salinity, dissolved oxygen, H_2S,NH_3,NO_2, etc. of water and redox potential of soil), rate of water exchange, presence of toxic bottom dwelling algae, the type of feed and its FCR ratio by the shrimps, phytoplankton bloom, physiological status of shrimps, etc. [13]. Most of the disease control methods are based on preventive measures. They are,

- Better husbandry practices,
- Use of balanced nutritional supplement,
- Implementing nursery setup to avoid mortality in culture ponds,
- Use of GMO stocks for culture,
- Use of herbal extracts as antibiotics and
- Use of vaccines or drugs.

Diseases can be prevented by adapting better animal handling practices and providing adequate amount of nutrient rich feed [14]. Vibriosis is controlled by rigorous water management through ROS systems and sanitation to prevent the entry of vibrio in the culture water and to reduce stress on the shrimps. Good site selection, pond design and pond preparation are also important. An increase in daily water exchanges and a reduction in pond biomass by partial harvesting are recommended to reduce mortalities caused by Vibriosis. Draining, drying and administering lime/dolomite to ponds following harvest is also recommended [15].

4. Conclusion

In spite of all these recent advancements to eradicate all the bacterial diseases in shrimps, still there is a void for complete eradication of these diseases. Various techniques and medicines are introduced to cure these bacterial infections, but still there are certain side effects for consumers, by introducing antibiotics and other medicines for respective infections. So when it comes to large scale like commercial farming, the efficacy of the above mentioned techniques for prevention and cure of cultured shrimps from bacterial diseases is low when compared to laboratory conditions.

Author details

Hethesh Chellapandian[1], Jeyachandran Sivakamavalli[1]*, A. Vijay Anand[2] and Balamuralikrishnan Balasubramanian[3]

1 Department of Biotechnology and Microbiology, National College, Tiruchirappalli, Tamilnadu, India

2 Department of Human Genetics and Molecular Biology, Bharathiyar University, Coimbatore, Tamilnadu, India

3 Department of Food Science and Biotechnology, College of Life Science, Sejong University, Seoul, South Korea

*Address all correspondence to: drjsvalli@nct.ac.in

References

[1] Jeyachandran S, Park K, Kwak I-S. Bacterial Disease Control Methods in Shrimp Farming Sector. Yeosu 59626, South Korea: Fisheries Science Institute, Chonnam National University

[2] Olafsen. Interaction between fish larvae and bacteria in marine aquaculture. 2001

[3] Lo C-F, Lee C-T, et al. The opportunistic marine pathogen *Vibrio parahaemolyticus* becomes virulent by acquiring a plasmid that expresses a deadly toxin. 2015

[4] Chen Y-Y, Chen J-C, Tseng K-C, Lin Y-C, Huang C-L. Activation of Immunity, Immune Response, Antioxidant Ability, and Resistance against *Vibrio alginolyticus* in White Shrimp *Litopenaeus vannamei* Decrease under Long-term Culture at Low pH. Keelung 202, Taiwan, ROC: Department of Aquaculture, National Taiwan Ocean University; 2015

[5] Chandrakala N, Priya S. Vibriosis in Shrimp Aquaculture A Review. Thanjavur, Tamilnadu, India: PG & Research Department of Zoology, Kundhavai Naacchiyaar Govt Arts College For Women(A); 2017

[6] Alavandi S, Vijayan K, Santiago T, Poornima M, Jithendran K, Ali S, et al. Evaluation of Pseudomonas sp.PM11 and Vibrio fluvialis PM17 on immune indices of tiger shrimp, Penaeus monodon. 2004

[7] Dash P, Avunje S, Tandel RS, Sandeep KP, Panigrahi A. Biocontrol of luminous vibriosis in shrimp aquaculture: A review of current approaches and future perspectives. 2017

[8] Hsu S, Chen J. The immune response of white shrimp *Penaeus vannamei* and its susceptibility to *Vibrio alginolyticus* under sulfide stress. 2007

[9] Rengpipat S, Tunyanun A, Fast AW, Piyatiratitivorakul S, Menasveta P. Enhanced growth and resistance to *Vibrio* challenge in pond-reared black tiger shrimp *Penaeus monodon* fed a Bacillus probiotic. 2003

[10] Culot A, Grosset N, Gautier M. Overcoming the challenges of phage therapy for industrial aquaculture: A review. 2019

[11] Abdul Hannan MD, Mahbubur Rahman MD, Nurunnabi Mondal MD, Suzan Chandra DEB, Chowdhury G, Tofazzal Islam MD. Molecular identification of Vibrio alginolyticus causing Vibriosis in shrimp and its Herbal remedy.

[12] Yasin IA, Hashizume A, Ido A, Takahashi T, Miura C, Miura T. Establishment of challenges study system for vibriosis of Japanese tiger prawn (*Marsupenaeus japonicus*) with a pathogenic *Vibrio penaeicida* strain. 2017

[13] Pérez-Sánchez T, Mora-Sánchez B, Luis Balcázar J. Biological approaches for disease control in aquaculture: Advantages, limitations and challenges. 2018

[14] Domínguez-Borbora C, Ardilesa V, Bermeoa M, Bolívar-Alvaradoa C, Tomaláa C, Sonnenholznera S, et al. The marine symbiont *Pseudovibrio denitrificans*, is effective to control pathogenic *Vibrio* spp. in shrimp aquaculture. 2019

[15] Hsu C-H, Chen J-C, Lin Y-C, Chen Y-Y, Liu P-C, Lin B-W, et al. White shrimp *Litopenaeus vannamei* that have received mixtures of heat-killed and formalin-inactivated *Vibrio alginolyticus* and *V. harveyi* exhibit recall memory and show increased phagocytosis and resistance to Vibrio infection. 2020

Section 2

Specific Infectious Pathologies

Chapter 10

Diabetic Foot Osteomyelitis: Frequent Pathogens and Conservative Antibiotic Therapy

Nicolas Vogel, Tanja Huber and Ilker Uçkay

Abstract

Chronic diabetic foot osteomyelitis (DFO) is a frequent complication in adult polyneuropathy patients with long-standing diabetes mellitus. Regarding the conservative therapy, there are several crucial steps in adequate diagnosing and approaches. The management should be performed in a multidisciplinary approach following the findings of recent research, general principles of antibiotic therapy for bone; and according to (inter-)national guidance. In this chapter we emphasize the overview on the state-of-the-art management regarding the diagnosis and antibiotic therapy in DFO. In contrast, in this general narrative review and clinical recommendation, we skip the surgical, vascular and psychological aspects.

Keywords: Diabetic foot osteomyelitis, remission, microbiology, diagnosis, antibiotic therapy

1. Introduction

Patients with diabetes mellitus are at risk of complications of several organ systems and immunological problems of the cellular and humoral pathways [1]. Frequent clinical complications are diabetic foot infections, including acutely the soft tissues, or chronically the bone: diabetic foot osteomyelitis (DFO). In adult patients there is a lifetime risk of 25% for foot infections and a 15 times higher risk of lower limb amputation. The latter is associated with a high associated mortality risk of 50% within five years [1, 2]. Understandably, these infections are leading to massive healthcare costs and antibiotic consumption [3]. In this chapter, we provide an overview over the current conservative (antibiotic) approach to chronic DFO; emphasizing the state-of-the-art of diagnostic procedures and antibiotic regimens for the conservative, internist management. To keep this chapter as short as possible, we skip the discussion of the different surgical procedures, diabetic foot soft tissue infections [4], treatment of necrosis and gangrene [5], the management of angiopathy, topical antibiotic use of ulcers, implant-related DFO, non-infectious complications in the diabetic foot [6], podiatry, or off-loading, for which a broader literature is available.

2. Pathophysiology

Several underlying mechanisms are leading to a chronic foot infection in adult diabetic patients [1, 7]. Of course, the immunological impairments are crucial for development of all sorts of infections, but there are more important factors contributing to the appearance of DFO, of which the neuropathy and vasculopathy are the most important cornerstones. In general, and as first step, foot ulcers are induced by pressure and further maceration of the skin [8]. Additionally, there might be a peripheral (microangiopathic) arterial disease (PAD), for which diabetes is an independent risk factor [9]. Wound healing may be impaired if blood flow is reduced. Data show the presence of PAD in about 30% of diabetic foot ulcers [10].

3. Diagnostic process

3.1 Clinical assessment

In general, the diagnosis and treatment of DFO should be embedded in a standardized multimodal and multidisciplinary approach. The first step is the clinical assessment in terms of the visual presence of infection: new induration, new warmth, new redness, tenderness, purulence and/or altered pain are the main findings. Besides the local signs of infection, there might be systemic repercussions with shivering, lymphangiopathy, and sepsis. Possible additional signs are delayed healing or granulation, putrid smell, or wound vulnerability. These latter symptoms are unspecific and can also occur in other differential diagnoses such as ischemia, acute gout or activated Charcot neuro-arthropathy [11, 12]. The only pathognomonic clinical sign for the external and visual diagnosis of DFO is the presence of fragments of bone discharging from a wound. This is only possible in advanced infections related to ulcers; and it is rare. Often, a DFO is suspected and later confirmed. Large, deep or chronic wounds (persisting for ≥3 months) or red and swollen toes ("sausage toe") raise the suspicion of DFO. Another simple diagnostic approach is the probe-to-bone test. The clinician uses a sterile blunt metal probe to determine, whether bone can be palpated through the diabetic foot ulcer. A negative test does not completely rule out DFO, while a positive test has an acceptable predictive value for deep bone infection [13, 14]. Although needle puncture of deep soft tissue does not reliably predict the results of bone cultures, puncture of the bone itself may be an easy way to obtain bone culture on the ward [15]. When DFO is suspected, two separate positive deep bony microbiological samples showing the same bacteria may sometimes additionally confirm DFO [16]. One or two weeks of "antibiotic-free window", before biopsy or surgery, are recommended to avoid false-negative results [17]. In contrast, the microbiological confirmation of DFO is not necessary when the infected area is amputated in toto [18]. All blood tests have no independent values in the mere confirmation of DFO, but might determine the initial, clinical severity of disease on admission.

3.2 Imaging

Upon the clinical suspicion of soft tissue infection and/or chronic ulcer in the polyneuropathy diabetic foot, the clinicians should also always exclude an underlying DFO; at minimum with an X-ray and once at the initial assessment. The X-ray can also be repeated if the lesions are not improving despite adequate therapy, local wound care and off-loading. In a usual approach, the X-ray should be the first imaging, in which signs of DFO can be detected such as osteopenia, periosteal reactions or erosions of the osseous borders [19, 20]. However, the overall sensitivity of the plain radiography in diagnosing DFO is low. One review cited a pooled sensitivity of 0.54 and a specificity of 0.68 [21]. If the X-ray cannot provide a definitive radiological diagnosis, guidelines frequently recommend MRI for diagnosing DFO with a specificity of 79% and a sensitivity of 93% [22, 23]. However, the MRI is no guarantee of correct radiological diagnosis of DFO [24]. In the MRI, we may find focal signs on T2-weighted images and a loss of signal intensity on T1-weighted images. Furthermore, there is the potential to use short tau inversion recovery sequences (STIR), in which we see high bone signal [25–27]. What is truly beneficial by using the MRI, is the possibility to detect bone marrow edema within 1–2 days after beginning of the bone infection [28, 29]. The MRI is a diagnostic tool for a more accurate diagnostic of DFO. However, we lack clinical data revealing that DFO diagnosed by MRI would have a better outcome than those diagnosed by X-ray and by clinical impression alone. For this latter question, we prospectively followed 390 DFO episodes in 186 adult patients for a median of 2.9 years and performed 318 standard conventional X-rays (median costs 100 Swiss Francs; 100 US$) and with 47 (12%) MRI scans (median costs 800 US$). Among them, 18 episodes were associated with positive findings in the MRI only, but lacked bone lesions in the previous X-ray two to three days ago. In the database, the median duration of systemic antibiotics was 28 days for MRI-only episodes and 30 days for X-ray-positive cases and we achieved overall remission in 25% of the MRI-managed cases compared to 27% of the cases with only a standard X-ray imaging on admission. When adjusting for the large case-mix, DFO episodes diagnosed by the MRI had no different remission rates [30].

3.3 Microbiological diagnostic

The microbiological diagnostic relies on specimens for culturing the involved pathogens. No expert recommends superficial wound swabs, because there is always an (inconstant) microbiome of multiple organisms in chronically open wounds. These superficial probes are frequently misleading, since they often represent colonizing species or contaminations [12] (unless the swab originates from mere pus). Clinicians should always aim for several deep samples of infected (intraoperative) tissues or bone. An optimal specimen would be deep, infected, and still vital tissue, with or without pus, to catch the anaerobic pathogens [12, 31]. The microbiological gold standard for DFO relies on a bone biopsy, which is also feasible outside of the operating theater; especially in patients with polyneuropathy, who feel almost no pain during the bed-side sampling [25]. The accuracy of the results is increased by taking at least two separate bone probes. If they show the same pathogen, we usually identify the pathogen of DFO [16]. Histology has no widely-accepted criteria for DFO. Characteristic findings are aggregates of inflammatory cells, bone lesions, fibrosis, and/or reactive bone formation. As with other orthopedic infections the results depend on the care with which intraoperative samples are obtained (to avoid contamination) and whether the patient was under active antibiotic therapy [32]. While newer molecular laboratory methods identify more pathogens from DFO, the IWGDF guidelines suggest sticking with conventional culture methods for the first-line identification [33]. This is because of their lower cost, the lack of evidence of any benefit to covering the additional isolates identified and the potential for incurring the adverse effects of unnecessarily broad-spectrum antibiotic therapy. Practically, the only serology with a theoretical use for diagnosing DFO are anti-streptolysin antibodies for beta-hemolytic streptococci. If they are positive [34], the clinicians can (retrospectively) diagnose a streptococcal infection, which might be more useful in acute and severe soft tissue diabetic foot infections than in chronic DFOs.

4. Microbiological therapy

4.1 Pathogens of DFO

Beside possible surgical intervention there is need for an antibacterial treatment. Choosing an active agent is always first empirical, and subsequently targeted to the microbiological culture results. Knowledge of the possible microorganisms is a precondition to an empirical therapy [35]. Dependent on the country, most isolates of DFO are *Staphylococcus aureus*, β-hemolytic streptococci, coagulase-negative staphylococci and Gram-negative pathogens such as *Pseudomonas aeruginosa* [36, 37]. Interestingly, the location of the infection is critical as well, so are calcaneal infections associated with *P. aeruginosa* in diabetic patients [19]. Unfortunately, despite the advocated greenish color of superficial *Pseudomonas* infections and a presumed characteristic smell of the infected wound, even long-standing clinicians cannot predict the presence of *P. aeruginosa* by visual and olfactory means alone. The microbiological laboratory assessment is still necessary [38]. Multi-resistant pathogens in DFO are increasing in frequency worldwide [39] such as extended-spectrum beta-lactamase-producing Gram-negative rods (ESBL). Compared to DFI without involvement of the bone a meta-analysis found a three times higher chance in DFO for isolating a multi-resistant pathogen [40]. Fungi are rarity. Enterococci are equally rare but relatively more prevalent in the infected diabetic foot compared to other osteoarticular infections in the body such as steptococci and staphylococci [41, 42]. It is important to recognize that in the DFO patient, we may retrieve any bacteria, including avirulent coagulase-negative staphylococci and corynebacteria. Unlike to other infections such as pneumonia or endocarditis, the causative pathogens can also change during the current therapy of DFO, by selection of new (more resistant) pathogens by the therapeutic antibiotics and iterative surgeries during treatment. Therefore, if ever there is surgery during ongoing systemic antibiotic treatment, we recommend to re-sample again. The incidence of such a new microbiological finding can be as high as 10% [43].

4.2 Antibiotic therapy

The systemic antibiotic therapy is – next to a possible surgery, iterative professional debridement, (podiatric) wound care, enhancement of the patient's compliance, and off-loading – always required, if the goal is the healing of DFO. A clear recommendation for a specific antimicrobial agent, or the general administration route, cannot be made. A lot of studies and meta-analyses failed to show a superiority of one specific drug against the others [44]. During the initial empirical treatment, we recommend to cover *S. aureus*. If the therapy fails to achieve a proper reduction of local inflammatory symptoms, then the therapy should be broadened to include (aerobic and anaerobic) Gram-negative bacteria [45]. In severe infections, (sub)tropical regions, or sepsis, a relatively broad empirical coverage targeting the local epidemiology of Gram-negative pathogens could be chosen [46] from the start. Further there is few data supporting parenteral therapy [47]. Of note, the microbiological culture results can lead to necessity of parenteral agents due to resistant pathogens.

Ideally, the DFO therapy is accompanied by professional debridement, or the resection of necrotic and infected bone (total amputation). A study of 50 patients with chronic toe DFO showed that patients with surgical resections had a significantly lower relapse rate. This was also witnessed in single-center survey with partial amputations [48]. In well-selected patients and neuropathic DFO cases without progressive ischemia, other studies report successful treatment without surgery, with selected remission rates of 60–70% [49, 50]. When surgery is not necessary for various reasons, a strictly conservative antibiotic therapy is very reasonable. Of note, the proportion of antibiotic-related side effects in randomized-controlled DFO trials may compromise up to 20–30% of all systemic antibiotic DFO regimens [49–55].

4.2.1 Biofilms

Clinicians often neglect the substantial role of bacterial biofilm in various infections, including the diabetic foot [35, 51]. Biofilm-forming bacteria are more refractory to host response and medical treatment and may be responsible for chronicity and complications. The proportion of biofilm-forming bacteria in DFO has been estimated at 30–60% [51]. In a clinical and microbiological study from Turkey [52], the assessed proportion of suspected biofilms among 339 diabetic foot wound isolates occurred in 34%. The multivariate regression analysis revealed two variables to be significant factors associated with biofilm: MDR micro-organism and XDR micro-organism [52]. New strategies are required in the management of wounds with biofilm to effectively destroy and even to prevent its formation.

One antibiotic might be associated with better outcomes in treating DFO biofilms: rifampin [53]. In analogy to implant-related staphylococcal infections, the antibiotic combination with rifampin may reveal a superior outcome. For example, Senneville et al. published a non-randomized observational study in 17 DFO patients treated with ofloxacin-rifampicin and achieved a remission in 88% of the cases [54]. Many other examples, especially from the US and France, are reported. We need the confirmation of the benefit of rifampicin use in DFO in future prospective-randomized trials.

4.3 Duration of antibiotic therapy

Because of a substantial risk for clinical failures according to every day's clinical experience, many physicians treat DFOs, on purpose, with a very long course of antimicrobial therapy, although guidelines limit the overall antibiotic prescription to 4–6 weeks only [33, 55]. Of note, this official guidance never had advocated a prolonged course. A retrospective evaluation with 1018 episodes of soft tissue infections and DFO failed to determine an optimal duration of systemic antibiotic administration regarding the remission, or failure, of diabetic foot infection [48]. A randomized controlled trial found that 6 weeks, compared with 12 weeks, of targeted antibiotic DFO therapy produced similar results [56]. This opinion is shared by other research groups [57, 58]. Today, a maximal duration of 6 weeks is the standard. If the is no remission after this period, clinicians should consider a new approach, which is surgical in the majority of cases. Maybe, the actual standard of 6 weeks might equally be too long for usual DFO cases. Recently, we published our experience of a randomized, controlled (RCT) pilot trial investigating shorter antibiotic administrations for DFO [55]. In this trial, a systemic antibiotic therapy of 3-weeks gave similar (and statistically non-inferior) incidences of remission and adverse events to a course of 6 weeks [55]. We also started the confirmatory RCT with 400 planned episodes in the Balgrist University Hospital in Zurich [59], by using a streamlined surgical approach, an initial radiological examination by magnetic resonance imaging and stratification between surgical versus totally antibiotic treatment approaches. If we confirm our pilot findings, the clinical implications, especially for improved antibiotic stewardship of in the field of DFO [60] might be substantial. Until further results are present, we agree with recommendations of up to six weeks of antibiotic therapy when residual infected bone is suspected or proven [25, 61–66].

4.3.1 Serum inflammatory parameters during the follow-up control of therapy

Clinicians frequently control serum C-reactive protein (CRP) levels during the therapy of DFO. This routine practice should be abandoned. There is often no immediate benefit. On the contrary, surprisingly high CRP blood levels usually trigger unnecessary exams (X-rays, angiology exams, superficial wound swabs, urinary cultures); even in absence of clinical indications. The worst consequence would be a prolongation of the scheduled antibiotic therapy, only basing on these CRP level. In our prospectively collected database [55], routine serum CRP samples, at different time points during ongoing antimicrobial therapy for (operated) DFO, failed to predict future clinical failures [58].

4.3.2 Duration of antibiotic therapy after surgical resection of DFO

After a complete surgical resection of all infected and necrotic bone, many experts only warrant a short very duration of antimicrobial therapy (2–5 days) to finish with a remaining soft tissue infection [18, 59, 60]. However, surgeons frequently doubt about the clinical absence of residual bone infection in the proximal amputation stump [63–65]. The IWGDF recommends sampling the marginal, remaining bone for evidence of residual infection; and advocates a up to 6 weeks of a consecutive, targeted antimicrobial therapy if the residual bone samples return with positive microbiological results [33]. This recommendation is cautious. We reported 482 DFO episodes with a median follow-up of two years after presumably curative total amputation [18]. According to this experience, neither the duration of the postsurgical antibiotic use, nor its immediate discontinuation, predicted future clinical failure [18]. Other research groups advocate that 5 days of a post-surgical antibiotic continuation are sufficient for a potential residual bone infection after amputation [64]. The residual cultures may also be false-negative, when receiving antibiotics, or false-positive when the samples are contaminated [33]. For example, colleagues from Basel, Switzerland, suggested that positive cultures, without a visual clinical confirmation of osteomyelitis and without concomitant histological confirmation, might overestimate the true rate of residual osteomyelitis, because of contamination at the time of surgery [66].

4.4 Administration route of antibiotic therapy

During the last decades, clinicians used a weeks'-long parenteral antibiotic therapy for all severe or moderate cases of DFO, usually with a switch to oral administration the hospitalized patient has been improving [67]. Today, we are living a change of paradigm in daily clinical life and start to consider oral regimens as efficacious as intravenous therapy in chronic DFO [48, 55, 67]. Therapy with oral antibiotic drugs is effective in non-bacteremic mild and moderate DFOs. A review of 93 DFO cases strongly supports the possibility of oral antibiotic regimens right from the start [68]. The same principle applies for other forms and localizations of chronic osteomyelitis [67]. Additional retrospective and prospective studies demonstrated the non-inferiority of oral antibiotic medication for DFO [60]. In our single-center cohort with a defined clinical diabetic foot infection pathway, oral β-lactam therapy did not alter the incidence of remission [67]. Spanish researchers conducted a prospective-randomized trial in DFO patients; with a strictly conservative antibiotic treatment of ninety days versus an approach with surgery plus antibiotics of ninety days. In the conservative arm, oral antibiotics were given very early in the course. Practically, the outcomes were equivalent [61]. The authors of this chapter ignore the existence of a prospective-randomized trial in favor of a long initial parenteral treatment for chronic, non-septic, DFO in adult patients. Finally, topical antibiotics have no place in the treatment of unresected, deep DFO [69].

4.5 Antibiotic stewardship and clinical pathways

DFO's are probably among the most frequent diseases leading to antibiotic overuse [60]. We think that the principles of antibiotic stewardship should also concern DFOs. We reviewed the literature on DFO [60] to assess the value of antibiotic stewardship in the management of DFO. According to this review, the three most effective measures could be: correct diagnosis of bone infection; use of antibiotic regimens with the narrowest spectrum; and, limiting the duration of antimicrobial treatment. Clinical pathways have been instituted for DFOs [70]. A multidisciplinary management regularly showed a significant reduction in amputation risks [71]. However, these multidisciplinary teams have also their limitations: 1) it is difficult to bring the team members together; 2) the number of patients requiring evaluation often exceeds the capacity of fixed regular meetings; 3) the meetings are time-consuming and key members may be absent. Theoretically, order-sets (especially if they are embedded within interactive electronic websites) [12] are tools to implement "bundles" of approaches and, hopefully, improve outcomes. However, the academic experience of these order sets must be further evaluated, especially in resource-poor settings. There are also many administrative approaches that might improve antibiotic stewardship in DFO. Governments can initiate diabetic foot centers [72], or regular workshops and public educational lectures. The access to regional or international guidelines must be encouraged [60].

5. Possible future research

We need many prospective, clinical trials targeting the reduction of unnecessary (systemic and topical) antibiotic use, assessing the value of antibiotic stewardship programs, and developing evidence-based guidance. We should also be interested in microbiomes and new therapies. We want to target unanswered questions and advance research in all aspects of DFO. For example, regarding neo-vascularization, one future hope lies in stem cells. Knowing that a subset of human monocytes expresses TIE-2, we could enhance neovascularization, since ischemia is a major concomitant problem to chronic DFO. We successfully extracted high numbers of proangiogenic TIE-2 monocytes from venous blood of diabetic patients without ischemia [73]. Likewise, current scientific achievements confirm the feasibility of amplifying adipose stem cells for angiogenesis from the abdominal fat of ischemic patients [74]. The implication of these findings in terms of autologous injections for therapeutic neo-angiogenesis will require further studies. DFO will remain a "never-ending challenge" [75].

6. Conclusions

We can treat DFO conservatively by (targeted) systemic antibiotic administration, proper wound debridement (if necessary), and adequate off-loading. With the conservative therapy, the progressive destruction of underlying bone can be arrested in probably 60–70% of episodes in well-selected, compliant patients without major bone destruction or advanced concomitant ischemia; at least for a short follow-up time. A clinical regular and close follow-up by specialized health-care workers is paramount, since clinical failures on the long-term are frequent;

especially in the reason for the initial chronic DFO has not been reversed. The secondary prevention of further infection episodes is important. Any systemic antimicrobial agent is suitable, and very probably in oral administration form from the start (unless there is a concomitant severe clinical systemic inflammation, bacteremia or sepsis). The duration of antibiotic therapy is currently fixed to six weeks, but further trials and evaluations reducing the overall duration to lesser time spans are under way [59].

Conflict of interest

The authors declare no conflict of interest.

Author details

Nicolas Vogel[1,2]*, Tanja Huber[3] and Ilker Uçkay[4]

1 Internal Medicine, Spital Zollikerberg, Zollikerberg, Switzerland

2 Internal Medicine, Balgrist University Hospital, Zurich, Switzerland

3 Hospital Pharmacy, Balgrist University Hospital, Zurich, Switzerland

4 Infectiology and Infection Control, Balgrist University Hospital, Zurich, Switzerland

*Address all correspondence to: nicolasvogel@yahoo.com

References

[1] Berbudi A, Rahmadika N, Tjahjadi AI, Ruslami R. Type 2 Diabetes and its Impact on the Immune System. Curr Diabetes Rev. 2020;16(5):442-449.

[2] Yammine K, Hayek F, Assi C. A meta-analysis of mortality after minor amputation among patients with diabetes and/or peripheral vascular disease. J Vasc Surg. 2020;72(6): 2197-2207.

[3] Association AD. Economic Costs of Diabetes in the U.S. in 2017. Diabetes Care. 2018;41(5):917-928.

[4] Tobalem M, Uçkay I. Images in clinical medicine. Evolution of a diabetic foot infection. N Engl J Med. 2013;369(23):2252.

[5] Al Wahbi A. Operative versus non-operative treatment in diabetic dry toe gangrene. Diabetes Metab Syndr. 2019;13(2):959-963.

[6] Gariani K, Waibel FWA, Viehöfer AF, Uçkay I. Plantar Fasciitis in Diabetic Foot Patients: Risk Factors, Pathophysiology, Diagnosis, and Management. Diabetes Metab Syndr Obes. 2020;13:1271-1279.

[7] Khanolkar MP, Bain SC, Stephens JW. The diabetic foot. QJM. 2008;101(9):685-695.

[8] Vinik AI, Nevoret ML, Casellini C, Parson H. Diabetic neuropathy. Endocrinol Metab Clin North Am. 2013;42(4):747-787.

[9] Association AD. Peripheral arterial disease in people with diabetes. Diabetes Care. 2003;26(12):3333-3341.

[10] Reiber GE, Vileikyte L, Boyko EJ, del Aguila M, Smith DG, Lavery LA, et al. Causal pathways for incident lower-extremity ulcers in patients with diabetes from two settings. Diabetes Care. 1999;22(1):157-162.

[11] Berli M, Vlachopoulos L, Leupi S, Böni T, Baltin C. Treatment of Charcot Neuroarthropathy and osteomyelitis of the same foot: a retrospective cohort study. BMC Musculoskelet Disord. 2017;18(1):460.

[12] Uçkay I, Gariani K, Pataky Z, Lipsky BA. Diabetic foot infections: state-of-the-art. Diabetes Obes Metab. 2014;16(4):305-316.

[13] Butalia S, Palda VA, Sargeant RJ, Detsky AS, Mourad O. Does this patient with diabetes have osteomyelitis of the lower extremity? JAMA. 2008;299(7):806-813.

[14] Aragón-Sánchez J, Lipsky BA, Lázaro-Martínez JL. Diagnosing diabetic foot osteomyelitis: is the combination of probe-to-bone test and plain radiography sufficient for high-risk inpatients? Diabet Med. 2011;28(2):191-194.

[15] Senneville E, Morant H, Descamps D, Dekeyser S, Beltrand E, Singer B, et al. Needle puncture and transcutaneous bone biopsy cultures are inconsistent in patients with diabetes and suspected osteomyelitis of the foot. Clin Infect Dis. 2009;48(7):888-893.

[16] Bernard L, Assal M, Garzoni C, Uçkay I. Predicting the pathogen of diabetic toe osteomyelitis by two consecutive ulcer cultures with bone contact. Eur J Clin Microbiol Infect Dis. 2011;30(2):279-281.

[17] Govaert GAM, Kuehl R, Atkins BL, Trampuz A, Morgenstern M, Obremskey WT, et al. Diagnosing Fracture-Related Infection: Current Concepts and Recommendations. J Orthop Trauma. 2020;34(1):8-17.

[18] Rossel A, Lebowitz D, Gariani K, Abbas M, Kressmann B, Assal M, et al. Stopping antibiotics after surgical amputation in diabetic foot and ankle infections-A daily practice cohort. Endocrinol Diabetes Metab. 2019;2(2): e00059.

[19] Waibel FWA, Uçkay I, Sairanen K, Waibel L, Berli MC, Böni T, et al. Diabetic calcaneal osteomyelitis. Infez Med. 2019;27(3):225-238.

[20] Álvaro-Afonso FJ, Lázaro-Martínez JL, Aragón-Sánchez J, García-Morales E, Cecilia-Matilla A, Beneit-Montesinos JV. Interobserver and intraobserver reproducibility of plain X-rays in the diagnosis of diabetic foot osteomyelitis. Int J Low Extrem Wounds. 2013;12(1):12-15.

[21] Newman LG, Waller J, Palestro CJ, Schwartz M, Klein MJ, Hermann G, et al. Unsuspected osteomyelitis in diabetic foot ulcers. Diagnosis and monitoring by leukocyte scanning with indium in 111 oxyquinoline. JAMA. 1991;266(9): 1246-1251.

[22] Lauri C, Tamminga M, Glaudemans AWJM, Juárez Orozco LE, Erba PA, Jutte PC, et al. Detection of Osteomyelitis in the Diabetic Foot by Imaging Techniques: A Systematic Review and Meta-analysis Comparing MRI, White Blood Cell Scintigraphy, and FDG-PET. Diabetes Care. 2017;40(8):1111-1120.

[23] Lipsky BA, Berendt AR, Cornia PB, Pile JC, Peters EJ, Armstrong DG, et al. 2012 Infectious Diseases Society of America clinical practice guideline for the diagnosis and treatment of diabetic foot infections. Clin Infect Dis. 2012;54(12):e132-e173.

[24] La Fontaine J, Bhavan K, Jupiter D, Lavery LA, Chhabra A. Magnetic Resonance Imaging of Diabetic Foot Osteomyelitis: Imaging Accuracy in Biopsy-Proven Disease. J Foot Ankle Surg. 2021;60(1):17-20.

[25] Lipsky BA, Peters EJ, Senneville E, Berendt AR, Embil JM, Lavery LA, et al. Expert opinion on the management of infections in the diabetic foot. Diabetes Metab Res Rev. 2012;28 Suppl 1:163-178.

[26] Gholamrezanezhad A, Basques K, Batouli A, Matcuk G, Alavi A, Jadvar H. Clinical Nononcologic Applications of PET/CT and PET/MRI in Musculoskeletal, Orthopedic, and Rheumatologic Imaging. AJR Am J Roentgenol. 2018;210(6):W245-WW63.

[27] Donovan A, Schweitzer ME. Use of MR imaging in diagnosing diabetes-related pedal osteomyelitis. Radiographics. 2010;30(3):723-736.

[28] Jaramillo D. Infection: musculoskeletal. Pediatr Radiol. 2011;41 Suppl 1:S127-S134.

[29] Lee YJ, Sadigh S, Mankad K, Kapse N, Rajeswaran G. The imaging of osteomyelitis. Quant Imaging Med Surg. 2016;6(2):184-198.

[30] Gariani K, Lebowitz D, Kressmann B, Gariani J, Uçkay I. X-Ray Versus Magnetic Resonance Imaging in Diabetic Foot Osteomyelitis: A Clinical Comparison. Curr Diabetes Rev. 2021;17(3):373-377.

[31] Charles PG, Uçkay I, Kressmann B, Emonet S, Lipsky BA. The role of anaerobes in diabetic foot infections. Anaerobe. 2015;34:8-13.

[32] Al-Mayahi M, Cian A, Lipsky BA, Suvà D, Müller C, Landelle C, et al. Administration of antibiotic agents before intraoperative sampling in orthopedic infections alters culture results. J Infect. 2015;71(5):518-525.

[33] Lipsky BA, Senneville É, Abbas ZG, Aragón-Sánchez J, Diggle M, Embil JM, et al. Guidelines on the diagnosis and

treatment of foot infection in persons with diabetes (IWGDF 2019 update). Diabetes Metab Res Rev. 2020;36 Suppl 1:e3280.

[34] Uçkay I, Ferry T, Stern R, Ambrosioni J, Gamulin A, Andrey D, et al. Use of serum antistreptolysin O titers in the microbial diagnosis of orthopedic infections. Int J Infect Dis. 2009;13(4):421-424.

[35] Ertuğrul B, Uçkay I, Schöni M, Peter-Riesch B, Lipsky BA. Management of diabetic foot infections in the light of recent literature and new international guidelines. Expert Rev Anti Infect Ther. 2020;18(4):293-305.

[36] Dang CN, Prasad YD, Boulton AJ, Jude EB. Methicillin-resistant Staphylococcus aureus in the diabetic foot clinic: a worsening problem. Diabet Med. 2003;20(2):159-161.

[37] Bowler PG, Davies BJ. The microbiology of infected and noninfected leg ulcers. Int J Dermatol. 1999;38(8):573-578.

[38] Uçkay I, Holy D, Schöni M, Waibel FWA, Trache T, Burkhard J, et al. How good are clinicians in predicting the presence of Pseudomonas spp. in diabetic foot infections? A prospective clinical evaluation. Endocrinol Diabetes Metab. 2021;4(2):e00225.

[39] Varaiya AY, Dogra JD, Kulkarni MH, Bhalekar PN. Extended-spectrum beta-lactamase-producing Escherichia coli and Klebsiella pneumoniae in diabetic foot infections. Indian J Pathol Microbiol. 2008;51(3):370-372.

[40] Chen Y, Ding H, Wu H, Chen HL. The Relationship Between Osteomyelitis Complication and Drug-Resistant Infection Risk in Diabetic Foot Ulcer: A Meta-analysis. Int J Low Extrem Wounds. 2017;16(3):183-190.

[41] Tumminello A, Dominguez D, Lebowitz D, Bartolone P, Betz M, Hannouche D, et al. Staphylococcus aureus versus streptococci in orthopaedic infections. Infect Dis (Lond). 2017;49(9):716-718.

[42] Uçkay I, Pires D, Agostinho A, Guanziroli N, Öztürk M, Bartolone P, et al. Enterococci in orthopaedic infections: Who is at risk getting infected? J Infect. 2017;75(4):309-314.

[43] Wuarin L, Abbas M, Harbarth S, Waibel F, Holy D, Burkhard J, et al. Changing perioperative prophylaxis during antibiotic therapy and iterative debridement for orthopedic infections? PLoS One. 2019;14(12):e0226674.

[44] Glaudemans AW, Uçkay I, Lipsky BA. Challenges in diagnosing infection in the diabetic foot. Diabet Med. 2015;32(6):748-759.

[45] Hatipoglu M, Mutluoglu M, Uzun G, Karabacak E, Turhan V, Lipsky BA. The microbiologic profile of diabetic foot infections in Turkey: a 20-year systematic review: diabetic foot infections in Turkey. Eur J Clin Microbiol Infect Dis. 2014;33(6): 871-878.

[46] Lipsky BA. Empirical therapy for diabetic foot infections: are there clinical clues to guide antibiotic selection? Clin Microbiol Infect. 2007;13(4):351-353.

[47] Li HK, Agweyu A, English M, Bejon P. An unsupported preference for intravenous antibiotics. PLoS Med. 2015;12(5):e1001825.

[48] Gariani K, Lebowitz D, von Dach E, Kressmann B, Lipsky BA, Uçkay I. Remission in diabetic foot infections: Duration of antibiotic therapy and other possible associated factors. Diabetes Obes Metab. 2019;21(2):244-251.

[49] Pittet D, Wyssa B, Herter-Clavel C, Kursteiner K, Vaucher J, Lew PD. Outcome of diabetic foot infections

treated conservatively: a retrospective cohort study with long-term follow-up. Arch Intern Med. 1999;159(8):851-856.

[50] Jeffcoate WJ, Lipsky BA. Controversies in diagnosing and managing osteomyelitis of the foot in diabetes. Clin Infect Dis. 2004;39 Suppl 2:S115-S122.

[51] Malik A, Mohammad Z, Ahmad J. The diabetic foot infections: biofilms and antimicrobial resistance. Diabetes Metab Syndr. 2013;7(2):101-107.

[52] Vatan A, Saltoglu N, Yemisen M, Balkan II, Surme S, Demiray T, et al. Association between biofilm and multi/extensive drug resistance in diabetic foot infection. Int J Clin Pract. 2018;72(3):e13060.

[53] Wilson BM, Bessesen MT, Doros G, Brown ST, Saade E, Hermos J, et al. Adjunctive Rifampin Therapy For Diabetic Foot Osteomyelitis in the Veterans Health Administration. JAMA Netw Open. 2019;2(11):e1916003.

[54] Senneville E, Yazdanpanah Y, Cazaubiel M, Cordonnier M, Valette M, Beltrand E, et al. Rifampicin-ofloxacin oral regimen for the treatment of mild to moderate diabetic foot osteomyelitis. J Antimicrob Chemother. 2001;48(6):927-930.

[55] Gariani K, Pham TT, Kressmann B, Jornayvaz FR, Gastaldi G, Stafylakis D, et al. Three versus six weeks of antibiotic therapy for diabetic foot osteomyelitis: A prospective, randomized, non-inferiority pilot trial. Clin Infect Dis. 2020.

[56] Tone A, Nguyen S, Devemy F, Topolinski H, Valette M, Cazaubiel M, et al. Six-week versus twelve-week antibiotic therapy for nonsurgically treated diabetic foot osteomyelitis: a multicenter open-label controlled randomized study. Diabetes Care 2015;38:302-307. Diabetes Care. 2015;38(4):735.

[57] Lazzarini L, Lipsky BA, Mader JT. Antibiotic treatment of osteomyelitis: what have we learned from 30 years of clinical trials? Int J Infect Dis. 2005;9(3):127-138.

[58] Pham TT, Wetzel O, Gariani K, Kressmann B, Jornayvaz FR, Lipsky BA, et al. Is routine measurement of the serum C-reactive protein level helpful during antibiotic therapy for diabetic foot infection? Diabetes Obes Metab. 2021;23(2):637-641.

[59] Waibel F, Berli M, Catanzaro S, Sairanen K, Schöni M, Böni T, et al. Optimization of the antibiotic management of diabetic foot infections: protocol for two randomized controlled trials. Trials. 2020;21(1):54.

[60] Uçkay I, Berli M, Sendi P, Lipsky BA. Principles and practice of antibiotic stewardship in the management of diabetic foot infections. Curr Opin Infect Dis. 2019;32(2):95-101.

[61] Lázaro-Martínez JL, Aragón-Sánchez J, García-Morales E. Antibiotics versus conservative surgery for treating diabetic foot osteomyelitis: a randomized comparative trial. Diabetes Care. 2014;37(3):789-795.

[62] Lesens O, Desbiez F, Theïs C, Ferry T, Bensalem M, Laurichesse H, et al. Staphylococcus aureus-Related Diabetic Osteomyelitis: Medical or Surgical Management? A French and Spanish Retrospective Cohort. Int J Low Extrem Wounds. 2015;14(3):284-290.

[63] Shiraev TP, Lipsky BA, Kwok TMY, Robinson DA. Utility of Culturing Marginal Bone in Patients Undergoing Lower Limb Amputation for Infection. J Foot Ankle Surg. 2019;58(5):847-851.

[64] Saltoglu N, Yemisen M, Ergonul O, Kadanali A, Karagoz G, Batirel A, et al. Predictors for limb loss among patient with diabetic foot infections: an observational retrospective multicentric

study in Turkey. Clin Microbiol Infect. 2015;21(7):659-664.

[65] Kowalski TJ, Matsuda M, Sorenson MD, Gundrum JD, Agger WA. The effect of residual osteomyelitis at the resection margin in patients with surgically treated diabetic foot infection. J Foot Ankle Surg. 2011;50(2):171-175.

[66] Mijuskovic B, Kuehl R, Widmer AF, Jundt G, Frei R, Gürke L, et al. Culture of Bone Biopsy Specimens Overestimates Rate of Residual Osteomyelitis After Toe or Forefoot Amputation. J Bone Joint Surg Am. 2018;100(17):1448-1454.

[67] Gariani K, Lebowitz D, Kressmann B, von Dach E, Sendi P, Waibel F, et al. Oral amoxicillin-clavulanate for treating diabetic foot infections. Diabetes Obes Metab. 2019;21(6):1483-1486.

[68] Embil JM, Rose G, Trepman E, Math MC, Duerksen F, Simonsen JN, et al. Oral antimicrobial therapy for diabetic foot osteomyelitis. Foot Ankle Int. 2006;27(10):771-779.

[69] Uçkay I, Kressmann B, Malacarne S, Toumanova A, Jaafar J, Lew D, et al. A randomized, controlled study to investigate the efficacy and safety of a topical gentamicin-collagen sponge in combination with systemic antibiotic therapy in diabetic patients with a moderate or severe foot ulcer infection. BMC Infect Dis. 2018;18(1):361.

[70] Catho G, De Kraker M, Waldispühl Suter B, Valotti R, Harbarth S, Kaiser L, et al. Study protocol for a multicentre, cluster randomised, superiority trial evaluating the impact of computerised decision support, audit and feedback on antibiotic use: the COMPuterized Antibiotic Stewardship Study (COMPASS). BMJ Open. 2018;8(6): e022666.

[71] Darbellay P, Uçkay I, Dominguez D, Mugnai D, Filtri L, Lew D, et al. Diabetic foot infection: a multidisciplinary approach. Rev Med Suisse. 2011;7(292):894-897.

[72] Cawich SO, Islam S, Hariharan S, Harnarayan P, Budhooram S, Ramsewak S, et al. The economic impact of hospitalization for diabetic foot infections in a Caribbean nation. Perm J. 2014;18(1):e101-e104.

[73] Uçkay I, Imhof BA, Kressmann B, Lew D, Lipsky BA, Sidibe A. Characterization of Proangiogenic Monocytes from Blood in Patients with Chronic Ischemic Diabetic Foot Ulcers and Controls. Stem Cells Dev. 2020;29(14):911-918.

[74] Uçkay I, Baquié M, Mosser S, Hervé MP, Bruyere-Cerdan P, Roux-Lombard P, et al. Regenerative Secretoma of Adipose-Derived Stem Cells from Ischemic Patients. J Stem Cell Res Ther 2019, 9:5.

[75] Peter-Riesch B. The Diabetic Foot: The Never-Ending Challenge. Endocr Dev. 2016;31:108-134.

Chapter 11

Infections in Neurosurgery and Their Management

Seyed Arad Senaobar Tahaei, Seyyed Ashkan Senobar Tahaei, Zoltan Mencser and Pal Barzo

Abstract

Surgical site and postoperative infections are common problems in surgical wards and treating them can be challenging and very complicated. It is important to understand different types of postoperative infections and their best management. In this chapter we try to emphasis on infections which are occurring in neurosurgical units and how to approach them. Foreign body infection is another challenge that happens in neurosurgical units, and it is vital to recognize these infections in time and start the treatment as soon as possible. Atypical infections occurrence is low therefore this problem is not addressed often in textbooks or in the literature, therefore atypical infections will be discussed in this chapter too. By discussing the most common postoperative complications and their best management profile, the authors here will try to widen the perspective of readers on infections in neurosurgical units in order to understand this problem better. Untreated infections or poorly treated infections can lead to sepsis and catastrophic results.

Keywords: post-operative infection, neurosurgical infection, CNS infections, septic cerebral embolization, subdural empyema, spondylodiscitis, epidural abscess, meningitis, atypical CNS infections, spinal infections

1. Introduction

1.1 General aspects

Central nervous system (CNS) infections are challenging in terms of correct and on time diagnosis, therefore treating them are quite complicated and require correct understanding of its origin, type of infection and severity of it. Here in this chapter, we will be discussing the most common CNS infections within the field of neurosurgery as well as their best treatment and patient management.

As a known fact, CNS infections can cause very mild to severe signs and symptoms as well as neurological deficits if left untreated or not treated properly. Identification of the primary source of infections are very important, as quite often seen, the source can be infected foreign bodies, or an infection originating somewhere else in the body. In surgical units, wound contamination and deficiencies in correct post-operative patient care are other common sources of infection.

In this chapter we will be discussing infectious diseases which are commonly seen in neurosurgical wards or infections which require neurosurgical interventions, therefore a vast majority of CNS infections which do not require surgical management and-or not occurring in neurosurgical wards are not discussed here.

Various risk factors contribute to the occurrence of infections, general risk factors such as existing co-morbidities (Diabetes mellitus (DM), Anemia, AIDS etc.), the use of immunosuppressant drugs, chronic existing infectious diseases and abnormalities of the immune system are among most common risk factors. Factors such as specific patient skin bacterial composition and local bacterial resistance patterns play an important role in post-operative surgical site infections. Indeed, the extend of aseptic practice and use of proper prophylactic antibiotics before/during surgery is another factor contributing to the occurrence/prevention of post-operative surgical site infection. However, there are studies where indicate that prophylactic use of antibiotics before surgery increase the rate of post-operative infections.

To minimize the risk for post-operative infections, it is recommended that a strict patient screening to be done in order to minimize risk factors which contribute to infections. Patients with higher blood glucose levels are monitored and their glucose profile and therapy are modified if needed, to achieve an acceptable blood glucose level. Patients on immunosuppressant drugs need greater attention pre-operatively and immunosuppressant drugs should be discontinued temporarily (if no contraindications) to minimize the risk of post-operative infections. Anemia should be corrected if present at the time of admission and screening for multi resistant bacteria should be done for every patient which is planned to undergo an elective surgery. All patients, regardless of their immune system and microbiological status should be given a proper Betadine bath the morning before the surgery, and proper prophylactic antibiotics should be administered intravenously, about 20 minutes before the skin incision is made. For longer procedures it is recommended to administer the prophylactic antibiotic once more while the surgery is going on. Proper wound closure, maintaining a good blood flow to the surgical site and proper fixation of existing wound drains with respect to the aseptic technique drastically can decrease the post-operative surgical site infection rate.

1.2 Pathogenesis

Understanding the pathomechanism of CNS infections and infection routes are necessary for proper diagnosis and proper treatment therefore in this section the basics to understand these infections are discussed. Since viral infections are not common in neurosurgical wards, and post-operative infections are mainly bacterial infections, we will be discussing the bacterial pathogenesis of the most common CNS infections here.

In general, bacterial infections reach the CNS by means of the hematogenous spread, but usually the organisms which are colonizing on the surface of the mucosal membranes of the nasopharyngeal cavities are responsible for most of the bacterial pre-operative infections of the CNS. These organisms can find their way to the nasal sinuses and then via the sinuses to the meninges and intracranial cavity. The blood brain barrier (BBB) is a very effective to repel and reduce the penetration of unwanted substances and organisms to the intracranial cavity, but sustained bacteremia and inflammatory and cytotoxic mediators of these organisms cause damage to the BBB and this in turn causes increase permeability of the BBB which is in fact the reason why these pathogenic organisms progress further and end up in the subdural and subarachnoid spaces. In most of cases the intracranial infections are originating from the adjacent ongoing inflammatory processes such as mastoiditis, otitis media, sinusitis and rhinitis [1].

The mucosal membranes in the oral and nasal cavities are lined with different types of bacteria in high quantities which are the normal flora of these mucus membranes, these organisms usually do not cause any CNS infections unless immunodeficiencies are present or these organisms find their way into the intracerebral space and start colonizing there. Skull base fractures are usually causing cerebrospinal fluid (CSF) leakage and this in return is facilitating the migration of bacteria from these adjacent places into the intracranial space causing various problems such as meningitis, cerebritis, intracerebral abscess, fistulas and subdural empyema formation. It is of great importance to mention that infection and inflammation of distant or adjacent organs can also be causing septic cerebral embolization which can be very challenging and hard to identify and differentiate from other lesions such as metastatic lesions or tuberculomas. Endocarditis and cardiac vegetations are among the common cause of septic cerebral embolization, but in general any distant or adjacent infection which spreads through the hematogenous pathway and causes septicemia can be causative of septic cerebral embolization.

The mechanism behind spinal infections is somewhat the same and the blood spine barrier which is the equivalent of BBB is having the same role in protection and isolation of the spinal cord. Spinal epidural abscess or empyema formations are mainly caused by hematogenous spread of bacteria, but besides this paravertebral injections, acupuncture and epidural catheters can be direct causes of bacterial colonization and formation of spinal epidural abscess and empyema. If the inflammation reaches the bony structures of the spinal column, then the term spondylitis is used to describe the latter. There are different forms of spondylitis, the most common type being spondylodiscitis which involves the inflammation of the vertebral body and the adjacent disco-ligamental system. Spondylodiscitis are usually complications of spine surgery but spontaneous forms of it in diabetic patients or patients who are on steroid or immunosuppressant therapy drugs can be found. The pathogenesis of these infections is also via the hematogenous spread and even simple infections such as urinary tract infections if left untreated can be a cause for septicemia and advancement of the infection to the spinal column.

1.3 Diagnosis

Diagnosing CNS infections require multiple tests and imaging, performing the right type of modality at the right time plays a crucial role in early and correct diagnosis. At early stages, infections of CNS can lack absolute neurological signs and only general inflammatory signs and symptoms are present, with progression of the infection, milder complains such as headaches and malaise appear and as the infection progresses further neurological signs and symptoms begin to appear as well. Most of the patients complain of headaches which are partly responsive to NSIADs, fatigue, nausea and vomiting, photosensitivity and with progression of the infection epileptic seizures and paresis can occur. In patients with spinal epidural abscess or severe spondylodiscitis, paraparesis with back pain which radiates to lower extremities can be the very first signs and symptoms of patients.

Depending on the patient's history, physical examination, signs and symptoms and laboratory findings, if a CNS infection is suspected then immediate action to confirm diagnosis should be done by performing supplementary tests such as imaging and lumbar puncture if necessary. CSF cell count as well as CSF biomarkers (such as IFN-γ, TNF-α, IL-2, IL-6, CD8, MIF, NfH-SM135, GFAP-SM126, S100B) analysis are necessary to confirm the presence of inflammatory process in CNS [2], but since these CSF findings in most of the inflammatory states are similar, a differential diagnosis becomes challenging based on the CSF cell analysis therefore further steps such as image acquisition is needed to be able to proceed further. The physical findings such as meningeal irritation signs (Brudzinski's and Kernig's sign) and photosensitivity are not enough for the establishment of any type of CNS infection; even in cases where beside the above mentioned signs and symptoms, pyrexia and increased inflammatory markers are present, a definite diagnosis of CNS infection cannot be made, because conditions like subarachnoid hemorrhage (SAH) can have the very same clinical findings, and the origin of pyrexia or elevated inflammatory factors can be something rather than the CNS. For establishing a diagnosis of CNS infection imaging techniques are necessary since without it other specific conditions such as SAH cannot be surely ruled out (despite positive CSF cell count for red blood cells (RBCs) as lumbar puncture (LP) can be traumatic) and abnormalities such as subdural empyema, cerebral abscess or fistulas cannot be detected.

MRI scans are the gold standard when it come to the imaging of the CNS, since the resolution and clarity of the MRI scans for soft tissue detection are much better and higher than CT scans, their use are more prominent in detection of CNS infections. CT scans are also capable of detecting abnormalities such as subdural empyema or cerebral abscess, but since the radiologic features of these conditions on CT scans are not very specific and very similar with other pathologies, once the suspicion of subdural empyema or cerebral abscess is raised, a contrast enhanced MRI should be done to confirm or rule out the diagnosis. In case of the spinal column infections and epidural abscess or empyema in the spine, MRI is the preferred choice due to its capability of detecting diffusion restriction both in bony structures and soft tissues as well as having a higher sensitivity and specificity for detecting lesions in the spinal canal.

2. Meningitis and its treatment

Meningitis is the term used to describe the inflammation of the meninges anywhere in the neural axis. The inflammation can be caused by viral, bacterial or even fungal pathogens, sterile meningitis is a form of inflammation of the leptomeninges where the patient is clinically having symptoms of meningitis, but leukocytosis is not seen in CSF analysis and no pathologic pathogen can be cultured from the CSF. The most common route of infection is usually the spread of pathogens via the hematogenous pathway after upper respiratory tract infections as well as transmission of bacteria from adjacent ongoing infections via the emissary veins from the nearby structures to the meninges (e.g. sinusitis, mastoiditis, odontogenic infections, otitis media), intra or post-operative contamination of the intracranial structures (e.g. after neurosurgical interventions) is another common way of transmission for these pathogens, skull base fractures are also a source for bacterial inoculation and can cause meningitis. In the following section we will be discussing the most common bacterial and viral pathogens causing meningitis.

2.1 Bacterial meningitis

Bacterial meningitis is a serious CNS infection which can be life threatening if left untreated or not treated properly. Various pathogens can cause meningitis in various age groups, in this section for the sake of simplicity we will be describing the most common adult pathogens and their treatments in details.

The common pathogens causing meningitis are, *Streptococcus pneumoniae*, Neisseria meningitidis, group B Streptococcus spp., *Listeria monocytogenes*, and Haemophilus influenzae. *Streptococcus pneumoniae* is usually causing meningitis in adults and children, neonates and infants are generally not infected by this microorganism. Patients who suffer from skull base fractures and have CSF leaks often develop meningitis due to S. pneumonia inoculation [3]. This so-called community acquired bacterial meningitis (CABM) is considered as a rare pathology with high mortality and morbidity rates. The prevalence of this disorder has decreased significantly in the past decades due to administration of conjugate vaccines and more efficient diagnostic methods and treatments. The most comm pathogens causing CABM are *S. pneumoniae*, N. meningitidis, L monocytogenes according to a study published by Tubiana et al. in 2020 [4].

The diagnosis of CABM is based on clinical findings, CSF analysis and complete blood count (CBC) findings, MRI scans can be useful for obtaining more information about the extent and severity of meningitis but not necessary for establishing the diagnosis. **Figure 1** shows alterations on brain MRI scans in a patient with severe meningococcal meningitis.

Once the diagnosis is confirmed, empirical broad-spectrum antibiotics based on local bacterial resistance should be started and afterwards modified based on antibiograms. For initial treatment third generation cephalosporins [4] alongside amoxicillin or ampicillin to cover treatment for L monocytogenes are recommended and once antibiotic susceptibility results are available then targeted therapy should be started with agents having higher CSF penetration; Steroids and C5 antibodies are also recommended, in case the ongoing infection is not responding well to systemic antibody treatment [5].

2.2 Post-operative

Post-operative meningitis or post neurosurgical meningitis (PNM) is a complication of cranial surgery, and its rate of occurrence is depending on multiple factors. We will be discussing the most common factors contributing to the occurrence of postoperative meningitis and its treatment. Surgeries are done in aseptic environment, careful disinfection of the surgical site and keeping the aseptic environment while performing the surgery is the most important factor in preventing postoperative meningitis. Studies have shown that shaving hair within the surgical site has little to no effect in decreasing postoperative infections [6], but regardless of this fact it is highly recommended to have surgical site free of hair in order to

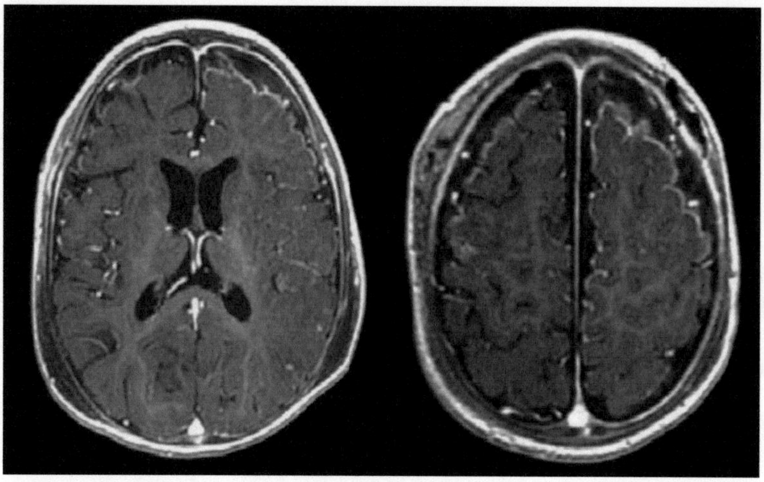

Figure 1.
Diffuse contrast enhancement of the arachnoid membrane and dura bilaterally in the fronto-temporal region is seen in a patient with meningococcal meningitis. The Arachnoiditis is a complication and sequel of untreated or very severe aggressive meningitis.

achieve better and easier access to the site. Prophylactic antibiotic administration is also an important key in preventing postoperative infections, however its use can be controversial as there are studies indicating that prophylactic antibiotic administration before surgery has little to no effect on preventing post-operative infections. The use of administration of antibiotics are usually depending on the existing local bacterial resistance patterns, individual skin flora, type and location of the surgery.

Usage of broad-spectrum antibiotics for cranial surgeries are not recommended simply because their use has not shown any advantage over other antibiotics; Cefazolin has been used for many years now for prophylactic purposes in cranial surgery. If multi resistant *Staphylococcus aureus* (MRSA) is present in the institute where the procedure is carried out or if the skin floral composition of the patient includes MRSA, then administration of Vancomycin is recommended supplementary to Cefazolin [7]. Since implanting foreign bodies both in cranial and spinal surgeries are quite often, it is important to handle the instruments and implants with care to maintain a fully aseptic environment.

One of the important factors contributing to prevention of the postoperative infections is wound closure and surgical wound management; An efficient watertight wound closure ensures proper anatomical closure of layers, minimizing the risk of infections in deeper layers and by proper management of the surgical wound the risk of superficial wound infection can be reduced drastically. It should be noted that patients scheduled for elective surgery should be screened for the presence of multi resistant bacteria in their flora. Patients with multi resistant bacterial composition should be isolated before and after surgery in order to decrease the transmission of the multi resistant bacteria to other patients and the medical staff. Disposable protective clothing should be used by medical staff in order to minimize the risk of transmission.

If signs and symptoms of surgical site wound infection are seen, a CBC and superficial and deep wound sampling for microbiological culturing are necessary. Empirical antibiotic treatment should be started and then modified based on the antibiogram results of culturing. After cranial surgery if signs and symptoms of meningitis are present, then LP should be performed for analysis. Slight elevations of WBC in CSF (up to 50 cells mm3) usually do not require prompt antibiotic treatment, symptomatic treatment for headache, nausea and vomiting and hydration are recommended, leukocytosis should be controlled and if a rise in WBCs count is seen then antibiotic treatment should be started. For values above 50 cells per mm3 empirical antibiotic should be considered and then modified based on culture results if needed. If severe leukocytosis in CSF is seen (above 1000 WBCs per mm3) or if systematic treatment is not achieving desired results, intrathecal antibiotic administration should be considered. Empirical treatment for PNM should include Vancomycin for the coverage of staphylococci and P. acnes, as well as a cephalosporin or carbapenem to cover gram negative bacteria and in particularly pseudomonas [8].

Postoperative meningitis after cranial surgeries can cause local osteomyelitis at the level of surgery and/or subdural empyema or cerebral abscess formation. These complications will be discussed in the upcoming sections.

2.3 Viral

Viral meningitis is not a common finding in neurosurgical wards, and its route of infection and treatment is usually different from PNM and bacterial routes, therefore this topic is not relevant to our discussion, and it will not be discussed here.

2.4 Sterile

Sterile meningitis is defined by irritation of the meninges without the presence of pathological organism. In sterile meningitis the cause of meningeal irritation is usually SAH and circulating red blood cells in the subarachnoid space which can damage the arachnoid granulations and cause meningeal irritation. Clinically signs and symptoms of sterile meningitis are similar to bacterial meningitis in terms of neck stiffness, photophobia, nausea, vomiting and headaches, but leukocytosis or pyrexia are not accompanying the above-mentioned signs. Damage of the arachnoid granulations by the RBCs can cause non-resorptive hydrocephalus following a SAH or a traumatic brain injury with intracranial hemorrhage.

If sterile meningitis is suspected clinically then a LP is performed for CSF analysis. CSF analysis generally reveals elevated number of RBCs with normal or slightly elevated WBCs and normal protein and glucose content. It is important to mention that the protein and glucose content of the CSF can be affected by other factors but in general CSF analysis in sterile meningitis reveals elevated RBCs count. Treatment of sterile meningitis in mild cases is just symptomatic treatment for headaches, nausea and vomiting whereas in moderate to severe cases, CSF drainage is necessary to wash out the RBCs in the subarachnoid space and clear out the CSF. Lumbar drains for continuous CSF drainage are used if there are no contraindications. External ventricular drains (EVD) can be used to clear out the CSF if a lumbar drain is contraindicated or cannot be used for any reason.

If Sterile meningitis is not treated, non-resorptive hydrocephalus occurs due to the fact that RBCs damage the Pacchionian granulations and CSF reabsorption becomes impaired. In these cases, hydrocephalus is treated by placing a ventriculo-peritoneal (V-P) shunt to divert the extra amount of CSF; if the abdominal cavity cannot be canulated due to ongoing inflammatory process or previous abdominal surgery and severe adhesions, then ventriculo-atrial or ventriculo-pleural shunts can be a substitution for the V-P shunt system.

3. Subdural empyema, cerebral abscess and septic cerebral emboli

Subdural empyema is the accumulation of pus in the subdural space which is usually a complication of cranial surgery and untreated postoperative meningitis. Purulent meningitis is another cause of subdural empyema, since primary purulent meningitis infection's rate has decreased drastically due to vaccinations and early diagnosis as well as antibiotic treatments, we will be focusing on postoperative meningitis and subsequently subdural empyema. Other pathologies such as chronic sinusitis, otitis media and mastoiditis, if left untreated contribute to formation of subdural empyema and mostly cerebral abscess formation. Odontogenic sources are also important to be mentioned, as often poor dental hygiene or invasive dental procedures are the origin of subdural empyema or cerebral abscess formation. Immunocompromised patients have a higher susceptibility for postoperative and primary infections, therefore they must be treated with care and normalization of their immune system prior to surgeries is required to prevent postoperative complications, for instance in cases where patients are on prolonged immunosuppressant drugs such as steroids due to chronic diseases, or other immunosuppressive drugs for treating autoimmune diseases, reduction of dose and even a complete halt of treatment for a temporary time should be considered if doing so does not interfere with the course of surgery or patient's primary treatment, reducing the dose of immunosuppressant drugs can be very effective in decreasing the PNM and in general postoperative infections.

Accumulation of pus in the subdural spaces irritates the meninges as well as the arachnoid membrane causing arachnoiditis, this in return can cause irritation of the cerebrum and cause cerebritis. If this process is not disrupted properly and intime, then cerebral abscess formation is occurring. With time as the abscess is maturing, it's wall thickens, and it gets bigger and bigger. The symptom presentation of patients can be very different and vary in a vast range, patients can have mild to severe meningitis signs or severe epileptic seizures and signs of increase intracranial pressure. In cases where an ongoing meningitis is not healed completely and it becomes chronic, the patient's signs and symptoms improve temporarily, but meantime the ongoing chronic cerebritis is leading to abscess formation. Depending on the site of abscess formation severe symptoms such as seizures, hemiparesis, agitation, aggressiveness and even loss of consciousness can occur (in accordance with lesion localization neurological deficits are present). **Figure 2** demonstrates a right sided temporal lesion with rim enhancement, perifocal edema and central diffusion restriction. The patient developed a sudden left sided hemiparesis due to the perifocal edema, and acute drainage and abscess excision was done to minimize neurological damage and complications.

Treatment of subdural empyema and cerebral abscess can be surgical or conservative, depending on their size and symptoms of the patient. Smaller abscesses or subdural empyemas can be treated with systematic antibiotics if they are not causing severe neurological deficits which are acute emergencies, such as hemiparesis, loss of consciousness, decreased arousal state and uncontrollable seizures.

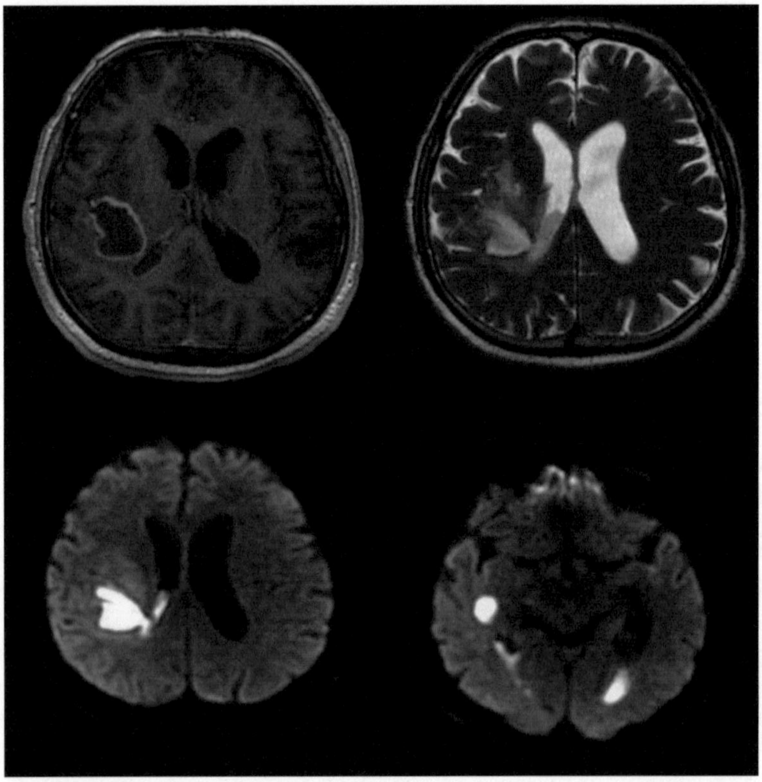

Figure 2.
Rim enhancement on T1 imaging (upper left) and perifocal edema on T2 (upper right) scans in this case are indicative for brain abscess. DWI sequences (lower images) show diffusion restriction in the areas as well as in the right lateral ventricle. It is to be noticed that the occipital horns of the lateral ventricles are also filled with pus and diffusion restriction can be seen there as well (lower right image).

If the above-mentioned symptoms are present, regardless of the size, surgical drainage and systemic antibiotic therapy should be started as soon as possible. In other scenarios where the mentioned symptoms are absent and the size of the abscess is not causing mass effect and midline shift, then proper antibiotic treatment can be the first line treatment, and if it fails or patient deterioration occurs, then surgical removal and drainage should be considered.

Figure 3 demonstrates a severe case of odontogenic subdural empyema which required immediate surgical drainage due to mass effect of the empyema and the neurological status of the patient. Multiple surgeries had to be carried out to achieve an acceptable level of drainage. In **Figure 4** post-operative scans show a significant reduction in contrast enhancement and no diffusion restriction can be seen on the DWI sequence. Surgical treatment was followed by intensive intravenous antibiotic treatment (intravenous Vancomycin, Ceftriaxone and Metronidazole).

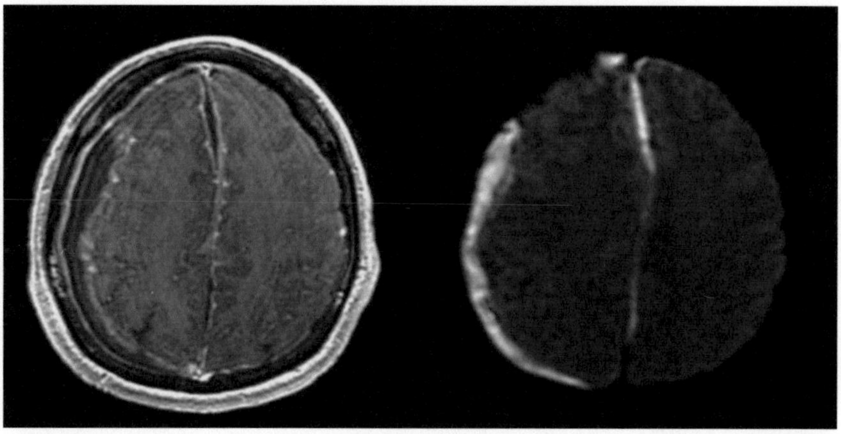

Figure 3.
Contrast enhanced T1 MRI scan (left side) shows contrast enhancement on the arachnoid membrane and dura diffusely on the right hemisphere. Next to the falx cerebri similar alteration are seen and cavitation between falx and dura is noticeable. On the right sided image, we can see diffusion restriction in the hypointense areas seen on T1 sequences. These alterations show accumulation of pus in the subdural space.

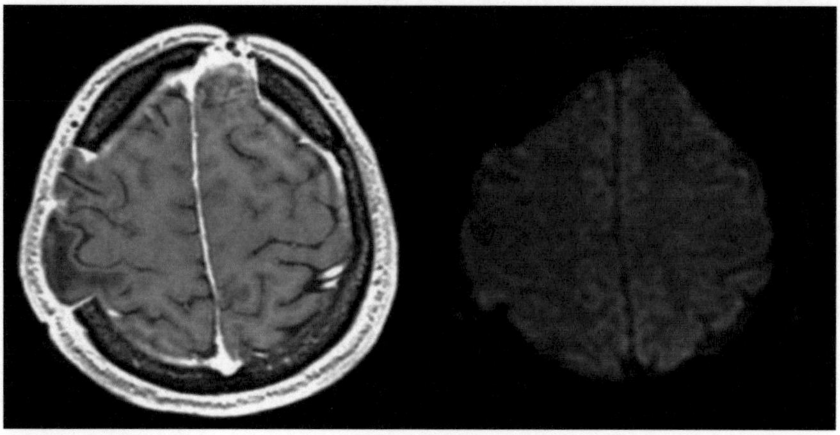

Figure 4.
Post-operative contrast enhanced T1 scan (left image) showing a significant decrease in contrast enhancement; Craniectomy site on the right fronto-temporal region and a burr hole on the left frontal region can be seen. DWI scans show no diffusion restriction.

Septic cerebral emboli are not common findings, and their diagnosis is quite challenging as they often resemble tumor like masses. Septic emboli usually originate from a distant organ via hematogenous spread and after seeding in the CNS they cause abscess formation. Cardiac vegetations are the most common cause of septic cerebral embolization and patients who have gone under valve replacements are at a greater risk of developing cardiac vegetations and consequently septic cerebral embolization. Differential diagnosis is the key point of a proper treatment here and the course of disease development plays a crucial role in differentiating septic cerebral emboli from other pathologies such as tumor masses or granulomas. A sudden onset of signs and symptoms with intracranial lesions should alert the physician for possibility of septic cerebral embolization and if ongoing inflammatory or infectious diseases or comorbidities such as DM, autoimmune disorders, existing mechanical heart valves are present then the probability of septic embolization significantly increases.

4. Foreign body infections

Implantation of foreign bodies in neurosurgery is quite often and so is their complications, but it should be taken into consideration that not all the foreign body implantations come with high infection rates. Aneurysm clips, coils and bone cement implantation have a much lower infection rate in comparison with shunt implantation, screws and rods, EVDs, cranioplasty flaps and deep brain stimulation (DBS) stimulators and electrodes. In both spinal and cranial surgery, there are a variety of pathologies which require implantation of foreign bodies for treatment, in this chapter we shall discuss the most common types of foreign body implantation which can result in a higher infection rate.

4.1 Cranioplasty flaps

Cranioplasty is defined by replacing a missing bone flap, either by means of 3D printed material, autologous bone graft, bone cement or titanium mesh. Regardless of indications for performing craniectomy followed by cranioplasty, the infection rates for this neurosurgical procedure compared to the other procedures is higher. In a broad-based study in 2019 by Ying Chen et al., it was revealed that after craniotomies (6.58% Infection rate), cranioplasties had the highest infection rate (5.89%) in neurosurgical procedures [9]. Infections in cranioplasty procedures can occur early or late in the post-operative period. Early onset of infection usually appears with symptoms of meningitis and quite often wound oozing and surgical site infection is seen as well. PNM is a common complication after neurosurgical procedures, and this is also true for cranioplasty procedures too, if the symptoms cannot be treated by antibiotics, and the bone flap is the source of infection with or without wound oozing, then the flap should be omitted as soon as possible to prevent subdural empyema or abscess formation. Once the ongoing inflammatory process is treated after removal of the bone flap, a minimum of 2 months is recommended before a newer skull reconstruction surgery is performed.

4.2 EVD

External ventricular drains may be the most frequently used implant in neurosurgery. There are different types of ventricular drains with different impregnations which offer a lower risk for EVD related meningitis and ventriculitis. Antibiotic coated or ionized silver particles impregnated EVDs lower the risk of EVD related infections similarly to the administration of intraventricular antibiotics via the EVD, however there are multiple factors contributing to the infection of EVDs, such as existing infection, lack of proper tunneling of EVD, multiple CSF sampling, leakage and improper isolation of the surgical site by the nursing staff [10]. EVDs quite often are inserted at bedside by neurosurgeons in intensive care units (ICU), where the environmental bacterial composition is quite different and more resistant and severe in terms of contagiosity compared to other sections of a hospital, therefore there is a higher chance of EVD infection if it is placed at the bed side and in ICU and this can be prevented by performing this procedure in an operation room where sterility is maximized. If an EVD becomes infected or colonized, then it should be removed, and a newer drain should be inserted in a different location if needed.

4.3 Shunts

Shunting CSF is one of the common procedures done routinely in neurosurgical wards, different variants of shunting are used for divergence of the CSF and they all include implantation of foreign bodies, therefore having similar high infection rates postoperatively. As V-P shunts are the most common used variant of the CSF divergence, we will be discussing only the complications of V-P shunts. The V-P shunt infection occurs at a rate of 5–10%, *Staphylococcus epidermidis* accounts for the majority of infections (60%) as well as *Staphylococcus aureus* (30%). The shunt

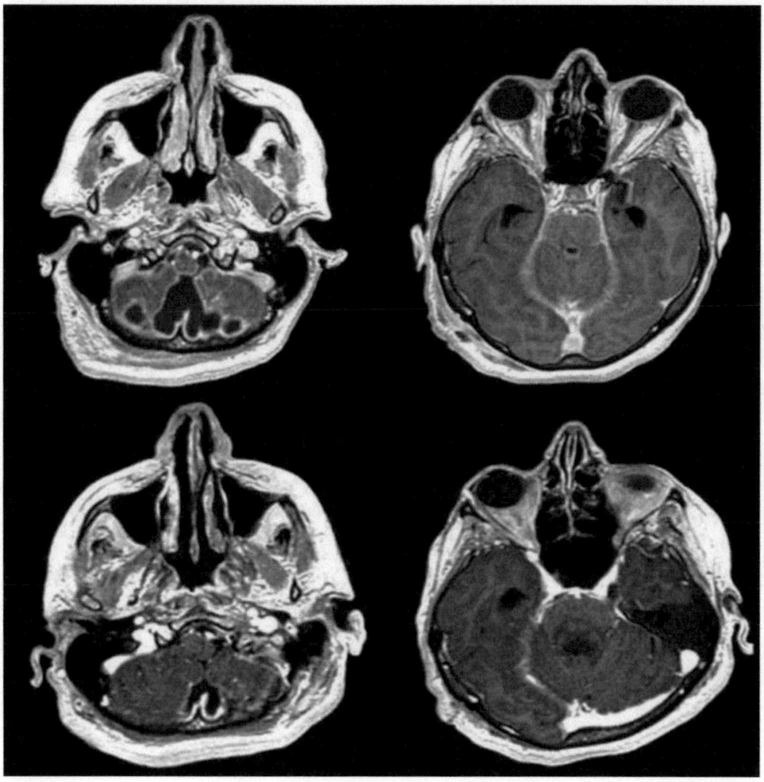

Figure 5.
Contrast enhancement on T1 scans (upper images) can be seen, rim enhancement and hypointense central compartment in the cerebellar region reveals multiplex abscess formation (upper left image). Contrast enhancement and dilation of aqueduct is seen, and this is indicative of intraventricular involvement of inflammation (upper right image). Lower pictures show regression of the inflammatory lesions after aggressive antibiotic treatment and removal of the V-P shunt system. Minimal contrast enhancement is seen between the two cerebellar hemispheres (lower left image).

infections usually occur within the first 6 months of implantation, the first month having the highest probability [11]. Factors such as contamination of shunt with skin flora during implantation, leakage, improper wound closure and ongoing intracerebral or abdominal inflammation at the time of surgery are the common causes of V-P shunt infections within the first month of implantation, long term complications of shunts are usually due to secondary infections. Peritonitis can be a severe complication of V-P shunt infection as well as a source for V-P shunt infection. Odontogenic infections often cause intracerebral inflammation and with the presence of V-P shunts, this can cause shunt failure and serious complications. **Figure 5** shows a case of V-P shunt infection after 3 years of implantation due to an ongoing untreated dental infection which had caused severe ventriculitis and multiple abdominal infected granulomas.

4.4 Deep brain stimulation and spinal cord stimulation

DBS surgeries are often used for treating movement disorders such as Parkinson's disease, dystonia, and essential tremor as well as psychiatric disorders such as obsessive–compulsive disorder. In the other hand as cases of chronic lumboischialgia and failed back surgery syndrome are rising, spinal cord stimulation surgeries are getting more attention. Both procedures involve implanting electrodes and neuromodulators in different sites, therefore these surgeries are carrying a high risk of infection. Infection rates are different in different areas and hospitals, in the literature the infection rate for DBS surgeries can be up to25%. As mentioned before *S. aureus* is the most common cause of neurosurgical infections and DBS and SCS surgeries are not an exclusion of this fact [12].

Intraoperative topical use of vancomycin has shown no advantage in preventing postoperative infections and its use intraoperatively remains controversial, in fact Bernstein et all in 2019 concluded that intraoperative topical use of vancomycin increases the risk of postoperative infection after electrode implantation [12].

Infection of brain electrodes can lead to abscess formation and spinal electrode infection can cause epidural abscess formation. Neuromodulators can also get infected and be a source for septic reactions.

4.5 Screws, rods and cages

The most common implants used in spine surgery are screws, rods and intervertebral cages. Different materials such as polypropylene-polyester, titanium, and polyetheretherketone (PEEK) are used in spinal surgeries and a study in 2019 revealed that the above-mentioned materials among all other materials used in neurosurgical procedures have the highest rate for infection [9]. Fusion surgeries require the removal of the intervertebral disk and implantation of an intervertebral cage, this in turn can cause spondylodiscitis which in turn can cause colonization and infection of the implanted screws and cages. The ongoing inflammation causes loosening of implanted screws, and this will lead to spine instability, therefore in such cases patients need to be immobilized, treated with antibiotics and revision surgery should be done when suitable. In addition, using thoracolumbar spinal orthosis (TLSO) braces can add some degrees of spine stability and fine patient mobilization can be allowed when wearing TLSO. Diagnosing is based on elevated inflammatory parameters on blood tests as well as contrast enhanced MRI scans to visualize the spinal canal and assess the extent of ongoing inflammation.

4.6 Treatment

Foreign body infection requires immediate attention and treatment; if left untreated it can cause severe intracranial or epidural inflammation and severe neurological deficits as well as sepsis and multi organ failure consequently. Diagnosing foreign body infection requires precise imaging, multiple repeated blood tests, culturing and patient examination. Once the diagnosis of foreign body colonization or infection has been made, broad spectrum empirical systemic antibiotic treatment should be started immediately and later on modified based on antibiograms. If the infection is caught in early phases and only mild symptoms are present and imaging modalities rule out presence of abscess or empyema and colonization of foreign bodies are not suspected then systematic or intrathecal antibiotic treatment might be enough to treat the infection, but in cases were abscess or empyema formation is already present on scans or CRP-PCT levels are not normalizing with antibiotic therapy, then removal or revision of the implanted foreign bodies are required.

Infected V-P shunts need to be removed and CSF divergence with EVD is preferred at a different site rather than the primary surgical site. In cases where deep brain electrodes need to be removed, patient management can become very challenging; for example, patients who suffer from Parkinson's disease and are non-responders to oral medication, will have severe disabilities if their neuro pacemaker was turned off suddenly and there was no pacing in the subthalamic nuclei. When infections are properly treated, then permanent electrodes, shunts or any other foreign body should be reimplanted if the patient's status and treatment require so.

5. Fungal and parasitic infections

Fungal and parasitic infections are not as common as bacterial infections in postoperative patients, therefore there is no solid information about fungal infection in postoperative patients in the field of neurosurgery. As a known fact patients who are immunocompromised are having a greater risk for developing any kind of infection, and fungal infections can be seen in these group of patients more often. Indeed, a prolonged antibiotic treatment increases the susceptibility of patients for developing fungal infections and this should be taken into consideration. Mycosis in the CNS can be hard to diagnose as often they resemble tumor masses on MRI or CT scans and their differentiation is quite challenging if the patient does not have any background for infection or does not present signs and symptoms of infection physically or on laboratory findings. A complication of ongoing fungal infection can be mycotic aneurysms which can rupture and be life threatening.

As in any other infectious disease, mycosis of the CNS should be treated immediately based on culture results. Surgical resection of fungal abscesses or granulomas might be necessary in severe cases where antifungal therapy is not yielding positive results or due to the mass effect and midline shift caused by these lesions in the brain.

6. Atypical infections

Atypical infections are quite rare and therefore very misleading, their diagnosis is very challenging and if not diagnosed correctly, the course of treatment can be very different and ineffective. The term atypical applies when the infection is caused by an organism which is not known to cause CNS infection or has not been reported yet, or infections which happen without any background or any obvious reason. Recently a case of septic cerebral embolus caused by Corynebacterium mucifaciens was described in a diabetic patient, C. mucifaciens is a normal flora of the skin and it can also be found in sterile body fluids [13]. Immunocompetent patients usually have a lower risk for atypical infections, but patients with defective immune system tend to have superinfections and even infections caused by organisms which normally do not cause any pathology. Course of disease development plays a crucial role in diagnosing these atypical infections, for example patients on prolonged antibiotic treatment, steroid treatment or immunosuppressants and in general immunocompromised patients should be considered for atypical strains of bacterial infection. If atypical strains are cultured or isolated in the abovementioned patient categories, they should not be precepted as contamination or false positive results but rather considered as atypical pathogens and they should be further investigated in order to confirm diagnosis.

The other scenario would be when a healthy immunocompetent individual suffers an atypical bacterial infection, this too should not be considered as false positive results or contamination, but rather it should be alarming as most immunocompromised patients are unaware of their condition are considered immunocompetent until such infections come along. This in turn does not mean that if a healthy individual is infected by atypical strains, then a defective immune system is the cause; this simply has to be investigated further to rule out any defects of the immune system and find the origin and primary cause of atypical infection. Healthy immunocompetent individuals can also be infected by atypical bacterial strains without any background or comorbidities playing along.

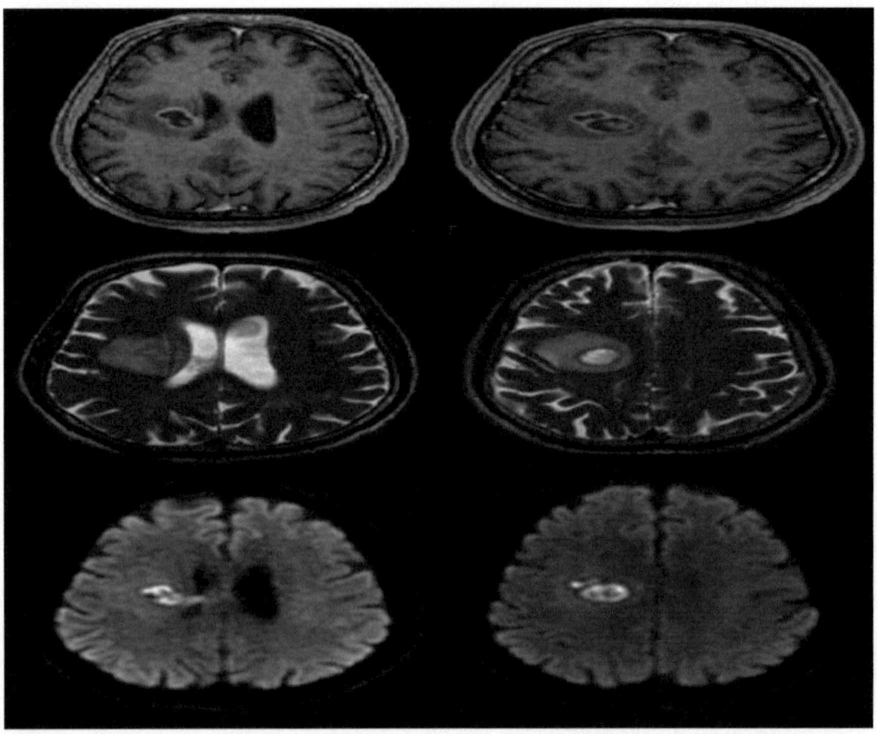

Figure 6.
T1 contrast enhanced images (upper images) show a cystic like lesion with perifocal edema and rim enhancement in the right temporal lobe, at the level of the internal capsule. T2 scans (middle images) reveal the extent of perifocal edema and the fluid content of the lesion. Diffusion restriction can be seen on DWI sequences (lower images) which is a typical finding for cerebral abscess.

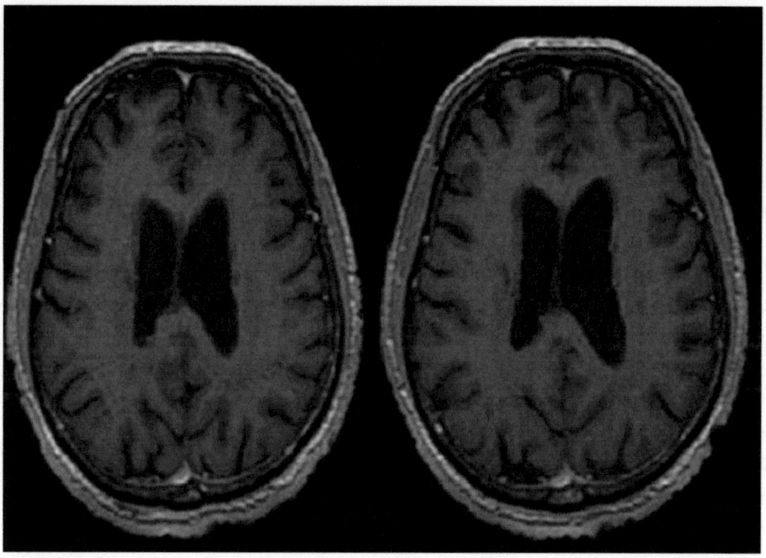

Figure 7.
Complete resolution of the lesion is seen after proper antibiotic treatment. The post gadolinium MRI scan was done for control purposes after 1 year.

Atypical bacterial infections should be reported so that, medical society all over the world can recognize the possibility of infection by these strains in immunocompetent or immunosuppressed individuals. Treatment of atypical strains remains the same as typical strains, except for if standard antibiotic treatment fails to control the infection, a more aggressive antibiotic treatment profile should be chosen.

Figure 6 shows the first ever reported case of cerebral embolus caused by C. mucifaciens by Tahaei et al. The radiographic findings are very typical for cerebral abscess or metastatic tumor lesions, and simply because the relevance of metastatic tumors and brain abscesses are much higher than septic emboli, the possibility of a cerebral septic embolus is often ignored, and they can be misdiagnosed and mistaken for tumors initially. A biopsy confirmed the diagnosis of septic cerebral embolus and proper antibiotic treatment based on antibiogram results were started after empiric treatment. In **Figure 7** the complete resolution of the septic embolus is seen after proper antibiotic treatment.

7. Spinal infections

They represent about 4% of all cases of osteomyelitis and 2–7% of all musculoskeletal infections. The incidence is between 1:20000 and 1:100000 and it has been increasing in the last decades [14–17].

Spinal infections can be extremely destructive and can cause instability and progressive neurological symptoms. Diagnosis of spinal infection is very challenging due to the fact that they mimic other noninfectious degenerative disorders [17].

7.1 Pathogenesis

Spinal infection can develop in three different ways:

- hematogenous spread

- direct inoculation
- spread of infection from an adjacent site

The sources of hematogenous infections are usually the skin, respiratory tract, genitourinary tract, gastrointestinal tract or the oral cavity through bacteremia. The extensive prevertebral venous plexus in the vertebral column provides a sophisticated anatomical background for spreading of bacterial infection. In adults, discitis mostly originates from one of the neighboring endplates, which are necrotized by a septic embolus, while the disc is infected secondarily. Spread from contiguous tissue is rare and mainly occurs in adjacent infections, including retropharyngeal abscess, esophageal ruptures, and infected implants [17, 18].

7.2 Microbial agents

The most common causative agents of spinal infections are *Staphylococcus aureus* and *Staphylococcus epidermidis*, gram negative organisms and in general anaerobe bacteria. In infants the most common agents are *Staphylococcus aureus*, *Streptococcus agalactiae* and *Escherichia coli* and in childhood *Staphylococcus aureus*, Staphylococcus pyogenes and Hemophilus influenzae. *Staphylococcus aureus* is the most common causative agent in hematogenous osteomyelitis in patients of all ages [19]. *Mycobacterium tuberculosis* can cause Pott's disease and skeletal tuberculosis which nowadays are extremely rare. Fungal origin of spinal infection is rarely found and particularly include Aspergillus spp., Candida spp., and *Cryptococcus neoformans* [17].

7.3 Classification of spinal infections

The spinal infections can be classified into the following categories:

a. Pyogenic infections

    i. Vertebral osteomyelitis

    ii. Discitis

    iii. Spondylodiscitis

    iv. Spinal epidural abscess

    v. Facet joint arthritis

b. Granulomatous infections

    i. Tuberculous infections

    ii. Fungal infections

    iii. Parasitic infections

c. Postoperative wound infection

d. Spinal infection in the immunocompromised patients

7.3.1 Pyogenic infections

The source of infections is usually the genitourinary, gastrointestinal and respiratory tract and in one-third of cases, the source is unknown. Patients who are on prolonged steroid treatments or immunosuppressants have a higher risk for pyogenic infections.

7.3.1.1 Vertebral osteomyelitis

Vertebral osteomyelitis most commonly occurs via the hematogenous route. The disease can progress to abscess formation and can involve the paravertebral structures and spinal canal. Risk factors are diabetes, renal failure, rheumatoid arthritis, AIDS, malignancy and old age. The most common bacterial agents responsible for vertebral osteomyelitis are *S. aureus*, Streptococcus sp., *P. aeruginosa*, *E. coli* and Proteus sp.

7.3.1.2 Discitis

This is an infection or inflammation of the intervertebral disc space. The infection starts at the endplates and spreads to the disc secondarily. *S. aureus* is the most common causative agent.

7.3.1.3 Spondylodiscitis

An infection and inflammation of the endplates of the vertebrae, as well as the joining intervertebral disc. It commonly occurs in sepsis, post-tonsillectomy, urinary tract, gastrointestinal and respiratory tract infections. The most common organisms are staphylococci (40–60%) and tuberculosis (20%). **Figure 8** demonstrates a case of active and healed spondylodiscitis in one patient.

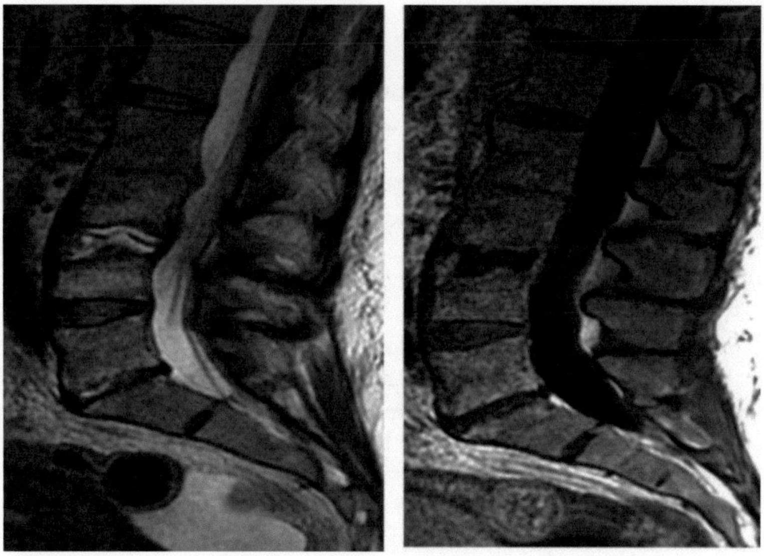

Figure 8.
Active spondylodiscitis at the level of LIII-IV and healed spondylodiscitis at the level of L II-III can be seen on both T1 and T2 sagittal images. Destruction of the disc and ossification of the two adjacent vertebral bodies are noted at the level of LII.

7.3.1.4 Spinal epidural abscess

Epidural abscesses are often complications of invasive spinal interventions, but spontaneous cases can also occur due to hematogenous spread or adjacent infected sites. The risk factors are diabetes mellitus, HIV, osteomyelitis, urinary tract infection, sepsis, soft tissue infections and spinal abnormality. *S. aureus* is the most common causative agent. The infection can come from contiguous areas, through hematogenous spread and from unknown distant locations as well [15, 17, 18].

Pain and muscle spasm are the most common symptoms of spine infection and the patient can be bedridden. In half of the cases, fever is the systemic manifestation of infection and early diagnosis is hindered by the fact that 30–70% of patients with spondylitis/spondylodiscitis do not show any signs of prior infection. Radicular pain and neurologic deficit are rare finding at the beginning but as a complication or progression of the situation serious neurological symptoms can occur [17].

Prevalence of spinal epidural abscess based on localization is 35% in thoracic region and 48% at lumbar region. Laboratory findings include elevated erythrocyte sedimentation rate and C-reactive protein, in about 40% of cases there are total or PMN leukocytosis [19]. X-ray shots are not very informative for diagnosing epidural abscesses, after 3–4 weeks the inflammation starts spreading around and degenerating the adjacent bony vertebra, and it is only then when destruction of bony parts can be visualized on X-ray shots; X-ray does not rule out the presence of a space occupying lesion in the spinal canal and therefore, post Gadolinium MRI scans are necessary to have a precise diagnosis. In cases where MRI scans are unavailable then CT scans or myelography can be done to gain more information. MRI scans remain the gold standard for confirming diagnosis when spinal epidural abscess formation is suspected. Epidural abscesses appear hypointense on T1 sequences and hyperintense on T2 and STIR sequences. Rim enhancement in post Gd scans can also be visualized. In **Figure 9** an epidural spinal abscess can be seen at the level of L IV – SI; Surgical excision and drainage of the abscess was done along with intensive iv. antibiotic treatment.

7.3.2 Granulomatous infection

Infectious diseases of spine which is caused by bacteria, fungi and parasites and it is accompanied by formation of granulomas. Granulomas are mixture of transformed macrophages, matrix and other inflammatory cells. Most cases are due to hematogenic spread of microorganisms to the spinal structures but spread from adjacent infected tissues are also a common pathway of infection [20].

7.3.2.1 Tuberculous infections

The spine is the most common site of skeletal tuberculosis and *Mycobacterium tuberculosis* is the most common causative agent. The lower thoracic spine is the segment frequently involved in tuberculous infections. The infections is a result of past hematogenous foci, contiguous disease or lymphatic spread from pleural disease, it gradually enlarges and spreads to involve two or more adjacent vertebrae by extension beneath the anterior longitudinal ligament or directly across the intervertebral disc.

X-ray shots reveal anterior wedging of two adjacent vertebral bodies with destruction of the intervening disc. On MRI scans post Gd sequences show subligamentous, Dural or discal contrast enhancement whereas T1 sequence shows a hypointense and T2 sequence a hyperintense marrow. Contrast enhanced MRI is the preferred modality of choice and if unavailable then contrast enhanced CT scans are the modality of choice.

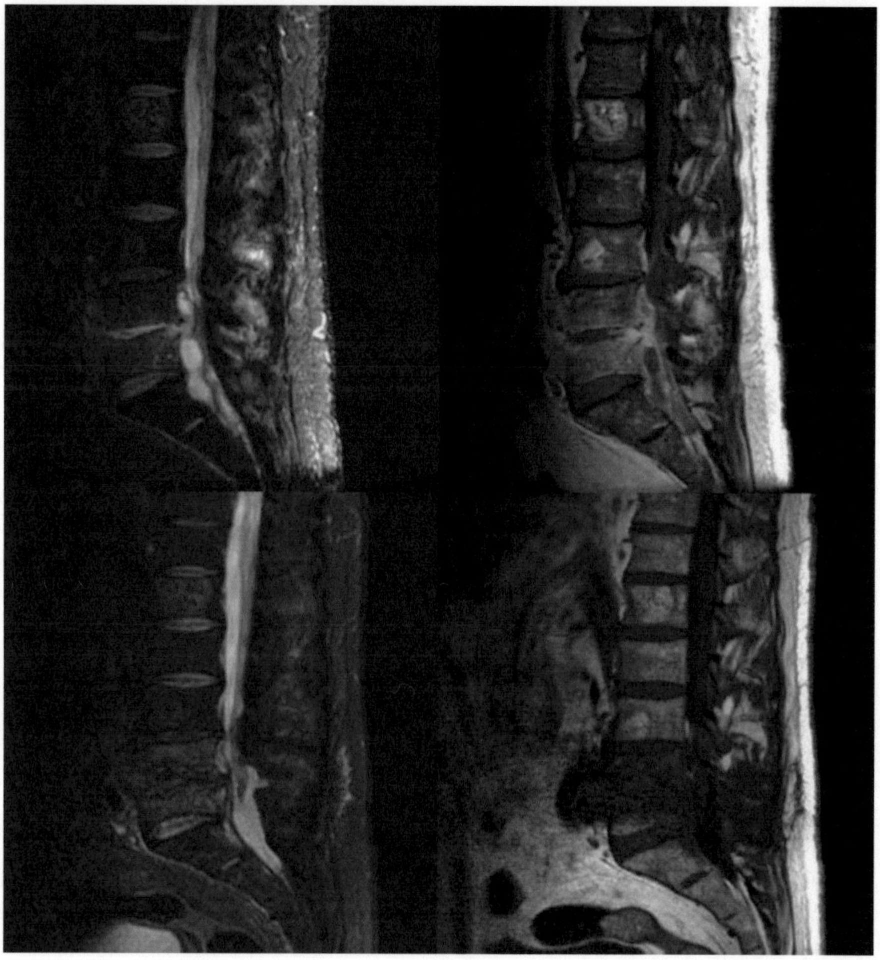

Figure 9.
A case of spontaneous epidural abscess formation, the patient was referred to the neurosurgical word due to progressive paraparesis; lab test results revealed leucocytosis and elevated CRP and PCT values. MRI scans show diffusion restriction (upper left image – STIR sequence) in the epidural region at the level of LIV-SI as well as LIV disc and LIV LV vertebral bodies, the post Gd T1 image (upper right) shows contrast enhancement of the lesion in the periphery. Control MRI scans after 6 weeks (lower images): On STIR (lower left image) sequence significant reduction of diffusion restriction is seen, T1 Contrast scan (lower right image) show no sign of contrast enhancement. The presence of hemangiomas at the level of LI and LIII vertebral bodies are noted.

7.3.2.2 Fungal infections

Fungal infections of the spine are rare and occur mainly as opportunistic infections in immunocompromised patients. They form noncaseating lesions. The common fungal agents causing fungal infections are Candida species, *Cryptococcus neoformans* and Aspergillus species. In fungal vertebral osteomyelitis epidemic fungi, such as Coccidiodes immitis and Blastomyces dermatitidis are the typical causative agents.

7.3.2.3 Parasitic infection

The parasites that have been reported to cause infections of the spine are Echinococcus granuosus (hydatid disease), Toxoplasma gondii (toxoplasmosis) and rarely Taenia solium (cysticercosis). The parasitic spine infection is extremely rare, and few cases have been reported in the literature.

7.3.2.4 Postoperative wound infection

Postoperative wound infections after spine surgeries are common complications and their occurrence rate vary depending on the type and site of surgery. Simpler surgeries such as lumbar microdiscectomy or sequestrectomy have lower rates of postoperative infection (~0.6–3%) whereas more complicated surgeries such as instrumented fusions have a higher occurrence rate (~6–18%). If left untreated or not diagnosed properly and in time, long term complications such as pseudoarthrosis, spinal deformities, chronic pain and even in severe cases sepsis and death can occur. Deep wound cultures accompanied by CBC and evaluation of CRP, PCT and ESR helps diagnosing postoperative SSIs. Picture modalities such as contrast enhanced MRI and CT scans are important in adding vital information for proper diagnosis, but they can also be very misleading [21].

Treatment of postoperative SSIs in spine surgery is no exception than other SSIs, early proper diagnosis, targeted antibiotic therapy and in severe cases surgical debridement and/or revision of surgery is needed to avoid long term complications. Sepsis and septic shock can be catastrophic outcomes of SSIs, therefore prompt response after diagnosing SSIs is a vital part of a good prognosis. Screening patients for multi resistant skin flora and proper bathing before surgery alongside with proper disinfection of the surgical site at the time of surgery and keeping an aseptic environment are modifiable factors which play an extensive role in SSIs. Factors such as prolonged steroid treatment, or use of immunosuppressant drugs, DM, chronic autoimmune diseases, alcoholism, malnutrition and acquired autoimmune defects are contributing to a higher rate of SSIs.

7.3.2.5 Spinal infection in the immunocompromised

As mentioned in Section 3, immunocompromised patients are at a greater risk for developing postoperative infections and spontaneous infections in general. The factors and strategies mentioned in Section 3 management and treating immunocompromised patients are all applicable for spine surgery as well. Patients with immune deficiencies should be considered for rare parasitic, fungal, and bacterial spine infections such as Cryptococcus, Mycobacterium and Echinococcus infections.

Figure 10 shows a case of spontaneous spondylodiscitis in a patient who was on chronic use of methylprednisolone tablets for treating rheumatoid arthritis.

7.3.2.6 Diagnosis of infection

ESR and CRP are both good indicators for determining inflammation in the body. ESR is more specific for tuberculosis infection, whereas CRP is an indicator for any inflammatory condition, including bacterial infections. Procalcitonin (PCT), a promising marker to distinguish between bacterial and nonbacterial infection, shows lower sensitivity than CRP in patients with spinal infection. Identification of the causative organism is essential, and if MRI or CT scans are suggestive of spinal infection then direct CT-guided biopsy or blood cultures should be obtained to identify the causative agent and clarify the diagnosis.

7.3.2.7 Imaging

The characteristics of spinal infection foci on picture modalities are as follow:

- X-ray: endplate irregularities and erosion in the vertebral endplates. Disadvantages: It is only after 2 to 4 weeks that the radiographs appreciate

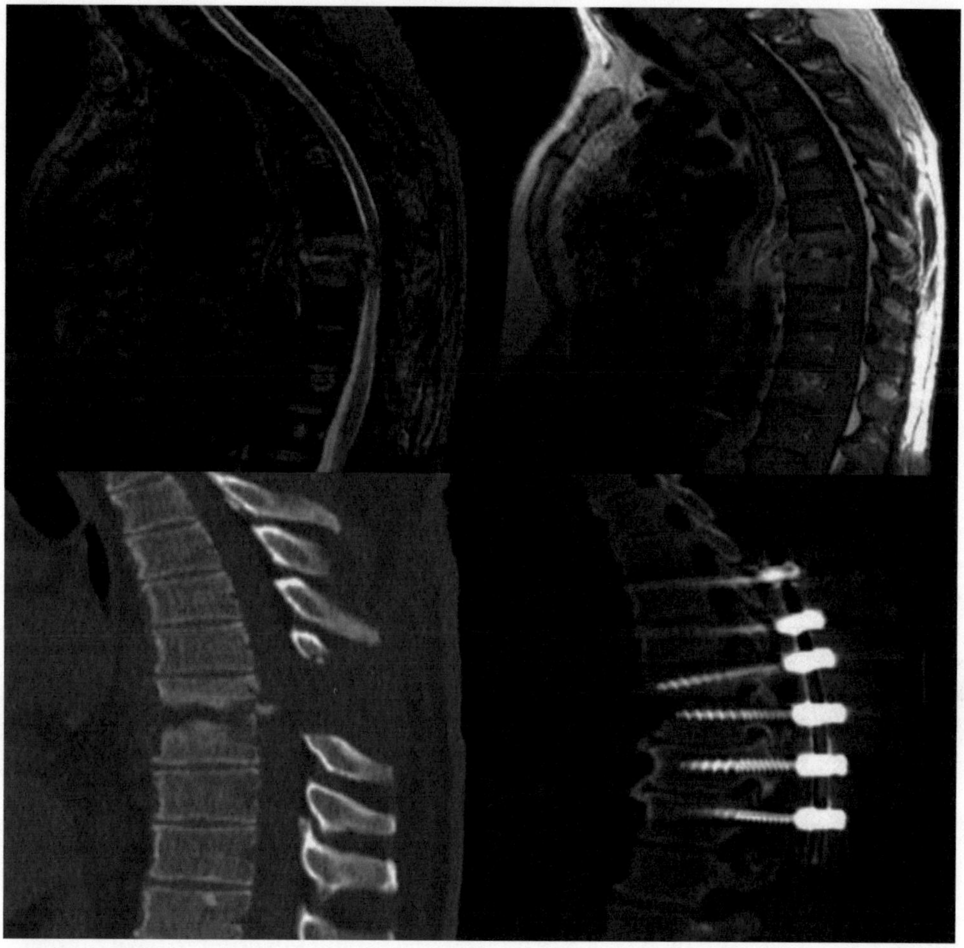

Figure 10.
A 40 years old male patient was brought to the emergency department due to sudden loss of lower extremities tone and severe paraparesis. Lab results were in favor of inflammatory process and the MRI scans have confirmed the diagnosis of spondylodiscitis. The STIR sequence (upper left image) shows diffusion restriction in the Th VIII-IX vertebral bodies as well as in the sub ligamental region which is causing spinal cord compression. Post Gd T1 sequence (upper right image) shows contrast enhancement of the lesion). The patient was admitted for acute surgery and first intraoperative CT scan (lower left image) shows the extent of posterior bony decompression (laminectomy) and the on the lower right image the final postoperative control scan is seen after percutaneous transpedicular fixation was done to achieve stability. It is important to mention that multiple lesions in the vertebral bodies were seen which typically assemble hemangiomas, but due to the complexity of this case and the fact that the patient was on prolonged steroid use, septic emboli and Pott's disease had to be ruled out. This was done by taking samples from the lesions and performing PCR, culturing, and sending samples for histopathological examination. All results were in favor of hemangiomas and an ongoing spondylodiscitis.

any changes. A positive radiograph may help in diagnosis, but a negative radiograph does not rule out the diagnosis of spinal infection.

- CT: Is the best way to demonstrate bone destruction and fragmentation. It can detect early changes like end-plate erosions, much sooner than radiography. It is superior in detecting bony fragments, new bone formation, bony sclerosis, and calcification. It can detect early changes like end-plate erosions, much sooner than radiography.

- MRI: It is considered the gold standard and is the most useful imaging modality in the evaluation of spinal infection. It can detect the form of increased vertebral marrow water content and micro destruction of trabecular bone. Typical findings in patients with spondylodiscitis are hypointense discs and vertebral bodies in T1-weighted images and hyperintense signals of the same structures in T2-weighted images. Although MRI is the gold standard in diagnosis of spinal infection, there is no pathognomonic finding on MRI that dependably discriminates between spinal infection and possible neoplasm [22].

Being a noninvasive and safe procedure follow-up MRI is good for assessing therapeutic-response and to guide clinical decisions. New MRI methods like diffusion-weighted imaging are useful in spinal cord abscess analysis. Contrast obtained pictures are a must in order to visualize the extent of epidural and meningeal inflammation. Diffusion tensor and fiber-tracking imaging methods are in use for assessing spinal cord integrity in long standing cord compression cases [19].

7.3.2.8 Management of spinal infections

Clinical picture and presentation of spinal infections vary widely, but usually the onset is insidious and axial back pain and spasm are the main symptoms. Fever, chills, weight loss, anorexia and malaise are not always present and neurological deficit presents usually late but may present acutely with epidural abscess formation causing paralysis or cauda equina syndrome. WBC, ESR and CRP are nonspecific, but may be helpful in monitoring the response to treatment.

X-ray and CT scan can show us the bony destruction, it takes a few weeks, but MRI is more sensitive and may show changes, early in the course of the disease. It can include bone marrow edema, endplate irregularity, fluid in the disc space, destruction of bone and adjacent disc, and epidural and/or paraspinal soft-tissue infection and abscess formation.

Nonsurgical Treatment consists of appropriate antibiotic treatment which can result in termination of the infection, but precise bacteriological diagnosis and culturing is required from blood culture or aspirated samples in order to have a target antibiotic therapy which is more efficient. It is important to start antibiotic therapy before significant bone destruction occurs, to avoid any long-standing unfavorable biomechanical consequences and spinal instabilities.

The following steps are required for diagnosing spinal infections correctly early in order to have the best maximized therapy:

1. Biopsy – to identify organism and to obtain its sensitivity (needle biopsy with cultures – percutaneously via transpedicular approach or CT guided biopsy)

2. antibiotics – once the tissue sample is obtained, empirical antibiotic therapy must be started using broad-spectrum antibiotics such as Clindamycin or Rifampicin for at least 6 weeks intravenously and then followed by 6–8 weeks of oral antibiotic treatment. Antibiotic treatment should be modified based on antibiograms if needed, to achieve the best targeted antibiotic therapy efficiency [23].

3. pain medication

4. Thoraco-lumbar spinal orthosis (TLSO) brace – to reduce pain.

Nonoperative treatment is more likely to yield good results if patients are younger than 60 years, having normal immunologic status and the treatment is started early in the course of the disease.

Monitoring response to treatment is crucial and factors like improvement in pain reduction, muscle spasm, general sense of wellbeing, as well as progressive drop in the inflammatory markers like ESR and CRP are good indicators of sufficient treatment. Repetition of MRI scans can be helpful, but in early phases of treatment (within 4 weeks), after starting antibiotic therapy, it can be misleading, due to the fact that the effect of the antibiotic therapy can only be detected on the tissues adjacent to the spine in this period of time. It is recommended to perform post Gd MRI scans after four weeks of continuous iv. antibiotic treatment [24].

When non invasive treatments fail to achieve proper results, surgical treatment needs to be considered in order to control the disease progression. The fundamental goals are drainage of the pus and debridement of granulation and bony stabilization if necessary. Most cases can be managed non-surgically with antibiotics and immobilization, especially if the patient lacks neurological symptoms and if the spine retains its stability. Accordingly, we have to treat the patient surgically when

1. there is progression of disease despite antibiotic therapy

2. spinal instability

3. spinal epidural abscess

4. antibiotic refractory chronic infection [25]

Decompression of neural elements, removal of inflammatory tissue and infected bone (to decrease bioburden) with instrumented fusion can give the best result.

8. Conclusion

Postoperative infections are common and challenging to treat. Understanding the nature of these infectious diseases and their management can increase survival rate and prevent catastrophic results. Treating these infections can be surgical or conservative depending on presenting signs and symptoms and severity of infection. Proper targeted antibiotic treatment alongside surgical interventions are necessary in most cases to achieve the best result. Untreated or poorly treated cases lead to septic reactions and multi organ failure. Screening patients for immunodeficiencies, comorbidities, and specific individual bacterial patterns can significantly reduce postoperative infection rates.

Conflict of interest

The authors declare no conflict of interest.

Author details

Seyed Arad Senaobar Tahaei[1*], Seyyed Ashkan Senobar Tahaei[2], Zoltan Mencser[1] and Pal Barzo[1]

1 Department of Neurosurgery, University of Szeged, Hungary

2 Department of Pharmacognosy, University of Szeged, Hungary

*Address all correspondence to: red.stradivarius@gmail.com

References

[1] Diseases I. CLASSIFICATION OF CENTRAL by Marko Pokorn. Brain. 2003;15(3):68-71.

[2] Ekmekci H, Ege F, Ozturk S. Cerebrospinal Fluid Abnormalities in Viral Encephalitis. Encephalitis. 2013;

[3] Archibald LK, Quisling RG. Textbook of Neurointensive Care. Textbook of Neurointensive Care. 2013.

[4] Tubiana S, Varon E, Biron C, Ploy MC, Mourvillier B, Taha MK, et al. Community-acquired bacterial meningitis in adults: in-hospital prognosis, long-term disability and determinants of outcome in a multicentre prospective cohort. Clin Microbiol Infect. 2020;26(9):1192-1200.

[5] Van De Beek D, Brouwer M, Hasbun R, Koedel U, Whitney CG, Wijdicks E. Community-acquired bacterial meningitis. Nat Rev Dis Prim. 2016;2.

[6] Broekman MLD, Van Beijnum J, Peul WC, Regli L. Neurosurgery and shaving: What's the evidence? A review. J Neurosurg. 2011;115(4):670-678.

[7] Liu W, Ni M, Zhang Y, Groen RJM. Antibiotic prophylaxis in craniotomy: A review. Neurosurg Rev. 2014;37(3):407-414.

[8] Hussein K, Bitterman R, Shofty B, Paul M, Neuberger A. Management of post-neurosurgical meningitis: narrative review. Clin Microbiol Infect [Internet]. 2017;23(9):621-8. Available from: doi:10.1016/j.cmi.2017.05.013

[9] Chen Y, Zhang L, Qin T, Wang Z, Li Y, Gu B. evaluation of neurosurgical implant infection rates and associated pathogens: Evidence from 1118 postoperative infections. Neurosurg Focus. 2019;47(2):1-10.

[10] Muralidharan R. External ventricular drains: Management and complications. Surg Neurol Int. 2015;6(7):S271–S274.

[11] Shunts V. Shunts, Neurosurgical short-term Memory. 2000;259-264.

[12] Bernstein JE, Kashyap S, Ray K, Ananda A. Infections in deep brain stimulator surgery. Cureus. 2019;11(8):1-8.

[13] Senaobar Tahaei SA, Mencser Z, Reisz Z, Barzo P. An unusual case (metastatic-like lesion) of septic cerebral embolus caused by Corynebacterium mucifaciens in a diabetic patient. J Investig Med High Impact Case Reports. 2020;8.

[14] Aagaard T, Roed C, Dahl B, Obel N. Long-term prognosis and causes of death after spondylodiscitis: A Danish nationwide cohort study. Infect Dis (Auckl). 2016;48(3):201-208.

[15] Artenstein AW, Friderici J, Holers A, Lewis D, Fitzgerald J, Visintainer P. Spinal epidural abscess in adults: A 10-year clinical experience at a tertiary care academic medical center. Open Forum Infect Dis. 2016;3(4):1-8.

[16] Kehrer M, Pedersen C, Jensen TG, Lassen AT. Increasing incidence of pyogenic spondylodiscitis: A 14-year population-based study. J Infect [Internet]. 2014;68(4):313-20. Available from: doi:10.1016/j.jinf.2013.11.011

[17] Spinal Infections and Trauma. Spinal Infect Trauma. 2011;

[18] Babinchak TJ, Riley DK, Rotheram EB. Pyogenic vertebral osteomyelitis of the posterior elements. Clin Infect Dis. 1997;25(2):221-224.

[19] Lener S, Hartmann S, Barbagallo GMV, Certo F, Thomé C,

Tschugg A. Management of spinal infection: A review of the literature. Acta Neurochir (Wien). 2018;160(3):487-496.

[20] Murray MR, Schroeder GD, Hsu WK. Granulomatous vertebral osteomyelitis: An update. J Am Acad Orthop Surg. 2015;23(9):529-538.

[21] Dowdell J, Brochin R, Kim J, Overley S, Oren J, Freedman B, et al. Postoperative spine infection: Diagnosis and management. Glob Spine J. 2018;8(4_suppl):37S-43S.

[22] Ratcliffe JF. Anatomic basis for the pathogenesis and radiologic features of vertebral osteomyelitis and its differentiation from childhood discitis. A microarteriographic investigation. Acta Radiol – Ser Diagnosis. 1985;26(2):137-143.

[23] Skaf GS, Fehlings MG, Ph D, Bouclaous CH. A BIWEEKLY PUBLICATION FOR CLINICAL NEUROSURGICAL Medical and Surgical Management of Pyogenic and Nonpyogenic Spondylodiscitis: Part I. 2004;26(19):1-6.

[24] Butler JS, Shelly MJ, Timlin M, Powderly WG, O'Byrne JM. Nontuberculous pyogenic spinal infection in adults: A 12-year experience from a tertiary referral center. Spine (Phila Pa 1976). 2006;31(23):2695-2700.

[25] Schoenfeld AJ, Wahlquist TC. Mortality, complication risk, and total charges after the treatment of epidural abscess. Spine J [Internet]. 2015;15(2):249-55. Available from: doi:10.1016/j.spinee.2014.09.003

Section 3

Sepsis Pathophysiology

Chapter 12

An Explainable Machine Learning Model for Early Prediction of Sepsis Using ICU Data

Naimahmed Nesaragi and Shivnarayan Patidar

Abstract

Early identification of individuals with sepsis is very useful in assisting clinical triage and decision-making, resulting in early intervention and improved outcomes. This study aims to develop an explainable machine learning model with the clinical interpretability to predict sepsis onset before 6 hours and validate with improved prediction risk power for every time interval since admission to the ICU. The retrospective observational cohort study is carried out using PhysioNet Challenge 2019 ICU data from three distinct hospital systems, viz. A, B, and C. Data from A and B were shared publicly for training and validation while sequestered data from all three cohorts were used for scoring. However, this study is limited only to publicly available training data. Training data contains 15,52,210 patient records of 40,336 ICU patients with up to 40 clinical variables (sourced for each hour of their ICU stay) divided into two datasets, based on hospital systems A and B. The clinical feature exploration and interpretation for early prediction of sepsis is achieved using the proposed framework, viz. the explainable Machine Learning model for Early Prediction of Sepsis (xMLEPS). A total of 85 features comprising the given 40 clinical variables augmented with 10 derived physiological features and 35 time-lag difference features are fed to xMLEPS for the said prediction task of sepsis onset. A ten-fold cross-validation scheme is employed wherein an optimal prediction risk threshold is searched for each of the 10 LightGBM models. These optimum threshold values are later used by the corresponding models to refine the predictive power in terms of utility score for the prediction of labels in each fold. The entire framework is designed via Bayesian optimization and trained with the resultant feature set of 85 features, yielding an average normalized utility score of 0.4214 and area under receiver operating characteristic curve of 0.8591 on publicly available training data. This study establish a practical and explainable sepsis onset prediction model for ICU data using applied ML approach, mainly gradient boosting. The study highlights the clinical significance of physiological inter-relations among the given and proposed clinical signs via feature importance and SHapley Additive exPlanations (SHAP) plots for visualized interpretation.

Keywords: sepsis, early prediction, machine learning, explainable AI, electronic health records, clinical informatics, critical care, model-based diagnosis

1. Introduction

Sepsis is an enigmatic clinical condition that occurs when the patient's body reacts adversely to infection and as a consequence develops organ dysfunction.

Sepsis can practically affect all organ systems however, the organs involved and the degree of dysfunction varies distinctly among patients and can even lead to death in most cases [1, 2]. In the early stages of the disease, the treatment of sepsis seems to be relatively easy with the availability of broad-spectrum antibiotics [3]. While in the later stages of the disease, diagnosis of sepsis becomes much easier but extremely hard to treat. Therefore, early diagnosis of sepsis is the need of the hour for better clinical management [4].

Current manual assessment of sepsis using screening tools, like the Sequential Organ Failure Assessment (SOFA) score for ICU-patients, are complex in terms of measured clinical signs and even lack adequate sensitivity [5, 6]. On the other hand, AI and machine learning-based automated clinical decision support systems that use easily accessible clinical data have reflected a significant improvement in agreement with these treatment protocols in ICUs by guiding physicians through predefined work-flows [7–11]. In the current era wherein we have abundant availability of electronic medical records (EMRs) has brought more feasibility to such automated realizations [12]. However, almost every machine learning (ML)-based AI model and automated decision support system lack proper explainability because of their uninterpretable black-box nature [13, 14]. This is where Explainable Artificial Intelligence (XAI) comes in rescue to address some of these restrictions imposed by a Black-box AI system by adding explainability. And thus assist clinicians in the interpretation of their diagnosis, and recommend future actions to be taken thereby improving the quality of predictions [15–17]. The development of such an explainable ML framework for sepsis onset prediction is an important and active area of investigation.

This work presents a novel clinical application of developing an explainable ML framework for sepsis onset prediction among ICU patients based on the physiological medical knowledge of given clinical signs, obtained via extensive analysis, and using popular gradient boosting ML techniques. The framework's design includes an optimal explainable gradient boosting architecture for clinical decision making that investigates questions of generalizability and interpretability of the proposed system.

2. Methods

An overview of the proposed methodology from raw data to explainable decision framework is shown in **Figure 1**.

2.1 Dataset and study population

The publically available training set consists of data from two cohorts [18]. Cohort A has 790,215 records of 20,336 patients. Cohort B has 761,995 records of 20,000 patients. Particularly, data for every patient record contains 40 clinical covariates i.e. 8 vital signs, 26 laboratory values, and 6 demographic values. The labeling of the patient data was done adhering to Sepsis-3 clinical criteria. **Table 1** presents the details of various clinical covariates used under study together with their missing information in percentage [18, 19].

2.2 Feature extraction

Feature extraction takes place on the imputed version of given clinical data that generates features sample-wise on an hourly time grid. Two types of features ware generated namely:

Physiological features: In literature, inter-relations among the clinical values have been proven to enhance the capability of anomaly detection tasks [7, 20]. By reviewing various studies that justify the clinical significance of well-established physiological inter-relations among the given clinical signs 10 such physiological relations are derived from the given covariates: Three Shock Indices firstly the well defined Shock Index (SIndex) using Systolic BP and the other two are its modified versions proposed in this study for Diastolic BP (DPBSIndex) [21] and Mean

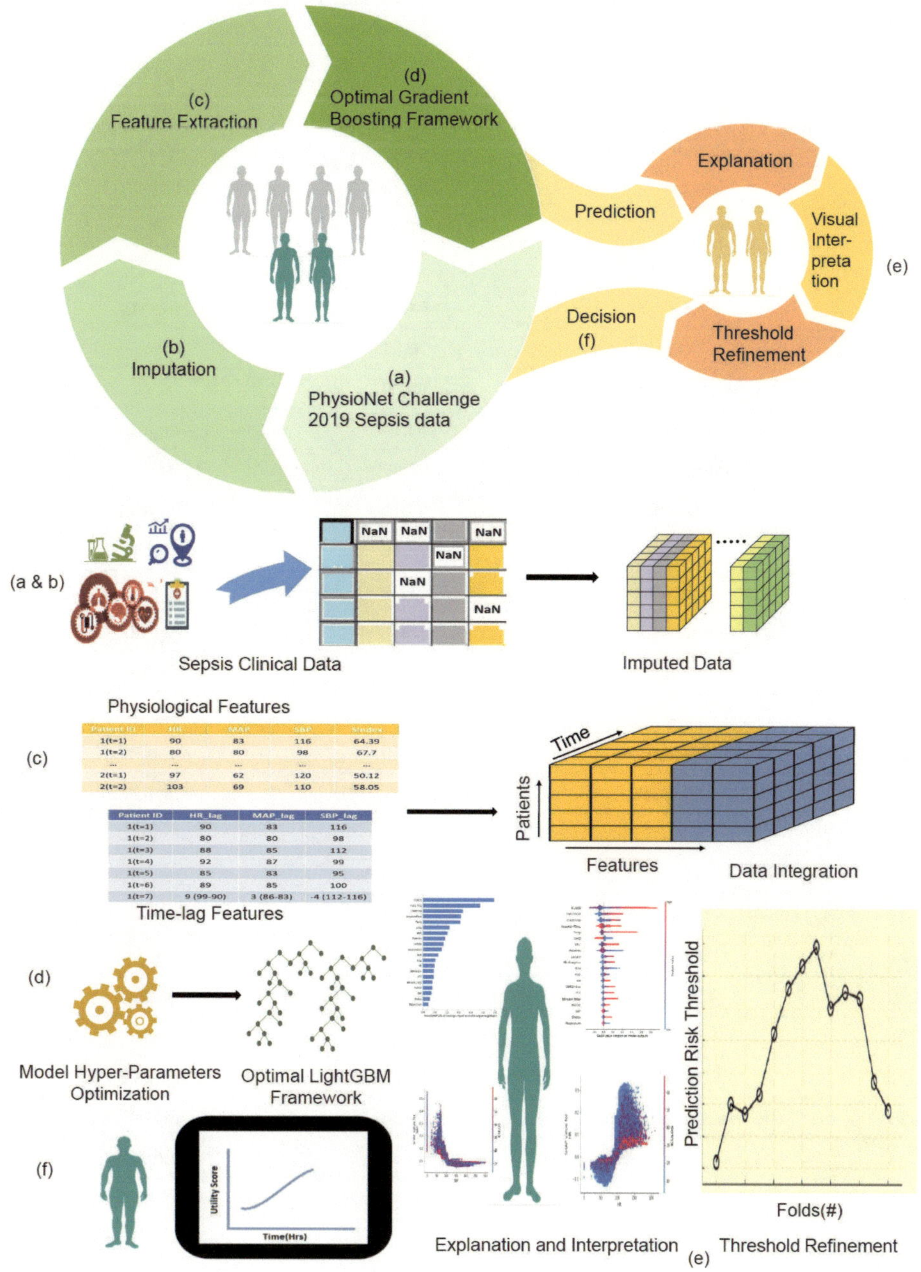

Figure 1.
Graphical overview: From given raw clinical data to explainable decision framework. (a & b) clinical data from two ICU cohorts is imputed. (c) Physiological inter-relations and time lag differences are computed as features. (d) an optimal sepsis onset prediction architecture is developed using LightGBM models via bayesian optimization. (e) the predictions are rendered to explanations and potentially their predictive power is increased by refining the threshold that drove the prediction at every time-point. (f) Final decision.

Sr. no.	Covariates	Missing values (%)	Units
1	Heart rate	9.8	beats/min
2	O_2Sat	13	%
3	Temperature	66	^oC
4	SBP	14.5	mm Hg
5	MAP	12.45	mm Hg
6	DBP	31.34	mm Hg
7	Resp	15.35	breaths/min
8	$EtCO_2$	96.28	mm Hg
9	Excess bicarbonate	95.57	mmol/L
10	Bicarbonate	94.81	mmol/L
11	FiO_2	91.66	%
12	pH	93.06	—
13	$PaCO_2$	94.44	mm Hg
14	SaO_2	96.54	%
15	Asparatate transaminase	98.37	IU/L
16	BUN	93.13	mg/dL
17	Alkaline phosphatase	98.39	IU/L
18	Calcium	94.11	mg/dL
19	Chloride	94.46	mmol/L
20	Creatinine	93.90	mg/dL
21	Direct bilirubin	99.8	mg/dL
22	Gl	82.89	mg/dL
23	Lactic acid	97.32	mg/dL
24	Magnesium	93.68	mmol/dL
25	Phosphate	93.98	mg/dL
26	Potassium	90.68	mmol/L
27	Total bilirubin	98.50	mg/dL
28	Troponin I	99.04	ng/mL
29	Hematocrit	91.14	%
30	Hemoglobin	92.61	g/dL
31	PTT	94.05	s
32	WBC	93.59	count/L
33	Fibrinogen concentration	99.34	mg/dL
34	Platelet count	94.05	count/mL
35	Age	—	yr
36	Gender	—	Male (1) or Female (0)
37	Unit 1	39.42	true (1) or false (0)
38	Unit 2	39.42	true (1) or false (0)
39	HospAdmTime	—	hours
40	LOS	—	hours

Sr. no.	Covariates	Missing values (%)	Units
41	SepsisLabel	—	septic (1) nonseptic (0).

Table 1.
Details of the various clinical variables used under study along with missing values information in percentage.

Sl. no	Abbreviation	Description	Formula
1	SIndex	Shock Index (SIndex) is the proportion of heart rate (HR) being divided by systolic blood pressure (SBP), normalized by age.	(HR/SBP)*Age
2	DBPSIndex	Diastolic Shock Index is the proportion HR being divided by systolic blood pressure (DBP), normalized by age.	(HR/DBP) *Age
3	MAPSIndex	It is defined as the proportion of HR being divided by Mean Arterial Pressure (MAP), normalized by age.	(HR/MAP) *Age
4	BUNCr	It is the ratio of Blood Urea Nitrogen(BUN) to Creatinine	BUN/ Creatinine
5	BILTCr	It is the ratio of Direct Bilirubin (Bilirubin_total) to Creatinine	Bilirubin_total/ Creatinine
6	SaO2 -FiO2	It is the ratio of oxygen saturation of arterial blood in percentage (SaO2) to the fraction of inspired oxygen (FiO2).	SaO2/FiO2
7	PaO2 -FiO2	It is defined as proportion of the partial pressure of oxygen PaO2 divided by the fraction of inspired oxygen (FiO2).	PaO2/FiO2
8	Pla_Age	It is the ratio of platelets to age	Platelets/Age
9	PP	Pulse Pressure (PP) is the difference between SBP and DBP	SBP-DBP
10	CO	Cardiac Output is the product of pulse pressure (PP) and HR.	PP * HR

Table 2.
Detailed definitions of the physiological features.

Arterial Pressure (MAPSIndex) [22] followed by ratios BUN/Creatinine (BUNCr) [7], Bilirubintotal/Creatinine (BILTcr), SaO2/FiO2 [23], PaO2/FiO2 [24], Platelets/ Age (PlaAge), the difference between SBP and DBP called Pulse Pressure (PP) [25], and lastly Cardiac Output (CO) [26]. **Table 2** gives a detailed description of Physiological features.

Time-Lag difference features: A set of 35 time-lag features are computed with 6 hours of time-lag difference among vital signs and lab values from the given 40 clinical variables excluding the last 5 demographic values.

Finally, the obtained 45 features are combined with the given 40 clinical signs, thereby increasing the final feature count to 85 features. The resultant feature set is then fed to train the proposed xMLEPS framework.

2.3 Implementation of xMLEPS

Together with Bayesian optimization and the refinement of prediction risk threshold an optimal disease onset detection method before six hours for sepsis called xMLEPS is developed. As shown in **Figure 1** the given clinical sepsis data has large amount of missing information (approximately 20%). So at the onset of the algorithm computation, filling of these missing values is carried out as as a pre-processing step. The data imputation to fill in the missing values is done by employing forward fill imputation on the given EHR clinical data. In the real-time scenario, the current missing values encountered are to be filled with previous available measurements. Thus only the previous clinical values of given EHR data are fetched for data imputation of current observation.

In this study, imputation is carried out into two rounds: first local imputation, for each individual record, and then global imputation for all the combined records together. In the case of local imputation, the trailing missing values in a row for a particular clinical covariate (or feature vector) are forward filled with the nearest past non-missing value in that row locally for the given record. Ipso facto, if the record encounters 'NaN' values, in the beginning, i.e. for the first alone measurement at t = 0, they are retained as it is initially and then later replaced with 'global mean' for that covariate row obtained by combining all records [19].

During model development, a ten-fold cross-validation scheme is employed wherein 10 LightGBM classifiers with the same complexity of model hyper-parameters obtained during Bayesian optimization are developed for the corresponding fold. The total feature set used to develop these models comprises of 85 features as described in *sub-Section 2.2*. Generally, hyper-parameter optimization aims at looking for the best hyper-parameter values to minimize the objective loss function. The hyper-parameter settings maximizing the custom-defined challenge metric- utility score on the subset of training data during the Bayesian optimization phase are later used to build models. These built models generate the predictions on the hold out 10% of validation data in each fold. The training process of the model in each fold stops when the utility score of the validation set does not show further improvements over 32 consecutive iterations, i.e. early stopping to best iteration is achieved to reset the model and thereby to avoid over-fitting.

The initial predictions generated by each optimal model on the corresponding validation data of each fold undergo refinement of the prediction risk threshold to enhance the utility score. The search space for the prediction risk thresholds lies in the range of 0 to 1 and is varied in steps of 0.05. Thus the threshold search space has 20 values. So the initial predictions of validation data of each fold are compared with each of these 20 values. After comparison, the threshold value that gives the maximum utility score for the set of predictions of that fold is said to be optimal. Such 10 optimum threshold values are later used by the corresponding models to refine the predictive power in terms of utility score for generated labels in each fold.

This LightGBM based gradient boosting framework serves with a specific processing method for sparse data which is important in our classification task with class imbalance problem [27]. For the interpretability of the proposed framework, the LightGBM uses its feature importance attribute to quantify each variable, and the explainability component is addressed by employing SHAP summary and dependency plots wherein the distribution of the variable importance is illustrated [28, 29].

3. Results

The proposed framework performs the prediction from the given patient-records to determine the risk of development of sepsis onset in the next 6 hours. This is achieved using a continuous-valued utility score as defined by challenge organizers for each prediction [18]. The utility function rewards or penalizes classifiers for their predictions within 12 hours before and 3 hours after sepsis onset time and was normalized as described in [18]. Using a ten-fold cross-validation scheme 10 LightGBM models are designed based on patient-wise stratified ten-folds each containing unique 10% of the entire training set. The hyper-parameters of the above models that minimize cross-validation loss are obtained by using automatic hyper-parameter optimization utility 'bayesopt' in Python [30, 31]. The underlying objective function formulated for the optimization is intended to maximize the AUROC. The given software utility finds optimal parameters automatically using Bayesian optimization. At the outset, the optimized models includes: 60 '*num_leaves*', 120 '*min _data_in_leaf*', '*max _depth*' of 2, '*learning_rate*' of 0.01, '*scale_pos_weight*' of 20, '*min _samples_split*' of 4.

Table 3 gives a summary of the results by the proposed framework on the entire training data in a ten-fold cross-validation scheme. Results also include performances of inter-cohort and baseline studies. To ensure that the models trained in the proposed study learn dependencies not only between the patient-records but also among the cohorts, we considered inter-cohort training and testing scheme. i.e. model trained with the data of cohort A was scored on cohort B data and vice versa. This certainly avoids the doubt of the over-fitting, thus increasing the robustness of the framework. Inter-cohort scores for A and B were 0.3191 and 0.3284 respectively.

3.1 Comparison of xMLEPS with baseline

Further, to emphasize the clinical relevance of the derived features under this proposed method, a comparative analysis of results is done by carrying out three baseline studies as shown in **Figure 2**.

As a part of comparative analysis three well-tuned baseline studies are performed: Firstly, the proposed method with feature set of 85 features is tested without optimal threshold refinement (default threshold value of 0.5 with no skill is used) in a 10-fold cross-validation scheme. In the second and third methods, the given 40 clinical variables only are directly fed to LightGBM models with and without refinement of optimal threshold respectively in a 10-fold cross-validation scheme. **Table 3** presents the results of these three baseline studies accordingly. As expected the proposed method xMLEPS outperforms these three studies. The third study carried out without derived features and optimal threshold refinement shows

Fold	AUROC	F1	Utility	Threshold
1	0.8456	0.1420	0.4234	0.35
2	0.8436	0.1501	0.4029	0.35
3	0.8605	0.2208	0.4452	0.40
4	0.8610	0.1737	0.4331	0.35
5	0.8568	0.1507	0.4069	0.35
6	0.8607	0.1290	0.4253	0.25
7	0.8628	0.1475	0.4302	0.25
8	0.8649	0.1294	0.4205	0.20
9	0.8648	0.1299	0.3973	0.20
10	0.8704	0.1285	0.4282	0.20
Average (Std)	0.8591 (0.0085)	0.1502 (0.0286)	0.4214 (0.0148)	—
Baseline 1	0.8560	0.1517	0.3870	—
Baseline 2	0.8502	0.1376	0.3509	—
Baseline 3	0.8124	0.1197	0.3198	—
xMLEPS	Set A (Training) and Set B (Test)		0.3191	
xMLEPS	Set B (Training) and Set A (Test)		0.3284	

Table 3.
Results summary of the proposed framework.

worst performance. Even for the first baseline study, results are significantly lower by 3% in terms of the utility score as compared to the proposed method.

3.2 Explanation and visualization of feature importance

The cumulative feature importance of the first top 50 features is shown in **Figure 3**. Here the LightGBM feature importance attribute is used for the gradient boosting framework developed. The approach used is to count the number of times a feature gets involved to split the dataset across all trees. The failure of such an approach is that it accounts for different impacts due to different splits. The next best approach is to attribute the gain achieved with the reduction in average training loss when using a feature for splitting. This "Gain" measure used for feature importance recovers the correct mutual information between feature inputs and label outputs [32]. The limitation of this approach is that it gets easily biased when greedy trees are built in the finite ensembles. So other methods are designed to compensate for the bias in feature selection using gain approach [33, 34].

SHAP summary plot with the 20 most important clinical features that cause sepsis onset identified by the xMLEPS framework is shown in **Figure 4(a)**. Here the approach used for the feature importance is to sort all the relevance scores across the entire population in decreasing order of mean relevance as computed for local, but considering only those individuals who were positive for sepsis. The mean relevance is displayed as blue horizontal bars in **Figure 4(a)**. While local explanations summary is shown in **Figure 4(b)**, wherein all the individual data points are displaced by mean relevance for sepsis and are colored by feature values. As shown from **Figure 4(b)** we can draw that the increase in the length of stay (ICULOS) and higher value of clinical ratio's like PaO2/FiO2, Shock indices: DBPSIndex and SIndex, etc. leads to the development of sepsis, whereas lower Platelets, DBP and Magnesium levels cause sepsis. These findings are found to be consistent with previous studies on it [7, 21, 35, 36].

Further, the impact of each feature and the interactions among them for sepsis development can also be illustrated using SHAP dependency plots. As an example, in **Figure 4(c)** the dependency plot showing the interaction of Heart rate with ICULOS is depicted. As seen the xMLEPS model seems to associate high heart rate values in the range 120–180 with increased ICULOS and hence causing sepsis.

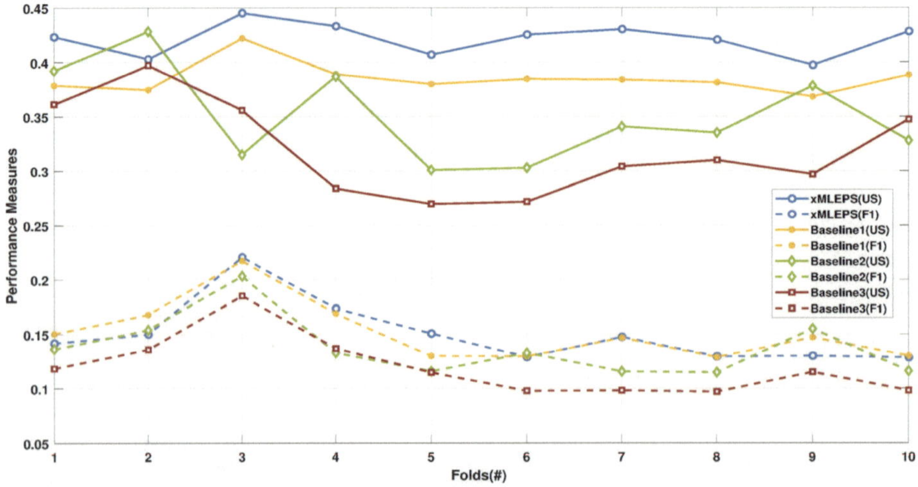

Figure 2.
Comparison of results by xMLEPS with the three base-line studies. US: Utility score, F1: F1 score.

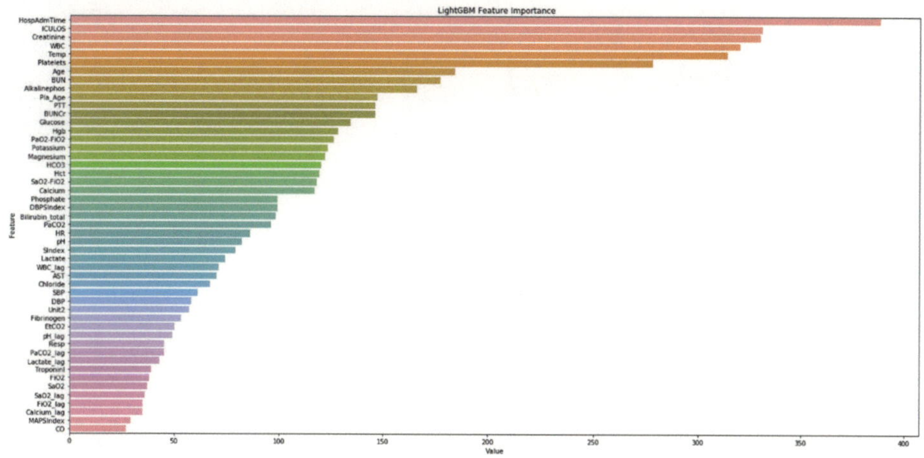

Figure 3.
Cumulative feature importance of the top 50 features using the feature importance attribute of LightGBM.

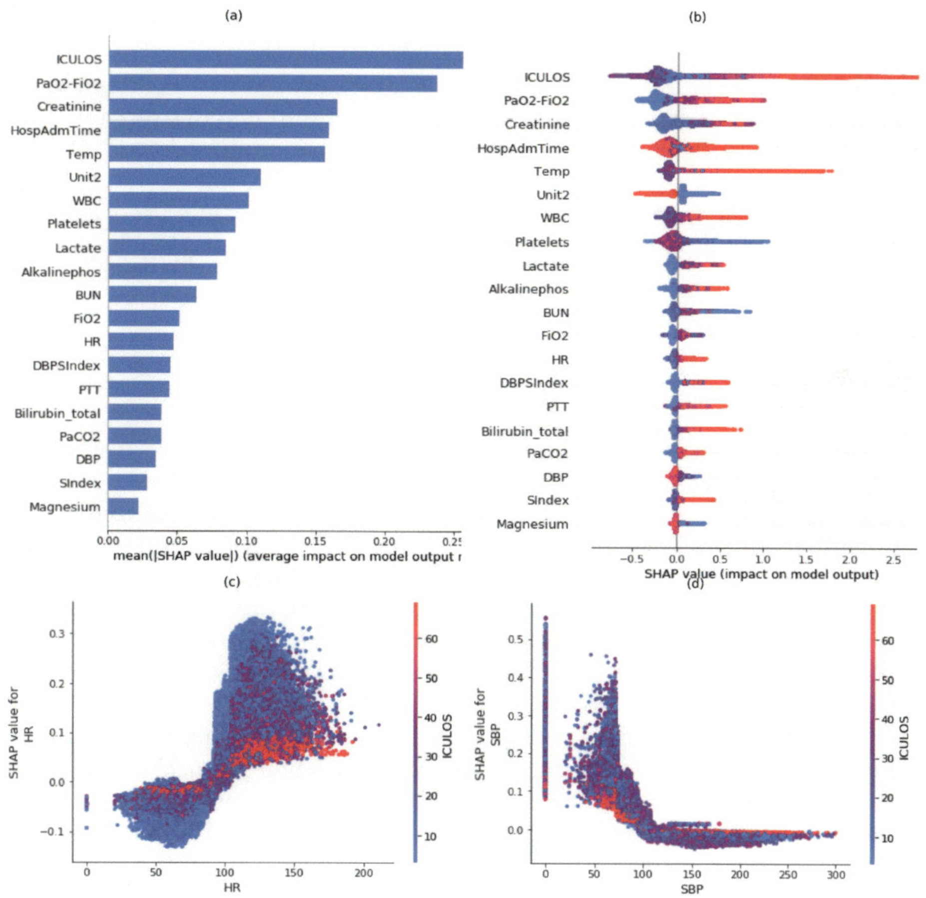

Figure 4.
Results from the SHAP explanation module showing the global feature importance together with local explanation summary. PaO_2: partial pressure of oxygen. FiO_2: fraction of inspired oxygen. HR: Heart Rate. DBP: Diastolic Blood Pressure. SBP: Systolic Blood Pressure. SIndex: Shock Index. DBPIndex: Diastolic Blood Pressure Shock Index. $PaCO_2$: Partial pressure of carbon dioxide. PTT: Partial thromboplastin time. WBC: Leukocyte count. BUN: Blood Urea Nitrogen.

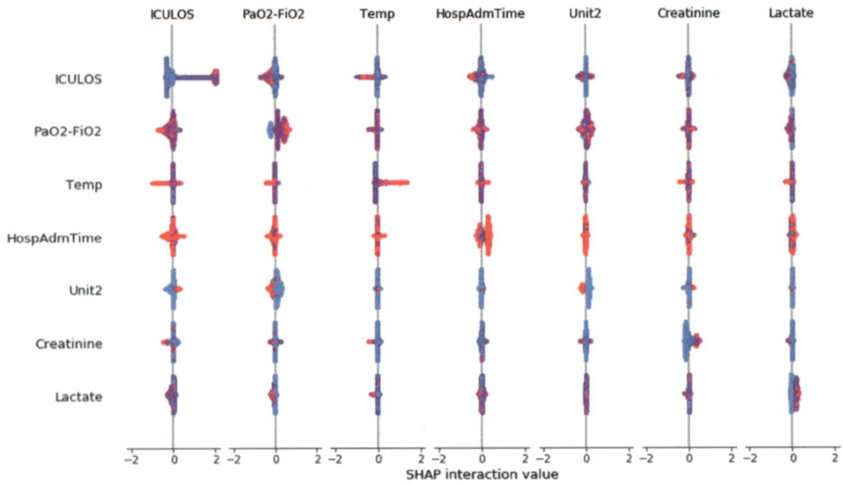

Figure 5.
Summary plot of a SHAP interaction value matrix.

Further **Figure 4(d)** shows lower values of SBP (approx. Below 90) is associated with increase ICULOS causing sepsis. A summary plot of a SHAP interaction value matrix is shown in **Figure 5** wherein the diagonal reflects the main effects, while across the diagonal show interaction effects. The explainable model will produce a high probability when it is confident about a decision, resulting in larger relevance scores due to the availability of more relevance for distributing backward. On the contrary, the model will output a lower probability when it is less confident about the patient to develop sepsis and as a result, yields lower relevant scores. This summary of scores distribution assists the clinicians with the hints to what to be expected from the designed model for clinical practice.

4. Discussion

This study justifies the clinical significance of the derived physiological interrelations among the clinical signs via feature importance and SHAP plots for visualized interpretation. Though SHAP values cannot be used as a generalized approach for early prediction of sepsis, they certainly help in generating relevant clinical hypotheses for desired events. The SHAP illustrations indeed assist in mitigating the concerns of the black-box issue associated with prediction models and might assist clinicians with a better understanding of the important features of the xMLEPS framework. The the proposed framework has the ability to establish the significance of the individual features contributing to enhance prediction of the utility score. Thus ensuring interpretablity of the framework to its clinical users. Furthermore, the proposed prediction framework, deploying clinical ICU data in the routine practice care can be potentially integrated into a computerized clinical decision support system instead of employing advanced molecular biomarkers.

The recent research literature relevant to early diagnosis of sepsis comes from the articles of various submission entries to PhysioNet Challenge 2019 [18]. This challenge aimed at the design and development of algorithms for early and automated prediction of sepsis onset with the optimal window definition of six hours before the actual clinical recognition of disease onset. The predictions of the machine learning algorithms were rewarded if they were able to detect true positives correctly up to 12 hours before disease onset and were slightly penalized if

Reference	Methodology	AUROC	Utility Score
Chang et al. [42]	Temporal Convolutional Networks (TCN)	—	0.4170
Li et al. [45]	A Time-phased model	—	0.4300
Morrill et al. [39]	A signature transform-based model	—	0.4340
Zabihi et al. [40]	XGBoost Ensemble models	0.8333	0.4280
Yang et al. [41]	Fusion-based XGBoost	0.8400	0.4300
Du et al. [46]	Gradient Boosting Scheme	0.8630	0.4090
Lee et al. [43]	Graph Convolutional Networks (GCN)	0.8170	0.3820
Lyra et al. [44]	Using Random forest classifier	0.8100	0.3760
Nesaragi and Patidar [38]	Ratio and Power-based features	0.8432	0.4013
Nesaragi et al. [19]	PMI-based Tensor factorization	0.8621	0.4519

Table 4.
Summary of the results obtained by our previous works and the submitted solutions to PhysioNet 2019 challenge under 5/10-fold cross-validation scheme using training data.

they were false positive. However predictions were strongly penalized if they were incorrect near disease onset. The reason for choosing the optimal prediction window to be six hours comes from the clinical fact that the ratio of observed median time to antimicrobial therapy is found to be 6 hours [37]. Furthermore, delay in each hour of treatment results in average decrease of survival rate of 7.6% [37].

The comparative analysis of the results obtained by the proposed method with our previous works [19, 38] and submission approaches [39–46] that reported the best results in the PhysioNet 2019 Challenge [18] is listed in **Table 4**. Most of these approaches utilized 5 or 10 fold cross-validation scheme and yielded utility scores in the range of 0.36–0.45.

This study supports the usage of the Utility score as an effective metric on ICU data for sepsis onset. However, experiments showed that even the F1 score gave reliable results aligning with utility score. i.e. the increase and decrease of F1 score follow accordingly with the Utility score. However, the bounds for utility score vary from −2 to 1 whereas the F1 Score has bounds from 0 to 1. The other conventional metrics namely AUROC, AUPRC, and Accuracy are insignificant to use with such a highly unbalanced dataset and are misleading for sepsis onset. Further, the fact that the interpretation of these results together with utility score is quite difficult cannot be ignored as mentioned by Roussel et al. [47].

The limitation of this study is, it constrains only to a two-center cohort design from the available training data, which might create doubt that the trained models may get over-fit towards the particular cohort data and it's patient-records. However, the analyzed ICU patient admissions originate from a diverse population covering the entire spectrum of ICU patients, and further, the validation in terms of inter-cohorts train-test approach along with optimum threshold refinement demonstrates the deployment of our framework in other ICUs.

5. Conclusion

This study presents xMLEPS – an explainable machine learning framework for the early prediction of sepsis using clinical data in the ICU setting. These predictive explanations justify the clinical significance of physiological inter-relations among the given clinical signs via visualized interpretation. And thus assist the clinicians in decision making for diagnosis and recommend future actions to be taken to improve the quality of predictions. This certainly ensures that the data-driven automated ML models have the potential to make the paradigm shift from conventional detection and treatment to an automated early prediction that prevents the failure of the organ system due to sepsis.

Conflict of interest

The authors declare no conflict of interest.

Author details

Naimahmed Nesaragi† and Shivnarayan Patidar*†
National Institute of Technology, Goa, India

*Address all correspondence to: shivnarayan.patidar@nitgoa.ac.in

† These authors contributed equally.

References

[1] M. Singer, C. S. Deutschman, C. W. Seymour, M. Shankar-Hari, D. Annane, M. Bauer, R. Bellomo, G. R. Bernard, J.-D. Chiche, C. M. Coopersmith, R. S. Hotchkiss, M. M. Levy, J. C. Marshall, G. S. Martin, S. M. Opal, G. D. Rubenfeld, T. van der Poll, J.-L. Vincent, D. C. Angus, The Third International Consensus Definitions for Sepsis and Septic Shock (Sepsis-3), JAMA 315 (2016) 801.

[2] L. Giesen, M. Singer, What Is Sepsis?, in: W. J. Wiersinga, C. W. Seymour (Eds.), Handbook of Sepsis, Springer International Publishing, Cham, 2018, pp. 3–14.

[3] H. Nishie, Guidelines for management of severe sepsis and septic shock, Okayama Igakkai Zasshi (Journal of Okayama Medical Association) 125 (2013) 153–157.

[4] C. W. Seymour, J. N. Kennedy, S. Wang, C.-C. H. Chang, C. F. Elliott, Z. Xu, S. Berry, G. Clermont, G. Cooper, H. Gomez, D. T. Huang, J. A. Kellum, Q. Mi, S. M. Opal, V. Talisa, T. van der Poll, S. Visweswaran, Y. Vodovotz, J. C. Weiss, D. M. Yealy, S. Yende, D. C. Angus, Derivation, Validation, and Potential Treatment Implications of Novel Clinical Phenotypes for Sepsis, JAMA 321 (2019) 2003.

[5] R. Goulden, M.-C. Hoyle, J. Monis, D. Railton, V. Riley, P. Martin, R. Martina, E. Nsutebu, qSOFA, SIRS and NEWS for predicting inhospital mortality and ICU admission in emergency admissions treated as sepsis, Emergency Medicine Journal 35 (2018) 345–349.

[6] V. Anand, Z. Zhang, S. S. Kadri, M. Klompas, C. Rhee, Epidemiology of Quick Sequential Organ Failure Assessment Criteria in Undifferentiated Patients and Association With Suspected Infection and Sepsis, Chest 156 (2019) 289–297.

[7] K. E. Henry, D. N. Hager, P. J. Pronovost, S. Saria, A targeted real-time early warning score (TREWScore) for septic shock, Science Translational Medicine 7 (2015) 299ra122–299ra122.

[8] J. Calvert, T. Desautels, U. Chettipally, C. Barton, J. Hoffman, M. Jay, Q. Mao, H. Mohamadlou, R. Das, High-performance detection and early prediction of septic shock for alcohol-use disorder patients, Annals of Medicine and Surgery 8 (2016 a) 50–55.

[9] J. S. Calvert, D. A. Price, U. K. Chettipally, C. W. Barton, M. D. Feldman, J. L. Hoffman, M. Jay, R. Das, A computational approach to early sepsis detection, Computers in Biology and Medicine 74 (2016 b) 69–73.

[10] S. Horng, D. A. Sontag, Y. Halpern, Y. Jernite, N. I. Shapiro, L. A. Nathanson, Creating an automated trigger for sepsis clinical decision support at emergency department triage using machine learning, PLOS ONE 12 (2017) e0174708.

[11] T. Desautels, J. Calvert, J. Hoffman, M. Jay, Y. Kerem, L. Shieh, D. Shimabukuro, U. Chettipally, M. D. Feldman, C. Barton, D. J. Wales, R. Das, Prediction of Sepsis in the Intensive Care Unit With Minimal Electronic Health Record Data: A Machine Learning Approach, JMIR Medical Informatics 4 (2016) e28.

[12] K. Kawamoto, C. A. Houlihan, E. A. Balas, D. F. Lobach, Improving clinical practice using clinical decision support systems: a systematic review of trials to identify features critical to success, BMJ 330 (2005) 765.

[13] F. Cabitza, R. Rasoini, G. F. Gensini, Unintended Consequences of Machine Learning in Medicine (2017) 2.

[14] D. Petkovic, L. Kobzik, C. Re, Machine learning and deep analytics for

biocomputing: call for better explainability, in: Biocomputing 2018, WORLD SCIENTIFIC, Kohala Coast, Hawaii, USA, 2018, pp. 623–627.

[15] R. Guidotti, A. Monreale, S. Ruggieri, F. Turini, F. Giannotti, D. Pedreschi, A Survey of Methods for Explaining Black Box Models, ACM Computing Surveys 51 (2019) 1–42.

[16] written on behalf of AME Big-Data Clinical Trial Collaborative Group, Z. Zhang, M. W. Beck, D. A. Winkler, B. Huang, W. Sibanda, H. Goyal, Opening the black box of neural networks: methods for interpreting neural network models in clinical applications, Annals of Translational Medicine 6 (2018) 216–216.

[17] S. Tan, M. Soloviev, G. Hooker, M. T. Wells, Tree Space Prototypes: Another Look at Making Tree Ensembles Interpretable, arXiv: 1611.07115 [cs, stat] (2020). ArXiv: 1611.07115.

[18] M. A. Reyna, C. S. Josef, R. Jeter, S. P. Shashikumar, M. B. Westover, S. Nemati, G. D. Clifford, A. Sharma, Early Prediction of Sepsis From Clinical Data: The PhysioNet/Computing in Cardiology Challenge 2019, Critical care medicine 48 (2020) 210–217. Publisher: Lippincott Williams & Wilkins.

[19] N. Nesaragi, S. Patidar, V. Aggarwal, Tensor learning of pointwise mutual information from ehr data for early prediction of sepsis, Computers in biology and medicine (2021) 104430.

[20] R. J. Delahanty, J. Alvarez, L. M. Flynn, R. L. Sherwin, S. S. Jones, Development and Evaluation of a Machine Learning Model for the Early Identification of Patients at Risk for Sepsis, Annals of Emergency Medicine 73 (2019) 334–344.

[21] G. A. Ospina-Tascón, J.-L. Teboul, G. Hernandez, I. Alvarez, A. I. Sánchez-Ortiz, L. E. Calderón-Tapia, R. Manzano-Nunez, E. Quiñones, H. J. Madriñan-Navia, J. E. Ruiz, J. L. Aldana, J. Bakker, Diastolic shock index and clinical outcomes in patients with septic shock, Annals of Intensive Care 10 (2020) 41.

[22] Y.-c. Liu, Modified shock index and mortality rate of emergency patients, World Journal of Emergency Medicine 3 (2012) 114.

[23] A. Linder, R. Arnold, M. Zindovic, I. Zindovic, A. Lange-Jendeberg, M. Paulsson, P. Nyberg, B. Christensson, P. Åkesson, Heparin-binding protein improves prediction of severe sepsis in the emergency department, Critical Care 17 (2013) P3.

[24] Y. Wang, H. Yang, L. Qiao, Z. Tan, J. Jin, J. Yang, L. Zhang, B. M. Fang, X. Xu, The predictive value of PaO2/FIO2 and additional parameters for in-hospital mortality in patients with acute pulmonary embolism: an 8-year prospective observational single-center cohort study, BMC Pulmonary Medicine 19 (2019) 242.

[25] A. Y. A. Amer, J. Vranken, F. Wouters, D. Mesotten, P. Vandervoort, V. Storms, S. Luca, B. Vanrumste, J.-M. Aerts, Feature Engineering for ICU Mortality Prediction Based on Hourly to Bi-Hourly Measurements, Applied Sciences 9 (2019) 3525.

[26] J.-L. Vincent, Understanding cardiac output, Critical Care 12 (2008) 174.

[27] G. Ke, Q. Meng, T. Finley, T. Wang, W. Chen, W. Ma, Q. Ye, T.-Y. Liu, Lightgbm: A highly efficient gradient boosting decision tree, in: Proceedings of the 31st International Conference on Neural Information Processing Systems, NIPS'17, Curran Associates Inc., Red Hook, NY, USA, 2017, p. 3149–3157.

[28] S. M. Lundberg, G. Erion, H. Chen, A. DeGrave, J. M. Prutkin, B. Nair, R.

Katz, J. Himmelfarb, N. Bansal, S.-I. Lee, Explainable AI for Trees: From Local Explanations to Global Understanding, arXiv:1905.04610 [cs, stat] (2019). ArXiv: 1905.04610.

[29] S. Lundberg, S.-I. Lee, A Unified Approach to Interpreting Model Predictions, arXiv:1705.07874 [cs, stat] (2017). ArXiv: 1705.07874.

[30] E. Brochu, V. M. Cora, N. de Freitas, A Tutorial on Bayesian Optimization of Expensive Cost Functions, with Application to Active User Modeling and Hierarchical Reinforcement Learning, arXiv:1012.2599 [cs] (2010). ArXiv: 1012.2599.

[31] J. Snoek, H. Larochelle, R. P. Adams, Practical bayesian optimization of machine learning algorithms, in: Proceedings of the 25th International Conference on Neural Information Processing Systems - Volume 2, NIPS'12, Curran Associates Inc., Red Hook, NY, USA, 2012, p. 2951–2959.

[32] G. Louppe, Understanding Random Forests: From Theory to Practice, arXiv: 1407.7502 [stat] (2015). ArXiv: 1407.7502.

[33] S. Chebrolu, A. Abraham, J. P. Thomas, Feature deduction and ensemble design of intrusion detection systems, Computers & Security 24 (2005) 295–307.

[34] V. A. Huynh-Thu, A. Irrthum, L. Wehenkel, P. Geurts, Inferring Regulatory Networks from Expression Data Using Tree-Based Methods, PLoS ONE 5 (2010) e12776.

[35] X. Li, Y. Kang, X. Jia, J. Wang, G. Xie, Tasp: A time-phased model for sepsis prediction, in: 2019 Computing in Cardiology (CinC), pp. Page 1–Page 4.

[36] D. W. Shimabukuro, C. W. Barton, M. D. Feldman, S. J. Mataraso, R. Das, Effect of a machine learning-based severe sepsis prediction algorithm on patient survival and hospital length of stay: a randomised clinical trial, BMJ Open Respiratory Research 4 (2017) e000234.

[37] A. Kumar, D. Roberts, K. E. Wood, B. Light, J. E. Parrillo, S. Sharma, R. Suppes, D. Feinstein, S. Zanotti, L. Taiberg, et al., Duration of hypotension before initiation of effective antimicrobial therapy is the critical determinant of survival in human septic shock, Critical care medicine 34 (2006) 1589–1596.

[38] N. Nesaragi, S. Patidar, Early prediction of sepsis from clinical data using ratio and power-based features, Critical Care Medicine 48 (2020) e1343–e1349.

[39] J. H. Morrill, A. Kormilitzin, A. J. Nevado-Holgado, S. Swaminathan, S. D. Howison, T. J. Lyons, Utilization of the signature method to identify the early onset of sepsis from multivariate physiological time series in critical care monitoring, Critical Care Medicine 48 (2020) e976–e981.

[40] M. Zabihi, S. Kiranyaz, M. Gabbouj, Sepsis Prediction in Intensive Care Unit Using Ensemble of XGboost Models.

[41] M. Yang, X. Wang, H. Gao, Y. Li, X. Liu, J. Li, C. Liu, Early Prediction of Sepsis Using Multi-Feature Fusion Based XGBoost Learning and Bayesian Optimization.

[42] Y. Chang, J. Rubin, G. Boverman, S. Vij, A. Rahman, A. Natarajan, S. Parvaneh, A multi-task imputation and classification neural architecture for early prediction of sepsis from multivariate clinical time series, in: 2019 Computing in Cardiology (CinC), IEEE, pp. Page1–Page4.

[43] B. T. Lee, O.-Y. Kwon, H. Park, K.-J. Cho, J.-M. Kwon, Y. Lee, et al., Graph convolutional networks-based noisy

data imputation in electronic health record, Critical Care Medicine 48 (2020) e1106–e1111.

[44] S. Lyra, S. Leonhardt, C. Hoog Antink, Early Prediction of Sepsis Using Random Forest Classification for Imbalanced Clinical Data.

[45] X. Li, X. Xu, F. Xie, X. Xu, Y. Sun, X. Liu, X. Jia, Y. Kang, L. Xie, F. Wang, et al., A time-phased machine learning model for real-time prediction of sepsis in critical care, Critical Care Medicine 48 (2020) e884–e888.

[46] J. A. Du, N. Sadr, P. d. Chazal, Automated prediction of sepsis onset using gradient boosted decision trees, in: 2019 Computing in Cardiology (CinC), pp. Page 1–Page 4.

[47] B. Roussel, J. Behar, J. Oster, A recurrent neural network for the prediction of vital sign evolution and sepsis in icu, in: 2019 Computing in Cardiology (CinC), pp. Page 1–Page 4.

Chapter 13

Organ Damage in Sepsis: Molecular Mechanisms

Grażyna Sygitowicz and Dariusz Sitkiewicz

Abstract

Sepsis is one of the most common reasons for hospitalisation. This condition is characterised by systemic inflammatory response to infection. International definition of sepsis mainly points out a multi-organ dysfunction caused by a deregulated host response to infection. An uncontrolled inflammatory response, often referred to as "cytokine storm", leads to an increase in oxidative stress as a result of the inhibition of cellular antioxidant systems. Oxidative stress, as well as pro-inflammatory cytokines, initiate vascular endothelial dysfunction and, in consequence, impair microcirculation. Microcirculation damage leads to adaptive modifications of cell metabolism. Moreover, mitochondrial dysfunction takes place which results in increased apoptosis and impaired autophagy. Non-coding RNA, especially miRNA and lncRNA molecules, may play an important role in the pathomechanism of sepsis. Altered expression of various ncRNAs in sepsis suggest, that these molecules can be used not only as diagnostics and prognostic markers but also as the target points in the pharmacotherapy of sepsis. The understanding of detailed molecular mechanisms leading to organ damage can contribute to the development of specific therapy methods thereby improving the prognosis of patients with sepsis.

Keywords: sepsis, cytokine storm, microcirculation, oxidative stress, RAS, ncRNA

1. Introduction

Sepsis was already known to ancient Greeks since the times of Hippocrates (460–370 BC) as a condition causing "rotting" of the body. Later, the Persian philosopher and physician Ibn Sina, or Avicenna (980–1037 AD) described for the first time sepsis as a "decay" of blood and tissues accompanied by fever. Sepsis is one of the most frequent causes of hospitalisation in Intensive Care Units. It constitutes a significant clinical problem, in many cases with a fatal outcome. Significant advances in critical care medicine have defined sepsis as an organ dysfunction syndrome. The incidence of this type of disorder is still constantly rising. Morbidity significantly correlates with the ageing of societies and presence of other comorbidities. The prognosis is worse when the mentioned correlations are strong and the patient is diagnosed too late. Although sepsis can occur in any age group, its risk is definitely greater in patients over 60 years of age. Moreover, sepsis is growing rapidly as a result of a poorly controlled, multidirectional response of the organism to an external factor, i.e. pathogen, and its further increase may be due to endogenous factors or coexisting diseases [1].

Sepsis starts with a period of hyperinflammation, in which the macrophages, monocytes, T-cells and neutrophils are activated and recruited to various organs.

The uncontrolled inflammatory response, so-called cytokine storm leads to many metabolic disorders associated with oxidative stress. The oxidative stress, but also proinflammatory cytokines, promote endothelial function disorders and, consequently, microcirculatory damages. At the final stage of cytokine storm a hypoinflammatory reaction develops, leading to multiple organ damages. These changes are underlined by mitochondrial function disorders, intensified oxidative stress and deregulation of apoptosis and autophagy processes. A neurohormonal activation, in the first place of the renin-angiotensin system (RAS), is an important element of the mechanisms leading to organ damage. Many studies have suggested that in sepsis, changes occur of the expression of various RNA molecules: long non-coding RNA (lncRNA) and microRNA (miRNA). The non-coding RNA fragments can thus play the role of molecular markers, both diagnostic, and prognostic, in the development of sepsis. The knowledge of the molecular mechanisms responsible for organ damages would enable a development of adequate and effective therapeutic methods, improving the prognosis for patients.

2. Cytokine storm in the course of sepsis

Cytokine storm is frequently described as an extremely dangerous immune response, being a positive feedback loop between cytokines and immune system cells [2]. That immune reaction provokes releasing of circulating proinflammatory cytokines, causing a direct threat to life. At the same time an increased activation occurs of the immune system cells as a result of, among other factors, action of various pathogens, autoimmune disorders, monogenic diseases or malignancies.

Proinflammatory cytokines, at the time of the beginning of the fight against pathogens by the immune system, send a signal to the lymphocytes and macrophages to start their transfer to the inflammation site. Cytokines activate also the cells to produce effector cytokines. All that cascade of interrelations frequently falls outside control, leading to hyperactivation of immune cells at a given site, damaging the organ involved in the inflammation. Remote organs also suffer damages but in the mechanism of cytokine release into the circulation, activating other immune system cells. Moreover, according to the literature data, it is believed that some inflammation mediators can be helpful for the monitoring of the inflammatory condition but also can be harmful for patient's organism [2]. That depends on the patient's health condition when the inflammation mediators are secreted into the bloodstream - whether the patient is in a physiological good condition or in a dysfunction state i.e. with upset immune system.

The course of cytokine storm itself can prognosticate the events being a consequence of the inflammatory condition but also suggests possible effects after administration of an appropriate treatment. Cytokine storm includes a number of immune system disorders with characteristic systemic signs of inflammation and multiple organ dysfunction, leading to damage in case of inadequate therapy. A plethora of factors are directly or indirectly involved in cytokine storm. The key factors include: interferon γ, interleukin-1, –6, –18, TNF-α and NFκB, but the transcription factor NFκB emerges to the foreground in view of its ability to induce expression of proinflammatory genes. NFκB and its protein inhibitor (IκB) are located in the cell cytoplasm. NFκB activation can occur due to the effect of many stimulators, such as: bacterial pathogens recognised by Toll-like receptor 4 (TLR-4) or proinflammatory cytokines recognised by their specific membrane receptors (e.g. TNF receptor) [3].

The inhibitor protein closely related to NFκB, being a heterodimer built from two subunits: p50 and p65, undergoes phosphorylation. The phosphorylation

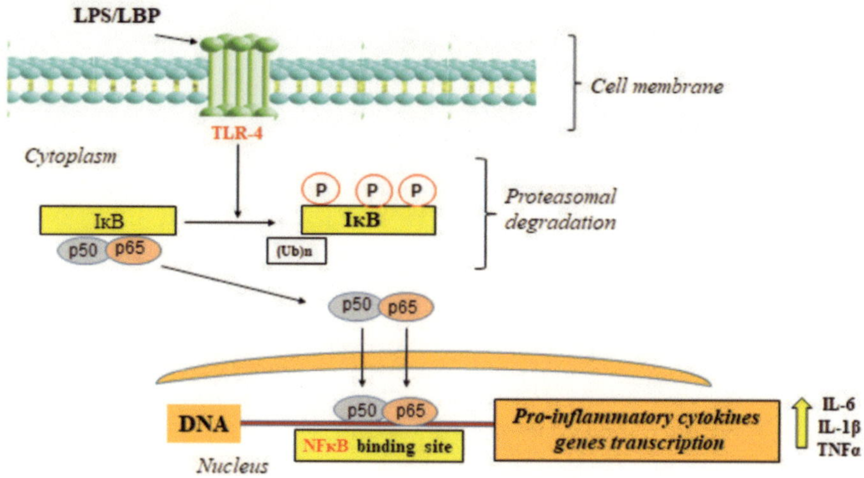

Figure 1.
NFκB activation pathway.

process is preceded by TLR-4 receptor activation by a lipopolysaccharide (LPS) complex with binding protein (LPS/LBP), leading to activation of redox-dependent kinases. Then, after ubiquitination, a degradation of the inhibitor occurs in proteasomes, as shown in **Figure 1**. At the same time, the p50:p65 dimer is released from its bond with IκB and transferred to the cell nucleus, where it regulates the expression of the genes of the proinflammatory molecules: TNFα, IL-1β, IL-6, MCP-1 (monocytic chemoattractant protein 1). The NFκB factor can also activate the expression of inducible nitric oxide synthase (iNOS) and cyclo-oxygenase-2 (COX-2). Such intensity of NFκB participation in immune system response, as well as in inflammatory reaction gives a possibility to consider that factor a candidate in the strategy of therapeutic management of multiple organ damage in sepsis [4].

3. Microcirculation and endothelial dysfunction in sepsis

Vascular endothelial cells constitute a dynamic vascular homeostasis regulator. They play not only the role of a barrier limiting the transportation of water, gases, proteins and cells between the intravascular and interstitial compartments, but also actively produce and release mediators, which regulate a wide range of physiological and pathological processes, including: vascular wall tension, angiogenesis, inflammatory condition and coagulation process. The activation and dysfunction of the endothelium are important elements of sepsis, and seem to play the key role in the sepsis phenotype as presented in **Figure 2**. During sepsis, endothelial cells become activated and dysfunctional, leading to haemostasis disturbances, increased migration of leucocytes, enhanced inflammatory condition, altered vascular wall tension and loss of the barrier function [5, 6]. The disturbed endothelial cell function can play a decisive role in microcirculation dysfunction. Microcirculatory changes in sepsis are characterised by heterogeneous perfusion of tissues due to absent or intermittent perfusion of the capillary vessels. Microcirculation heterogeneity in sepsis can disturb tissue oxygenation and lead to insufficient oxygen supply even in the presence of maintained total blood flow to organs. Such microcirculation disorders create favourable conditions for perfusion impairment, insufficient oxygen supply to tissues and then for organ failure.

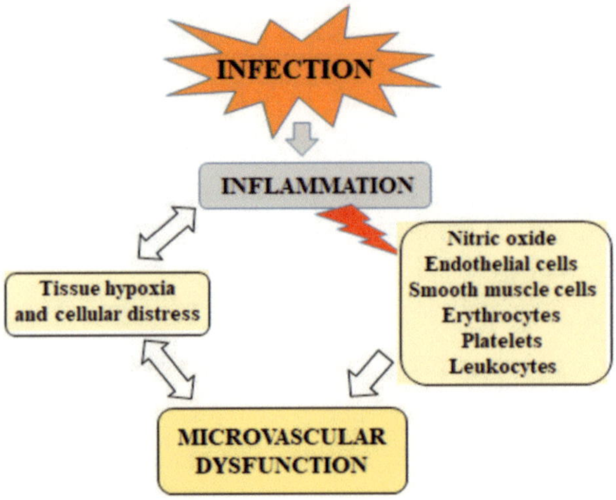

Figure 2.
Pathophysiology of microcirculatory change in sepsis.

Endothelial cells, receiving metabolic and physical signals regulate the microcirculatory flow through local releasing of vasodilating substances, particularly nitric oxide (NO), which modulate the tonus of vascular smooth muscles. NO is an activator of soluble guanylyl cyclase, the enzyme responsible for production of cGMP, a mediator of smooth muscle cell relaxation. For that reason, NO is considered the key factor of maintaining and autoregulation of homeostasis and microcirculation patency. During sepsis, the NO system is significantly disturbed – iNOS is non-homogeneously expressed in various vascular spaces, what results in pathological blood flow in the microcirculation.

Endothelial cells usually promote antithrombotic properties and prevention of thrombocyte activation and aggregation. Endothelium also participates in the major pathogenetic pathways of diseases associated with a coagulopathy in sepsis, including, in the first place, in tissue factor (TF)-mediated generation of thrombin, and in dysfunctional and impaired fibrinolysis. A natural antithrombotic protein – protein C is activated on endothelial cell surface, while thrombin binds to thrombomodulin (TM) – a transmembrane glycoprotein. In sepsis, the C protein system is weakened, possibly due to reduced synthesis and increased protein C consumption and reduced protein C activation as a consequence of reduced endothelial expression of thrombomodulin. In sepsis, an internalisation and degradation of TM occurs, leading to formation of inactive soluble fragments as illustrated in **Figure 3**. Under these

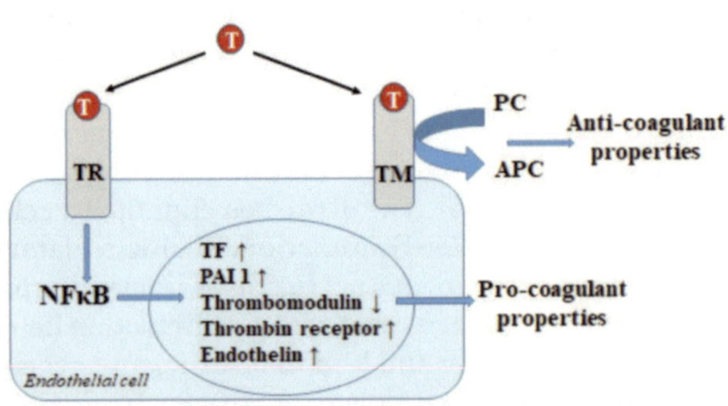

Figure 3.
Change of endothelial cell properties after thrombin receptor stimulation.

conditions the interaction between thrombin and thrombin receptor leads to a change of endothelial phenotype from antithrombotic to a prothrombotic phenotype.

In sepsis, the tissue factor can be released not only by monocytes and macrophages but also by endothelial cells. The TF pathway inhibitor, mainly expressed by endothelial cells, is functionally inhibited by reduced synthesis of glycosaminoglycans on endothelial surfaces. Furthermore, platelets, the aggregation of which leads to the development of thrombocytic thrombi, are a strong amplifier of the coagulation cascade. Thrombus formation can be additionally facilitated by the factors released from neutrophils undergoing apoptosis. The formation of microvascular thrombi can cause tissue ischaemia and multiple organ failure.

4. Renin-angiotensin system in sepsis

The renin-angiotensin system (RAS) is one of the most important hormonal mechanisms controlling haemodynamic stability through regulation of blood pressure, fluid volume and sodium-potassium balance as shown in **Figure 4**. Changes in the concentrations of molecules which form RAS contribute to arterial hypertension development. Renin is synthesised in the kidneys as inactive form and released into the bloodstream, where pro-renin is proteolytically transformed into its active form. Active renin catalyses angiotensinogen breakdown, generating angiotensin I (Ang I). Ang I is decomposed through angiotensin-converting enzyme (ACE) to angiotensin II (Ang II), the main effector in RAS (**Figure 4**). Ang I is also transformed through neutral endopeptidase (NEP) into angiotensin (1–7), another active peptide, which remains in opposition to Ang II (**Figure 4**). Angiotensin (1–7) can be also produced by Ang II splitting by angiotensin-converting enzyme 2 (ACE2), reducing thus Ang II concentration [7].

The mechanisms of RAS effect on sepsis development is presented in **Figure 5**. RAS participates in the pathogenesis of sepsis through equilibration of the modulation of the inflammation-related pathways. Through binding to AT1R, Ang II can increase the abundance of inflammatory mediators, increase vascular permeability and stimulate the expression of chemoattractants and adhesive molecules and also lead to recruitment of inflammatory cells. Moreover, the activation of the ERK 1/2, JNK, p38MAPK and NF-κB pathways is also involved in the intensification of inflammatory reaction by Ang II.

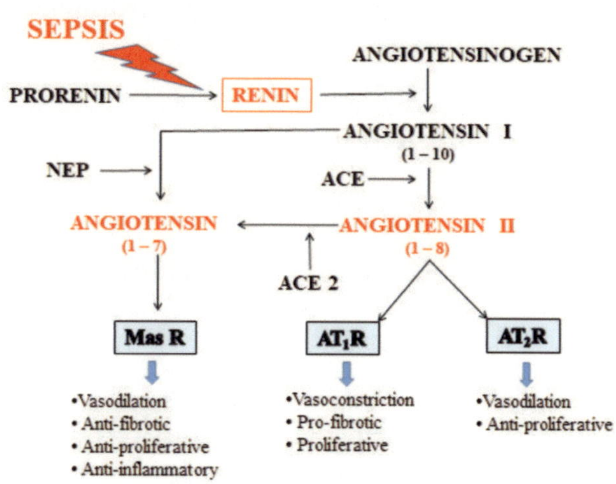

Figure 4.
Renin-angiotensin system.

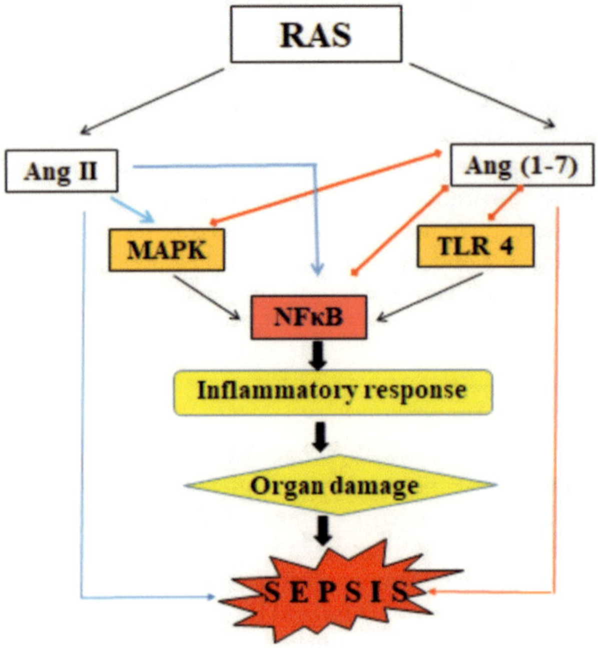

Figure 5.
The mechanisms of RAS effect on sepsis development, blue line - promote; red line - inhibit.

Ang (1–7) can inhibit the activity of these signalling pathways and thus can inhibit the inflammatory reaction in sepsis. Many studies have provided evidence that RAS interventions can alleviate sepsis and associated organ function disorders through inhibition of the above mentioned inflammation-related pathways. ACE2 exerts a protective effect against acute respiratory distress syndrome (ARDS) caused by sepsis, through inhibition of TLR4, ERK1/2, JNK and NF-κB pathways. Ang (1–7) inhibited the p38MAPK pathway in order to protect mice against sepsis-induced skeletal muscle atrophy and liver damage. AT1R blockade can exert a protective effect against sepsis-induced multiple organ damage (SIMD) through inhibition of the MAPK and NF-κB pathways. Moreover, angiotensin I-converting enzyme inhibitors (ACEIs) and sartans (angiotensin receptor blockers, ARBs) decrease the release of proinflammatory cytokines, pro-oxidants and proapoptotic factors and thus alleviate the damages caused by sepsis.

5. Oxidative stress and mitochondria in sepsis

5.1 Generation of reactive oxygen species (ROS)

The internal mitochondrial membrane is a vast, impermeable structure containing enzymatic complexes of the respiratory chain (I – IV) and ATP synthase system (complex V). The transportation of electrons through respiratory chain complexes is accompanied by translocation of protons (H^+) to the intermembrane space and development of potential difference on either side of the membrane.

That process includes development of reactive oxygen species (ROS) as a consequence of electron "escape" and mono-electron reduction of oxygen to 0_2. radical. That reaction occurs in the I and III complexes of the respiratory chain as presented in **Figure 6**. The developing oxygen free radicals are transferred both

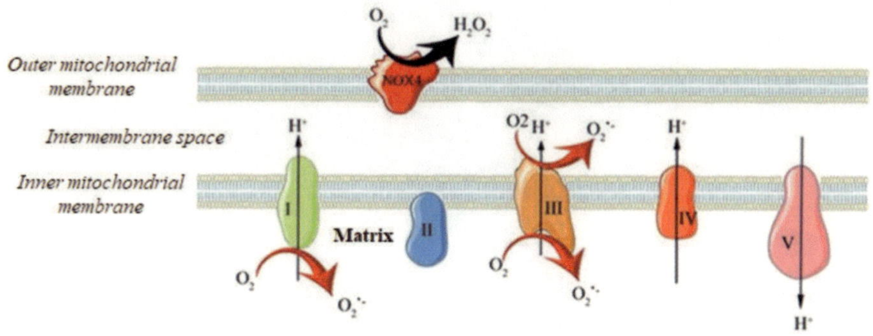

Figure 6.
ROS production in mitochondria.

to the mitochondrial matrix and intermembrane space. The outer mitochondrial membrane is the site of location of NADPH, which generates hydrogen peroxide (H_2O_2). The ROS produced in the mitochondria cause damages of the mitochondrial proteins and mitochondrial DNA (mtDNA). These damages lead to the development of a mega-channel, enabling outflow of cytochrome C into the cytosol, with consequent initiation of apoptosis process. An increased permeability of the inner mitochondrial membrane creates also a possibility of transportation of many small molecules. Mitochondrial ROS affects also many processes both under normal and pathological conditions, what as shown in **Figure** 7 can modulate vital cell functions.

5.2 Generation of reactive nitrogen species (RNS)

In sepsis, besides ROS production in the mitochondria, increased synthesis of nitric oxide (NO) is also an important element of oxidative stress. NO is produced by various cells, such as: activated macrophages, neutrophils or lymphocytes. Many molecules involved in septic inflammatory process, such as: tumour necrosis factor-α (TNFα) interferon γ (IFNγ) or interleukin-1β (IL-1β) also participate in the induction of type II NO synthase (iNOS) through activation of IκB degradation and transcription of *iNOS* gene.

An adequate nitric oxide production is a prerequisite of normal vascular structure and function. Muscle cells and haematopoietic cells are an important source of NO. Numerous inflammatory mediators participate in the induction and activation of the isoform of calcium-independent nitric oxygen synthase (iNOS). In order to prevent NO overproduction during sepsis, an administration of NOS inhibitors was suggested. NOS inhibition, however, has a limited therapeutic efficacy in view of intensification of organ dysfunction, which results in a high mortality rate. This is most likely related to the double role of iNOS in sepsis [8].

In particular cases, besides NO production, iNOS catalyses also the formation of reactive nitrogen species (RNS). NO reacts with superoxide anion to form peroxynitrite anion ($ONOO^-$), which oxidises and nitrosylates various biological targets. Peroxynitrite can be a potential mediator of the cytotoxic effect of NO.

During sepsis, iNOS can become an important source of RNS as a consequence of enzyme decoupling. Decoupled iNOS is a source of superoxide anion, which is rapidly broken down by superoxide dismutase (SOD), and hydrogen peroxide (H_2O_2) is produced. Moreover, the availability of NO is reduced in view of its rapid reaction with the peroxide. During sepsis, three main factors can contribute to iNOS decoupling: suboptimal tetrahydrobiopterin (BH_4) concentration, insufficient

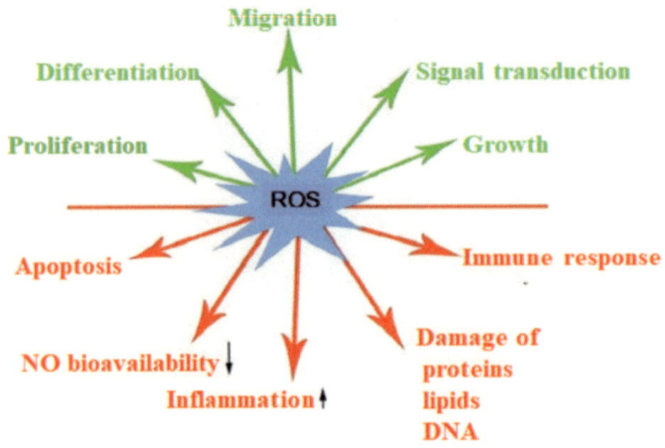

Figure 7.
The role of ROS in normal and pathological conditions.

concentration of L-arginine substrate and also increased production of asymmetric dimethylarginine (ADMA, endogenous NOS inhibitor) [8].

5.3 Cellular antioxidant systems

Cells have developed protective mechanisms counteracting mitochondrial dysfunction. The most important of them include: a system of endogenous antioxidants, dynamic changes of mitochondria and also processes of removal of damaged organelles and biogenesis of new ones. To counteract oxidative damage, mitochondria contain high concentrations of antioxidants, i.e. substances, which, when present in low concentrations, reduce the level and/or protect the substrates against their oxidative modification. ROS uptake is the function of the antioxidants. Two types of antioxidants can be distinguished: enzymatic and non-enzymatic. The important antioxidant enzymes include superoxide dismutase (SOD), catalase and glutathione peroxidise (GPx). SOD catalyses conversion of $O_2^{\cdot}$ to H_2O_2 and oxygen. In mammalian cells two forms of SOD are present: CuZnSOD (SOD 1) and MnSOD (SOD 2). SOD 1 requires presence of copper and zinc as cofactors and is mainly present in cytosol, while SOD 2 is manganese-dependent and is mainly found in mitochondria. The hydrogen peroxide produced as a result of a reaction catalysed by SOD is then detoxicated by catalase or GPx. In the reaction catalysed by catalase, water and oxygen are produced. GPx converts H_2O_2 into water in a reaction, in which glutathione (GSH) is oxidised to glutathione disulfide (GSSG) and then reduced to GSH by glutathione reductase (GR). Both GPx and GR require the presence of selenium to reach their full activity.

The important non-enzymatic antioxidants include vitamins, enzymatic cofactors and many endogenous substances. The antioxidant vitamins include vitamin A, C and E, which mainly act as compounds scavenging free radicals. As mentioned above, microelements such as manganese, copper, zinc, and selenium are important elements of the antioxidant systems. Endogenous antioxidant substances include in the first place bilirubin albumin, ferritin and melatonin.

5.4 Mitochondrial dynamics

Mitochondria are dynamic organelles undergoing constant regular cycles of fusion and breakdown. The fusion of damaged mitochondria and then asymmetric breakdown are the mechanism leading to regaining of the functionality of the basic components. The damaged elements present in the organelles can be grouped, as a result of fusion, in one mitochondrium. Asymmetric breakdown leads to creation of functionally efficient organelles and of mitochondria, in which all damages are accumulated. These dysfunctional mitochondria are eliminated by autophagy [9].

Mitochondrial fusion and breakdown are strictly balanced processes. Both an uncontrolled fusion and breakdown can constitute an extreme threat to the cell function and lead to cell death. At present, the data on mitochondrial fusion and breakdown in critical conditions are scarce. An increased level of markers presenting the mitochondrial dynamics was found in *post mortem* liver biopsies but not *in vivo* in critically ill patients. In an animal model, in rabbits, which had a significant dysfunction of the hepatic and renal mitochondria, the level of mitochondrial fusion protein of the inner membrane (optic atrophy protein-1) was only significantly increased in the liver. A reduction was also observed of the concentration of mitofusin-2, involved in the fusion of the outer mitochondrial membrane. The breakdown markers remained unchanged in both organs. The results of those studies may suggest that the ability of the mitochondria to fuse and break down differs between the organs.

The elimination of dysfunctional mitochondria requires replenishing of their population through biogenesis. Mitochondrial biogenesis depends on nuclear and mitochondrial transcription systems. Peroxisome proliferator-activated receptor gamma-activator 1 alpha (PGC-1α) has been identified as the key element of the biogenesis process. It activates the nuclear respiratory factors 1 and 2 (NRF1, NRF2), which induce important transcription factors, such as mitochondrial transcription factor A (TFAM) and nuclear-encoded mitochondrial proteins – subunits of respiratory chain complexes. That complex transcription programme causes mtDNA replication and synthesis of new proteins indispensable for development of new mitochondria. That programme is extremely metabolically expensive, since it requires a huge energy expenditure.

In animal sepsis models increased levels were observed of hepatic markers of mitochondrial biogenesis: PGC-1α, NRF1 and TRAM, which was associated with regaining of metabolic activity and improvement of the clinical condition. No differences were found in the levels of hepatic and renal mitochondrial biogenesis markers in rabbits, which were in critical condition but survived, compared to the animals, which failed to survive the experiment. In patients surviving a sepsis, no changes in mitochondrial protein synthesis were observed *in vivo*, in spite of an increase of the mRNA level of mitochondrial transcription factors.

6. Apoptosis in sepsis

Apoptosis plays a significant role in the pathophysiology of sepsis. The role of a potential factor involved in immunosuppression and mortality in sepsis has been ascribed to lymphocyte apoptosis. An increased apoptosis of T and B cells was observed in patients dying of sepsis. The results of clinical studies have confirmed the observations, which demonstrated a significant increase of lymphocyte apoptosis in the model of cecal ligation and puncture (CLP)-induced sepsis in mice. Although death of adaptative immune system cells, limiting thus the inflammatory reaction, may be beneficial for the body, but the presence of intense apoptosis of immune cells leads to a reduced possibility of defence during invasion of pathogens. It seems that lymphocyte apoptosis, leading to immune response impairment, can predispose to septic death. That suggestion has been confirmed by the results of studies in transgenic mice with increased expression of antiapoptotic Bcl-2 protein. In the model of CLP-induced sepsis a protective effect of Bcl-2 on T-cells has

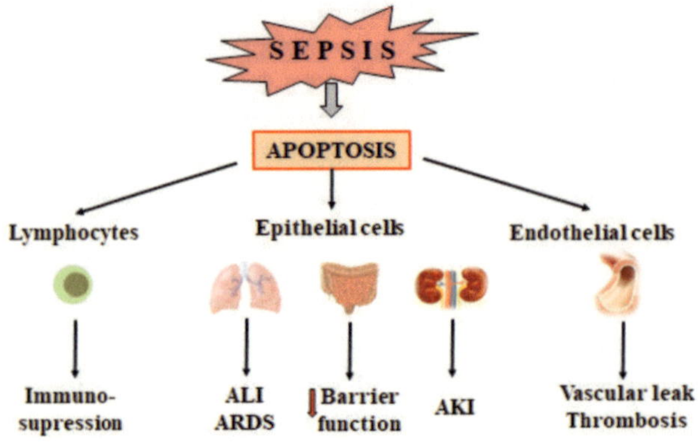

Figure 8.
Apoptosis of various cells in sepsis and its consequences for organ function.

been demonstrated, which increased the survival. That suggests that apoptosis of immune cells plays a significant role in the development of sepsis and is of decisive importance for its possible unfavourable course. The role of a apoptosis of various cells in sepsis and its consequences for organ function is presented in **Figure 8**.

In experimental sepsis models, also an intense apoptosis has been observed of interstitial cells, such as intestinal and pulmonary epithelial cells. A defect of intestinal epithelial cells can lead to a significant impairment of their barrier function and to facilitation of bacterial translocation into blood and/or lymphatic system. That results in an increased antigen presentation and massive immune response, which have a direct effect on the survival.

Apoptosis of pulmonary epithelial cells leads to the development of acute lung injury (ALI). That pathology is directly caused not only by inflammation or trauma but also by haemorrhagic shock and multibacterial sepsis. The silencing of Fas receptors on the membranes of pulmonary epithelial cells in mice with haemorrhagic shock, leads to ALI reduction through blocking of their apoptosis and, thus, inhibition of histological remodelling of the lungs.

7. mTOR and autophagy in sepsis

The mTOR pathway plays an important role in promoting sepsis progression. TLR4 activation through LPS binding increases mTOR activity. In a clinical study in 106 patients with sepsis an activation of HIF-1α and mTOR genes was observed in peripheral blood leucocytes. An injection of LPS to mice caused an activation of mTOR signalling in macrophages and led to an increase of inflammatory renal injury followed by fibrosis. An activation of mTOR pathway by LPS in rats resulted in a blood pressure reduction and heart rate acceleration and also in an increase of the level of inflammatory markers in the tissues of the kidneys, heart and blood vessels. In both mentioned animal models, an administration of rapamycin and mTOR inhibitor significantly reversed the harmful effects of LPS. The inhibition of mTOR in sepsis can be partly explained by activation of the autophagy process.

Autophagy is a degradation system, preserved in an evolutionary way in the cells, and it participates in maintaining of intracellular homeostasis. The process of autophagy includes formation of autophagosomes, fusion of autophagosome-lysosomes and development of degradation products. In sepsis, autophagy is a recognised protective adaptative mechanism limiting cell injury and apoptosis [10, 11]. Autophagy not only eliminates damaged protein aggregates and organelles, but also eliminates bacteria and pathogens present in the cytoplasm. Some special bacteria, such as *Staphylococcus aureus,* can avoid selective autophagy through activation of cell kinases of the host.

The main role of autophagy in sepsis illustrates in **Figure 9**. Autophagy promotes pathogen elimination directly by phagocytosis, regulation of antigen presentation, activation of immune cells and secretion of type I interferon. It inhibits the immune response through degradation of inflammasomes. It prevents immunosuppression through inhibition of apoptosis and elimination of damaged mitochondria. It affects the metabolism through regulation of mitochondrial functions and participation of AMPK and mTOR in the regulation of autophagy activity. That effect is, however, limited. In the case of severe sepsis, even a significant increase of autophagy fails to reverse the overwhelming inflammatory reaction. The body of evidence gathered, suggest that autophagy dynamically changes to become insufficient and non-adaptative at later stages of sepsis. Dynamic changes of autophagy during sepsis was shown in **Figure 10**. That deficit is associated with mTOR signalling regulation, while ineffectiveness of elimination of dysfunctional organelles and toxic intracellular material causes an overwhelming accumulation of danger-associated molecular patterns (DAMPs).

Both autophagy and mTOR pathway are promoted at the initial stages of sepsis. At later sepsis stages a long-lasting drop of autophagy is observed, contributing to organ dysfunction and reduced lymphocyte count, what is important for inflammatory dysregulation, apoptosis and mitochondrial disorders. Two separate animal models demonstrated that autophagy regulation through rapamycin administration reversed the heart damage observed during sepsis. These studies have shown that mTOR is the main inhibitor of autophagy.

Autophagy has been proposed as a potential therapeutic goal, particularly during evident immunosuppression and then in the phase of sepsis, as a way of immune homeostasis restoration. It seems that autophagy promotion can be a novel

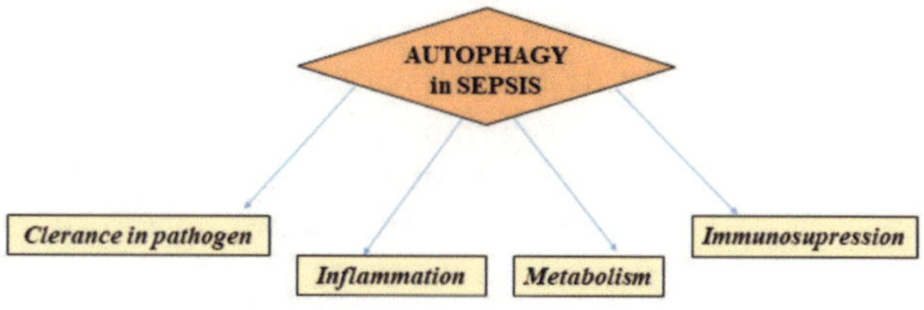

Figure 9.
The main role of autophagy in sepsis.

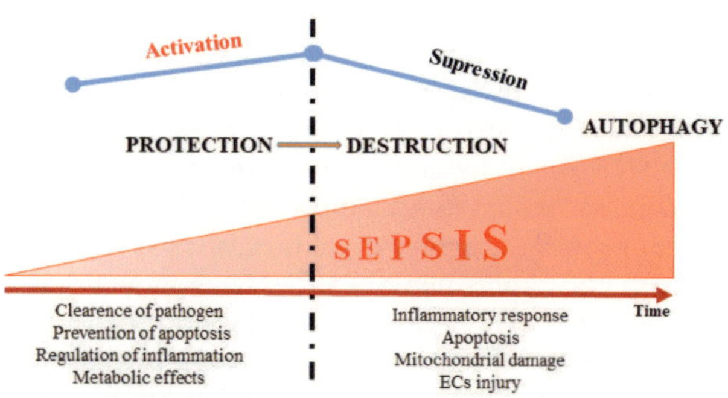

Figure 10.
Dynamic changes of autophagy during sepsis.

and effective intervention in order to reduce organ dysfunction caused by insufficient and non-adaptative autophagy during severe sepsis.

8. Non-coding RNAs in sepsis

Non-coding RNAs are responsible for the regulation of many cell signalling pathways. The molecules include long non-coding RNA (lncRNA) and microRNA (miRNA), participating in many biological processes, such as apoptosis, mitochondrial dysfunction and innate immunity.

All cells synthesise RNA molecules of 21 to 25 nucleotide length, called miRNA. The molecules of miRNA bind to complementary sequences at 3′ ends of target mRNAs and are able to post-transcriptionally regulate the expression of many genes. They can, therefore, exert protective or harmful effects in various immune system-related disorders and affect the levels of proinflammatory cytokines: TNFα and IL-1β through signalling pathways including p38 mitogen-activated protein kinase (MAPK) and MAPK 1 phosphatase (MKP-1). Many studies have demonstrated significant differences in the expression of some miRNAs in septic patients. It was suggested, therefore, that miRNAs may serve as biomarkers in the diagnostic process or risk stratification, and even can be a therapeutic target in the treatment of sepsis.

The lncRNA family includes molecules of protein-non-coding RNAs containing about 200 nucleotides and consists of over 60,000 individually catalogued members. lncRNAs have many functions and activities such as: regulation of gene expression, changing chromatin arrangement, modification of histones and alternative gene splicing, which suggest their possible role in the pathogenesis of various diseases and disorders.

8.1 MicroRNA

MicroRNA molecules play an important role in the regulation of adaptative and innate immune responses in the pathogenesis of sepsis as presented in **Table 1**. The molecules affect the development of regulatory T-cells and also T-helper cells, which are indispensable for immune response optimisation. During sepsis the immune system of the host seems to be both in the state of immunosuppression, but also, at the same time can be in a proinflammatory state [12].

In proinflammatory state, many cytokines, including TNFα, are overexpressed. miRNAs can control TNFα production both at translation and transcription levels. miR-181 has been shown to regulate TNFα synthesis through intensification of TNFα mRNA degradation. It has been also observed that a significantly reduced miR-125b expression was accompanied by a higher TNFα expression in the monocytes of newborns after LPS stimulation. Besides that, miRNAs can also regulate the TNF pathway and mediate inflammatory reactions. It has been suggested that miR-511 is a regulator of TNF receptor protein synthesis and, thus, it affects the sensitivity of cells to TNF. An effect of miR-511 is therefore possible, protecting against TNF-dependent endotoxic shock syndrome. It has been also demonstrated that the levels of other proinflammatory cytokines, such as IL-6, are significantly increased in septic patients. Experimental studies have shown that miR-146a expression is correlated with an increased IL-6 concentration in septic patients. Many studies have demonstrated that miRNA molecules are able to regulate inflammatory reactions through their effect on the Toll-like receptor 4 (TLR4) signalling pathway. The TLR4-induced signalling activates in the first place NFκB, the key transcription factor modulating the expression of proinflammatory and

miRNAs	Expression in Sepsis	Observed effects of miRNAs
miR-150	down	miR-150 levels in both leukocytes and plasma correlated with the severity of sepsis and could be used as a marker of early sepsis. Plasma ratio of levels of miR-150/IL-18 could be used for assessing the severity of sepsis
miR-31	down	miR-31 down regulation in CD4+ T cells contributes to immunosuppression in sepsis patients via promoting TH2 skewing humans T cells
miR-27a	down	miR-34a, miR-15a, and miR-27a are correlated with shock development in severe sepsis patients; they also target cell cycle regulation, apoptosis, cell layer permeability, and inflammatory pathways humans plasma
miR-25	down	A correlation between levels of miR-25 and the severity of sepsis was observed; surviving patients had higher levels of this biomarker compared with non-surviving subjects; decreased levels of miR-25 were associated with the concentrations of oxidative stress indicators in sepsis
miR-15a	up	Upregulated miR-15a down regulated the LPS induced inflammatory pathway
miR-16	up	Upregulated miR-16 down regulated the LPS induced inflammatory pathway
miR-574-5p	up	Serum level was correlated with the death of sepsis patients; the combined analysis of miR-574-5p, SOFA humans serum scores, and the sepsis stage on the day of diagnosis provided a good predictor for sepsis prognosis
miR-297	up	serum miR-297 level was higher in survivors than non-survivors among septic patients
miR-143	up	serum miR-143 levels were significantly higher in sepsis than in SIRS and healthy controls

Table 1.
Selected miRNAs involved in human sepsis.

immunoregulatory factors. Some miRNA molecules, such as miR-155, miR-125 and miR-146a play the main role in the negative modulation of the TLR4/NFκB inflammatory cascade, but also in innate immunity. The expression of miR-155 and also many other miRNA molecules depends on NFκB, since it has been shown that LPS stimulation of THP-1 monocytes induces the expression of miR-146a and miR146b. The miR146a molecule directly regulates the expression of TNF receptor-associated factor 6 (TRAF6) and IL-1 receptor-associated kinase 1 (IRAK1), which are important adaptor molecules in the TLR4 signalling pathway. miR-146a plays also a significant role in the *in vitro* tolerance of monocytes to endotoxins. That effect can be, however, reversed by miR-146a suppression. It has been recently reported that the NFκB/DICER signalling pathway inhibits TNFα synthesis through production of mature forms of miR-130 and miR-125b, which regulate TNFα mRNA. The presented miRNA effects seem particularly important in the aspect of the critical role of TLR4-induced pathway in sepsis.

8.2 lncRNAs and sepsis

The molecules of lncRNA play an important role in biological processes and their dysregulation is associated with various disorders [13]. The experimental studies presented in **Table 2**, were conducted in order to assess the correlation between sepsis and expression of lncRNA molecules. It has been demonstrated that lncRNA expression is changed in human monocytes, cardiomyocytes and renal canalicular epithelial cells during development of sepsis or after exposure to LPS.

lncRNAs	Expression in Sepsis	Observed effects of lncRNAs
NEAT1	up	Circulating lncRNA NEAT1 was related to severity, increased risk, and unfavourable prognosis in sepsis patients
ANRIL/miR-125a axis	up	lnc-ANRIL/miR-125a axis could serve as a biomarker for prognosis, severity, and inflammation in sepsis patients
ITSN1-2	up	High expression of ITSN1-2 is associated with disease severity and inflammation in sepsis patients.
TUG1	down	Decreased TUG1 expression may induce sepsis related AKI by modulating the NF-kB pathway and regulating the miR-142-3p/SIRT1 axis (*humans in vitro*)
MALAT1	down	IL-6 induced upregulation of MALAT1 in LPS treated cardiomyocytes, and MALAT1 could promote the expression of TNF-a at least partly bySAA3 in response to LPS treatment in cardiomyocytes (*mice in vitro*)
HULC	down	Upregulation of lncRNA HULC is required for the pro-inflammatory response during LPS induced sepsis (*mice in vitro*)

Table 2.
Selected lncRNAs involved in sepsis.

In spite of many studies on that topic, sepsis still remains a complex clinical condition, the pathophysiology of which has not been fully elucidated. Non-coding RNAs offer a chance for early diagnosis and monitoring of patients in Intensive Care Units.

9. Conclusions and perspectives

Uncontrolled inflammation, immune disorders, oxidative stress, apoptosis, mitochondrial damage and also endothelial function disorders play the key role in sepsis and organ dysfunction associated with it. Sepsis releases a series of signalling cascades, starting with recognition of the whole spectrum of pathogen-associated molecular patterns (PAMPs) and organ damage-associated molecular patterns (DAMPs). Each stage of the signalling pathways participating in the release of inflammatory mediators is extremely important for the course of the disease and can be a target point in the therapeutic strategy in septic patients. The general agreement present as yet, concerning the inflammatory response only mediated by the TLR4/NFκB pathway is not so obvious any longer. Administration of anti-inflammatory drugs, including corticosteroids, or antagonists of TNFα and IL-1, failed to produce the expected effects in septic patients.

The target points in the treatment of sepsis can also be the molecules of non-coding RNA (ncRNA). Recent studies have suggested, among other findings, that the miRNA-23b molecule prevents the development of myocardial dysfunction in late sepsis. It seems therefore, that research in the field of development of drugs targeted at ncRNA molecules can be the future of antiseptic pharmacotherapy.

The new SARS-CoV-2 coronaviral disease has aroused interest in viral sepsis. Although bacteria are the predominant pathogens in sepsis, a viral sepsis cannot be disregarded. According to the literature reports, the percentage of septic patients with negative results of blood cultures for bacterial pathogens reaches 42% [14, 15]. In COVID-19 patients a septic shock and multiple organ dysfunction may develop. In view of absence of specific drugs, the current therapeutic strategies include isolation of patients, controlling of infections and maintaining normal organ functioning. The SARS-CoV-2 infection depends on the host's cell factors. Recent studies have demonstrated that COVID-19 virus uses the angiotensin 2-converting enzyme (ACE2) and serine protease TMPRSS2 to penetrate into host's cells. That suggests a possibility of administration of protease inhibitors as effective drugs blocking the transmission of the virus [16]. The studies on viral sepsis caused by COVID-19 could help to indicate also other target points for drugs, which would reduce the damages of the lungs and other organs.

Conflict of interest

The authors declare no conflict of interest.

Author details

Grażyna Sygitowicz and Dariusz Sitkiewicz*
Department of Clinical Chemistry and Laboratory Diagnostics, Medical University of Warsaw, Poland

*Address all correspondence to: dariusz.sitkiewicz@gmail.com

References

[1] Kumar V. Sepsis roadmap: what we know, what we learned, and where we are going. Clin Immunol 2020; 210: 108264. DOI: 10.1016/j.clim.2019.108264

[2] Fajgenbaum DC, June CH. Cytokine Storm. NEJM 2020; 383(23): 2255-2273. DOI: 10.1056/NEJMra2026131

[3] Kumar V. Toll-like receptors in sepsis-associated cytokine storm and their endogenous negative regulators as future immunomodulatory targets. Int Immunopharmacol 2020; 89: 107087. DOI: 10.1016/j.intimp.2020.107087

[4] Mitchell S, Vargas J, Hoffmann A. Signaling via the NFκB system. WIREs Syst Biol Med. 2016; 8: 227-241. DOI: 10.1002/wsbm.1331

[5] Miranda M, Balarini M, Caixeta D, Bouskela E. Microcirculatory dysfunction in sepsis: pathophysiology, clinical monitoring, and potential therapies. Am J Physiol Heart Circ Physiol 2016; 311: H24-H35. DOI: 10.1152/ajpheart.00034.2016

[6] Lipinska-Gediga M. Endothelium as a part of septic multiple organ dysfunction syndrome (Mods) – Is Endocan an Answer? J Clin Cell Immunol 2015; 6:1. DOI: 10.4172/2155-9899.1000304

[7] Ning L, Rong J, Zhang Z, Xu Y. Therapeutic approaches targeting renin-angiotensin system in sepsis and its complications. Pharmacol Res 2021; 167: 105409. DOI: 10.1016/j.phrs.2020.105409

[8] Sharawy N, Lenmann C. Molecular mechanisms by which iNOS uncouplin can induce cardiovascular dysfunction during sepsis: Role of posttranslational modifications (PTMs). Life Sci 2020; 255: 117821. DOI: 10.1016/j.lfs.2020.117821

[9] Sygitowicz G, Sitkiewicz D. Molecular mechanisms of organ damage in sepsis: an overview. Braz J Infect Dis 2020: 24(6): 552-560. DOI: 10.1016/j.bjid.2020.09.004

[10] Feng Y, Liu B, Zheng X, Chen L, Chen W, Fang Z. The prospective role of autophagy in sepsis. Microbial Pathogenesis 2019; 131: 106-111. DOI: 10.1016/j.micpath.2019.03.039

[11] Li Y, Suo L, Fu Z, Li G, Zhang J. Pivotal role of endothelial cell autophagy in sepsis. Life Sci 2021; 276: 119413. DOI: 10.1016/j.lfs.2021.119413

[12] Essandoh K, Fan G-Ch. Role of extracellular and intracellular microRNAs in sepsis. Bioch Bioph Acta 2014; 1842: 2155-2162. DOI: 10.1016/j.bbadis.2014.07.021

[13] Hashemian SM, Pourhanifeh MH, Fadaei S, Velayati AA, Mirzaei H, Hamblin MR. Non-coding RNAs and exosomes: The role in the pathogenesis of sepsis. Mol Ther Nucleic Acids 2020: 4, 21: 51-74. DOI: 10.1016/j.omtn.2020.05.012

[14] Ljungstrom LR, Jacobsson G, Chesson BEB, Andersson R, Enroth H. Respiratory viral infections are underdiagnosed in patients with suspected sepsis. Eur J Clin Microbiol Infect Dis 2017; 36: 1767-1776. DOI: 10.1007/s10096-017-2990-z

[15] Phua J, Ngerng WJ, See KCh, Tay ChK, Kiong T, Lim HaF, Chew MY, Yip HS, Tan A, Khalizah HJ, Capistrano R, Lee KH, Mukhopadjyay A. Characteristics and outcomes of culture-negative versus

culture-positive severe sepsis. Crit Care 2013; 17: R202. DOI: 10.1186/cc12896

[16] Hoffmann M, Kleine-Weber H, Schroeder S, Kruger N, Herrier T, Erichsen S, Schiergens TS, Herrier G, Wu NH, Nitsche A, Muller MA, Drosten C, Pohlmann S. SARS-CoV-2 cell entry depends on ACE2 and TMPRSS2 and is blocked by a clinically proven protease inhibitor. Cell 2020; 181: 271-280. DOI: 10.1016/j.cell.2020.02.052

Chapter 14

Inflammatory Mediators Leading to Edema Formation through Plasma Membrane Receptors

Guilherme Teixeira and Robson Faria

Abstract

Edema is a swelling from liquid accumulation in body tissues. Injuries in tissues or organs may cause this disorder leading to chemical mediators releasing and triggering the inflammatory process. Inflammatory mediators, when released in response to injuries, promote biological reactions at the affected site. Furthermore, plasma membrane receptors modulate the inflammatory chemical agent synthesis and release. Pattern recognition receptors, such as Toll Like is an example of plasma membrane receptors associated with chemical agents recognizing and cascade amplification. Therefore, these plasma membrane proteins exhibit essential roles during injuries and immunologic response. Thus, this review discusses the plasma membrane receptors modulation in the inflammatory area, focusing on edema formation.

Keywords: membrane receptors, edema, inflammation, cytokines, vascular permeability

1. Introduction

Edema is characterized as a swelling caused by an increase of fluids in the interstitial space. Interstitial liquid deregulation causes liquid accumulation in the body with harmful consequences to tissues and organs [1, 2]. The physiologist Ernest Starling defined the interaction between the fluids forces in blood vessels. The fluid movement (FM) in the blood vessel is correlated with blood vessel wall permeability (constant Kf) and the difference between hydrostatic pressure variations (ΔP) and colloid osmotic pressure ($\Delta\pi$) forces [1, 3]. The following mathematical equation (Starling's equation) describes this interaction: $FM = Kf. (\Delta P- \Delta\pi)$.

The liquid retention becomes harmful to tissues affecting the cellular balance and homeostasis. Several factors induce this phenomenon: hormones, plasma proteins, inflammation, infectious diseases, and disturbs in some organs [3–5]. After an injury, inflammatory mediators cause physiological reactions in the lesioned region. Some of these inflammatory molecules include interleukins (IL-1β, IL-6, and IL-18), tumor necrosis factor-alpha (TNF-α), vasodilators, arachidonic acid metabolites, nitric oxide (NO), among others [6–8]. The inflammatory agent overproduction mediates increase in vascular permeability and leukocyte recruitment, causing edema formation and hyperalgesia [2, 9].

Membrane receptors are a group of functional proteins located in the plasma and organelles membranes. These receptors are able to trigger intracellular chemical cascades [10]. Approaches in the pharmacological field investigated several plasma membrane receptors modulating inflammation [11], such as the purinergic system, TRP channels, and pattern recognition receptors (PRRs), are commonly associated with inflammatory pathways [12–16]. Therefore, this chapter will address the plasma membrane receptors modulation on inflammatory agents and subsequent edema formation.

2. Inflammation and edema: influence in the vascular permeability

Inflammation is a natural defense mechanism to Pathogen-associated molecular pattern (PAMPs) or Damage-associated molecular pattern (DAMPs) involving cells and blood vessels. In this process, local and immune cells (macrophages, neutrophils, and lymphocytes) promote the release of pro-inflammatory mediators, such as those mentioned earlier. Although the inflammatory response is a natural mechanism, this process may become harmful to tissues and organs when persistently stimulated [17, 18]. The inflammation course and edema formation are linked because edema is one of inflammation cardinal signs [2].

After a trauma or injury, intracellular components are released, modifying the inflammatory site characteristics (**Figure 1**). Migrant and local cells, such as mast cells and basophils, release vasoactive amines, serotonin, and histamine. These molecules initially cause increase in blood vessel permeability and vasodilation [19–21]. Thus, these vascular changes cause liquid leakage from the vascular environment. Plasma protein, such as albumin, in the extravascular medium may modulate the vascular pressures. The press alteration favors the fluid and electrolyte passage to interstitial space generating swelling [3, 22].

Coagulation factor activation, such as the Hangeman factor, induces bradykinin and proteases synthesis stimulation. Bradykinin is a kinin involved in vascular permeability and other vascular mechanisms [23–25]. Additionally, the complement system fragments exhibit a crucial role in the immunity and vascular processes. The anaphylatoxins, such as C3a, C4a, and C5a, act on leukocyte recruitment and also in bradykinin signaling [23, 26–29].

The pro-inflammatory cytokines participate in pain mechanisms and also promotes increase in vascular permeability [23]. Stamacovic [30] described cytokines participating in the central nervous system inflammation and Blood–brain barrier

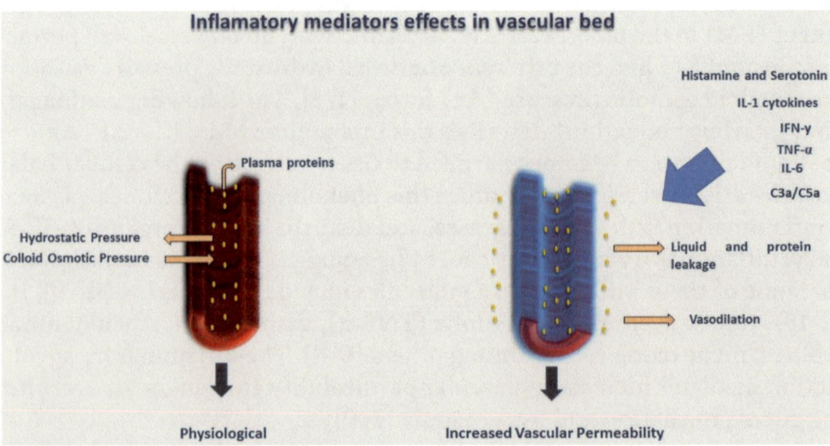

Figure 1.
Inflammatory mediators are acting on vascular permeability.

permeability. The increase in IL-1β, IL-6, and TNF-α may cooperate for brain edema emergence. Martin et al. [31] showed vascular increase induced by IL-1 and IFN-y in Wistar rats. IL-1β is very approached in a mechanism involving nociception and sensibility to pain, as well as bradykinin [32, 33]. Furthermore, increase of IL-1β and TNF-α induct arachidonic acid metabolites [34]. Arachidonic acid metabolites like prostaglandins, leukotrienes, prostacyclin, and thromboxane also mediate vascular changes [35]. Prostaglandins is directly involved in the modulation of pain mechanisms [9, 36].

IL-18 is another IL-1 family member involved in pain mechanisms. The IL-1β and IL-18 synthesis possess similarities in their signaling [37]. Pilat and colleagues' study involving the IL-18 inhibition [38] showed nociception reduction in a neuropathic pain model. Besides, IL-18 is also notorious as the IFN-y-inducing factor [37, 39].

Additionally, inflammatory mediators modulate inflammatory diseases, and some data confirms this actuation in organ pathophysiology such as lung, liver, heart, and others [40–43]. Thus, vital organ disturbs promote vascular fluids imbalance. Additional data about cytokines modulation at vascular mechanisms can be found in the following works [23, 44, 45].

3. Membrane receptors participation in the inflammation and edema pathophysiology modulation

Scientific advances provide new discoveries about plasma membrane receptors function and identity. Molecules impermeable to the membrane can selectivity cross to the intracellular environment through these receptors. Many receptors characteristics are investigated in the physicochemical field, including biophysical properties and structure. Membrane receptors generally have three classifications: receptors coupled to enzymes such as tyrosine kinase (RTKs), G protein-coupled receptors (GPCRs), and ion channels [46]. Interestingly, there is a group of membrane proteins that are widely addressed in scientific research for modulating inflammatory mediators release and search for new anti-inflammatory drugs. Based on this, the following topics exhibit some of studied plasma membrane receptors related to the inflammatory response.

3.1 Toll-like receptors

The host defense against infections and tissue damage is a complex mechanism. In this process, the cells must recognize PAMPs and DAMPs to initiate a specific intracellular response against infectious agents, such as viruses and bacteria or dangerous signs, such as burn injuries [47].

The Toll-Like Receptors (TLRs) are a group of membrane proteins involved in inflammation and immunity. They act on PRRs expressed in macrophages, neutrophils, and dendritic cells [47, 48]. TLRs compose the interleukin 1 receptors superfamily (IL-1Rs) with slight structural differences. Ten TLRs subtypes were described in humans (TLR1–10), although other species may exhibit variations.

TLRs are located in different compartments in the cell. For instance, the subtypes 1, 2, 4, 5, and 6 are located at the cell plasma membrane, whereas subtypes 3, 7, 8, 9, and 10 are in the intracellular compartment, located in endosomes. [RF1] TLR2 and TLR4 are the best-studied receptors of this family [49, 50].

TLRs, when activated, are essential for the host response to harmful agents, since these receptors modulate the inflammatory mediators release. The factor nuclear kappa β (NF-kβ) and mitogen-activated protein kinase (MAPKs) are classical pathways activated by Toll-Like Receptors (**Figure 2**) [48]. When stimulated

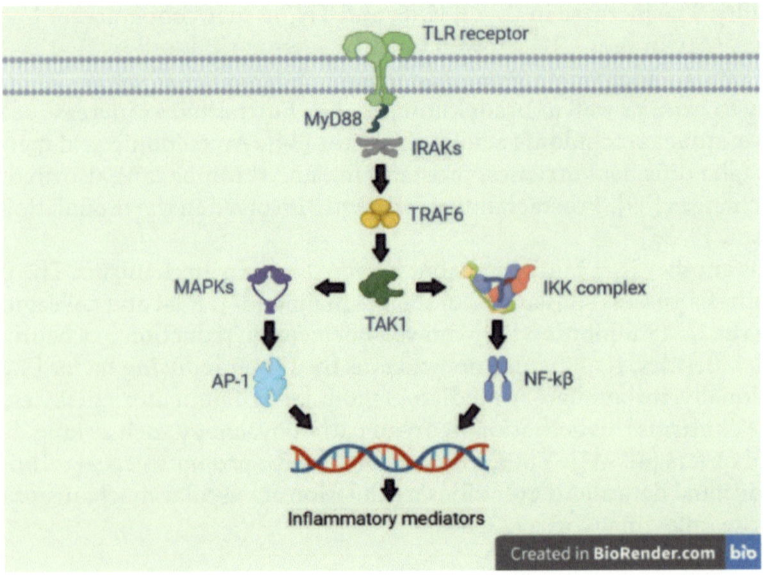

Figure 2.
Plasma membrane TLR signaling pathway. TLR receptor activation triggers AP-1 and NF-kβ transcription factors.

by a ligand, such as lipopolysaccharides (LPS), TLRs transduces the signal through adaptor molecules in the intracellular environment. Myeloid differentiation primary response 88 (MyD88) is an adaptor molecule of the interleukin- 1 receptor-associated kinases (IRKs) signaling with subsequent TNF receptor-associated factor 6 (TRAF6) activation. TRAF6 activates the growth factor β-activated kinase 1 (TAK1), which triggers an enzymatic complex associated with NF-kβ translocation to the cell nucleus. TAK1 signaling also activates the MAPKs pathway with activator protein 1 (AP-1) nuclear factor translocation. This pathway leads to various pro-inflammatory mediators transcription, such as cytokines (IL-1 family, IL-6, TNF-α), **COX-2** stimulation (prostaglandin E2), and interferons [50, 51].

TLR activation may exhibit a crucial role in edema formation through inflammatory mediator production (**Table 1**). In a recent paper, Okada and colleagues [55] described brain edema reduction in a subarachnoid hemorrhage model (SAH) mouse after treatment with TAK-242, a TLR4 receptor inhibitor. The molecular mechanism by which this occur was not evaluated. However, the pathophysiology development of brain edema shows association with TLR4 function. In liver diseases, such as acute liver failure, astrocyte swelling is a notable characteristic that promotes brain edema formation. Interestingly, NF-kβ and MAPKs-induced cytokine release are crucial mechanisms for astrocyte swelling development [56, 57]. Jayakumar et al. [58] have demonstrated LPS and cytokines-induced astrocyte swelling increase. These data suggest TLR4 may be a target in the brain edema pathophysiology. **Table 1** represent more data about TLR receptors in the inflammatory context.

3.2 Histamine receptors

Histamine constitutes an essential molecule in cell biology, edema pathophysiology, and the inflammatory process. The histamine synthesis occurs with the amino acid L-histidine decarboxylation through the histidine decarboxylase enzyme (HDC). Other inflammatory mediators can lead to increase HDC activity, such as IL-1 cytokines [60]. Histamine synthesis occurs in different body cells, although this production primordially occurs in mast cells and basophils [61]. In these cells, histamine is

Receptor	Ligand	Involvement in inflammation and edema	References
TLR1	Tri-acyl lipopeptides	TLR1 works together with TLR2 as a heterodimer. This subtype also mediates the intracellular cytokines transcription	[47, 52]
TLR2	Peptidoglycan	TLR2 signaling intracellular transcription of inflammatory mediators Cytokine gene expression such as IL-1β, TNF-α, and IL-6 decrease in TLR2 Knock out mice in vascular injury model TLR2 plays a role in mast cells degranulation and cytokine release stimulated by peptidoglycan	[47, 53, 54]
TLR4	LPS	TLR4 activation leads to inflammatory mediators transcription involved in pain and edema, such as **COX-2** metabolites, IL-1 cytokines, and TNF-α LPS induces astrocyte swelling and brain edema pathogenesis. TLR4 also increases TNF-α and IL-1β in LPS-induced mast cells	[47, 50, 54–58]
TLR5	Flagellin	TLR5 can be activated by high mobility group box 1 (HMGB1), a protein that plays a role in inflammation. The HMGB1 action on TLR5 induced the pro-inflammatory mediators intracellular signaling. TLR5 also plays a protective role in intestinal cells.	[47, 52, 59]
TLR6	Di-acyl lipopeptides	TLR6 functions are interacting with TLR2 and TLR4 as a heterodimer.	[47, 52]

Table 1.
Plasma membrane TLRs modulate inflammatory mediators.

stored in cytoplasmatic granules and released according to the stimulus presented. Histamine interacts with GPCRs membrane receptors classified as histamine receptors (HRs) and divided into four subtypes: HR1, HR2, HR3, and HR4 (**Table 2**) [61].

The histamine action is remarkable in the vascular modulation mechanism, including vascular permeability increase. HRs actuate as a second messenger, leading to intracellular signal and cytokine synthesis [68]. A study by Delaunois and co-authors [69] showed a protective HR3 agonist role in pulmonary edema stimulated by inflammation-promoting molecules. In addition, HR3 stimulation appears to play a significant role in perfusion in post-burn tissues [70]. HRs also participate in the mechanisms related to antinociception [61].

Among HRs, HR4 has become a new antihistamines studies target. The HR4 activation triggers MAPK, which leads to pro-inflammatory mediators synthesis [60]. Coruzzi and collaborates [66] showed promising results in inhibiting paw edema by HR4 in acute inflammation. After carrageenan-induced edema, two selective HR4 inhibitors, JNJ7777120, and VUF6002, respectively, were evaluated. Inhibition by JNJ7777120 after two hours of carrageenan induction has shown notable values compared to VUF6002. Another study using JNJ7777120 described the anti-nociceptive role in a pain inflammation model through HR4 antagonism. Additionally, HR4 inhibition decreases neutrophilic influx to stimulated area pretreated with JNJ7777120 [67]. These findings suggest HR4 with a crucial role in edema and pain mechanism.

3.3 Serotonin receptors

Diseases involving the psychiatric area have been widely addressed in scientific research, such as depression. [RF2] Factors involving mood and mental disorders,

Receptor	Ligand	Involvement in inflammation and edema	References
HR1	Histamine	HR1 is involved in allergic response HR1 influences MPAK signaling and modulates Th1 response.	[61–63]
HR2	Histamine	HR2 modulates Th2 response HR2 regulates IL-10 and antinociceptive activity	[61, 62, 64]
HR3	Histamine	HR3 exhibits an essential role in neuronal inflammation and neuropathic pain. HR3 inhibition has been shown to be beneficial in inflammation and edema stimulated by formalin	[61, 65]
HR4	Histamine	HR4 also participates in MAPK signaling. HR4 inhibition shows to reduce neutrophil infiltration, edema, and hyperalgesia in acute inflammation	[60, 63, 66, 67]

Table 2.
Histamine receptors.

include serotonin, a critical functional amine in this disease. Interestingly, serotonin regulates inflammatory signaling, playing a role in vascular permeability. Therefore, serotonin becomes a multifunctional molecule modulating many body processes [71–73].

5-hydroxytryptamine (5-HT), serotonin is synthesized from the amino acid tryptophan. The enzymes tryptophan hydroxylase and tryptophan decarboxylase are responsible for 5-HT production. Serotonin may be found in various body tissues, such as enterochromaffin, platelets, brain, and lung [71]. 5-HT interacts with membrane receptors (5-HT receptors), divided into seven families (5-HT1–7), where these receptors are GPCRs, except for 5HT3, which belongs to ion channels. These receptors possess fourteen subtypes: 5-HT1 (A, B, D, E, and F), 5-HT2 (A, B, and C), 5-HT3 (A, B), 5-HT4, 5-HT5 (A), 5-HT6, and 5-HT7 [74, 75].

The 5-HT role in other systems has been studied over the years. During inflammation, 5-HT plays an essential role in vascular permeability, as well as histamine, in addition to participating in pro-inflammatory mediator production [72]. In this context, serotonergic receptor subtypes act on inflammation process biochemistry. 5-HT7 is influential in peripheral inflammatory modulation, according to Albayrak and co-authors [76]. The 5-HT7 participates in the nociception mechanism with other 5-HT receptors, such as 5-HT1 and 5-HT2 [77, 78]. The 5-HT2 subtype (A) subtype also modulates the inflammatory process. Nishiyama studies [79] have demonstrated a role for 5-HT2A in cytokines synthesis during an inflammation model induced by endotoxin shock. The 5-HT2A inhibition reduced TNF-α, IL-1β, IL-8, and IL-6 levels. Interestingly, IL-10 levels (cytokine with anti-inflammatory function) increased due to 5-HT2A inhibition. Additionally, 5-HT2A shows to play a function in body temperature control [80]. These data demonstrate a relevant role for 5-HT2A receptors in inflammation pathophysiology (**Table 3**).

3.4 Purinergic receptors

The purinergic system is a group of transmembrane proteins activated by extracellular purine ligands, such as adenosine and other derivatives, adenosine triphosphate and diphosphate (ATP and ADP). Interestingly, when the ATP molecule is found in elevated concentration in the extracellular environment (eATP), this nucleotide may become a DAMP and regulates the inflammatory process. Purinergic receptors are formed by two groups (P1 and P2) differing in structure and activation ligands on mammalian cells [93, 94].

Receptor	Ligand	Involvement in inflammation and edema	References
5-HT1	Serotonin	5-HT1 receptors stimulation induces a role in neurogenic inflammation Intrathecal 5-HT1A, 5-HT1B, and 5-HT1D receptor agonists administration decreased the peripheral inflammatory edema induced by carrageenan.	[81, 82]
5-HT2	Serotonin	5-HT2A subtype inhibition increased IL-10 in inflammation induced by shock with endotoxins. 5-HT2A receptor activation decrease TNF-α-induced inflammation 5-HT2A regulates the body temperature 5-HT2B subtype shows the immunomodulatory function in dendritic cells	[79, 80, 83, 84]
5-HT3	Serotonin	5-HT3 inhibition decreased inflammatory cytokines and neutrophilic action in a colitis model 5-HT3 decreases pain in carrageenan-induced inflammation	[72, 85, 86]
5-HT4	Serotonin	Spinal 5-HT4 receptor antagonism decreased hyperalgesia effects 5-HT4 induced IL-1β and IL-8 release in mature dendritic cells.	[72, 87, 88]
5-HT5	Serotonin	Intrathecal administration appears to show an anti-nociceptive role for spinal 5-HT5A receptors	[89, 90]
5-HT6	Serotonin	Like 5-HT4, 5-HT6 receptor antagonism is also beneficial in hyperalgesia	[87, 91]
5-HT7	Serotonin	5-HT7 receptor stimulation has an anti-inflammatory role in the periphery carrageenan-induced inflammation 5-HT7 agonist decreased **COX-2** levels. Like 5-HT4, 5-HT7 activation also induces IL-1β and IL-8 secretion in dendritic cells.	[76, 88, 92]

Table 3.
Serotonin receptors.

The adenosine molecule activates the P1 group and possesses four subtypes (A1, A2a, A2b, and A3). The P1 group comprises GPCRs receptors, and the P2 group is extensive and divided into two families, P2X and P2Y. The P2X receptors form ATP-activated ion channel receptors with seven subtypes (P2X1–7). P2Y receptors are GPCRs, like the P1 group. Interestingly, ATP and their derivatives activate the P2Y receptors, although, pyrimidine molecules, such as uridine diphosphate (UDP and UDP-glucose), also modulate some subtypes activation. This family consists in eight subtypes (P2Y1, P2Y2, P2Y4, P2Y6, P2Y11, P2Y12, P213, and P2Y14) in mammals. The purinergic receptors participate in inflammation and immune response and are expressed in several tissues [14].

In the purinergic group, the receptor of great scientific notoriety is the P2X7 receptor (P2X7R), addressed in several mechanisms, such as cell death and inflammatory cytokines release [14]. P2X7R have the capacity to increase membrane permeability for large solutes after prolonged ATP activation. The prolonged P2X7R stimulation induces a pore opening that allows the molecules of up to 900 Da. This mechanism highlights the P2X7R as a pore-forming protein, similar to other membrane receptors, such as some TRP channels [95].

However, a striking P2X7R feature is the participation in the maturation of IL-1 cytokine family (IL-1β and IL-18) release. The IL-1β and IL-18 production and maturation require two signaling mechanisms, one mediated by pattern recognition receptors (via TLRs family activation) and a second by a danger signal, such as eATP. The activation of TLRs induces nuclear transcription through NF-kβ of the immature forms of these cytokines (ProIL-1β and ProIL-18), concluding the first stage.The eATP activates the P2X7R, beginning the cascade signaling that compose the Nod-like receptor protein-3 (NLRP3) inflammasome complex with subsequent IL-1β and IL-18 maturation and release [48, 96]. The following figure illustrates this mechanism more clearly (**Figure 3**).

The IL-1β inhibition in inflammation and pain has been addressed in several inflammation studies. Experiments in vivo using P2X7R antagonist have demonstrated improvements in the swelling caused by inflammation in a model of paw edema [97, 98]. The pain sensibility mechanism is linked to vascular permeability, causing edema [2]. Furthermore, P2X7R inhibition reduces pro-inflammatory cytokines, such as IL-1β and other mediators, since the P2X7R is responsible for these mechanisms [96]. Additionally, the P2X4 receptor has participated in IL-1β and IL-18 signaling based on Chen et al. [99]. Further, other purinergic receptors data in edema and inflammation have already been approached in the literature (**Table 4**).

3.5 TRP channels

The physiological mechanisms of pain and temperature stimuli indicate the transient receptor potential (TRP) as a target in this regard [110]. The TRP channels superfamily is constituted of transmembrane cationic ionotropic receptors. In mammals, six subfamilies classify the TRP channels into two groups. The first group: TRPC (canonical), TRPV (vanilloid), TRPA (ankyrin), and TRPM (melastatin). The second group is composed of TRPML (mucolipin) and TRPP (polycystic). This chapter will discuss the most addressed subfamilies in the scientific literature: TRPV, TRPM, and TRPA based on their involvement in inflammation and pain. These subfamilies are classified in TRPV1–6, TRPM1–8, and TRPA1 receptors [111, 112].

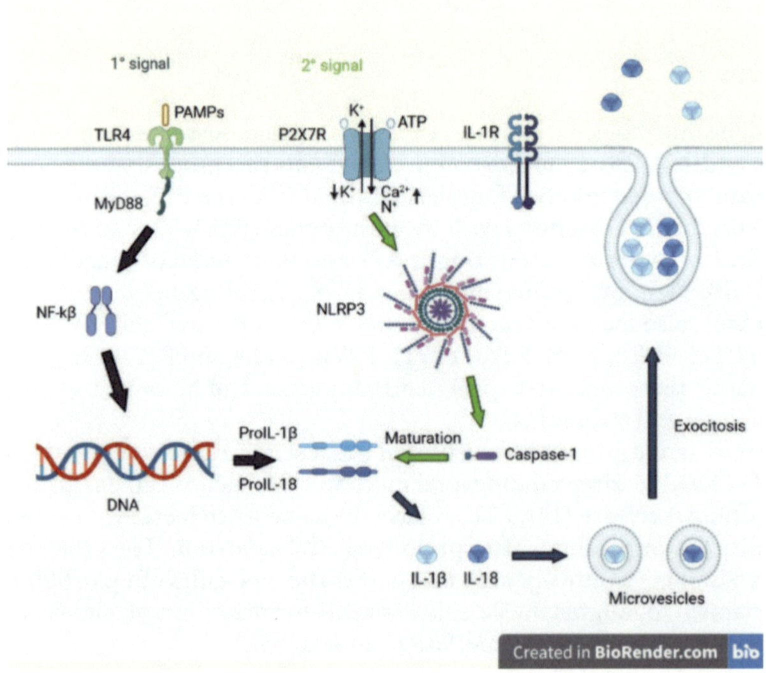

Figure 3.
IL-1β and IL-18 synthesis after P2X7R activation. The first signaling occurs with the ProIL-1β and ProIL-18 transcription after TLRs receptor activation (TLR4). The second signal arrives with the eATP stimulating the P2X7R. The receptor activation induces the NLRP3 inflammasome complex, and finally, IL-1β and IL-18 conversion for mature form.

Receptor	Ligand	Involvement in inflammation and edema	References
A1R	Adenosine	A1R receptor stimulation increased leukocyte recruitment and edema formation in acute pancreatitis disease. A1R participates in pulmonary inflammation and influence vascular permeability through inflammatory cytokines release in monocytes and neutrophils	[100, 101]
A2R	Adenosine	A2aR decreases cytokine synthesis (IFN-γ, IL-4, and IL-2) in lymphocytes and influence platelet aggregation. A2bR mediates several pro-inflammatory cytokines (IL-1β, TNF-α) synthesis In contrast, A2bR also exerts an anti-inflammatory action, as observed for IL-10 release in macrophages.	[101]
A3R	Adenosine	A3R stimulation induces histamine and serotonin release and inflammation in rat paw. A3R seems to mediate benefits in control hyperalgesia	[102, 103]
P2X4R	ATP	P2X4 induces IL-1β and IL-18 cytokines maturation through NRLP3 inflammasome P2X4R is involved in prostaglandin E2 release and pain	[14, 99, 104]
P2X7R	ATP	P2X7R activation produces cytokines, such as IL-1β and IL-18 maturation through NRLP3 inflammasome and TNF-α P2X7R regulates prostaglandin E2 release P2X7R antagonism reversed edema and hyperalgesia P2X7R stimulation leads to vascular bed inflammation through IL-1β release	[14, 96–98, 105, 106]
P2YR	ATP/UDP/ UDP-glucose	P2Y1R, P2Y2R, and P2Y6R are associated with leukocyte chemotaxis. P2Y1R, together with P2Y12R, have a function in platelet aggregation Like P2X7R, P2Y6R activation in endothelial cells promotes vascular inflammation and fluids leakage.	[107–109]

Table 4.
Purinergic receptors.

TRPV1 is the most studied TRP channel because of its noxious heat and inflammation perception. TRPV1 is a pore-forming protein, like P2X7R and other TRPs, such as TRPV2–4, TRPA1, and TRPM8 (**Table 5**). All these channels promote pore opening, and molecules flux up to 900 Da [117]. Capsaicin is one TRPV1 receptor agonist and plays a critical role in nociception pathogenesis [124].

The TRPV1 receptor (heat sensor) together with TRPA1 (cold sensor) can modulate the neuropeptide molecules release like substance P. This molecule encompasses many biochemical processes involved in inflammation, such as histamine and serotonin released by mast cells, which leads to increased vascular permeability and hyperalgesia [113]. Hoffmeister and co-authors [125] described a reversion in edema and pain caused by monosodium urate crystals after TRPV1 inhibition. These findings may be associated with the mechanism mentioned above with TRPV1 participation. Additionally, TRPV1 and TRPA1 receptor inhibition

Receptor	Ligand	Involvement in inflammation and edema	References
TRPV1	Capsaicin/Protons/Heat sensor	TRPV1 channel is involved in the release of the neuropeptide like substance P in sensory fibers Capsaicin administration showed painful effects in mouse paws, which were diminished by TRPV1 inhibitors TRPV1 increased intracellular Ca^{+2} concentration inducing the cytokines transcription such as IL-1β and TNF-α through the NF-kβ pathway In the endotoxin-induced lung injury model, TRPV1 reduced the pro-inflammatory cytokines levels	[113–116]
TRPV4	4α-Phorbol 12,13-didecanoate/ Osmotic sensor	TRPV4 activation in vascular endothelial cells caused an increase in vascular permeability. TRPV4 is sensitive to hypo-osmotic stress in chondrocytes	[117–119]
TRPA1	Allyl Isothiocyanate (AITC)/ Cold sensor	Like TRPV1 channels, TRPA1 acts on neuropeptides molecules regulation and nociception. TRPA1 induced edema in an acute inflammation model using AITC TRPA1 stimulation by AITC has been shown to influence the **COX-2** regulation in HEK 293 cells	[113, 116, 120]
TRPM8	Menthol/Eucalyptol/Cold sensor	TRPM8 channels inhibited edema and inflammation by decreasing pro-inflammatory cytokines (TNF-α and IL-1β) Menthol produced analgesic effects on inflammatory pain through the TRPM8 channel	[16, 121–123]

Table 5.
Transient receptors potential.

decreased pro-inflammatory cytokines levels, such as TNF-α, IL-1β, and IL-6 in an endotoxin-induced lung injury model [114]. Interestingly, Li et al. [115] demonstrated TRPV1 activation associated with NF-kβ phosphorylation through the intracellular Ca^{2+} influx. Based on this data, TRPV1 receptors play a critical role in the modulation of the pro-inflammatory cytokines.

Another notorious receptor involved in the low temperatures detection in conjunction with TRPA1 is the TRPM8 receptor. TRPM8 exhibits an essential role in neuropathic pain and anti-inflammatory effects [111]. TRPM8 is the most studied receptor in cold physiology. TRPM8 activation reverses the hyperalgesia caused by TRPV1 and TRPA1 stimuli [16]. Experiments using eucalyptol, a TRPM8 agonist, show promising results in reducing pro-inflammatory cytokines in paw edema [121]. Studies with cold therapy can have analgesic and anti-edema effects [122]. These findings make the TRPM8 receptor a target in this context.

3.6 Other receptors involved

A large quantity of plasma membrane receptors modulates the inflammation and immune response processes. In this work, we discuss the membrane receptor groups as therapeutic targets for inflammation and edema processes. The connection between the receptor systems is vast, and the response can vary according to the stimulus. Thus, other receptors can fit this context, such as cholinergic, dopaminergic, and adrenergic receptors. These are other examples of membrane receptors that can also be addressed in this context [126–128].

Additionally, bradykinin also promotes a role in vascular permeability. Bradykinin receptors divide into B1, and B2 (GPCRs) play a crucial role in edema pathogenesis [129, 130]. Further, cytokines receptors are also involved in inflammation mechanisms, such as IL-1 family and TNF-α receptor [131].

4. Therapeutic perspective of membrane receptors for inflammatory diseases

The inflammatory process (edema, cell migration, pain, and other) treatment mainly uses non-steroidal anti-inflammatory drugs (NSAIDs) and corticosteroids.

Receptor	Compound	Disease	Clinical study	Results	References
TLR4	NI-0101	Rheumatoid arthritis (RA)	Phase II	Insufficient therapeutic effects	[133]
HR4	JNJ-39758979	Asthma	Phase IIa	Potential in patients with eosinophilic inflammation	[134]
	Toreforant	RA	Phase IIa and IIb	No improvement in Phase IIb study	[135]
		Eosinophilic asthma	Phase IIa	No significant effects on the applied dose	[136]
	ZPL-3893787	Atopic dermatites (DA)	Phase IIa	Improvement in skin lesions	[137]
P2X7R	AZD9056	RA	Phase IIa and IIb	Insufficient therapeutic effects	[138]
		Crohn's disease (DC)	Phase IIa	Good effects in improving symptoms in moderate and severe DC	[139]
	CE-224.535	RA	Phase IIa	Insufficient therapeutic effects	[140]
TRPV1	JNJ-38893777	Not available	Phase I	Tolerable and safe for future investigations	[141]
	PAC-14028	DA	Phase IIb	Effectiveness for the treatment of mild and moderate AD	[142]

Table 6.
Receptor antagonist compounds highlighted in clinical trials for inflammatory diseases.

NSAIDs inhibit eicosanoid metabolites produced for the COX pathway, whereas corticosteroids are based on hormones released by the endocrine glands [132]. On the other hand, the more serious problem with these drugs is their prolonged use in treatments, presenting toxicity to organs. Based on this, the membrane receptors discussed in this chapter are promisor candidates for inflammation treatment. In addition, some classes possess agonists and antagonists commercially available among these receptors, such as 5-HT receptors and HRs.

Interestingly, clinical trials have already been realized and described in the literature concerning other membrane receptor types for reducing inflammatory diseases and their symptoms (**Table 6**). Therefore, we highlight four receptors discussed in this chapter with great potential in modulating the inflammation (TLR4, HR4, P2X7R, and TRPV1).

5. Conclusion

The inflammation field encompasses broad aspects, such as chemical mediators (cytokines, vasoactive amines, and lipid mediators), pain, and edema. The plasma membrane receptors influence on the inflammatory process is widely explored in scientific research. Concerning data discussed in this chapter, membrane receptors are promising and directly involved in the inflammatory mediators modulation in the edema and hyperalgesia pathophysiology. Thus, these new data open a horizon in the search for new pharmacological targets with anti-edema and analgesic effects in the therapeutic perspective of the inflammatory process.

Acknowledgements

We grateful the Coordination of Superior Level Staff Improvement (CAPES) – Finance Code 001, Oswaldo Cruz Institute (IOC), and Post-graduation of Sciences and Biotechnology PPBI), and Federal Fluminense University (UFF). This work was supported by CNPq (National Council of Research of Brazil) (RXF holds a grant with Fellowship Process Number 308755/2018-9), CP holds a grant from the Brazilian agency CNPq. FAPERJ (Research Support Foundation of the State of Rio de Janeiro) (JCNE (Young Scientist from Our State) with Fellowship process number E-26/203.246/2017) and Emergent Group of Research from Rio de Janeiro (E-26/211.025/2019).

Conflict of interest

The authors declare no conflict of interest.

Notes/thanks/other declarations.

Place any other declarations, such as "Notes", "Thanks", etc. in before the References section. Assign the appropriate heading.

Author details

Guilherme Teixeira* and Robson Faria
Laboratório de Avaliação e Promoção da Saúde Ambiental, Instituto Oswaldo Cruz (IOC), CEP, Rio de Janeiro Fiocruz, Brazil

*Address all correspondence to: gpegas67@gmail.com

References

[1] Barbosa Coelho E. Mecanismos de formação de edemas. Medicina. 2004. p. 189-98.

[2] Diskin CJ, Stokes TJ, Dansby LM, Carter TB, Radcliff L, Thomas SG. Towards an understanding of oedema. Br Med J. 1999;318:1610-3.

[3] Scallan J, Huxley VH, Korthuis RJ. Capillary Fluid Exchange: Regulation, Functions, and Pathology. San Rafael (CA): Morgan & Claypool Life Sciences; 2010. Chapter 4, Pathophysiology of Edema Formation.

[4] Lund T, Onarheim H, Reed RK. Pathogenesis of edema formation in burn injuries. World J Surg. 1992;16:2-9.

[5] Kao SJ, Yang FL, Ksu YH, Chen HI. Mechanism of fulminant pulmonary edema caused by enterovirus 71. Clin Infect Dis. 2004;38:1784-8.

[6] Hotamisligil GS. Inflammation and metabolic disorders. Nature. 2006;444: 860-7.

[7] Black PH. Stress and the inflammatory response: A review of neurogenic inflammation. Brain Behav Immun. 2002;16:622-53.

[8] White M. Mediators of inflammation and the inflammatory process. J Allergy Clin Immunol. 1999;103:S378-81.

[9] Williams TJ, Morley J. Prostaglandins as potentiators of increased vascular permeability in inflammation. Nature. 1973;246:215-7.

[10] Gordon S, Plüddemann A, Mukhopadhyay S. Plasma membrane receptors of tissue macrophages: functions and role in pathology. J Pathol. 2020;250:656-66.

[11] Bianchi ME. DAMPs, PAMPs and alarmins: all we need to know about danger. J Leukoc Biol. 2007;81:1-5.

[12] Creagh EM, O'Neill LAJ. TLRs, NLRs and RLRs: a trinity of pathogen sensors that co-operate in innate immunity. Trends Immunol. 2006;27:352-257.

[13] Burnstock G. P2X ion channel receptors and inflammation. Purinergic Signal. 2016;12:59-57.

[14] Burnstock G, Verkhratsky A. Receptors for Purines and Pyrimidines BT - Purinergic Signalling and the Nervous System. In: Burnstock G, Verkhratsky A, editors. Purinergic Signalling and the Nervous System [Internet]. Berlin, Heidelberg: Springer Berlin Heidelberg; 2012. p. 119-244.

[15] Bujak JK, Kosmala D, Szopa IM, Majchrzak K, Bednarczyk P. Inflammation, Cancer and Immunity—Implication of TRPV1 Channel. Front Oncol. 2019;9:1-16.

[16] Liu B, Fan L, Balakrishna S, Sui A, Morris JB, Jordt SE. TRPM8 is the principal mediator of menthol-induced analgesia of acute and inflammatory pain. Pain. 2013;154:2169-77.

[17] Fujiwara N, Kobayashi K. Macrophages in inflammation. Curr Drug Targets Inflamm Allergy. 2005;4:281-6.

[18] Lima RR, Costa AMR, Souza RD de, Gomes-Leal W. Inflamação em doenças neurodegenerativas. Rev Para Med. 2007;21:29-34.

[19] Majno G, Palade GE. Studies on inflammation. 1. The effect of histamine and serotonin on vascular permeability: an electron microscopic study. J Biophys Biochem Cytol. 1961;11:571-605.

[20] Abdulkhaleq LA, Assi MA, Abdullah R, Zamri-Saad M, Taufiq-Yap YH, Hezmee MNM. The crucial roles of inflammatory mediators in inflammation: A review. Vet World. 2018;11:627-35.

[21] Benly P. Role of histamine in acute inflammation. J Pharm Sci Res. 2015;7: 373-6.

[22] Claesson-Welsh L. Vascular permeability - The essentials. Ups J Med Sci. 2015;120:135-43.

[23] Liew PM, Yong YK. Role of vascular permeability and its signaling cascade in inflammation. Songklanakarin J. Sci. Technol. 2019;41:1204-10.

[24] Imamura T, Dubin A, Moore W, Tanaka R, Travis J. Induction of vascular permeability enhancement by human tryptase: Dependence on activation of prekallikrein and direct release of bradykinin from kininogens. Lab Investig. 1996;74:861-70.

[25] Oschatz C, Maas C, Lecher B, Jansen T, Björkqvist J, Tradler T, et al. Mast Cells Increase Vascular Permeability by Heparin-Initiated Bradykinin Formation In Vivo. Immunity. 2011;34: 258-68.

[26] Damerau B, Vogt W. Effect of hog anaphylatoxin (C5a) on vascular permeability and leukocyte emigration in vivo. Naunyn Schmiedebergs Arch Pharmacol. 1976;295:237-241.

[27] Jose PJ, Forrest MJ, Williams TJ. Human C5a des Arg increases vascular permeability. J Immunol. 1981;127: 2376-80.

[28] Sacks SH. Complement fragments C3a and C5a: The salt and pepper of the immune response. Eur J Immunol. 2010;40:668-70.

[29] Bossi F, Peerschke EI, Ghebrehiwet B, Tedesco F. Cross-talk between the complement and the kinin system in vascular permeability. Immunol Lett. 2011;140:7-13.

[30] Stamatovic SM, Dimitrijevic OB, Keep RF, Andjelkovic A V. Inflammation and brain edema: New insights into the role of chemokines and their receptors. Acta Neurochir Suppl. 2006;96:444-50.

[31] Martin S, Maruta K, Burkart V, Gillis S, Kolb *H. IL*-1 and IFN-gamma increase vascular permeability. Immunology. 1988;64:301-5.

[32] Ren K, Torres R. Role of interleukin-1β during pain and inflammation. Brain Res Rev. 2009;60:57-64.

[33] Dray A, Perkins M. Bradykinin and inflammatory pain. Trends Neurosci. 1993;16:99-104.

[34] Feng L, Xia Y, Garcia GE, Hwang D, Wilson CB. Involvement of reactive oxygen intermediates in cyclooxygenase-2 expression induced by interleukin-1, tumor necrosis factor-α, and lipopolysaccharide. J Clin Invest. 1995;95:1669-75.

[35] Okiji T, Morita I, Sunada I, Murota S. Involvement of arachidonic acid metabolites in increases in vascular permeability in experimental dental pulpal inflammation in the rat. Arch Oral Biol. 1989;34:523-8.

[36] Kawabata A. Prostaglandin E2 and pain - An update. Biol Pharm Bull. 2011;34:1170-3.

[37] Gracie JA, Robertson SE, McInnes IB. Interleukin-18. J Leukoc Biol. 2003;73: 213-24.

[38] Pilat D, Piotrowska A, Rojewska E, Jurga A, Ślusarczyk J, Makuch W, et al. Blockade of IL-18 signaling diminished neuropathic pain and enhanced the efficacy of morphine and buprenorphine. Mol Cell Neurosci. 2016;71:114-24.

[39] Nakamura K, Okamura H, Wada M, Nagata K, Tamura T. Endotoxin-induced serum factor that stimulates gamma interferon production. Infect Immun. 1989;57:590-5.

[40] Mehra VC, Ramgolam VS, Bender JR. Cytokines and

cardiovascular disease. J Leukoc Biol. 2005;78:805-18.

[41] Agostoni P, Cattadori G, Bianchi M, Wasserman K. Exercise-induced pulmonary edema in heart failure. Circulation. 2003;108:2666-71.

[42] Andreucci M, Federico S, Andreucci VE. Edema and acute renal failure. Semin Nephrol. 2001;21:251-6.

[43] Galea J, Armstrong J, Gadsdon P, Holden H, Francis SE, Holt CM. Interleukin-1 beta in coronary arteries of patients with ischemic heart disease. Arterioscler Thromb Vasc Biol. 1996;16:1000-6.

[44] Krüger-Genge A, Blocki A, Franke RP, Jung F. Vascular Endothelial Cell Biology: An Update. Int J Mol Sci. 2019;20:1-22.

[45] Sprague AH, Khalil RA. Inflammatory cytokines in vascular dysfunction and vascular disease. Biochem Pharmacol. 2009;78:539-52.

[46] Bolander FF. CHAPTER 7 - Membrane Receptors. In: Bolander FFBT-ME (Third E, editor. San Diego: Academic Press; 2004. p. 147-213.

[47] Takeda K, Kaisho T, Akira S. Toll-like receptors. Annu Rev Immunol. 2003;21:335-76.

[48] Moresco EM, LaVine D, Beutler B. Toll-like receptors. Curr Biol. 2011:12;21: R488-93.

[49] Nabar NR, Shi CS, Kehrl JH. Signaling by the Toll-Like Receptors Induces Autophagy Through Modification of Beclin 1: Molecular Mechanism. In: Immunology: Immunotoxicology, Immunopathology, and Immunotherapy. 2018. p. 75-84.

[50] Santos EGFBBDBDSVASJN Dos. Receptores Toll-Like : ativação e regulação da resposta imune Toll-Like Receptors : regulation of the immune responses. RGO - Rev Gaúcha Odontol. 2011;59:483-90.

[51] Li H, Yoon JH, Won HJ, Ji HS, Yuk HJ, Park KH, Park HY, Jeong TS. Isotrifoliol inhibits pro-inflammatory mediators by suppression of TLR/NF-κB and TLR/MAPK signaling in LPS-induced RAW264.7 cells. Int Immunopharmacol. 2017;45:110-119.

[52] Wang Y, Zhang S, Li H, Wang H, Zhang T, Hutchinson MR, Yin H, Wang X. Small-Molecule Modulators of Toll-like Receptors. Acc Chem Res. 2020;53:1046-1055.

[53] Shishido T, Nozaki N, Takahashi H, Arimoto T, Niizeki T, Koyama Y, Abe J, Takeishi Y, Kubota I. Central role of endogenous Toll-like receptor-2 activation in regulating inflammation, reactive oxygen species production, and subsequent neointimal formation after vascular injury. Biochem Biophys Res Commun. 2006;345:1446-53.

[54] Supajatura V, Ushio H, Nakao A, Akira S, Okumura K, Ra C, Ogawa H. Differential responses of mast cell Toll-like receptors 2 and 4 in allergy and innate immunity. J Clin Invest. 2002; 109:1351-9.

[55] Okada T, Lei L, Nishikawa H, Nakano F, Nakatsuka Y, Suzuki H. TAK-242, Toll-Like Receptor 4 Antagonist, Attenuates Brain Edema in Subarachnoid Hemorrhage Mice. Acta Neurochir Suppl. 2020;127:77-81.

[56] Jayakumar AR, Tong XY, Ruiz-Cordero R, Bregy A, Bethea JR, Bramlett HM, Norenberg MD. Activation of NF-κB mediates astrocyte swelling and brain edema in traumatic brain injury. J Neurotrauma. 2014 Jul;31: 1249-57.

[57] Rama Rao KV, Jayakumar AR, Norenberg MD. Brain edema in acute liver failure: mechanisms and concepts. Metab Brain Dis. 2014;29:927-36.

[58] Jayakumar AR, Tong XY, Ospel J, Norenberg MD. Role of cerebral endothelial cells in the astrocyte swelling and brain edema associated with acute hepatic encephalopathy. Neuroscience. 2012;218:305-16.

[59] Das N, Dewan V, Grace PM, Gunn RJ, Tamura R, Tzarum N, Watkins LR, Wilson IA, Yin H. HMGB1 Activates Proinflammatory Signaling via TLR5 Leading to Allodynia. Cell Rep. 2016;17:1128-1140.

[60] Jutel M, Akdis M, Akdis CA. Histamine, histamine receptors and their role in immune pathology. Clin Exp Allergy. 2009;39:1786-800.

[61] Obara I, Telezhkin V, Alrashdi I, Chazot PL. Histamine, histamine receptors, and neuropathic pain relief. Br J Pharmacol. 2020 Feb;177:580-599.

[62] Branco ACCC, Yoshikawa FSY, Pietrobon AJ, Sato MN. Role of Histamine in Modulating the Immune Response and Inflammation. Mediators Inflamm. 2018;2018:9524075.

[63] Beermann S, Bernhardt G, Seifert R, Buschauer A, Neumann D. Histamine H(1)- and H(4)-receptor signaling cooperatively regulate MAPK activation. Biochem Pharmacol. 2015;98:432-9.

[64] Elenkov IJ, Webster E, Papanicolaou DA, Fleisher TA, Chrousos GP, Wilder RL. Histamine potently suppresses human IL-12 and stimulates IL-10 production via H2 receptors. J Immunol. 1998;161:2586-93.

[65] Cannon KE, Leurs R, Hough LB. Activation of peripheral and spinal histamine H3 receptors inhibits formalin-induced inflammation and nociception, respectively. Pharmacol Biochem Behav. 2007;88:122-9.

[66] Coruzzi G, Adami M, Guaita E, de Esch IJ, Leurs R. Antiinflammatory and antinociceptive effects of the selective histamine H4-receptor antagonists JNJ7777120 and VUF6002 in a rat model of carrageenan-induced acute inflammation. Eur J Pharmacol. 2007;563: 240-4.

[67] Hsieh GC, Chandran P, Salyers AK, Pai M, Zhu CZ, Wensink EJ, Witte DG, Miller TR, Mikusa JP, Baker SJ, Wetter JM, Marsh KC, Hancock AA, Cowart MD, Esbenshade TA, Brioni JD, Honore P. H4 receptor antagonism exhibits anti-nociceptive effects in inflammatory and neuropathic pain models in rats. Pharmacol Biochem Behav. 2010;95:41-50.

[68] O'Mahony L, Akdis M, Akdis CA. Regulation of the immune response and inflammation by histamine and histamine receptors. J Allergy Clin Immunol. 2011 Dec;128:1153-62.

[69] Delaunois A, Gustin P, Garbarg M, Ansay M. Modulation of acetylcholine, capsaicin and substance P effects by histamine H3 receptors in isolated perfused rabbit lungs. Eur J Pharmacol. 1995;277:243-50.

[70] Räntfors J, Cassuto J. Role of histamine receptors in the regulation of edema and circulation postburn. Burns. 2003;29:769-77.

[71] Mohammad-Zadeh LF, Moses L, Gwaltney-Brant SM. Serotonin: a review. J Vet Pharmacol Ther. 2008;31:187-99.

[72] Sommer C. Serotonin in pain and analgesia: actions in the periphery. Mol Neurobiol. 2004;30:117-25.

[73] Cole HW, Brown CE, Magee DE, Magee C, Roudebush RE, Bryant HU. Serotonin-induced paw edema in the rat: pharmacological profile. Gen Pharmacol. 1995;26:431-6.

[74] Nichols DE, Nichols CD. Serotonin receptors. Chem Rev. 2008;108:1614-41.

[75] Hou YW, Xiong P, Gu X, Huang X, Wang M, Wu J. Association of Serotonin

Receptors with Attention Deficit Hyperactivity Disorder: A Systematic Review and Meta-analysis. Curr Med Sci. 2018;38:538-551.

[76] Albayrak A, Halici Z, Cadirci E, Polat B, Karakus E, Bayir Y, Unal D, Atasoy M, Dogrul A. Inflammation and peripheral 5-HT7 receptors: the role of 5-HT7 receptors in carrageenan induced inflammation in rats. Eur J Pharmacol. 2013;715:270-9.

[77] Brenchat A, Zamanillo D, Hamon M, Romero L, Vela JM. Role of peripheral versus spinal 5-HT(7) receptors in the modulation of pain undersensitizing conditions. Eur J Pain. 2012;16:72-81.

[78] Nascimento EB Jr, Seniuk JG, Godin AM, Ferreira WC, Dutra MB, Oliveira AC, Bastos LF, Fiebich BL, Coelho MM. Peripheral 5-HT1B and 5-HT2A receptors mediate the nociceptive response induced by 5-hydroxytryptamine in mice. Pharmacol Biochem Behav. 2011;99:598-603.

[79] Nishiyama T. Acute effects of sarpogrelate, a 5-HT2A receptor antagonist on cytokine production in endotoxin shock model of rats. Eur J Pharmacol. 2009 Jul;614:122-7.

[80] Voronova IP, Khramova GM, Kulikova EA, Petrovskii DV, Bazovkina DV, Kulikov AV. 5-HT2A receptors control body temperature in mice during LPS-induced inflammation via regulation of NO production. Pharmacol Res. 2016;103:123-31.

[81] Kajekar R, Gupta P, Shepperson NB, Brain SD. Effect of a 5-HT1 receptor agonist, CP-122,288, on oedema formation induced by stimulation of the rat saphenous nerve. Br J Pharmacol. 1995;115:1-2.

[82] Daher JB, de Melo MD, Tonussi CR. Evidence for a spinal serotonergic control of the peripheral inflammation in the rat. Life Sci. 2005;76:2349-59.

[83] Yu B, Becnel J, Zerfaoui M, Rohatgi R, Boulares AH, Nichols CD. Serotonin 5-hydroxytryptamine(2A) receptor activation suppresses tumor necrosis factor-alpha-induced inflammation with extraordinary potency. J Pharmacol Exp Ther. 2008 Nov;327(2):316-23.

[84] Szabo A, Gogolak P, Koncz G, Foldvari Z, Pazmandi K, Miltner N, Poliska S, Bacsi A, Djurovic S, Rajnavolgyi E. Immunomodulatory capacity of the serotonin receptor 5-HT2B in a subset of human dendritic cells. Sci Rep. 2018;8:1765

[85] Mousavizadeh K, Rahimian R, Fakhfouri G, Aslani FS, Ghafourifar P. Anti-inflammatory effects of 5-HT receptor antagonist, tropisetron on experimental colitis in rats. Eur J Clin Invest. 2009;39:375-83.

[86] Eschalier A, Kayser V, Guilbaud G. Influence of a specific 5-HT3 antagonist on carrageenan-induced hyperalgesia in rats. Pain. 1989;36:249-255.

[87] Pineda-Farias JB, Barragán-Iglesias P, Valdivieso-Sánchez A, Rodríguez-Silverio J, Flores-Murrieta FJ, Granados-Soto V, Rocha-González HI. Spinal 5-HT4 and 5-HT6 receptors contribute to the maintenance of neuropathic pain in rats. Pharmacol Rep. 2017;69:916-923.

[88] Idzko M, Panther E, Stratz C, Müller T, Bayer H, Zissel G, Dürk T, Sorichter S, Di Virgilio F, Geissler M, Fiebich B, Herouy Y, Elsner P, Norgauer J, Ferrari D. The serotoninergic receptors of human dendritic cells: identification and coupling to cytokine release. J Immunol. 2004;172:6011-9.

[89] Liu QQ, Yao XX, Gao SH, Li R, Li BJ, Yang W, Cui RJ. Role of 5-HT receptors in neuropathic pain: potential therapeutic implications. Pharmacol Res. 2020;159:104949.

[90] Avila-Rojas SH, Velázquez-Lagunas I, Salinas-Abarca AB, Barragán-Iglesias P, Pineda-Farias JB, Granados-Soto V. Role of spinal 5-HT5A, and 5-HT1A/1B/1D, receptors in neuropathic pain induced by spinal nerve ligation in rats. Brain Res. 2015;1622: 377-85.

[91] Castañeda-Corral G, Rocha-González HI, Araiza-Saldaña CI, Ambriz-Tututi M, Vidal-Cantú GC, Granados-Soto V. Role of peripheral and spinal 5-HT6 receptors according to the rat formalin test. Neuroscience. 2009;162:444-52.

[92] Quintero-Villegas A, Valdés-Ferrer SI. Role of 5-HT7 receptors in the immune system in health and disease. Mol Med. 2019;26:2.

[93] Burnstock G. Pathophysiology and therapeutic potential of purinergic signaling. Pharmacol Rev. 2006;58:58-86.

[94] Trautmann A. Extracellular ATP in the immune system: more than just a "danger signal". Sci Signal. 2009;2:pe6.

[95] Alves LA, Ferreira LB, Pacheco PF, Mendivelso EAC, Teixeira PCN, Faria RX. Pore forming channels as a drug delivery system for photodynamic therapy in cancer associated with nanoscintillators. Oncotarget. 2018;9:25342-25354.

[96] Di Virgilio F, Dal Ben D, Sarti AC, Giuliani AL, Falzoni S. The P2X7 Receptor in Infection and Inflammation. Immunity. 2017;47:15-31.

[97] Gonzaga DT, Oliveira FH, Salles JP, Bello ML, Rodrigues CR, Castro HC, et al. Synthesis, biological evaluation and molecular modeling studies of new thiadiazole derivatives as potent P2X7 receptor inhibitors. Front Chem. 2019;7: 1-15.

[98] Dell'Antonio G, Quattrini A, Dal Cin E, Fulgenzi A, Ferrero ME. Relief of inflammatory pain in rats by local use of the selective P2X7 ATP receptor inhibitor, oxidized ATP. Arthritis Rheum. 2002;46:3378-85.

[99] Chen K, Zhang J, Zhang W, Zhang J, Yang J, Li K, He Y. ATP-P2X4 signaling mediates NLRP3 inflammasome activation: a novel pathway of diabetic nephropathy. Int J Biochem Cell Biol. 2013;45:932-43.

[100] Satoh A, Shimosegawa T, Satoh K, Ito H, Kohno Y, Masamune A, Fujita M, Toyota T. Activation of adenosine A1-receptor pathway induces edema formation in the pancreas of rats. Gastroenterology. 2000;119:829-36.

[101] Effendi WI, Nagano T, Kobayashi K, Nishimura Y. Focusing on Adenosine Receptors as a Potential Targeted Therapy in Human Diseases. Cells. 2020;9:785.

[102] Sawynok J, Zarrindast MR, Reid AR, Doak GJ. Adenosine A3 receptor activation produces nociceptive behaviour and edema by release of histamine and 5-hydroxytryptamine. Eur J Pharmacol. 1997;333:1-7.

[103] Chen Z, Janes K, Chen C, Doyle T, Bryant L, Tosh DK, Jacobson KA, Salvemini D. Controlling murine and rat chronic pain through A3 adenosine receptor activation. FASEB J. 2012;26: 1855-65.

[104] Ulmann L, Hirbec H, Rassendren F. P2X4 receptors mediate PGE2 release by tissue-resident macrophages and initiate inflammatory pain. EMBO J. 2010;29: 2290-300.

[105] Barberà-Cremades M, Baroja-Mazo A, Gomez AI, Machado F, Di Virgilio F, Pelegrín P. P2X7 receptor-stimulation causes fever via PGE2 and IL-1β release. FASEB J. 2012;26:2951-62.

[106] Chiao CW, Tostes RC, Webb RC. P2X7 receptor activation amplifies lipopolysaccharide-induced vascular

hyporeactivity via interleukin-1 beta release. J Pharmacol Exp Ther. 2008;326: 864-70.

[107] Eltzschig HK, Sitkovsky MV, Robson SC. Purinergic signaling during inflammation. N Engl J Med. 2012; 367:2322-33.

[108] Le Duc D, Schulz A, Lede V, Schulze A, ThorD, Brüser A, Schöneberg T. P2Y Receptors in Immune Response and Inflammation. Adv Immunol. 2017;136:85-121.

[109] Riegel AK, Faigle M, Zug S, Rosenberger P, Robaye B, Boeynaems JM, Idzko M, Eltzschig HK. Selective induction of endothelial P2Y6 nucleotide receptor promotes vascular inflammation. Blood. 2011;117:2548-55.

[110] Venkatachalam K, Montell C. TRP channels. Annu Rev Biochem. 2007;76: 387-417.

[111] Samanta A, Hughes TET, Moiseenkova-Bell VY. Transient receptor potential (TRP) channels. In: Subcellular Biochemistry. 2018. p. 141-65.

[112] Nilius B, Owsianik G. The transient receptor potential family of ion channels. Genome Biol. 2011;12:218.

[113] Aubdool AA, Brain SD. Neurovascular aspects of skin neurogenic inflammation. J Investig Dermatol Symp Proc. 2011;15:33-9.

[114] Liu Z, Wang P, Lu S, Guo R, Gao W, Tong H, Yin Y, Han X, Liu T, Chen X, Zhu MX, Yang Z. Liquiritin, a novel inhibitor of TRPV1 and TRPA1, protects against LPS-induced acute lung injury. Cell Calcium. 2020;88:102198.

[115] Li C, Bo L, Liu Q, Liu W, Chen X, Xu D, Jin F. Activation of TRPV1-dependent calcium oscillation exacerbates seawater inhalation-induced acute lung injury. Mol Med Rep. 2016;13:1989-98.

[116] Sałat K, Filipek B. Antinociceptive activity of transient receptor potential channel TRPV1, TRPA1, and TRPM8 antagonists in neurogenic and neuropathic pain models in mice. J Zhejiang Univ Sci B. 2015;16:167-78.

[117] Ferreira LGB, Faria RX. TRPing on the pore phenomenon: What do we know about transient receptor potential ion channel-related pore dilation up to now? Journal of Bioenergetics and Biomembranes. 2016;48:1-12

[118] Phan MN, Leddy HA, Votta BJ, Kumar S, Levy DS, Lipshutz DB, Lee SH, Liedtke W, Guilak F. Functional characterization of TRPV4 as an osmotically sensitive ion channel in porcine articular chondrocytes. Arthritis Rheum. 2009;60:3028-37.

[119] Peng S, Grace MS, Gondin AB, Retamal JS, Dill L, Darby W, Bunnett NW, Abogadie FC, Carbone SE, Tigani T, Davis TP, Poole DP, Veldhuis NA, McIntyre P. The transient receptor potential vanilloid 4 (TRPV4) ion channel mediates protease activated receptor 1 (PAR1)-induced vascular hyperpermeability. Lab Invest. 2020;100:1057-1067.

[120] Moilanen LJ, Laavola M, Kukkonen M, Korhonen R, Leppänen T, Högestätt ED, Zygmunt PM, Nieminen RM, Moilanen E. TRPA1 contributes to the acute inflammatory response and mediates carrageenan-induced paw edema in the mouse. Sci Rep. 2012;2:380.

[121] Caceres AI, Liu B, Jabba SV, Achanta S, Morris JB, Jordt SE. Transient Receptor Potential Cation Channel Subfamily M Member 8 channels mediate the anti-inflammatory effects of eucalyptol. Br J Pharmacol. 2017;174: 867-879.

[122] Wright B, Kronen PW, Lascelles D, Monteiro B, Murrell JC, Robertson S, Steagall PVM, Yamashita K. Ice therapy:

cool, current and complicated. J Small Anim Pract. 2020;61:267-271.

[123] Liu B, Fan L, Balakrishna S, Sui A, Morris JB, Jordt SE. TRPM8 is the principal mediator of menthol-induced analgesia of acute and inflammatory pain.

[124] Frias B, Merighi A. Capsaicin, Nociception and Pain. Molecules. 2016;21:797.

[125] Hoffmeister C, Trevisan G, Rossato MF, de Oliveira SM, Gomez MV, Ferreira J. Role of TRPV1 in nociception and edema induced by monosodium urate crystals in rats. Pain. 2011;152: 1777-1788.

[126] Rosas-Ballina M, Tracey KJ. Cholinergic control of inflammation. J Intern Med. 2009;265:663-79.

[127] Beck GCh, Brinkkoetter P, Hanusch C, Schulte J, van Ackern K, van der Woude FJ, Yard BA. Clinical review: immunomodulatory effects of dopamine in general inflammation. Crit Care. 2004;8:485-91.

[128] Kolmus K, Tavernier J, Gerlo S. β2-Adrenergic receptors in immunity and inflammation: stressing NF-κB. Brain Behav Immun. 2015;45:297-310.

[129] Hall JM. Bradykinin receptors. Gen Pharmacol. 1997;28:1-6.

[130] Haddy FJ. The Mechanism of Bradykinin Edema. In: Sicuteri F., e Silva M.R., Back N. (eds) Bradykinin and Related Kinins. Advances in Experimental Medicine and Biology, vol 8. Springer, Boston, MA. 1970. p.283-289.

[131] Dinarello CA. The IL-1 family of cytokines and receptors in rheumatic diseases. Nat Rev Rheumatol. 2019;15: 612-632.

[132] Vane J, Botting R. Inflammation and the mechanism of action of anti-inflammatory drugs. FASEB J [Internet]. 1987;1:89-96.

[133] Monnet E, Choy EH, McInnes I, Kobakhidze T, de Graaf K, Jacqmin P, et al. Efficacy and safety of NI-0101, an anti-toll-like receptor 4 monoclonal antibody, in patients with rheumatoid arthritis after inadequate response to methotrexate: a phase II study. Ann Rheum Dis [Internet]. 2020;79:316—323.

[134] Kollmeier AP, Greenspan A, Xu XL, Silkoff PE, Barnathan ES, Loza MJ, et al. Phase 2a, randomized, double-blind, placebo-controlled, multicentre, parallel-group study of an H4R-antagonist (JNJ-39758979) in adults with uncontrolled asthma. Clin Exp Allergy [Internet]. 2018;48:957-69.

[135] Thurmond RL, Greenspan A, Radziszewski W, Xu XL, Miao Y, Chen B, et al. Toreforant, A Histamine H4 Receptor Antagonist, in Patients with Active Rheumatoid Arthritis Despite Methotrexate Therapy: Results of 2 Phase II Studies. J Rheumatol [Internet]. 2016;43:1637-42.

[136] Kollmeier AP, Barnathan ES, O'Brien C, Chen B, Xia Y (Karen), Zhou B, et al. A phase 2a study of toreforant, a histamine H4 receptor antagonist, in eosinophilic asthma. Ann Allergy, Asthma Immunol [Internet]. 2018 Nov 1;121:568-74.

[137] Werfel T, Layton G, Yeadon M, Whitlock L, Osterloh I, Jimenez P, et al. Efficacy and safety of the histamine H4 receptor antagonist ZPL-3893787 in patients with atopic dermatitis. J Allergy Clin Immunol [Internet]. 2019 May 1;143:1830-1837.e4.

[138] Keystone EC, Wang MM, Layton M, Hollis S, McInnes IB. Clinical evaluation of the efficacy of the P2X7 purinergic receptor antagonist AZD9056 on the signs and symptoms of rheumatoid arthritis in patients with active disease despite treatment with methotrexate or sulphasalazine. Ann Rheum Dis. 2012;71:1630-5.

[139] Eser A, Colombel J, Rutgeerts P, Vermeire S, Vogelsang H, Braddock M, et al. Safety and Efficacy of an Oral Inhibitor of the Purinergic Receptor P2X7 in Adult Patients with Moderately to Severely Active Crohn's Disease: A Randomized Placebo-controlled, Double-blind, Phase IIa Study. Inflamm Bowel Dis. 2015;21:224W_2253.

[140] Stock TC, Bloom BJ, Wei N, Ishaq S, Park W, Wang X, et al. Efficacy and safety of CE-224,535, an antagonist of P2X7 receptor, in treatment of patients with rheumatoid arthritis inadequately controlled by methotrexate. J Rheumatol. 2012;39:720-7

[141] anitpisitkul P, Mayorga A, Shalayda K, De Meulder M, Romano G, Jun C, et al. Safety, Tolerability and Pharmacokinetic and Pharmacodynamic Learnings from a Double-Blind, Randomized, Placebo-Controlled, Sequential Group First-in-Human Study of the TRPV1 Antagonist, JNJ-38893777, in Healthy Men. Clin Drug Investig [Internet]. 2015;35: 353—363.

[142] Lee YW, Won C-H, Jung K, Nam H-J, Choi G, Park Y-H, et al. Efficacy and safety of PAC-14028 cream - a novel, topical, nonsteroidal, selective TRPV1 antagonist in patients with mild-to-moderate atopic dermatitis: a phase IIb randomized trial. Br J Dermatol [Internet]. 2019;180:1030—1038.

Chapter 15

Intestinal Barrier Dysfunction, Bacterial Translocation and Inflammation: Deathly Triad in Sepsis

Bercis Imge Ucar and Gulberk Ucar

Abstract

Sepsis, as a complex entity, comprises multiple pathophysiological mechanisms which bring about high morbidity and mortality. The previous studies showed that the gastrointestinal tract is damaged during sepsis, and its main symptoms include increased permeability, bacterial translocation (BT), and malabsorption. BT is the invasion of indigenous intestinal bacteria via the gut mucosa to other tissues. It occurs in pathological conditions such as disruption of the intestine's ecological balance and mucosal barrier permeability, immunosuppression, and oxidative stress through transcellular/paracellular pathways and initiate an excessive systemic inflammatory response. Thereby, recent clinical and preclinical studies focus on the association between sepsis and intestinal barrier dysfunction. This chapter overviews the current knowledge about the molecular basis of BT of the intestine, its role in the progress of sepsis, detection of BT, and actual therapeutic approaches.

Keywords: bacterial translocation, intestinal barrier, inflammation, sepsis, multiple organ failure

1. Introduction

Sepsis has been announced to be a global health priority by the World Health Organization as in 2017, 48.9 million sepsis cases and 11 million sepsis-related deaths were reported worldwide [1, 2]. However, although significant progress has been made regarding the mechanism of sepsis, treatment modalities still have not gone beyond fluid resuscitation, vasopressors, antibiotics, and palliative care, after all [1, 3].

Sepsis is a perilous condition caused by the dysregulated and hyperactive host response to the pathogen. This response leads to an inflammation out of control and eventually multiple organ dysfunction syndrome (MODS), which is the primary cause of sepsis-related deaths. The propulsive force of the severe consequences of sepsis, such as MODS, is the intestines due to its potential to provoke systemic immune response via the injured intestinal epithelia losing its barrier function, and cannot prevent the pathogens and toxins to confined intraluminally and secreting and releasing the pro-inflammatory cytokines into the circulation [1, 3–9]. In this chapter, we aimed to cover the fate of the intestinal barrier (IB) and bacterial translocation (BT) during sepsis along with diagnostic methods and potential therapeutic options for IB dysfunction in the light of this information.

2. Structure and functions of the IB

The mammalian IB is responsible for fulfilling two primary tasks: to absorb the ingested nutrients and to prevent the microorganisms, toxins, allergens, as well as luminal pro-inflammatory factors from passing through the luminal surface of the intestines into the circulatory system [6, 10–13].

The gastrointestinal tract, which consists of the mouth, esophagus, stomach, small and large intestines, calls for a single layer epithelial lining with its partners in crime, such as cells of innate and adaptive immune system, forming a multifunctional system to fulfill its barrier function [11].

In the name of intestinal homeostasis, "some" (capital S should be replaced with lowercase "s". ome of the complex functions should be performed alongside the absorption of the nutrients like to prevent the trespassing of the pathogens, toxins, or allergens limiting the pathogenic bacterial growth to maintain the balance of the luminal microbiota, detoxification of the endotoxins, and immune response on demand as it is the largest lymphoid organ of the body by a multilayer morpho-functional barrier [9, 14] (for a recent review, *see* reference [13]).

2.1 First line of defense: commensal microbiota as the biological barrier

Human beings are in a symbiotic relationship with millions of bacteria, fungi, and viruses colonized in our gastrointestinal tract [12, 15, 16]. This host-commensal relationship, which starts at birth, even in-utero [17–19], maintains the intestinal homeostasis as a biological barrier and responsible for the differentiation, growth, and integrity of the intestinal epithelium [12, 15, 16]. Most of the species of commensal bacteria are obligate anaerobes, and the rest are facultative anaerobes and aerobic bacteria (**Table 1**) [16, 20]. The majority of the anaerobic bacteria are found in the colon as the oxygen tension is relatively low, whereas the aerobic bacteria are prone to reside in the small intestines [21]. The bacterial population in the proximal small intestines and the colon are around 10^4 ml^{-1} and ~10^7 ml^{-1}, respectively [22].

These coexisting symbiotic bacteria demonstrate immunologic and metabolic functions and protect the intestines from pathogenic bacteria growth via alimentary competition and colonization suppression. They help ferment and digest carbohydrates and synthesize vitamin B and K, along with short-chain fatty acids, which will then become the energy source for the intestinal epithelium. They are also responsible for the deconjugation of bile acids which will then reenter the enterohepatic circulation [12, 16].

Obligate anaerobes	Facultative anaerobes
Bifidobacterium	*Lactobacillus*
Clostridium	*Bacillus*
Eubacterium	*Streptococcus*
Bacteroides	*Staphylococcus*
Fusobacterium	*Escherichia coli*
Peptococcus	*Klebsiella*
Peptostreptococcus	*Pseudomonas aeruginosa*

Table 1.
The intestinal microbiota: Most common commensal anaerobic bacteria species in the human intestines (95% of them are obligate and 5% are facultative anaerobes) [16].

The intestinal immune system is modulated via the collaboration between the gut microbiota with the adaptive and innate immune systems, which is carried out by interacting pathogen-associated molecular patterns (PAMPs) with the specific receptors in the intestinal immune cells [12, 16].

2.2 Second line of defense: intestinal alkaline phosphatase (IAP)

IAP, one of four of the human alkaline phosphatase family, is an intestinal epithelial cell-derived enzyme constantly staying active intraluminally and in the mucosal lining to ease the gut's inflammatory response triggered by PAMPs. This way, it regulates the pH balance of the duodenal surface via bicarbonate secretion, helps the absorption of the long-chain fatty acids, defends the brush border membrane against the members of the intestinal microbiota. IAP also dephosphorylates bacterial endotoxin lipopolysaccharide (LPS) and pro-inflammatory nucleotides. Hence, it prevents the inhibition of the commensal microorganisms, as they are affected by the excessive luminal ATP by removing the phosphate groups from adenosine di- and triphosphate. LPS, which causes a systemic immune response and septic shock, is located on the wall of gram-negative bacteria and shows these effects by binding to toll-like receptor 4 (TLR4) thanks to its Lipid A moiety. TLR4 is expressed both in myeloid-borne immune cells (dendritic cells (DCs), macrophages, and monocytes) and in non-immune cells (i.e., endothelial cells) [23]. When dephosphorylated Lipid A moiety binds to TLR4, LPS shifts to a TLR4 antagonist, diminishes the pro-inflammatory cytokines, and activates nuclear factor-kappa-B (NF-κB), thereby minimizing the inflammatory response. It was previously shown that even being exposed to a lethal dose of E.coli, 80% of the mice survived with the help of IAP treatment. Thus, it was concluded that microbiota dysbiosis, intestinal inflammatory response, and transmigration of bacteria are inevitable in the absence of IAP [5, 14, 24, 25].

2.3 Third line of defense: the mucous layer

The first layer of the mechanical barrier is the mucosal layer which comprises water (95%), soluble glycoproteins (1–10%), nucleic acids, electrolytes, and antibodies. Mucin, a highly glycated protein, is secreted by goblet cells (specialized epithelial cells located in the villi), and with the help of other secreted proteins, they organize into a coherent mucus layer [11, 14].

Bacteria are responsible for the degradation of the mucus, and the balance between the secretion and the erosion of this layer determines the functionality of the IB. It was previously shown that this highly glycated structure of mucin feeds commensal bacteria, such as *Akkermansia muciniphila*, which is a gram-negative bacteria and gets protection from the potential pathogenic growth in return [26]. A previous study, in which bacterial adherence was coherently found to be elevated in the intestinal epithelia of the Mucin 2−/− mice leading to mucosal barrier dysfunction [14].

The outer intestinal mucosal layer is much looser and thicker in comparison with the inner layer. Therefore, the inner layer restrains the transmigration of the bacteria as it is tightly attached to intestinal epithelia to block the direct contact between epithelial cells and the bacteria. Contrarily, the outer layer retains the commensal microbiota elements to eliminate the opportunistic activity of pathogenic bacteria. For that reason, consistent usage of pro- and prebiotic preparations is reported to boost the number of commensal microbiota in order to promote mucosal barrier function [14].

Besides, the anionic residues like sialic acid or sulfate groups at the N-terminal of the mucin glycoprotein promote convergence of the cationic immune molecules, which serve as a chemical defense mechanism [27].

2.4 Fourth line of defense: physical barrier composed of the intestinal epithelial layer and submucosal capillary endothelial cells

The second mechanical barrier is the polarized single layer of gut epithelial cells (enterocytes-responsible for the absorption, goblet-specialized in mucus production, enteroendocrine cells-responsible for the secretion of the intestinal hormones, Paneth cells-responsible for expressing the microbicidal proteins and peptides among other properties, and microfold cells (M cells)) besides submucosal capillary endothelial cells [21, 28, 29], which act as a selectively permeable interface allowing the transmigration of the essential nutrients, water, electrolytes, and immune factors, and preventing the transfer of luminal pathogenic microorganisms, antigens, and toxins to the circulatory system [4, 12–14, 30]. This feature of selectivity is coordinated by the paracellular pathway regulated by desmosomes, adherens junctions, and tight junctions (TJs), located at the apicolateral membrane junction, lateral membrane, and basolateral membrane, respectively, and the transepithelial pathway, which is maintained mainly by the selective transporters allowing the uptake of the nutrients [13, 14, 28, 31] (for a recent review about mechanobiology of TJs, see reference [32]).

2.5 Fifth line of defense: antibacterial peptides

Hence their vast Golgi and endoplasmic reticulum system Paneth cells known for their cytoplasmic eosinophilic granules, [33], which are exclusively found in the crypts of the small intestine and they the secretory cells of the intestinal mucosa specialized in the secretion of the antimicrobial peptides, which are crucial modulators of innate immunity, as well as with neuropeptides and hormones [14, 34].

α-defensin, a ubiquitous antimicrobial peptide found in the intestine, along with β-defensin, has bactericidal activity, particularly against both the gram-negative and gram-positive bacteria, and any disturbance in the existence of these peptides is shown to increase predisposition to inflammatory bowel disease [14, 34].

Apart from defensins, other antimicrobial proteins such as phospholipase A_2 and lysozyme are also secreted from Paneth cells in case of an interaction with bacteria or bacterial antigen [34].

Besides these Paneth cell-driven antimicrobial activities, immunoglobulin A (IgA), which is secreted by plasma immune cells through lamina propria (transcytosis) [5, 14, 35–37], also contribute to the fifth line of defense in the IB. IgA either binds directly to the potential pathogenic microorganism and toxins to counter the unwanted colonization or epithelial injury or binds and interacts with immune complexes within the lamina propria to clear out these complexes to soothe the systemic inflammatory responses [14]. It also pumps the already translocated bacteria and antigens in the lamina propria back into the lumen [38].

The previous experimental studies on the B cell-deficient mice (as the IgA secreting plasma cells are differentiated from B cells) and the polymeric immunoglobulin receptor (pIgR) knockout mice (as the transcytosis of IgA to the intestinal lumen is conducted by pIgR) noted intestinal inflammation due to faded IgA-operated adaptive immune response is seen in both mice groups [14, 39].

2.6 Sixth line of defense: immune barrier as “the largest lymphoid organ”

As the largest immunological organ [40], the gut’s innate and adaptive immune system is in continuous interaction with the biological barrier to prevent the conversion of intestinal microbiota into pathobiota. The immune barrier consists of different types of cells, which are members of the gut-associated lymphoid tissue (GALT) like intraepithelial lymphocytes (IELs), natural killer cells (NK cells), innate lymphoid cells (ILCs), mast cells, and M cells (**Table 2**) [9, 12, 41, 42].

Cell type	Location	Structure and functions
IELs	Within the intestinal epithelium (between intestinal lumen and lamina propria)	T cells specialized in destroying the transformed, damaged, necrotic, or infected intestinal epithelial cells with their cytotoxic activities regulate the growth and proliferation of the enterocytes. They directly contact the antigens, microbiota, and potential pathogens, and during this interaction, interleukin-15 (IL-15) activates IELs and causes them to express cytokines like IL-2, IL-4, IL-1 and interferon-gamma (IFNγ) excessively. Although IELs are mostly T cells, they possess unconventional properties compared to other T cells due to their unique location and tasks. These functions are usually in favor of the intestine as they react immediately to the pathogenic microorganism or antigen, block the initial attempt of trespassing and invasion, and inhibit unnecessary inflammatory reactions against innocuous antigens. Nevertheless, they may mistaken self-antigens from the pathogenic antigens in a chaotic inflammatory milieu and trigger a pathological autoimmune response. There are two types of IELs: "type a" (induced IELs) and "type b" (natural IELs). Type a (induced) IELs are either CD8αβ heterodimer (Major-Histocompatibility-Complex (MHC) class I-restricted) or CD4+ (MHC class II-restricted) T cells, which express an αβ T cell receptor (αβTCR). They arise from the naive T cells and are activated postthymically (in secondary lymph nodes). After contact with the peripheral antigen as a tissue-resident memory, T cells accumulate in the gut. Type b (natural) IELs are CD8αα homodimer-T cells (do not express CD8β), expressing either a γδTCR or an αβTCR, which are thymically derived and activated by the self-antigens (they can be detected in-utero) and migrate to intestinal epithelium for further differentiation. The adult human jejunum predominantly contains type a IELs expressing CD8αβ along with αβTCR, while the ileal and colonic IELs mainly express αβTCR without CD4 and CD8 expression. Also, IELs are recruited in the small intestines via interacting with E-cadherin through their hallmark marker CD103 (αE integrin).
M cells	Peyer's patches	M cells contact the luminal antigens via their irregular short microvilli located on the apical surface and translocate the pathogens to the lymphocytes, or the antigen-presenting cells (APCs) are carried out by the intraepithelial pockets under the basolateral surface, which provides acquired immunity via interaction between the CD4+ T cells and the presented peptide epitopes of the pathogens.
ILCs	Scattered both in the epithelium and the stroma	ILCs are the coordinators of mucosal immunity as they regulate other functions of the other cells that are part of innate and adaptive immunity, and they also secrete certain effector cytokines. These functions together serve to orchestrate the innate immune response during infection, tissue damage, and inflammation in order, so the gut homeostasis is maintained. Based on their cytokine production, they are classified into three groups: Type 1 ILCs (ILC1s): NK cells. They exclusively express IFNγ and no other Th-17 cell-associated cytokines. NK cells are widely in contact with the microorganisms or the microbial components due to their location, and they also interact with immune cells such as DCs, T cells, macrophages, and fibroblasts, and epithelial cells. Intestinal NK cells recruit peripheral NK cells via IFNγ production. Type 2 ILCs (ILC2s): Cells located in the lower respiratory system along with the gut and mesentery. They produce TH2-associated cytokines. Type 3 ILCs (ILC3s): Cells that produce Th-17 cytokines (IL-17 and IL-22; cytokines associated with gut inflammation and immunity to extracellular bacteria). Besides, DCs, modulated by the resident commensal bacteria, stimulate secretion of the antibacterial peptides from induced intestinal epithelial cells by activating ILC3s.

Table 2.
Intestinal immune cells: Different types of the cells of "the largest lymphoid organ" contribute to IB function [9, 12, 21, 41–46].

These cells reside in the intestinal mucosal lymphoid structures of GALT, including the intestinal epithelium, isolated lymphoid follicles (responsible for the local IgA response), and mesenteric lymph nodes the lamina propria and Peyer's patches (5–10% of the follicle-associated epithelial cells) [21, 43, 44, 47] (for a recent review, *see* reference [48]).

ILCs, innate lymphoid cells; ILEs, intraepithelial lymphocytes; M cells, microfold cells; NK, natural killer; Th-17 cell, T helper-17 cell.

3. Mechanism of IB dysfunction in sepsis

All of the aforementioned layers of the IB are the sole protectors of the body, acting as a barrier between 40 trillion luminal microorganisms [49] and the body. Thus they carry a heavy burden in terms of maintaining intestinal homeostasis. Therefore, luminal content should be deliberately compartmentalized, and filtered selectively via preserving intestinal integrity, otherwise increased gut permeability provokes the activation of mucosal immunity via promoting BT along with translocating endotoxins and other pro-inflammatory antigens from lumen to the circulation [3, 5, 9, 14]. This catastrophic cascade can be seen during any infection or any incident triggering local and systemic inflammatory response generating impairment of IB integrity such as sepsis, shock, trauma, abdominothoracic vascular surgery, transplantation, severe burn, and intestinal/mesenteric ischemia and reperfusion [50–52].

3.1 BT

The concept of BT was first described in 1966 [53] and further expanded in 1979 [54] as the transportation of indigenous bacteria through the intestinal wall into the mesenteric lymph nodes and other sterile organs. Translocation of PAMPs, which are small molecular motifs (i.e., LPS, peptidoglycan, and bacterial DNA) located in the microorganism, are added to this definition later on [12]. The mechanism behind the BT are diverse.

3.1.1 Imbalance of the intestinal flora

Intestinal microbiota can be affected by diverse factors, including gastrointestinal secretions, antibiotics, secreted IgA (sIgA), bile salts, and peristalsis of the intestines. Overgrowth of the microbiota upsets the protective features of the beneficial intestinal bacteria and disrupts the first line of defense of the IB resulting in BT.

3.1.2 Dysfunction of mucosal immune function

Under physiological conditions, IgA secreted by the plasma cells has a feature of encapsulation of bacteria to prevent their trespassing and encapsulation of viruses invading the cells. It also has features enhancing the effects of lysozyme and complements. However, pathological processes inhibit the functionality of IgA, including encapsulation ability, as well as their concentration via a declined number of plasma cells secreting the IgA. This will eventually cause BT.

3.1.3 Increased intestinal permeability

Pathological processes such as conditions causing immunocompromisation or immunosuppression, MODS, severe burn injury generate BT via overgrowth of intestinal microbiota, immune dysfunction of the body together with the physical intestinal injury, particularly in the mucosal barrier. Oxygen depletion (caused by shock, mesenteric ischemia, cardiovascular surgery, transplant surgery) [50], acidosis, nitric oxide (NO), as exaggerated NO production by inducible NO synthase (iNOS) disturbs mitochondrial functions and cellular respiration, resulting in decreased ATP synthesis and accelerated apoptosis which causes mucosal injury, inflammatory mediators (IFN-γ, IL-4, tumor necrosis factor-α (TNF-α), platelet-activating factor (PAF), reactive oxygen species (ROS)) and endotoxins (causes edema in the submucosa, decreases the intestinal blood flow, villi necrosis) are primary factors in charge of the injured intestinal mucosal barrier and increase the intestinal permeability and BT consequently [38].

3.2 Who is the victim? Who is the criminal?

Sepsis is a hazardous organ dysfunction with high mortality and morbidity rate. The main characteristic of sepsis is "dysregulated host response to infection" [55], which will eventually bring about microvascular injury, problematic perfusion, cellular hypoxia, and finally, shock [2–5, 15].

Intestines are usually referred to as the "star of the show" during sepsis as they are accused of causing MODS [4, 7, 9, 12], yet sepsis (and septic shock) also disrupts the intestines by impairing the perfusion of the intestinal mucosa, epithelial edema, initiation of excessive apoptosis and necrosis of the gut epithelia [56], coagulation-associated local dysregulation, and cause hyperpermeability, microbiota transformation into pathobiota, BT and loss of absorptive functions [3].

3.2.1 Systemic inflammatory response

As an exaggerated inflammatory response is implicated in the pathophysiology of sepsis, involvement of inflammatory cells along with pro-inflammatory cytokines in this process is inevitable [2–5, 15, 55].

Upregulation of the adhesion molecules in the endothelial layer of the gut, induced by damage-associated molecular patterns (DAMPs) and PAMPs, leads to migration of the neutrophils, monocytes, and macrophages to the intestinal tissue. Pro-inflammatory cytokines released from these recruited cells initiate local and systemic inflammation [5, 14]. In addition, escalated activated macrophage infiltration into the artery walls inaugurates atherogenesis [14].

Besides, pattern recognition receptors (PRR) of PAMPs (including TLRs and NLRs) recognize the cell wall components of the bacteria via TLRs. TLR4 recognizes gram-negative bacteria, whereas TLR2 recognizes gram-positive bacteria. At this point, LPS-induced TLR4 activates signaling pathways either by activation of mitogen-activated protein kinase (MAPK) and NF-κB via MyD88-dependent signaling pathways or the TIR-domain-containing adapter-inducing IFN-β (TRIF)-dependent (MyD88-independent) by TLR4 endocytosis [23]. In the MyD88-dependent pathway, nuclear translocation of NF-κB encourages the transcription of pro-inflammatory genes such as IL-1 α/β, IL-6, IL-18, and TNF-α, whereas, in the TRIF-dependent pathway, nuclear translocation of IFN regulatory factor 3 (IRF3) promotes IFN-inducible genes and the type I IFNs [14, 23, 57].

TLR4 cannot bind LPS per se, needs a cofactor, CD14, which hands the LPS to TLR4 [14], and controls the LPS-induced endocytosis of TLR4 apart from the signaling pathways mentioned above [23, 58].

Although these reactions initially manifest as local inflammation, the process ultimately transforms into a "cytokine storm" [5, 14]. On the contrary, both the MyD88-dependent and TRIF-dependent signaling pathways produce pro- and anti-inflammatory mediators (IL-10) synchronously [23]. Thus, although it has been presumed that extinguishing the hyperinflammation is beneficial in septic patients, an overbalance of anti-inflammatory activity causes an inadequate response to primary infection and makes the patient prone to secondary infections [5, 59, 60].

Additionally, TLR4 manages intestinal cell turnover. During sepsis, elevated cytokine levels shift the balance between proliferation and apoptosis of the crypt and villus in favor of apoptosis and necrosis of the intestinal mucosa, which increases the intestinal permeability as a consequence of decreased villus height, increased release of DAMPs which feed the inflammatory process and brings about ulcer development along with hemorrhage and acceleration in intestinal impairment [4, 5, 56]. The elevated levels of pro-inflammatory cytokines are also shown to reduce the thickness of the mucus layer, the adherence of the mucus layer, and the luminal coverage [4, 52].

Besides, several studies reported that M cells located in the villi provide antigens a channel to mucosal lymphoid tissue, which is a trap where they encounter antigen-presenting cells (APCs). APCs present them with the help of MHC class II to CD4+T-cells [61]. In addition to that, DCs interact with T cells and B cells and selectively generate pro- and anti-inflammatory immune responses mostly through LPS-induced TLR-associated pathways (for a recent review, *see* reference [23]).

Inflammatory host response during sepsis may alter the layers of the IB and cause intestinal hyperpermeability and BT, and these alterations modulate the changes in the expression of the proteins of the TJs such as transmembrane proteins (occludin, junctional adhesion molecules, claudins) and peripheral proteins like zonula occludens-1 (ZO-1), which is in a relationship with actin-myosin complex of the cytoskeleton [11]. Furthermore, TNF-α, IL-6, and IL-1β levels can be elevated via activation of myosin light chain kinase (MLCK), an enzyme phosphorylating the myosin regulatory light chain and leading to hyperpermeability and create a positive feedback mechanism of MLCK activation through ZO-1 and occludin alterations. Aggravated systemic inflammation because of the increased permeability leads to a futile cycle [4].

3.2.2 Sepsis-induced self-digestion of the gut

Pancreatic enzymes are shown to cause multiple organ failure via autophagy [62]. Sepsis-induced ischemia of the gut exacerbates self-digestion and causes mucosal barrier damage leading to the release of DAMPs and pro-inflammatory cytokines from intestinal epithelial cells [5, 63].

Proteases, including pancreatic enzymes in the intestines, also activate the pro-metalloproteinases (MMPs) under ischemic conditions. Enzymatic activity of MMPs destructs intercellular junctions via proteolytic cleavage of junctional proteins' ectodomain, therefore increasing the intestinal permeability. Additionally, MMPs can digest the endothelial basal membrane [64].

Besides, LPS can induce expression of MMP7, and Paneth cells' degranulation, which promotes gut hyperpermeability, while MMP7 itself enhances local intestinal inflammation and intestinal damage via activation of α-defensin, subsequently stimulating the release of IL-6 from ileal epithelia and macrophages. Furthermore, it was previously confirmed that MMP7 and MMP13 are correlated with loss of intestinal integrity, inflated BT, and the development of multiple organ dysfunction [5].

After all, it has been reported in several studies that the inhibition of pancreatic enzymes protects the sepsis-induced intestinal autophagy and improves the overall progress [64, 65].

DOI: http://dx.doi.org/10.5772/intechopen.99554

3.2.3 Intestinal circulatory problems during sepsis

25% of the total cardiac output (up to 35% during digestion) is normally diverted to splanchnic vasculature [5]. Intestinal hypoperfusion can be caused by various reasons like mesenteric ischemia, abdominothoracic vascular surgery, shock, severe burns, transplantation surgery, necrotizing enterocolitis, sepsis, and septic shock [50], because of the redistribution of blood to protect the vital organs [38]. Intestines are highly sensitive to hypoperfusion as the enterocytes have the highest turnover rate among other fixed-cell populations in the body, with a lifespan of 2–6 days [3, 66]. Thus, hypoperfusion causes damage to the intestinal mucosal barrier [5]; moreover, the inflammation as a response to hypoperfusion caused by the ischemia/reperfusion further injures the intestines [3], resulting in loss of IB integrity, BT accompanied by systemic inflammatory response via release of pro-inflammatory cytokines [5, 50, 67].

In addition to that, vasodilation emerges as the pro-inflammatory cytokines (IFN-γ, TNF-α, IL-4, platelet-activating factor) affect vascular smooth musculature and endothelium, as well as capillary leakage, venous stasis, and ultimately diminished cardiac output, and hypoperfusion is seen [38, 68, 69]. Furthermore, compensatory mechanisms, such as the renin-angiotensin-aldosterone system, provokes the release of vasoconstriction and contribute to hypoperfusion. Also, regulatory features of the microvasculature (arterioles, venules, and capillaries) related to perfusion and oxygen distribution are lost due to sepsis-induced hyperinflammation and its inevitable outcome, ROS [38, 69–71].

3.2.4 Coagulopathy

Disseminated intravascular coagulation (DIC) is still an up-to-date challenge as of the significant lethal problems of sepsis. It is suggested that both intravascular and extravascular fibrin formation are seen in sepsis-associated DIC due to coagulation activation combined with fibrinolysis inhibition [72].

In sepsis, activation of coagulation is driven mainly by the tissue factor (TF) pathway, in which TF is derived from endothelial cells, monocytes, neutrophils, and liver, whereas suppression of fibrinolysis is coordinated by plasminogen activator inhibitor-1 (PAI-1) [5]. "Activation of coagulation": Neutrophil activation, caused either by direct contact with the pathogen or damaged cell- or bacteria-originated small molecules cause neutrophils initially to release a significant amount of TF [73, 74]. Later on, elastase is released from the neutrophils as well. Elastase has the ability to inhibit plasminogen together with the TF pathway, which is a crucial coagulation suppressor system [75, 76]. Neutrophil extracellular traps (NETs), which are released from neutrophils in order to trap and eliminate the microbes, also contribute to alterations in the coagulation via activation of Factor XII due to their negatively charged surfaces, fibrin formation, and competitively blocking the binding sites of tissue plasminogen activator (tPA) for clot degradation by fibrin cleavage [77–80] This explains the persevere on-going of the post-sepsis micro- and macro-thrombosis events [81]. "Inhibition of fibrinolysis": Sepsis-associated DIC differs from malignancy-associated one, since it is characterized by intensive suppression of fibrinolysis via overproduction of PAI-1, instead of the consumption of coagulation factors, od and differs from fibrinolytic phenotype DIC, as the consequential effects of this suppression in sepsis-associated DIC lead to tissue hypoperfusion resulted in organ dysfunction. Hence, the fibrin-related markers are not safe to use to assess the severity of sepsis as hypofibrinogenemia is uncommon [81, 82].

Besides, antibody-mediated action in the presence of pathogens can activate the complement system during sepsis. Coagulation system is also affected by the activated complement factors via generating an epithelial surface to facilitate clot formation. Activated C3 also activates platelets through the alternative pathway for stimulating aggregation, while activated C5 stimulates endothelial and inflammatory cells, inducing TF expression [83, 84]. In reverse, activated coagulation system can also impact the complement system. TCC production via activation of C5 is achieved by thrombin. Additionally, plasmin can also activate C3 and C5, forby other proteases of the coagulation cascade activate several complement factors like IXa, Xa, XIa, and XIIA [85]. These factors collectively disturb intestinal microcirculation and intestinal physiology and recruit the immune cells throughout the incidence of sepsis-associated DIC [5].

4. Diagnostic techniques

It is pretty challenging to diagnose or assess the IB function directly due to the invasiveness of intestinal tissue sampling. However, there are some methods or biomarkers that indirectly assess IB function. The measurement of biomarkers in urine, blood, or feces generally needs simple, non-invasive test methods.

4.1 Tissue culture methods

The tissue culture methods are based on the direct detection of intestinal bacteria in extraintestinal tissues. The mesenteric lymph nodes (MLN), extraintestinal tissues, swabs of the intestinal wall serosa or abdominal cavity, blood, and lymph are subjected to bacterial culture. Living bacteria are isolated, counted, and detected using microscopy. Direct detection has tremendous importance; however, many factors may interfere with the measurement [38]. For the culture of MLN, lymph nodes are suggested to be excised and be homogenized in saline. The homogenate can be inoculated onto Columbia blood agar and cysteine lactose electrolyte deficient media.

BT can also be measured by identifying intestinal bacteria from MLN, which is normally sterile [86]. For the culture of MLN, a lymph node from the mesentery of the terminal ileum is suggested to be excised at laparotomy and be homogenized in saline. Then, the homogenate can be inoculated onto Columbia blood agar and cysteine lactose electrolyte-free media.

4.2 Use of labeled bacteria

Radioactive tracers or plasmids are used to label bacteria for their in vivo detection. This method can detect the bacteria which is attached to intestinal mucosa-associated lymphoid tissue. However, this method can be used primarily in scientific research labs due to its cost and technical requirements.

Fluorescence and isotopes labeling methods are recently in use. PUC19 plasmid was constructed in the 1980s and was used extensively in molecular cloning and discrimination of gene recombination [87]. In this method, the plasmid vector carries the ampicillin resistance gene; the plasmid contains polyclonal restriction endonuclease sites, which discriminates against the positive bacteria. Thus, the PUC19 plasmid is introduced as an ideal tracer for demonstrating BT.

4.3 PCR techniques

Intestinal BT can be demonstrated by isolating bacterial DNA in patients' blood or body fluids and then amplifying and sequencing them. The PCR detection method is more sensitive, has a higher positive rate, and can specifically detect certain bacteria when compared to blood culture methods. PCR technic is also a valuable tool for detecting BT in patients with undetected infectious focus. The disadvantage of this method is that only the presence of bacterial debris can be detected, the viability and quantity of the bacteria cannot be determined, and drug sensitivity tests cannot be performed. The quantification of total bacterial 16S rDNA in plasma is used to assess human and animal systemic microbial translocation *in vivo* and thus is a great tool to study the role of systemic microbial products in disease pathogenesis and mucosal barrier function. The bacterial 16S rDNA assay can analyze 90% of bacterial strains, including Gram-positive and Gram-negative bacteria. However, the use of this assay is highly challenging because of its high technical demands and the risk of contamination [88].

4.4 Detection of endotoxin

Lipopolysaccharide (LPS), the integral component of the outer membrane of all gram-negative bacteria are shown to lead to BT. Since sepsis leads to intestinal submucosal edema and impairs the integrity of the mucosal barrier resulting in an imbalance of gut microflora and increased bacterial endotoxin-induced mucosal injury, endotoxin detection in the blood is a good marker of BT [38, 89].

Endotoxins can be detected in biological fluids by the Limulus amoebocyte lysate assay. Methods using fluorescence phage recombinant technology are also introduced [90].

4.5 Measurement of IB function

Several methods are used for the measurement and the evaluation of intestinal permeability and barrier function, such as the measurements of transepithelial resistance and assessment of macromolecular flux across isolated segments of GI tissue or colonic biopsies in Ussing chambers, measurement of permeability using fluorescein isothiocyanate (FITC)-dextran permeability in cell lines, morphological measurements of the TJ components, measurement of dilution potentials, and polyethylene glycol (PEG) profiling to assess the pore pathways [91, 92].

4.6 Intestinal permeability

Methods used to measure intestinal permeability are based on detecting the passage of the molecules across the intestinal epithelium. Several markers can be used alone or in combination to assess intestinal fluxes. Large molecules, lipophilic compounds, and nutrients generally prefer the transcellular route by passing through the intestinal epithelial cells by endocytosis, passive diffusion, or membrane transporters. On the other hand, ions and small hydrophilic molecules prefer the paracellular transport pathway. Thus, molecular size and structure are significant determinants of intestinal permeability [93].

Cell culture-based models using Caco-2 or HT-29 cell lines assess electrical resistance and intestinal flux in vivo. In contrast, differential urinary excretion tests with the use of chromium-labeled EDTA (51Cr-EDTA), polyethylene glycols (PEG), or non-metabolizable sugars such as lactulose and mannitol are frequently used to measure in vivo intestinal permeability [94]. Lactulose can cross the membrane via the paracellular pathway, while mannitol can easily cross the intestinal epithelium through transcellular and paracellular routes. Multi-sugar tests are offered to assess intestinal permeability simultaneously [28, 95]. Ovalbumin, horseradish peroxidase, dextrans, and fluorescently labeled microorganisms are used to measure the intestinal permeability in the blood [96]. Claudin protein levels can be measured in urine samples for intestinal TJ loss since claudins play a critical role in regulating the paracellular barrier pathway [97].

4.7 Urinary biomarkers

Markers of microbial translocation, inflammation (IL-6), and intestinal damage as well as fatty acid-binding proteins (FABP) and glutathione S-transferases (GSTs), which can be determined using ELISA technics, are suggested as significant biomarkers demonstrating intestinal epithelial cell damage. Fatty acid-binding proteins (FABPs) are small intracellularly or membrane-localized proteins released in the extracellular space in their soluble extracellularly from early after a cell or tissue damage. There are three main types of FABP. Liver-type FABP, intestinal-type FABP, and ileal FABP. During intestinal cell damage, intestinal-type FABP (I-FABP) is released from the enterocytes in the systemic circulation and excreted through the kidney [98]. Therefore, it has been suggested that I-FABP is an early biomarker to detect impairment of IB and injury in sepsis [99–101].

GSTs are cytosolic enzymes released when the cell membrane is damaged and play a crucial role in the detoxification of xenobiotics. Hence, α-GSTs are introduced as intestinal biomarkers [95].

4.8 Fecal biomarkers

Inflammatory molecules such as calprotectin in feces are proposed as a fecal biomarker reflecting the impaired IB function [102]. Calprotectin is a small protein in the leukocytes and is released in the lumen upon neutrophilic infiltration of the gut mucosa during inflammation and can be detected using ELISA technics.

5. Therapeutic options for the improvement of the IB dysfunction in sepsis

Although it has been known that BT is strongly associated with the progress of sepsis and septic morbidity, no decisive clinical therapy is proposed for the repair of the impaired IB and the treatment of sepsis [14]. However, some strategies such as modulation of the IB, inhibiting immoderate bacterial growth, regulating the effects of immune mediators, endotoxins, and NO, preventing oxidative stress, and improving intestinal ischemia and reperfusion injury were reported the severity of sepsis-associated BT [38].

5.1 Selective elimination of pathogenic bacteria

Removal of pathogenic bacteria, including gram-negative bacilli and symbiotic anaerobic bacteria, by the treatment with non-absorbed oral antibiotics such as polymyxin E, polymyxin B, amphotericin B, and tobramycin were suggested to reduce mortality [103, 104]. Although the treatment with non-absorbable antibiotics was believed to reduce the incidence of infection by pathogenic gram-negative bacteria and improve mortality rates, antibiotic resistance appeared as a limiting factor [105]. Since sepsis is an acute disease with high morbidity and mortality in intensive care units leads to intestinal flora disturbance, induces IB impairment, causes BT, systemic inflammation, and MODS; broad-spectrum antibiotics are frequently used in severe sepsis treatment [106]. Antibiotics are reported to affect the inflammatory process and ameliorate intestinal microcirculation in sepsis [107].

It was recently demonstrated that broad-spectrum antibiotics prevent BT to distant organs such as the liver and lungs in septic rats [108]. There is, however, evidence that broad-spectrum antibiotics can lead to an imbalance in the intestinal micro ecological environment, promote BT in sepsis, and cause drug resistance and pathogenicity, especially when MODS develops [109]. High-dose antibiotic therapy is also suggested to promote the translocation of native symbiotic bacteria and induce an inflammatory response, leading to late-onset sepsis [110]. It was concluded that metronidazole, an antibacterial and antiprotozoal drug used to treat giardiasis, anaerobic infections, and inflammatory bowel disease, reduces colonic bacterial counts and improves intestinal inflammation by suppressing cellular immunity [111]. Erythromycin was shown to increase gastric motility by affecting the motilin receptors in smooth muscle cells of the stomach, facilitating gastric emptying and decreasing the acidity and residual gastric fluid volume [112]. Treatment with antibiotic combinations (vancomycin, neomycin, and polymyxin b) prevented the translocation of intestinal bacteria to the pancreas by inhibiting the pancreatic NLRP3 pathway and inhibiting intestinal-pancreatic inflammatory responses [113].

5.2 Modulation of immune function and oxidative stress

During the attack of pathogenic bacteria, which destroys the IB or at decreased IAP conditions and increased LPS levels, the TJs are disintegrated. Macrophages are activated to produce pro-inflammatory cytokines, which also activate macrophages in circulation and cause the transportation of bacteria and LPS into the blood circulation [14, 114]. As previously mentioned, both the quantity and the functions of the secreted IgA diminish during pathological conditions [38]. Oral sIgA supplementation was shown to increase local sIgA levels in the intestine. Epithelial growth factor is suggested to promote the regeneration of intestinal mucosal epithelial cells, maintain the normal structure of intestinal mucosa, protect the intestinal mucosal immune barrier, and prevent BT [115]. Studies indicated that glutamine and growth hormone supplementations reduce intestinal BT and regulate inflammatory pathways [38].

Exogenous IAP administration was suggested to improve the IB function, while oral or enteral administration of IAP ameliorated the disintegrated IB [116, 117]. It was recently reported that high fat, Western-type diet-induced IB dysfunction, improved glucose intolerance, and orally administered IAP improved severe ulcerative colitis patients [118]. Since it was reported that anti-TNFα antibodies and inhibition of myosin light chain kinase (MLCK) prevented the impaired barrier function, treatment with these antibodies and inhibitors was suggested to reduce the severity of inflammatory bowel diseases. As IL-13 induces the disruption of barrier function by upregulation of claudin-2 expression, inhibition of IL-13 or claudin-2 seems to be proper targets for the treatment of BT [14]. The antimicrobial peptide cathelicidin-BF (C-BF) inhibited small IB dysfunction in the LPS-induced septic model in rodents [119].

Curcumin reduces the LPS/IL-1β-induced impairment of TJs [120], while berberine decreases the effects of LPS-mediated signaling through the Wnt/beta-catenin pathway to restore intestinal permeability in a rat model of sepsis [121]. It was suggested that cortisol reduces the expression of TJ proteins by alleviating the glucocorticoid receptor (GR) binding to the occludin and increases paracellular permeability and lubiprostone prevents stress-induced IB dysfunction [122]. A new GR agonist, 16α-hydroxytrametenolic acid (from edible mushrooms), is suggested to ameliorate the barrier dysfunction through PI3K/Akt/NF-κB signaling pathway [123]. Metformin is introduced to be beneficial for the protection of IB dysfunction by the inhibition of JNK activation through the AMPKα1-dependent signaling pathway [124]. Treatment with resveratrol increased the expression of sirtuin-1 in obese septic mice and decreased the inflammatory response. Sirtuins also play a significant role during the late onset of septic "hypo-inflammation"; SIRT-2 inhibition in obese septic mice preserved a decreased microvascular inflammation and protected against thrombotic events [125]. Tezosentan, a non-selective ETA and ETB receptor antagonist, improved intestinal microcirculation in intestinal ischemia–reperfusion injury by reversing the BT and cellular disintegrate of the intestinal mucosa [50]. Allopurinol, vitamin C, coenzyme A, Quercetin, *Ginkgo biloba* extract, and N-acetyl cysteine are suggested to inhibit ROS production, protect the cell membrane, and intestinal mucosa against ROS-related damage [38]. Rhubarb, the edible petioles of species and hybrids (culinary rhubarb) of Rheum in the family Polygonaceae, was shown to reduce intestinal BT and intestinal mucosal permeability through ROS scavenging and protection of the intestinal mucosa integrity [126]. Huoxue Jiedu Ling, a mixture of wormwood, *salvia miltiorrhiza*, white-headed weng, rhubarb, and licorice, is suggested to inhibit intestinal BT and reduces the oversecretion of cytokines by macrophages [127]. Shen-Fu Decoction (SFD), a traditional Chinese herb formulation, has been widely used to treat sepsis in China. A recent study showed that SFD significantly prevented intestine and liver damage, relieved sepsis-induced intestinal permeability and inflammation, ameliorated sepsis-induced impaired intestinal permeability by regulating the expression of ZO-1, Occludin, Claudin-1, and p-VASP [128].

5.3 Probiotics

The World Health Organization (WHO) describes *probiotics* as "live microorganisms which when administered in adequate amounts confer a health benefit on the host" [129]. The most known microorganisms used as probiotics are the Lactobacillus, Bifidobacterium genera, Enterococcus, Streptococcus, and Escherichia, which have been suggested to benefit some gastrointestinal disorders by ameliorating the gut microbiota ecosystem [130]. *Prebiotics* are non-digestible food component fibers selectively inducing the growth and activity of probiotic bacteria, and *synbiotics* are described as the mixtures of probiotics and prebiotics, which are expected to be more beneficial in many pathological conditions. These microecological regulators promote the intestinal flora by inhibiting the colonization of exogenous bacteria and excessive growth of endogenous pathogenic bacteria, maintaining the ecological balance in the intestine, and reducing BT [131]. In addition, it is believed that probiotics produce bacteriocins to kill pathogens, synthesize IgA and reduce inflammation by stimulating regulatory lymphocytes through interleukin (IL)-10 and transforming growth factor signaling [132]. It was reported that *Lactobacillus rhamnosus* GG pretreatment in a septic mouse model effectively reduced mortality, possibly by improving intestinal permeability and modulating microbiota dysbiosis [133]. Studies showed that supplementation of Bifidobacterium breve strain Yakult and *Lactobacillus casei* strain Shirota as probiotics and galactooligosaccharides as prebiotics reduced the incidence of infectious complications such as enteritis, pneumonia, and bacteremia in patients with severe SIRS compared to those who did not receive synbiotics [134]. Synbiotics are a potential treatment option for sepsis patients since the complications of enteritis, and ventilation-associated pneumonia was significantly decreased in the patients treated with synbiotics [135]. However, the application of probiotics on sepsis has been limited due to the theoretical risk of aggravating bacteremia in patients with critical illnesses [136].

5.4 Fecal microbiota transplantation

Clinical studies showed that sepsis is influenced by gut microbiota disruption [137]. Fecal microbiota transplantation (FMT) is the administration of fecal material from a healthy donor into a patient's intestinal tract with an altered gut microbiota to restore its functions. Randomized controlled trials showed that FMT is successfully applied in treating recurrent *C. difficile* infections. In addition, it helped restore bacterial communities in cecal crypts crucial in protecting intestinal stem cells, preserving immunological pathways by enhancing the expression of toll-like receptors and introduce the short-chain fatty acids, bile acids, eukaryotic, and prokaryotic viruses to the intestinal ecosystem [138, 139]. It has been postulated that if the symbiosis between the commensal bacteria and the human host becomes imbalanced, the innate and adaptive immune systems are disturbed [140]. Protective anaerobes are lost in fecal specimens with severe sepsis, indicating that pathobiota may dysregulate the immune system during sepsis [137]. Thus, FMT provides the restoration of intensive care unit-associated dysbiosis and intestinal decolonization of multidrug-resistant (MDR) organisms.

Furthermore, the introduction of symbiotic bacteria may decrease the antibiotic resistance genes present in the microbiome [139]. Treatment with FMT provides a complete reversal of dysbiosis, decreases the levels of inflammatory mediators, and normalizes T helper-(Th-)1/Th2 and Th1/Th17 ratios. However, since MDR is a leading cause of sepsis complications in intensive care unit patients, FMT has been evaluated in different case series. Results cannot be easily analyzed because of the high risk of bias in smaller studies, results of different studies cannot be conclusive because of different patient populations (with the most common organisms are carbapenem-resistant Enterobacteriaceae, vancomycin-resistant Enterococci, and extended-spectrum β-lactamase-producing bacteria, and Pseudomonas, methicillin-resistant *S. aureus*, and Acinetobacter [141].

6. Conclusion

Sepsis is a severe life-threatening organ dysfunction resulting from a systemic inflammatory response to infection. BT occurs more frequently in patients with intestinal obstruction, endogenous infections, endotoxemia, and impaired immune system, which is the cause of subsequent sepsis and ultimately leads to multiple organ dysfunction. The present chapter focused on sepsis-induced dysfunction of the IB leading to BT and multiple organ dysfunction. In addition, the underlying molecular mechanisms of BT in sepsis, diagnosis, and assessment of BT and therapeutic approaches were also discussed. Elucidating the factors affecting BT may lead to implementing interventions that contribute to improved patient outcomes. Unfortunately, there are no proven beneficial therapeutic options to prevent sepsis-induced BT yet; however, attempts at selective gut decontamination, the use of pre-or probiotics, new regimes for antibiotic prophylaxis, and fecal microbiota transplantation, to patient care will provide significant improvement for the treatment of sepsis.

Author details

Bercis Imge Ucar[1]* and Gulberk Ucar[2]

1 Department of General Surgery, Faculty of Medicine, Kutahya Health Sciences University, Kutahya, Turkey

2 Department of Biochemistry, Faculty of Pharmacy, Hacettepe University, Ankara, Turkey

*Address all correspondence to: bercis.imge@gmail

References

[1] Gai X, Wang H, Li Y, Zhao H, He C, Wang Z, Zhao H. Fecal microbiota transplantation reconstructs the gut microbiota of septic mice and protects the intestinal mucosal barrier. bioRxiv. 2020 Jan 1.

[2] Rudd KE, Johnson SC, Agesa KM, Shackelford KA, Tsoi D, Kievlan DR, Colombara DV, Ikuta KS, Kissoon N, Finfer S, Fleischmann-Struzek C. Global, regional, and national sepsis incidence and mortality, 1990-2017: analysis for the Global Burden of Disease Study. The Lancet. 2020 Jan 18;395(10219):200-11.

[3] Longhitano Y, Zanza C, Thangathurai D, Taurone S, Kozel D, Racca F, Audo A, Ravera E, Migneco A, Piccioni A, Franceschi F. Gut Alterations in Septic Patients: A Biochemical Literature Review. Reviews

[4] Sun J, Zhang J, Wang X, Ji F, Ronco C, Tian J, Yin Y. Gut-liver crosstalk in sepsis-induced liver injury. Critical Care. 2020 Dec;24(1):1-8.

[5] Haussner F, Chakraborty S, Halbgebauer R, Huber-Lang M. Challenge to the intestinal mucosa during sepsis. Frontiers in immunology. 2019 Apr 30;10:891

[6] Zheng D, Zhou H, Wang H, Zhu Y, Wu Y, Li Q, Li T, Liu L. Mesenchymal stem cell-derived microvesicles improve intestinal barrier function by restoring mitochondrial dynamic balance in sepsis rats. Stem Cell Research and Therapy. 2021 Dec;12(1):1-21.

[7] Appiah MG, Park EJ, Darkwah S, Kawamoto E, Akama Y, Gaowa A, Kalsan M, Ahmad S, Shimaoka M. Intestinal Epithelium-Derived Luminally Released Extracellular Vesicles in Sepsis Exhibit the Ability to Suppress TNF-a and IL-17A Expression in Mucosal Inflammation. International journal of molecular sciences. 2020 Jan;21(22):8445.

[8] Meng M, Klingensmith NJ, Liang Z, Lyons JD, Fay KT, Chen CW, Ford ML, Coopersmith CM. Regulators of intestinal epithelial migration in sepsis. Shock (Augusta, Ga.). 2019 Jan;51(1):88.

[9] Sun Y, Ford ML, Coopersmith CM. Gut Immunity–Homeostasis and Dysregulation in Sepsis. Journal of Translational Critical Care Medicine. 2019 Jul 1;1(3):89

[10] Hamad AA, Yaseen HA, Taylor-Robinson AW. Dissecting the Molecular Mechanisms of Intestinal Bacterial Translocation to Facilitate Definition of its Proposed Role in Systemic Sepsis. Iraqi Journal of Medical Sciences. 2014 Apr 1;12(2).

[11] Van Looveren K, Wallaeys C, Libert C. Potential of glucocorticoids to treat intestinal inflammation during sepsis. Current opinion in pharmacology. 2020 Aug 1;53:1-7.

[12] Assimakopoulos SF, Triantos C, Thomopoulos K, Fligou F, Maroulis I, Marangos M, Gogos CA. Gut-origin sepsis in the critically ill patient: pathophysiology and treatment. Infection. 2018 Dec;46(6):751-60.

[13] Thoo L, Noti M, Krebs P. Keep calm: the intestinal barrier at the interface of peace and war. Cell death and disease. 2019 Nov 7;10(11):1-3.

[14] Ghosh SS, Wang J, Yannie PJ, Ghosh S. Intestinal barrier dysfunction, LPS translocation, and disease development. Journal of the Endocrine Society. 2020 Feb;4(2):bvz039.

[15] Iacob S, Iacob DG. Infectious threats, the intestinal barrier, and its trojan horse: dysbiosis. Frontiers in microbiology. 2019 Aug 7;10:1676.

[16] Vaishnavi C. Translocation of gut flora and its role in sepsis. Indian journal of medical microbiology. 2013 Oct 1;31(4):334-42.

[17] Stras SF, Werner L, Toothaker JM, Olaloye OO, Oldham AL, McCourt CC, Lee YN, Rechavi E, Shouval DS, Konnikova L. Maturation of the human intestinal immune system occurs early in fetal development. Developmental cell. 2019 Nov 4;51(3):357-73.

[18] Park JE, Jardine L, Gottgens B, Teichmann SA, Haniffa M. Prenatal development of human immunity. Science. 2020 May 8;368(6491): 600-3.

[19] Li Y, Toothaker JM, Ben-Simon S, Ozeri L, Schweitzer R, McCourt BT, McCourt CC, Werner L, Snapper SB, Shouval DS, Khatib S. In utero human intestine harbors unique metabolome, including bacterial metabolites. JCI insight. 2020 Nov 5;5(21).)

[20] Chung H, Pamp SJ, Hill JA, Surana NK, Edelman SM, Troy EB, Reading NC, Villablanca EJ, Wang S, Mora JR, Umesaki Y. Gut immune maturation depends on colonization with a host-specific microbiota. Cell. 2012 Jun 22;149(7):1578-93.2 Jun 2

[21] Mowat AM, Agace WW. Regional specialization within the intestinal immune system. Nature Reviews Immunology. 2014 Oct;14(10):667-85.2;14

[22] Dethlefsen L, Eckburg PB, Bik EM, Relman DA. Assembly of the human intestinal microbiota. Trends in ecology and evolution. 2006 Sep 1;21(9):517-239(7):157

[23] Ciesielska A, Matyjek M, Kwiatkowska K. TLR4 and CD14 trafficking and its influence on LPS-induced pro-inflammatory signaling. Cellular and Molecular Life Sciences. 2020 Oct 15:1-29.8-

[24] Singh SB, Carroll-Portillo A, Coffman C, Ritz NL, Lin HC. Intestinal alkaline phosphatase exerts anti-inflammatory effects against lipopolysaccharide by inducing autophagy. Scientific reports. 2020 Feb 20;10(1):1-5.93

[25] Lallès JP. Intestinal alkaline phosphatase: novel functions and protective effects. Nutrition reviews. 2014 Feb 1;72(2):82-94.

[26] Reunanen J, Kainulainen V, Huuskonen L, Ottman N, Belzer C, Huhtinen H, de Vos WM, Satokari R. Akkermansia muciniphila adheres to enterocytes and strengthens the integrity of the epithelial cell layer. Applied and environmental microbiology. 2015 Jun 1;81(11): 3655-62.

[27] Pierre JF, Busch RA, Kudsk KA. The gastrointestinal immune system: implications for the surgical patient. Current problems in surgery. 2016 Jan;53(1):11.

[28] Vancamelbeke M, Vermeire S. The intestinal barrier: a fundamental role in health and disease. Expert review of gastroenterology and hepatology. 2017 Sep 2;11(9):821-34.

[29] Cramer JM, Thompson T, Geskin A, LaFramboise W, Lagasse E. Distinct human stem cell populations in small and large intestine. PloS one. 2015 Mar 9;10(3):e0118792.

[30] Abraham MN, Kelly AP, Brandwein AB, Fernandes TD, Leisman DE, Taylor MD, Brewer MR, Capone CA, Deutschman CS. Use of organ dysfunction as a primary outcome variable following cecal ligation and puncture: recommendations for future studies. Shock. 2020 Aug 1;54(2):168-82.

[31] Groschwitz KR, Hogan SP. Intestinal barrier function: molecular regulation

and disease pathogenesis. Journal of allergy and clinical immunology. 2009 Jul 1;124(1):3-20.

[32] Citi S. The mechanobiology of tight junctions. Biophysical reviews. 2019 Oct;11(5):783-93.

[33] Lehrer RI, Bevins CL, Ganz T. Defensins and other antimicrobial peptides and proteins. Mucosal immunology. 2005:95.

[34] Shroyer NF, Kocoshis SA. Anatomy and physiology of the small and large intestines. InPediatric Gastrointestinal and Liver Disease 2011 Jan 1 (pp. 324-336). WB Saunders.

[35] Hooper LV, Littman DR, Macpherson AJ. Interactions between the microbiota and the immune system. science. 2012 Jun 8;336(6086):1268-73.

[36] Macpherson AJ, Uhr T. Induction of protective IgA by intestinal dendritic cells carrying commensal bacteria. Science. 2004 Mar 12;303(5664):1662-5.

[37] Mach J, Hshieh T, Hsieh D, Grubbs N, Chervonsky A. Development of intestinal M cells. Immunological reviews. 2005 Aug;206(1):177-89.

[38] Wang YH. Current progress of research on intestinal bacterial translocation. Microbial Pathogenesis. 2021 Mar 1;152:104652.

[39] Johansen FE, Kaetzel CS. Regulation of the polymeric immunoglobulin receptor and IgA transport: new advances in environmental factors that stimulate pIgR expression and its role in mucosal immunity. Mucosal immunology. 2011 Nov;4(6):598-602.

[40] Gatt M. The role of the gut in sepsis. Surgery (Oxford). 2015 Nov 1;33(11):534-41.

[41] Zhang CX, Wang HY, Chen TX. Interactions between Intestinal Microflora/Probiotics and the Immune System. BioMed research international. 2019 Nov 20;2019.

[42] Cheroutre H, Lambolez F, Mucida D. The light and dark sides of intestinal intraepithelial lymphocytes. Nature Reviews Immunology. 2011 Jul;11(7):445-56.

[43] Shi N, Li N, Duan X, Niu H. Interaction between the gut microbiome and mucosal immune system. Military Medical Research. 2017 Dec;4(1):1-7.

[44] Montalban-Arques A, Chaparro M, Gisbert JP, Bernardo D. The innate immune system in the gastrointestinal tract: role of intraepithelial lymphocytes and lamina propria innate lymphoid cells in intestinal inflammation. Inflammatory bowel diseases. 2018 Jul 12;24(8):1649-59

[45] Albert-Bayo M, Paracuellos I, González-Castro AM, Rodríguez-Urrutia A, Rodríguez-Lagunas MJ, Alonso-Cotoner C, Santos J, Vicario M. Intestinal mucosal mast cells: key modulators of barrier function and homeostasis. Cells. 2019 Feb;8(2):135.

[46] Guan Q, Xiao C, Zhang M. Immune Regulatory Cells in Inflammation, Infection, Tumor, Metabolism, and Other Diseases 2019.

[47] Stahl MG, Belkind-Gerson J. Development of the gastrointestinal tract. In: Wyllie R, Hyams JS, Kay M, editors. Pediatric Gastrointestinal and Liver Disease. Elsevier; 2021. p. 2-10.e2.

[48] Kayisoglu Ö, Schlegel N, Bartfeld S. Gastrointestinal epithelial innate immunity—regionalization and organoids as new model. Journal of Molecular Medicine. 2021 Feb 4:1-4.

[49] Otani S, Coopersmith CM. Gut integrity in critical illness. Journal of intensive care. 2019 Dec;7(1):1-7.

[50] Ucar BI, Erikci A, Kosemehmetoglu K, Ozkul C, Iskit AB, Ucar G, Zeren S. Effects of endothelin receptor blockade and COX inhibition on intestinal I/R injury in a rat model: Experimental research. International Journal of Surgery. 2020 Nov 1;83:89-97.

[51] Farhadi A, Banan AL, Fields J, Keshavarzian AL. Intestinal barrier: an interface between health and disease. Journal of gastroenterology and hepatology. 2003 May;18(5):479-97.

[52] Chang M, Alsaigh T, Kistler EB, Schmid-Schönbein GW. Breakdown of mucin as barrier to digestive enzymes in the ischemic rat small intestine. PloS one. 2012 Jun 29;7(6):e40087.

[53] Wolochow H, Hildebrand GJ, Lamanna C. Translocation of Microorganisms across the Intestinal Wall of the Rat: Effect of Microbial Size and Concentration [with Discussion]. The Journal of infectious diseases. 1966 Oct 1;116(4):523-8.

[54] Berg RD, Garlington AW. Translocation of certain indigenous bacteria from the gastrointestinal tract to the mesenteric lymph nodes and other organs in a gnotobiotic mouse model. Infection and immunity. 1979 Feb;23(2):403-11.

[55] Singer M, Deutschman CS, Seymour CW, Shankar-Hari M, Annane D, Bauer M, Bellomo R, Bernard GR, Chiche JD, Coopersmith CM, Hotchkiss RS. The third international consensus definitions for sepsis and septic shock (Sepsis-3). Jama. 2016 Feb 23;315(8):801-10.

[56] Hotchkiss RS, Swanson PE, Freeman BD, Tinsley KW, Cobb JP, Matuschak GM, Buchman TG, Karl IE. Apoptotic cell death in patients with sepsis, shock, and multiple organ dysfunction. Critical care medicine. 1999 Jul 1;27(7):1230-51.

[57] Diamond CE, Khameneh HJ, Brough D, Mortellaro A. Novel Perspectives on Non-Canonical Inflammasome Activation. ImmunoTargets and therapy. 2015 Jul 24;4:131-41.

[58] Zanoni I, Ostuni R, Marek LR, Barresi S, Barbalat R, Barton GM, Granucci F, Kagan JC. CD14 controls the LPS-induced endocytosis of Toll-like receptor 4. Cell. 2011 Nov 11;147(4):868-80.

[59] Otto GP, Sossdorf M, Claus RA, Rödel J, Menge K, Reinhart K, Bauer M, Riedemann NC. The late phase of sepsis is characterized by an increased microbiological burden and death rate. Critical care. 2011 Aug;15(4):1-8.

[60] van Vught LA, Klouwenberg PM, Spitoni C, Scicluna BP, Wiewel MA, Horn J, Schultz MJ, Nürnberg P, Bonten MJ, Cremer OL, van der Poll T. Incidence, risk factors, and attributable mortality of secondary infections in the intensive care unit after admission for sepsis. Jama. 2016 Apr 12;315(14):1469-79.

[61] Wosen JE, Mukhopadhyay D, Macaubas C, Mellins ED. Epithelial MHC class II expression and its role in antigen presentation in the gastrointestinal and respiratory tracts. Frontiers in immunology. 2018 Sep 25;9:2144.

[62] Schmid-Schönbein GW, Hugli TE. A new hypothesis for microvascular inflammation in shock and multiorgan failure: self-digestion by pancreatic enzymes. Microcirculation. 2005 Jan 1;12(1):71-82.

[63] Peoc'h K, Nuzzo A, Guedj K, Paugam C, Corcos O. Diagnosis biomarkers in acute intestinal ischemic injury: so close, yet so far. Clinical Chemistry and Laboratory Medicine (CCLM). 2018 Mar 1;56(3):373-85.

[64] Altshuler AE, Kistler EB, Schmid-Schönbein GW. Autodigestion: proteolytic degradation and multiple organ failure in shock. Shock (Augusta, Ga.). 2016 May;45(5):483.

[65] DeLano FA, Hoyt DB, Schmid-Schönbein GW. Pancreatic digestive enzyme blockade in the intestine increases survival after experimental shock. Science translational medicine. 2013 Jan 23;5(169):169ra11-.

[66] Williams JM, Duckworth CA, Burkitt MD, Watson AJ, Campbell BJ, Pritchard DM. Epithelial cell shedding and barrier function: a matter of life and death at the small intestinal villus tip. Veterinary pathology. 2015 May;52(3):445-55.

[67] Deitch EA. Bacterial translocation or lymphatic drainage of toxic products from the gut: what is important in human beings?. Surgery. 2002 Mar 1;131(3):241-4.

[68] Morelli A, Passariello M. Hemodynamic coherence in sepsis. Best Practice and Research Clinical Anaesthesiology. 2016 Dec 1;30(4):453-63.

[69] Kumar V. Inflammasomes: Pandora's box for sepsis. Journal of inflammation research. 2018;11:477.

[70] Thorburn T, Aali M, Lehmann C. Immune response to systemic inflammation in the intestinal microcirculation. Front. Biosci. (Landmark Ed). 2018 Jan 1;23:782-95.

[71] Boisrame-Helms J, Kremer H, Schini-Kerth V, Meziani F. Endothelial dysfunction in sepsis. Current Vascular Pharmacology. 2013 Mar 1;11(2):150-60.

[72] Wang L, Bastarache JA, Ware LB. The coagulation cascade in sepsis. Current pharmaceutical design. 2008 Jul 1;14(19):1860-9.

[73] Nakamura S, Imamura T, Okamoto K. Tissue factor in neutrophils: yes. J Thromb Haemost. 2004;2(2): 214-7.

[74] Okamoto K, Tamura T, Sawatsubashi Y. Sepsis and disseminated intravascular coagulation. Journal of intensive care. 2016 Dec;4(1):1-8.

[75] Barrett CD, Moore HB, Banerjee A, Silliman CC, Moore EE, Yaffe MB. Human neutrophil elastase mediates fibrinolysis shutdown through competitive degradation of plasminogen and generation of angiostatin. The journal of trauma and acute care surgery. 2017 Dec;83(6):1053.

[76] Massberg S, Grahl L, von Bruehl ML, Manukyan D, Pfeiler S, Goosmann C, Brinkmann V, Lorenz M, Bidzhekov K, Khandagale AB, Konrad I. Reciprocal coupling of coagulation and innate immunity via neutrophil serine proteases. Nature medicine. 2010 Aug;16(8):887-96.

[77] Brinkmann V, Reichard U, Goosmann C, Fauler B, Uhlemann Y, Weiss DS, Weinrauch Y, Zychlinsky A. Neutrophil extracellular traps kill bacteria. science. 2004 Mar 5;303(5663):1532-5.

[78] Fuchs TA, Brill A, Wagner DD. Neutrophil extracellular trap (NET) impact on deep vein thrombosis. Arteriosclerosis, thrombosis, and vascular biology. 2012 Aug;32(8):1777-83.

[79] von Brühl ML, Stark K, Steinhart A, Chandraratne S, Konrad I, Lorenz M, Khandoga A, Tirniceriu A, Coletti R, Köllnberger M, Byrne RA. Monocytes, neutrophils, and platelets cooperate to initiate and propagate venous thrombosis in mice in vivo. Journal of Experimental Medicine. 2012 Apr 9;209(4):819-35.

[80] Fuchs TA, Brill A, Duerschmied D, Schatzberg D, Monestier M, Myers DD,

Wrobleski SK, Wakefield TW, Hartwig JH, Wagner DD. Extracellular DNA traps promote thrombosis. Proceedings of the National Academy of Sciences. 2010 Sep 7;107(36):15880-5.

[81] Samuels JM, Moore HB, Moore EE. Coagulopathy in severe sepsis: interconnectivity of coagulation and the immune system. Surgical infections. 2018 Feb 1;19(2):208-15.

[82] Iba T, Levy JH, Warkentin TE, Thachil J, van der Poll T, Levi M. Diagnosis and management of sepsis-induced coagulopathy and disseminated intravascular coagulation. Journal of thrombosis and haemostasis: JTH. 2019 Nov;17(11):1989-94.

[83] Kurosawa S, Stearns-Kurosawa DJ. Complement, thrombotic microangiopathy and disseminated intravascular coagulation. Journal of intensive care. 2014 Dec;2(1):1-8.

[84] Hamad OA, Bäck J, Nilsson PH, Nilsson B, Ekdahl KN. Platelets, complement, and contact activation: partners in inflammation and thrombosis. Current Topics in Innate Immunity II. 2012:185-205.

[85] Huber-Lang M, Sarma JV, Zetoune FS, Rittirsch D, Neff TA, McGuire SR, Lambris JD, Warner RL, Flierl MA, Hoesel LM, Gebhard F. Generation of C5a in the absence of C3: a new complement activation pathway. Nature medicine. 2006 Jun;12(6):682-7.

[86] Magnotti LJ, Upperman JS, Xu DZ, Lu Q, Deitch EA. Gut-derived mesenteric lymph but not portal blood increases endothelial cell permeability and promotes lung injury after hemorrhagic shock. Annals of surgery. 1998 Oct;228(4):518.

[87] Fu WL, Xiao GX, Yue XL, Hua C, Lei MP. Tracing method study of bacterial translocation in vivo. World journal of gastroenterology. 2000 Feb 15;6(1):153.

[88] Yokoyama Y, Fukaya M, Mizuno T, Ebata T, Asahara T, Nagino M. Clinical importance of "occult-bacterial translocation" in patients undergoing highly invasive gastrointestinal surgery: A review. Surgery Today. 2020 Aug 28:1-8.

[89] Vaishnavi C, Kochhar R, Kaur S, Singh G. Estimation of endotoxin in infected bile from patients with biliary diseases. Tropical gastroenterology: official journal of the Digestive Diseases Foundation. 2006 Jan 1;27(1):22-5.

[90] Su W, Ding X. Methods of endotoxin detection. Journal of laboratory automation. 2015 Aug;20(4):354-64.

[91] Galipeau HJ, Verdu EF. The complex task of measuring intestinal permeability in basic and clinical science. Neurogastroenterology and Motility. 2016 Jul;28(7):957-65.

[92] Camilleri Á, Madsen K, Spiller R, Van Meerveld BG, Verne GN. Intestinal barrier function in health and gastrointestinal disease. Neurogastroenterology and Motility. 2012 Jun;24(6):503-12.

[93] Farré R, Vicario M. Abnormal barrier function in gastrointestinal disorders. Gastrointestinal Pharmacology. 2016:193-217.

[94] Menard S, Cerf-Bensussan N, Heyman M. Multiple facets of intestinal permeability and epithelial handling of dietary antigens. Mucosal immunology. 2010 May;3(3):247-59.

[95] Grootjans J, Thuijls G, Verdam F, Derikx JP, Lenaerts K, Buurman WA. Non-invasive assessment of barrier integrity and function of the human gut. World Journal of Gastrointestinal Surgery. 2010 Mar 27;2(3):61.

[96] Stappaerts J, Brouwers J, Annaert P, Augustijns P. In situ perfusion in rodents to explore intestinal drug absorption: challenges and opportunities. International journal of pharmaceutics. 2015 Jan 30;478(2):665-81.

[97] Wu J, He C, Bu J, Luo Y, Yang S, Ye C, Yu S, He B, Yin Y, Yang X. Betaine attenuates LPS-induced downregulation of Occludin and Claudin-1 and restores intestinal barrier function. BMC veterinary research. 2020 Dec;16(1):1-8.

[98] Lau E, Marques C, Pestana D, Santoalha M, Carvalho D, Freitas P, Calhau C. The role of I-FABP as a biomarker of intestinal barrier dysfunction driven by gut microbiota changes in obesity. Nutrition and metabolism. 2016 Dec;13(1):1-7.

[99] Thuijls G, Derikx JP, van Wijck K, Zimmermann LJ, Degraeuwe PL, Mulder TL, Van der Zee DC, Brouwers HA, Verhoeven BH, van Heurn LE, Kramer BW. Non-invasive markers for early diagnosis and determination of the severity of necrotizing enterocolitis. Annals of surgery. 2010 Jun 1;251(6):1174-80.

[100] Sikora M, Stec A, Chrabaszcz M, Waskiel-Burnat A, Zaremba M, Olszewska M, Rudnicka L. Intestinal fatty acid binding protein, a biomarker of intestinal barrier, is associated with severity of psoriasis. Journal of clinical medicine. 2019 Jul;8(7):1021.

[101] Machado MC, Barbeiro HV, da Silva FP, de Souza HP. Circulating fatty acid binding protein as a marker of intestinal failure in septic patients. Critical Care. 2012 Dec;16(6):1-2.

[102] Ikhtaire S, Shajib MS, Reinisch W, Khan WI. Fecal calprotectin: its scope and utility in the management of inflammatory bowel disease. Journal of gastroenterology. 2016 May 1;51(5):434-46.

[103] Kell MR, Barry BD, Redmond HP. Systemic inflammatory response syndrome: a new direction?. Irish journal of medical science. 2003 Mar 1;172(1):7-8.

[104] De Rosa S, Cutuli SL, Ferrer R, Antonelli M, Ronco C. Polymyxin B hemoperfusion in COVID-19 Patients with endotoxic shock: Case Series from EUPHAS II registry. Artificial Organs. 2020 Dec 30.

[105] Oostdijk EA, de Smet AM, Blok HE, Thieme Groen ES, van Asselt GJ, Benus RF, Bernards SA, Frénay IH, Jansz AR, de Jongh BM, Kaan JA. Ecological effects of selective decontamination on resistant gram-negative bacterial colonization. American journal of respiratory and critical care medicine. 2010 Mar 1;181(5):452-7.

[106] Gotts JE, Matthay MA. Sepsis: pathophysiology and clinical management. Bmj. 2016 May 23;353.

[107] Al-Banna NA, Pavlovic D, Bac VH, Utpatel K, Janke E, Rippke JN, Borowiak M, Cerny V, Spassov A, Johnston B, Issekutz TB. Acute administration of antibiotics modulates intestinal capillary perfusion and leukocyte adherence during experimental sepsis. International journal of antimicrobial agents. 2013 Jun 1;41(6):536-43.

[108] Wen ZL, Zhang LD, Liu SZ, Liu J, Chen YZ, Chen DC. Effect of broad-spectrum antibiotics on bacterial translocation in burned or septic rats. Chinese medical journal. 2019 May 20;132(10):1179.

[109] Oostdijk EA, Kesecioglu J, Schultz MJ, Visser CE, De Jonge E, van Essen EH, Bernards AT, Purmer I, Brimicombe R, Bergmans D, van Tiel F. Notice of retraction and replacement: Oostdijk et al. effects of decontamination

of the oropharynx and intestinal tract on antibiotic resistance in ICUs: a randomized clinical trial. JAMA. 2014; 312 (14): 1429-1437. Jama. 2017 Apr 18;317(15):1583-4.

[110] Knoop KA, McDonald KG, Kulkarni DH, Newberry RD. Antibiotics promote inflammation through the translocation of native commensal colonic bacteria. Gut. 2016 Jul 1;65(7):1100-9.

[111] Bjarnason I, Hayllar J, Smethurst P, Price A, Gumpel MJ. Metronidazole reduces intestinal inflammation and blood loss in non-steroidal anti-inflammatory drug induced enteropathy. Gut. 1992 Sep 1;33(9):1204-8.

[112] Czarnetzki C, Elia N, Frossard JL, Giostra E, Spahr L, Waeber JL, Pavlovic G, Lysakowski C, Tramèr MR. Erythromycin for gastric emptying in patients undergoing general anesthesia for emergency surgery: a randomized clinical trial. JAMA surgery. 2015 Aug 1;150(8):730-7.

[113] Jia L, Chen H, Yang J, Fang X, Niu W, Zhang M, Li J, Pan X, Ren Z, Sun J, Pan LL. Combinatory antibiotic treatment protects against experimental acute pancreatitis by suppressing gut bacterial translocation to pancreas and inhibiting NLRP3 inflammasome pathway. Innate immunity. 2020 Jan;26(1):48-61.

[114] Bellot P, Francés R, Such J. Pathological bacterial translocation in cirrhosis: pathophysiology, diagnosis and clinical implications. Liver International. 2013 Jan;33(1):31-9.

[115] Hollander D, Kaunitz JD. The "Leaky Gut": Tight Junctions but Loose Associations?. Digestive diseases and sciences. 2020 May;65(5):1277.

[116] Kaliannan K, Hamarneh SR, Economopoulos KP, Alam SN, Moaven O, Patel P, Malo NS, Ray M, Abtahi SM, Muhammad N, Raychowdhury A. Intestinal alkaline phosphatase prevents metabolic syndrome in mice. Proceedings of the National Academy of Sciences. 2013 Apr 23;110(17):7003-8.

[117] Hamarneh SR, Kim BM, Kaliannan K, Morrison SA, Tantillo TJ, Tao Q, Mohamed MM, Ramirez JM, Karas A, Liu W, Hu D. Intestinal alkaline phosphatase attenuates alcohol-induced hepatosteatosis in mice. Digestive diseases and sciences. 2017 Aug;62(8):2021-34.

[118] Ghosh SS, He H, Wang J, Korzun W, Yannie PJ, Ghosh S. Intestine-specific expression of human chimeric intestinal alkaline phosphatase attenuates Western diet-induced barrier dysfunction and glucose intolerance. Physiological reports. 2018 Jul;6(14):e13790.

[119] Song D, Zong X, Zhang H, Wang T, Yi H, Luan C, Wang Y. Antimicrobial peptide Cathelicidin-BF prevents intestinal barrier dysfunction in a mouse model of endotoxemia. International immunopharmacology. 2015 Mar 1;25(1):141-7.

[120] Wang J, Ghosh SS, Ghosh S. Curcumin improves intestinal barrier function: modulation of intracellular signaling, and organization of tight junctions. American Journal of Physiology-Cell Physiology. 2017 Apr 1;312(4):C438-45.

[121] He Y, Yuan X, Zuo H, Sun Y, Feng A. Berberine exerts a protective effect on gut-vascular barrier via the modulation of the Wnt/beta-catenin signaling pathway during sepsis. Cellular Physiology and Biochemistry. 2018;49(4):1342-51.

[122] Zong Y, Zhu S, Zhang S, Zheng G, Wiley JW, Hong S. Chronic stress and intestinal permeability: Lubiprostone

regulates glucocorticoid receptor-mediated changes in colon epithelial tight junction proteins, barrier function, and visceral pain in the rodent and human. Neurogastroenterology and Motility. 2019 Feb;31(2):e13477.

[123] Xu H, Wang Y, Jurutka PW, Wu S, Chen Y, Cao C, Chen G, Tian B, Wang S, Cheng S. 16α-Hydroxytrametenolic acid from Poria cocos improves intestinal barrier function through the glucocorticoid receptor-mediated PI3K/Akt/NF-κB pathway. Journal of agricultural and food chemistry. 2019 Sep 13;67(39):10871-9.

[124] Deng J, Zeng L, Lai X, Li J, Liu L, Lin Q, Chen Y. Metformin protects against intestinal barrier dysfunction via AMPKα1-dependent inhibition of JNK signalling activation. Journal of Cellular and Molecular Medicine. 2018 Jan;22(1):546.

[125] Wang X, Buechler NL, Yoza BK, McCall CE, Vachharajani VT. Resveratrol attenuates microvascular inflammation in sepsis via SIRT-1-Induced modulation of adhesion molecules in ob/ob mice. Obesity. 2015 Jun;23(6):1209-17.

[126] Wang L, Cui YL, Zhang Z, Lin ZF, Chen DC. Rhubarb monomers protect intestinal mucosal barrier in sepsis via junction proteins. Chinese medical journal. 2017 May 20;130(10):1218.

[127] Liang X, Zhou M, Ge XY, Li CB, Fang SP, Tang L, Shao DH, Xu G. Efficacy of traditional Chinese medicine on sepsis: a systematic review and Meta-Analysis. International journal of clinical and experimental medicine. 2015;8(11):20024.

[128] Liu F, Liu J, Liu Y, Zhang Y, Ding X. Shen-Fu Decoction could ameliorate intestinal permeability by regulating the intestinal expression of tight junction proteins and p-VASP in septic rats. Journal of Ethnopharmacology. 2021 Mar 25;268:113562.

[129] Mack DR. Probiotics: Mixed messages. Canadian Family Physician. 2005 Nov 10;51(11):1455.

[130] Reddy VS, Patole SK, Rao S. Role of probiotics in short bowel syndrome in infants and children—a systematic review. Nutrients. 2013 Mar;5(3):679-99.

[131] Gharajalar SN, Kazemi-Darabadi S, Lajimi HV, Shahbazfar AA. The Roles of Lactobacillus Acidophilus and Pectin in Preventing Postoperative Sepsis and Intestinal Adaptation in a Rat Model of Short Bowel Syndrome. Probiotics and Antimicrobial Proteins. 2021 Mar 14:1-8.

[132] Jo SG, Noh EJ, Lee JY, Kim G, Choi JH, Lee ME, Song JH, Chang JY, Park JH. Lactobacillus curvatus WiKim38 isolated from kimchi induces IL-10 production in dendritic cells and alleviates DSS-induced colitis in mice. Journal of Microbiology. 2016 Jul;54(7):503-9.

[133] Chen L, Li H, Li J, Chen Y, Yang Y. Lactobacillus rhamnosus GG treatment improves intestinal permeability and modulates microbiota dysbiosis in an experimental model of sepsis. International journal of molecular medicine. 2019 Mar 1;43(3):1139-48.

[134] Shimizu K, Yamada T, Ogura H, Mohri T, Kiguchi T, Fujimi S, Asahara T, Yamada T, Ojima M, Ikeda M, Shimazu T. Synbiotics modulate gut microbiota and reduce enteritis and ventilator-associated pneumonia in patients with sepsis: a randomized controlled trial. Critical care. 2018 Dec;22(1):1-9.

[135] Ávila PR, Michels M, Vuolo F, Bilésimo R, Burger H, Milioli MV, Sonai B, Borges H, Carneiro C, Abatti M, Santana IV. Protective effects of fecal microbiota transplantation in sepsis are independent of the modulation of the intestinal flora. Nutrition. 2020 May 1;73:110727.

[136] Lamprecht G, Heininger A. Current aspects of sepsis caused by bacterial translocation. Zentralblatt fur Chirurgie. 2012 Jun 18;137(3):274-8.

[137] Bassetti M, Bandera A, Gori A. Therapeutic potential of the gut microbiota in the management of sepsis. Annual Update in Intensive Care and Emergency Medicine 2020. 2020:293-304.

[138] Xu MQ, Cao HL, Wang WQ, Wang S, Cao XC, Yan F, Wang BM. Fecal microbiota transplantation broadening its application beyond intestinal disorders. World journal of gastroenterology: WJG. 2015 Jan 7;21(1):102.

[139] Keskey R, Cone JT, DeFazio JR, Alverdy JC. The use of fecal microbiota transplant in sepsis. Translational Research. 2020 Jul 7.

[140] Littman DR, Pamer EG. Role of the commensal microbiota in normal and pathogenic host immune responses. Cell host and microbe. 2011 Oct 20;10(4):311-23.

[141] Gargiullo L, Del Chierico F, D'Argenio P, Putignani L. Gut microbiota modulation for multidrug-resistant organism decolonization: present and future perspectives. Frontiers in microbiology. 2019 Jul 25;10:1704.

Chapter 16

Assessment and Management of Hypoperfusion in Sepsis and Septic Shock

Zohair Al Aseri

Abstract

Diagnosis of organ hypoperfusion in patient with sepsis is not always straightforward which makes septic shock definition, diagnosis, and early treatment are major challenges that emergency physicians and intensivist must deal with in their daily practice. Normal blood pressure does not always mean good organ perfusion, which means patient might develop septic shock, yet they are not hypotensive. There are several indices that could be used in combination to diagnose and manage hypoperfusion in patients with septic shock. Fluid resuscitation and vasopressor administration along with infection sources control are the cornerstones in septic shock management. This chapter will cover indices that can be used to diagnose hypoperfusion, type and amount of fluid and vasopressor that can be used in resuscitating septic shock patients.

Keywords: septic shock, hypoperfusion, fluid resuscitation, vasopressor

1. Introduction

Sepsis is defined as life-threatening condition caused by a dysregulated host response to infection, resulting in organ dysfunction while septic shock is circulatory, cellular, and metabolic abnormalities in septic patients, presenting as fluid-refractory hypotension requiring vasopressor therapy with associated tissue hypoperfusion [1]. Septic shock has high mortality rate and constitutes 20% of all global deaths [2]. Mortality associated with septic shock range from 24–41% [3–6]. Increased morbidities and decreased functional status of septic shock patients after hospital discharge are major concerns and related to poor management [7]. Management of Septic shock include early recognition, source control with antibiotic and surgical intervention if needed, adequate perfusion and vital organ support including renal and respiratory support [8]. Patient in the early stage of septic shock required individualized fluid resuscitation and early administration of vasopressor to ensure tissue perfusion.

2. Indices of Hypoperfusion

Progression of sepsis to septic shock occur very quickly and leads to hypoperfusion, end organ failure and death. **Figure 1** summaries the pathophysiology of sepsis and septic shock [9–11]. Hemodynamic, clinical and laboratory indices could be used to determine the level of hypoperfusion and its response to resuscitation. **Table 1** summaries the perfusion indices of and their targets during resuscitation.

IntechOpen

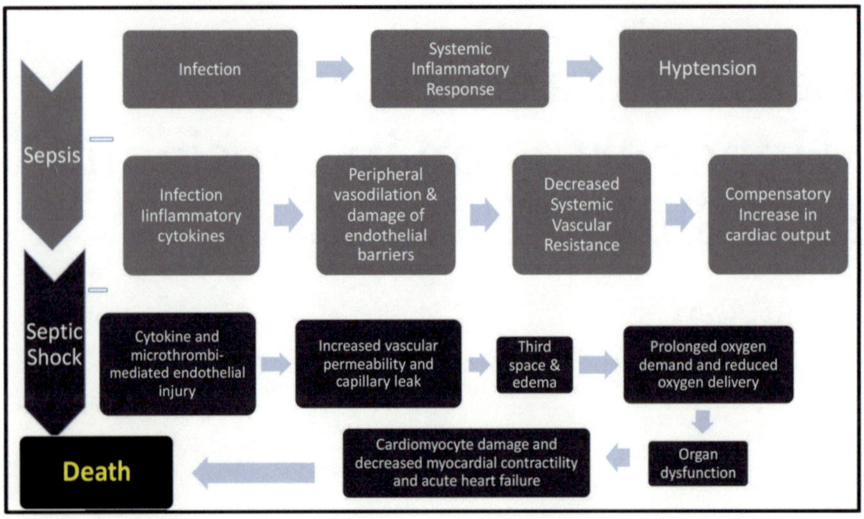

Figure 1.
Pathophysiology of sepsis and septic shock.

Index	Target
Heart Rate	60–90 Beats per minute
Mean arterial pressure MAP	≥65 mmHg
Diastolic arterial pressure (DAP)	≥50 mmHg
Skin examination	Normal color worminess
Temperature	≥ 36oC
Capillary Refill Time (CRT)	< 3 seconds
Urine Output (OUP)	≥ 0.5 ml/kg/hour
Central Venous Pressure (CVP)	< 6–8 mmHg in spontaneous breathing > 12–15 mmHg in ventilated patient
Serum Lactate	< 2.2 mmol/L

Table 1.
Indices of hypoperfusion and their targets.

2.1 Heart rate

Tachycardia is common sign of septic shock, and it predicts poor prognosis of septic shock patient. It is caused by stimulation of α- and β-adrenergic receptors increases in response to venodilattion and could be also related high temperature. Tachycardia is a sign impaired arterial tone [12]. It increases oxygen consumption, decreases diastolic filling and coronary perfusion, and increases arrhythmia [13]. Patients with septic shock and persistent tachycardia despite resuscitation measures has high mortality and morbidity rate [14].

2.2 Blood pressure

Blood pressure is easy to measure and monitor. Blood pressure is determined by cardiac output, systemic vascular resistance, and arterioles pressure and coronary perfusion and heart flow depend upon diastolic arterial pressure (DAP) [15].

Hypotension reflects decrease cardiac output, but it could be a delayed sign of hypoperfusion, and its absence does not necessarily rule out hypoperfusion. Hypotension triggers resuscitation. Low diastolic arterial pressure, in septic shock indicates impaired arterial tone. Optimizing blood pressure is one of the goals of fluid resuscitation and associated with better outcome [16]. Prolonged hypotension, low mean arterial pressure (MAP) and DAP associated with high mortality in septic shock patient [17, 18]. Normal MAP and DAP should be targeted to improve survival of septic shock patients [15]. No evidence what the best target level of DBP is but common approach is to titrate vasopressors in septic shock to keep DAP ≥50 mmHg [19]. Resuscitation should target MAP of 65 mmHg per the septic shock guidelines [20]. Hypoperfusion may persist even when pressure is restored so personalization approach to target blood pressure should consider other indices of perfusion [21].

2.3 Skin changes

Skin examination including its color, blanching and worminess is one of the most important physical examination to determine level of skin perfusion which reflect vital organ perfusion. Anterior aspect of the knee is one body area that commonly examined for skin perfusion Mottling score is one of indices of hypoperfusion and associated with worse outcome regardless of vasopressor use [22, 23]. Normalization of skin color and disappearance of mottled skin are targets of resuscitation and related to higher survival rate of septic shock patient [24, 25].

2.4 Skin temperature

Skin temperature is one of the most accessible markers of skin perfusion and hence tissue perfusion [26]. Hypothermia in circulatory shock is associated with impaired outcome [27].

2.5 Capillary refill time (CRT)

CRT is the time taken to regain distal capillary bed color after blanching by pressure. Normally should be less than 3 seconds. It has been shown in in study of 783 critically ill patients that CRT is sensitive sign of decrease cardiac output measured by echocardiogram [28]. Capillary refill time is one of the best indices of adequate perfusion [29, 30]. And could be used as screening tool to predict sick patient that might need admission to critical care area. In one study, CRT and lactate are similar in predict survival [31]. In other study prolonged CRT associated with decrease perfusion of the liver, kidneys, gut and spleen [32]. CRT more than 4 seconds associated with higher mortality rate of septic shock patients [33]. In a randomized controlled study of septic shock patients with high lactate level but with a normal CRT had lower day-28 mortality when compared to prolonged CRT and high lactate level and survival of patients is higher with when resuscitation is guided by capillary refill time but not lactate levels [34]. When CRT used as index as optimal resuscitation it led to decrease mortality rate and should be used to guide fluid resuscitation in septic shock patient [34–36]. Septic shock patients failing to normalize their CRT after the first fluid bolus in ED had high mortality [37].

2.6 Passive leg raise

Passive Leg Raise (PLR) Can assist in identifying preload dependence. Utilization of the passive leg raise as index of resuscitation lead to reduce net fluid balance, acute kidney injury and pulmonary edema and may improve outcomes [38].

PLR became more popular and easier to use in different sitting including emergency department sitting [39].

By moving the patient from a semi-recumbent position, lowering the trunk and raising the patient's legs to 45°, an amount of ~300 mL of blood is transferred to the ventricles, thereby increasing the cardiac preload. If CO increases of at least 10% compared to baseline, the patient is considered preload responsive, thus capable of displaying a CO increase following administration of fluid. The change in cardiac output changes in is measured by thermodilution, echocardiography, pulse contour analysis or pulse pressure variation. Passive leg rising is shifts venous blood from the legs to the intrathoracic compartment. This response can predict the response to a fluid challenge. Passive leg-raise test is accurate and has excellent sensitivity and specificity, for that it is recommended to determine fluid responsiveness [20, 40]. A meta-analysis of 21 studies and 991 adult patients showed that a 10% 2% increase in cardiac output with PLR predicted fluid responsiveness [41].

2.7 Urine output

Oliguria which is urine output less than 0.5 ml/kg/hour is one of the main triggers for fluid challenges in septic shock patient [16]. Oliguria is one of signs of acute renal failure which is an independent risk factor associated with increased mortality during sepsis. Low UOP may reflect low renal perfusion pressure. UOP 30–50 mL/h in adult patient with septic shock should prompt further fluid resuscitation or other measures to increase cardiac output in a non–fluid-responsive patient [42]. UOP should not be taken alone as fluid resuscitation may not increase urinary output and cause positive fluid balance in patients with septic shock [20].

2.8 Central venous pressure (CVP)

Venodilation and hypovolemia cause decrease in ventricular preload which is signaled by decrease in central venous pressure. CVP reflect the right atrial pressure [43]. CVP alone is a poor variable to predict fluid responsiveness [44, 45]. The target CVP is < 6–8 mmHg in spontaneous breathing patient and > 12–15 mmHg in mechanically ventilated patient [46].

2.9 Lactate

Lactates reflect the onset of anaerobic metabolism. In experimental conditions, lactate increases when oxygen consumption increased and oxygen delivery decreased. Lactate also elevated in beta-adrenergic stimulation, leading to an accelerated glycolysis and liver failure. Lactate >2 mmol/L associated tissue hypoperfusion (lactate >2 mmol/L) [47]. Clinical studies show high lactate levels are associated with a high mortality, independently of its cause [48]. Lactate is easy to measure and can be used in emergency department triage and as a goal of early sepsis therapy [49]. Repeating lactate measurements is a trigger of resuscitation [20]. Lactate-guided resuscitation has emerged after the observation that the higher the decrease in lactate levels, the best the outcome [50].

Indices of hypoperfusion are combinations of pressure and flow measurements and clinical markers. They should be taken together and not to rely only on one index to diagnose and mange hypoperfusion [51].

3. Fluid resuscitation of septic shock patient

Crystalloid intravenous fluid either ringer lactate or 0.9% normal saline is the first and the main step in restoring hemodynamic instability. Septic shock patient in the initial stage should be considered fluid responsive and receive fluid bolus [52]. Not all septic shock patient will respond to the initial fluid resuscitation, hence additional pharmaceutics intervention is needed to augment of fluid resuscitation to restore the hemodynamic and improve organ perfusion [53, 54]. Fast intravenous (IV) crystalloid infusion has a slower redistribution rate. Interstitial distribution is hypothesized to be greater in sepsis than in healthy volunteers due to sepsis pathophysiology [55] (**Figure 1**). The maximal effect of IV crystalloid bolus achieves at one minute and return to baseline after 30 minutes. Only one third of septic shock patient will have risen in MAP after fluid challenge [56, 57]. Amount of IV fluid resuscitation in patients with septic shock is not known. In one retrospective study found large amount of fluid more than 5 liter per day associated with increase mortality rate and need of ventilatory support [58, 59]. 50% 0f septic shock patients will be non-fluid responsive, where a condition where the administration of more fluid bolus may lead to fluid accumulation, impaired oxygen delivery, and worsening hypoperfusion [60]. How fast fluid should be administered in septic shock resuscitation is not known. Mainly retrospective studies shows failure to complete 30 mL/kg of IV crystalloid over 3 hours was associated with increased mortality [61]. In multi-center study found IV fluid administration within six hours was associated with decreased mortality [62]. regarding type of fluid in resuscitating septic shock patient, the current guideline recommends both sodium chloride and balanced crystalloids [20]. Studies within the critically ill have shown lower risk of in-hospital or 30-day mortality, AKI, or major adverse kidney event in the first 30 days with the use of balanced crystalloids over sodium chloride solutions [63, 64]. SMART trial, compared the two solutions in 15,802 critically ill patients, reported a lower rate of death from any cause, renal-replacement therapy, or renal failure with using balanced crystalloids versus normal saline [63]. In secondary analysis of SMART study among 1,641 patients were admitted to the medical ICU with a diagnosis of sepsis, balanced crystalloids was associated with a lower 30-day in-hospital mortality rate, renal failure, and a higher number of vasopressor free days compared with use of saline [64]. Amount of fluids resuscitation should be decided to minimize the complication of over resuscitation as pulmonary edema, brain edema, abdominal compartment syndrome and third space edema which will lead resulting in end-organ hypoperfusion by decrease oxygen delivery, capillary blood flow and lymphatic drainage. Which explain worse outcomes in shock with a positive fluid balance [55, 65, 66]. Collapsible inferior vena cava can along with other hypoperfusion indices can be used to monitor fluid and resuscitation of septic shock patient [67]. Resuscitation of septic shock patient with high volume of normal saline is associated with hyperchloremia, AKI, multiorgan dysfunction, and high mortality [68, 69]. Fixed amount of fluid hardly suitable for all septic shock patients, Teboul and Monnet proposed to administer crystalloid about 10 mL/kg within the first 30 to 60 min and monitor patient [52]. If patient develop any signs of respiratory failure stop further boluses. In case CRT is still prolonged, tachycardia or low blood pressure reading, skin mottling increase in the infusion rate [70].

Perfusion indices should be used to individualize fluid administration approach in balanced crystalloid is recommended over normal slain in septic shock resuscitation.

4. Vasopressors in septic shock management

Vasopressor increases systemic vascular resistance (SVR), cardiac output CO, and heart rate (HR) and rapidly restore organ perfusion [71]. Vasopressors either catecholamine- or non-catecholamine-based agents. Dopamine, norepinephrine, epinephrine, and phenylephrine are catecholamine-based vasopressors while vasopressin is a non-catecholamine-based vasopressors [72]. Norepinephrine is the first-line vasopressor for patients with septic shock [20]. Early vasopressors administration in septic shock patients revert the severely impaired arterial tone and associated with lowest mortality rate occurred when vasoactive agents were started 1 to 6 hours of septic shock identification [20, 73–76]. CENSER trial shows early NE administration is associated with increased shock control over the first 6 hours [76]. Addition of vasopressin to norepinephrine in the few hours of shock when doses of norepinephrine dose is ≥1 μg/Kg/min, may decrease mortality, arrhythmia, hypotension and need for renal replacement therapy [77, 78]. Addition of vasopressin to norepinephrine is more effective in early septic shock management and reach MAP target faster and lower incidence of atrial fibrillation [79, 80]. Possible complication of vasopressor includes dysrhythmias tachycardia or atrial fibrillation. Hyperlactatemia and hyperglycemia [80, 81]. Peripheral administration of vasopressors includes extravasation and peripheral ischemia given their potent vasoconstrictive properties [82]. Extravasation was uncommon if vasopressors are administered peripherally for less than 22 hours. Peripheral administration of vasopressors in upper arm using 20 gauge or larger is safe and feasible in the initial hours of resuscitation [82–84]. Vasopressor treatment can be initiated on a peripheral venous line with non-invasive BP monitoring, and shifted, as soon as possible, to central venous catheter with arterial pressure monitoring [85].

Early norepinephrine administration should be started in septic shock patient with slow response to fluid resuscitation. Vasopressin is recommended in when norepinephrine dose is ≥1 μg/Kg/min.

5. Conclusion

Septic shock is life threatening condition complicated with hypoperfusion, Indices of hypoperfusion are combinations of pressure and flow measurements and clinical markers. Indices should be taken together and not to rely only on one index to diagnose and mange hypoperfusion. Perfusion indices should be used to individualize fluid administration approach in balanced crystalloid is recommended over normal slain in septic shock resuscitation. Early norepinephrine administration should be started in septic shock patient with slow response to fluid resuscitation. Vasopressin is recommended in when norepinephrine dose is ≥1 μg/Kg/min.

Author details

Zohair Al Aseri
Department of Emergency Medicine and Critical Care, College of Medicine, King Saud University, Riyadh, Saudi Arabia

*Address all correspondence to: zalaseri@ksu.edu.sa

References

[1] Singer M, Deutschman CS, Seymour CW, et al. The Third International Consensus Defi nitions for Sepsis and Septic Shock (Sepsis-3). JAMA 2016; 315(8):801-810. doi:10.1001/jama.2016.0287

[2] Rudd KE, Johnson SC, Agesa KM, Shackelford KA, Tsoi D, Kievlan DR, et al. Global, regional, and national sepsis incidence and mortality, 1990-2017: analysis for the Global Burden of Disease Study. Lancet. 2020 Jan 18;395(10219): 200-211. doi: 10.1016/ S0140-6736(19)32989-7.

[3] Sprung CL, Annane D, Keh D, Moreno R, Singer M, Freivogel K, et al. Hydrocortisone therapy for patients with septic shock. N Engl J Med. 2008 Jan 10. 358(2):111-124.

[4] Ranieri VM, Thompson BT, Barie PS, Dhainaut JF, Douglas IS, Finfer S, et al. Drotrecogin alfa (activated) in adults with septic shock. N Engl J Med. 2012 May 31. 366(22):2055-2064.

[5] Levy MM, Artigas A, Phillips GS, Rhodes A, Beale R, Osborn T, et al. Outcomes of the Surviving Sepsis Campaign in intensive care units in the USA and Europe: a prospective cohort study. Lancet Infect Dis. 2012 Dec. 12(12):919-924.

[6] Opal SM, Laterre PF, Francois B, LaRosa SP, Angus DC, Mira JP, et al. Effect of eritoran, an antagonist of MD2-TLR4, on mortality in patients with severe sepsis: the ACCESS randomized trial. JAMA. 2013 Mar 20. 309(11):1154-1162.

[7] Meyer N, Harhay MO, Small DS, Prescott HC, Bowles KH, Gaieski DF, Mikkelsen ME. Temporal Trends in Incidence, Sepsis-Related Mortality, and Hospital-Based Acute Care After Sepsis. Crit Care Med. 2018 Mar;46(3):354-360. doi: 10.1097/CCM.0000000000002872.

[8] De Backer D, Dorman T. Surviving Sepsis Guidelines: a continuous move toward better care of patients with sepsis. Journal of the American Medical Association 2017;317:807-808.

[9] Gotts JE, Matthay MA. Sepsis: pathophysiology and clinical management. BMJ. 2016 May 23;353:i1585. doi: 10.1136/bmj.i1585.

[10] Angus DC, van der Poll T. Severe Sepsis and Septic Shock. N Engl J Med 369(9):840- 851, 2013.

[11] Russell JA, Rush B, Boyd J. Pathophysiology of Septic Shock. Crit Care Clin 34(1):43-61, 2018.

[12] Magder S. The meaning of blood pressure. Crit Care. 2018 Oct 11;22(1):257. doi: 10.1186/ s13054-018-2171-1.

[13] Rudiger A, Singer M. Mechanisms of sepsis-induced cardiac dysfunction. Crit Care Med. 2007 Jun;35(6):1599-1608. doi: 10.1097/01.CCM. 0000266683.64081.02.

[14] Domizi R, Calcinaro S, Harris S, Beilstein C, Boerma C, Chiche JD, D'Egidio A, et al. Relationship between norepinephrine dose, tachycardia and outcome in septic shock: A multicentre evaluation. J Crit Care. 2020 Jun;57:185-190. doi: 10.1016/j.jcrc.2020.02.014. Epub 2020 Feb 28.

[15] Magder SA. The highs and lows of blood pressure: toward meaningful clinical targets in patients with shock. Crit Care Med 2014;42(5):1241-1251.

[16] Cecconi M, Hofer C, Teboul JL, etal. Fluid challenges in intensive care:the FENICE study: a global inception cohort

study. Intensive Care Med 2015; 41: 1529 – 1537.

[17] Varpula M, Tallgren M, Saukkonen K, Voipio-Pulkki LM, Pettilä V. Hemodynamic variables related to outcome in septic shock. Intensive Care Med 2005;31:1066-1071.

[18] Vincent JL, Nielsen ND, Shapiro NI, Gerbasi ME, Grossman A, Doroff R, et al. Mean arterial pressure and mortality in patients with distributive shock: A retrospective analysis of the MIMIC-III database. Ann Intensive Care 2018;8:107.

[19] Benchekroune S, Karpati PC, Berton C, Nathan C, Mateo J, Chaara M, et al. Diastolic arterial blood pressure: a reliable early predictor of survival in human septic shock. J Trauma 2008;64(5):1188-1195. https://doi.org/10.1097/TA.0b013e31811f3a45.

[20] Rhodes A, Evans LE, Alhazzani W, Levy MM, Antonelli M, Ferrer R, Kumar A, Sevransky JE, Sprung CL, Nunnally ME, et al. Surviving Sepsis Campaign: International Guidelines for Management of Sepsis and Septic Shock: 2016. Crit Care Med 45(3):486-552, 2017.

[21] Kato R, Pinsky MR. Personalizing blood pressure management in septic shock. Ann Intensive Care 2015;5(1):41.

[22] Ait-Oufella H, Lemoinne S, Boelle PY, Galbois A, Baudel JL, Lemant J, et al. Mottling score predicts survival in septic shock. Intensive Care Med 2011;37:801-807.

[23] Ait-Oufella H, Bourcier S, Alves M, Galbois A, Baudel JL, Margetis D, et al. Alteration of skin perfusion in mottling area during septic shock. Ann Intensive Care 2013;3:31.

[24] Jouffroy R, Saade A, Tourtier JP, Gueye P, Bloch-Laine E, Ecollan P, et al. Skin mottling score and capillary refill time to assess mortality of septic shock since pre-hospital setting. Am J Emerg Med 2019;37:664-671.

[25] Dumas G, Lavillegrand JR, Joffre J, Bigé N, de-Moura EB, Baudel JL, et al. Mottling score is a strong predictor of 14-day mortality in septic patients whatever vasopressor doses and other tissue perfusion parameters. Crit Care 2019;23:211.

[26] Ait-Oufella H, Bakker J. Understanding clinical signs of poor tissue perfusion during septic shock. Intensive Care Med 2016;42:2070-2072.

[27] Bourcier S, Pichereau C, Boelle PY, Nemlaghi S, Dubée V, Lejour G, et al. Toe-to-room temperature gradient correlates with tissue perfusion and predicts outcome in selected critically ill patients with severe infections. Ann Intensive Care 2016;6:63.

[28] Hiemstra B, Koster G, Wiersema R, et al. The diagnostic accuracy of clinical & examination for estimating cardiac index in critically ill patients: the Simple Intensive Care Studies-I. Intensive Care Med 2019; 45:190-200.

[29] 29. Lima A,van Bommel J, Sikorska K,etal.The relation of near-infrared spectroscopy with changes in peripheral circulation in critically ill patients. Crit Care. Med 2011; 39:1649-1654.

[30] Lima A, van Genderen ME, Klijn E, Bakker J, van Bommel J. Peripheral vasoconstriction influences thenar oxygen saturation as measured by near-infrared spectroscopy. Intensive Care Med. 2012 Apr;38(4):606-611. doi: 10.1007/s00134-012-2486-3. Epub 2012 Feb 14

[31] Mongkolpun W, Orbegozo D, Cordeiro CPR, Franco CJCS, Vincent JL, Creteur J. Alterations in Skin Blood Flow at the Fingertip Are Related to Mortality

in Patients With Circulatory Shock. Crit Care Med. 2020 Apr;48(4):443-450. doi: 10.1097/CCM.0000000000004177.

[32] Brunauer A, Koköfer A, Bataar O, Gradwohl-Matis I, Dankl D, Bakker J, et al. Changes in peripheral perfusion relate to visceral organ perfusion in early septic shock: A pilot study. J Crit Care. 2016 Oct;35:105-109. doi: 10.1016/j.jcrc.2016.05.007. Epub 2016 May

[33] Hernández G, Ospina-Tascón GA, Damiani LP, Estenssoro E, Dubin A, Hurtado J, et al. Effect of a Resuscitation Strategy Targeting Peripheral Perfusion Status vs Serum Lactate Levels on 28-Day Mortality Among Patients With Septic Shock: The ANDROMEDA-SHOCK Randomized Clinical Trial. JAMA. 2019 Feb 19;321(7):654-664. doi: 10.1001/jama.2019.0071

[34] Kattan E, Hernández G, Ospina-Tascón G, Valenzuela ED, Bakker J, Castro R; ANDROMEDA-SHOCK Study Investigators and the Latin America Intensive Care Network (LIVEN). A lactate-targeted resuscitation strategy may be associated with higher mortality in patients with septic shock and normal capillary refill time: a post hoc analysis of the ANDROMEDA-SHOCK study. Ann Intensive Care. 2020 Aug 26;10(1):114. doi: 10.1186/s13613-020-00732-1.

[35] Zampieri FG, Damiani LP, Bakker J, Ospina-Tascón GA, Castro R, Cavalcanti AB, et al. Effects of a Resuscitation Strategy Targeting Peripheral Perfusion Status versus Serum Lactate Levels among Patients with Septic Shock. A Bayesian Reanalysis of the ANDROMEDA-SHOCK Trial. Am J Respir Crit Care Med. 2020 Feb 15;201(4):423-429. doi: 10.1164/rccm.201905-0968OC.

[36] Kattan E, Ospina-Tascón GA, Teboul JL, Castro R, Cecconi M, Ferri G, et al. ANDROMEDA-SHOCK Investigators. Systematic assessment of fluid responsiveness during early septic shock resuscitation: secondary analysis of the ANDROMEDA-SHOCK trial. Crit Care. 2020 Jan 23;24(1):23. doi: 10.1186/s13054-020-2732-y.

[37] Lara B, Enberg L, Ortega M, Leon P, Kripper C, Aguilera P, Kattan E, et al. Capillary refill time during fluid resuscitation in patients with sepsis-related hyperlactatemia at the emergency department is related to mortality. PLoS One. 2017 Nov 27;12(11):e0188548. doi: 10.1371/journal.pone.0188548.

[38] Douglas IS, Alapat PM, Corl KA, Exline MC, Forni LG, Holder AL, et al. Fluid Response Evaluation in Sepsis Hypotension and Shock: A Randomized Clinical Trial. Chest. 2020 Oct;158(4):1431-1445. doi: 10.1016/j.chest.2020.04.025. Epub 2020 Apr 27.

[39] Monnet X, Teboul JL. Passive leg raising: five rules, not a drop of fluid! Crit Care. 2015 Jan 14;19(1):18. doi: 10.1186/s13054-014-0708-5.

[40] Monnet X, Marik P, Teboul JL. Passive leg raising for predicting fluid responsiveness: a systematic review and meta-analysis. Intensive Care Med 2016; 42(12):1935-1947. doi:10.1007/s00134-015-4134-1

[41] Bentzer P, Griesdale DE, Boyd J, MacLean K, Sirounis D, Ayas NT. Will this hemodynamically unstable patient respond to a bolus of intravenous fluids? JAMA. 2016;316(12):1298-1309.

[42] Godin M, Murray P, Mehta RL. Clinical approach to the patient with AKI and sepsis. Semin Nephrol. 2015;35(1):12-22. doi:10.1016/j.semnephrol.2015.01.003

[43] De Backer D, Vincent JL. Should we measure the central venous pressure to guide fluid management? Ten answers

to 10 questions. Crit Care. 2018 Feb 23;22(1):43. doi: 10.1186/s13054-018-1959-3.

[44] Marik PE, Cavallazzi R. Does the central venous pressure predict fluid responsiveness? An updated meta-analysis and a plea for some common sense. Crit Care Med. 2013 Jul;41(7):1774-1781. doi: 10.1097/CCM.0b013e31828a25fd.

[45] Cecconi M, Aya HD. Central venous pressure cannot predict fluid-responsiveness. Evid Based Med. 2014;19:63. doi: 10.1136/eb-2013-101496.

[46] Eskesen TG, Wetterslev M, Perner A. Systematic review including re-analyses of 1148 individual data sets of central venous pressure as a predictor of fluid responsiveness. Intensive Care Med. 2016;42:324-332. doi: 10.1007/s00134-015-4168-4

[47] Rimachi R, Bruzzi de Carvahlo F, Orellano-Jimenez C, Cotton F, Vincent JL, et al. Lactate/pyruvate ratio as a marker of tissue hypoxia in circulatory and septic shock. Anaesth Intensive Care 2012;40:427-432.

[48] Casserly B, Phillips GS, Schorr C, Dellinger RP, Townsend SR, Osborn TM, et al. Lactate measurements in sepsis-induced tissue hypoperfusion: Results from the Surviving Sepsis Campaign database. Crit Care Med 2015;43:567-573.

[49] Jones AE, Shapiro NI, Trzeciak S, Arnold RC, Claremont HA, Kline JA, et al. Lactate clearance vs. central venous oxygen saturation as goals of early sepsis therapy: A randomized clinical trial. JAMA 2010;303:739-746.

[50] Bakker J, De Backer D, Hernandez G. Lactate-guided resuscitation saves lives: We are not sure. Intensive Care Med 2016;42:472-474.

[51] Hernandez G, Luengo C, Bruhn A, Kattan E, Friedman G, Ospina-Tascon GA, et al. When to stop septic shock resuscitation: clues from a dynamic perfusion monitoring. Ann Intensive Care. 2014 Oct 11;4:30. doi: 10.1186/s13613-014-0030-z.

[52] Monnet X, Teboul JL. Prediction of fluid responsiveness in spontaneously breathing patients. Ann Transl Med. 2020 Jun;8(12):790. doi: 10.21037/atm-2020-hdm-18.

[53] Marik PE, Lemson J. Fluid responsiveness: an evolution of our understanding. Br J Anaesth. 2014 Apr;112(4):617-620. doi: 10.1093/bja/aet590. Epub 2014 Feb 16.

[54] Dugar S, Choudhary C, Duggal A. Sepsis and septic shock: Guideline-based management. Cleve Clin J Med. 2020 Jan;87(1):53-64. doi: 10.3949/ccjm.87a.18143. Epub 2020 Jan 2

[55] Bissell BD, Mefford B. Pathophysiology of Volume Administration in Septic Shock and the Role of the Clinical Pharmacist. Ann Pharmacother. 2020 Apr;54(4):388-396. doi: 10.1177/1060028019887160. Epub 2019 Nov 6.

[56] Aya HD, Ster IC, Fletcher N, Grounds RM, Rhodes A, Cecconi M. Pharmacodynamic Analysis of a Fluid Challenge. Crit Care Med. 2016 May;44(5):880-891. doi: 10.1097/CCM.0000000000001517.

[57] Monge García MI, Guijo González P, Gracia Romero M, Gil Cano A, Oscier C, Rhodes A, et al. Effects of fluid administration on arterial load in septic shock patients. Intensive Care Med. 2015 Jul;41(7):1247-1255.

[58] Marik PE, Linde-Zwirble WT, Bittner EA, Sahatjian J, Hansell D. Fluid administration in severe sepsis and septic shock, patterns and outcomes: an

analysis of a large national database. Intensive Care Med 43(5):625-632, 2017.

[59] Seymour CW, Gesten F, Prescott HC, Friedrich ME, Iwashyna TJ, Phillips GS, et al. Time to Treatment and Mortality during Mandated Emergency Care for Sepsis. N Engl J Med 2017;376(23):2235-2244.

[60] Monnet X, Teboul JL. My patient has received fluid. How to assess its efficacy and side effects? Ann Intensive Care. 2018 Apr 24;8(1):54. doi: 10.1186/s13613-018-0400-z.

[61] Kuttab HI, Lykins JD, Hughes MD, Wroblewski K, Keast EP, Kukoyi O, et al. Evaluation and Predictors of Fluid Resuscitation in Patients With Severe Sepsis and Septic Shock. Crit Care Med 2019;47(11):1582-1590.

[62] Levy MM, Gesten FC, Phillips GS, Terry KM, Seymour CW, Prescott HC, et al. The Results of the New York State Initiative. Am J Respir Crit Care Med 2018;198:1406-1412.

[63] Semler MW, Self WH, Wanderer JP, Ehrenfeld JM, Wang L, Byrne DW, et al. SMART Investigators and the Pragmatic Critical Care Research Group. Balanced Crystalloids versus Saline in Critically Ill Adults. N Engl J Med. 2018 Mar 1;378(9):829-839. doi: 10.1056/NEJMoa1711584. Epub 2018 Feb 27.

[64] Brown RM, Wang L, Coston TD, Krishnan NI, Casey JD, Wanderer JP, et al. Balanced Crystalloids versus Saline in Sepsis. A Secondary Analysis of the SMART Clinical Trial. Am J Respir Crit Care Med. 2019 Dec 15;200(12):1487-1495. doi: 10.1164/rccm.201903-0557OC.

[65] Tigabu BM, Davari M, Kebriaeezadeh A, Mojtahedzadeh M. Fluid volume, fluid balance and patient outcome in severe sepsis and septic shock: A systematic review. J Crit Care 2018;48:153-159.

[66] Sakr Y, Rubatto Birri PN, Kotfis K, Nanchal R, Shah B, Kluge S, et al. Intensive Care Over Nations Investigators. Higher Fluid Balance Increases the Risk of Death From Sepsis: Results From a Large International Audit. Crit Care Med. 2017 Mar;45(3):386-394. doi: 10.1097/CCM.0000000000002189.

[67] Vallabhajosyula S, Ahmed AM, Sundaragiri PR. Role of echocardiography in sepsis and septic shock. Ann Transl Med 2020; 8(5):150-150.

[68] Suetrong B, Pisitsak C, Boyd JH, Russell JA, Walley KR. Hyperchloremia and moderate increase in serum chloride are associated with acute kidney injury in severe sepsis and septic shock patients. Crit Care. 2016 Oct 6;20(1):315. doi: 10.1186/s13054-016-1499-7.

[69] Yeh P, Pan Y, Sanchez-Pinto LN, Luo Y. Hyperchloremia in critically ill patients: association with outcomes and prediction using electronic health record data. BMC Med Inform Decis Mak. 2020 Dec 15;20(Suppl 14):302. doi: 10.1186/s12911-020-01326-4.

[70] Jozwiak M, Hamzaoui O, Monnet X, Teboul JL. Fluid resuscitation during early sepsis: a need for individualization. Minerva Anestesiol. 2018 Aug;84(8):987-992. doi: 10.23736/S0375-9393.18.12422-9. Epub 2018 Feb 14.

[71] Saugel B, Malbrain MLNG, Perel A. Hemodynamic monitoring in the era of evidence- based medicine. Crit Care 2016;20(1):401.

[72] Manolopoulos PP, Boutsikos I, Boutsikos P, Iacovidou N, Ekmektzoglou K. Current use and advances in vasopressors and inotropes support in shock. J Emerg Crit Care Med 2020; 4(0):20-20.

[73] Levy MM, Evans LE, Rhodes A. The Surviving Sepsis Campaign Bundle:

2018 Update. Crit Care Med. 2018 Jun;46(6):997-1000. doi: 10.1097/CCM.0000000000003119.

[74] Colon Hidalgo D, Patel J, Masic D, Park D, Rech MA. Delayed vasopressor initiation is associated with increased mortality in patients with septic shock. J Crit Care. 2020 Feb;55:145-148. doi: 10.1016/j.jcrc.2019.11.004. Epub 2019 Nov 9.

[75] Permpikul C, Tongyoo S, Viarasilpa T, Trainarongsakul T, Chakorn T, Udompanturak S. Early Use of Norepinephrine in Septic Shock Resuscitation (CENSER). A Randomized Trial. Am J Respir Crit Care Med. 2019 May 1;199(9):1097-1105. doi: 10.1164/rccm.201806-1034OC.

[76] Li Y, Li H, Zhang D. Timing of norepinephrine initiation in patients with septic shock: a systematic review and meta-analysis. Crit Care. 2020 Aug 6;24(1):488. doi: 10.1186/s13054-020-03204-x.

[77] Hammond DA, Cullen J, Painter JT, McCain K, Clem OA, Brotherton AL, et al. Efficacy and Safety of the Early Addition of Vasopressin to Norepinephrine in Septic Shock. J Intensive Care Med. 2019 Nov-Dec;34(11-12):910-916. doi: 10.1177/0885066617725255. Epub 2017 Aug 18.

[78] Gordon AC, Mason AJ, Thirunavukkarasu N, Perkins GD, Cecconi M, Cepkova M, et al. VANISH Investigators. Effect of Early Vasopressin vs Norepinephrine on Kidney Failure in Patients With Septic Shock: The VANISH Randomized Clinical Trial. JAMA. 2016 Aug 2;316(5):509-518. doi: 10.1001/jama.2016.10485.

[79] Russell JA, Walley KR, Singer J, Gordon AC, Hébert PC, Cooper DJ, et al. VASST Investigators. Vasopressin versus norepinephrine infusion in patients with septic shock. N Engl J Med. 2008 Feb 28;358(9):877-887. doi: 10.1056/NEJMoa067373.

[80] McIntyre WF, Um KJ, Alhazzani W, Lengyel AP, Hajjar L, Gordon AC, Lamontagne F, et al. Association of vasopressin plus catecholamine vasopressors vs catecholamines alone with atrial fibrillation in patients with distributive shock a systematic review and meta-Analysis. JAMA 319(18):1889-1900, 2018.

[81] De Backer D, Biston P, Devriendt J, Madl C, Chochrad D, Aldecoa C, et al. SOAP II Investigators. Comparison of dopamine and norepinephrine in the treatment of shock. N Engl J Med. 2010 Mar 4;362(9):779-789. doi: 10.1056/NEJMoa0907118.

[82] Tian DH, Smyth C, Keijzers G, Macdonald SP, Peake S, Udy A, et al. Safety of peripheral administration of vasopressor medications: A systematic review. Emerg Med Australas. 2020 Apr;32(2):220-227. doi: 10.1111/1742-6723.13406. Epub 2019 Nov 7.

[83] Cardenas-Garcia J, Schaub KF, Belchikov YG, Narasimhan M, Koenig SJ, Mayo PH. Safety of peripheral intravenous administration of vasoactive medication. J Hosp Med 2015;10(9):581-585. https://doi.org/10.1002/jhm.2394.

[84] Lewis T, Merchan C, Altshuler D, Papadopoulos J. Safety of the peripheral administration of vasopressor agents. J Intensive Care Med 2019;34(1):26-33. https://doi. org/10.1177/0885066616686035.

[85] Ospina-Tascón GA, Hernandez G, Alvarez I, Calderón-Tapia LE, Manzano-Nunez R, Sánchez-Ortiz AI, et al. Effects of very early start of norepinephrine in patients with septic shock: a propensity score-based analysis. Crit Care. 2020 Feb 14;24(1):52. doi: 10.1186/s13054-020-2756-3.

Chapter 17

Sepsis Associated Acute Kidney Injury

Titik Setyawati, Ricky Aditya and Tinni Trihartini Maskoen

Abstract

AKI is a syndrome consisting of several clinical conditions, due to sudden kidney dysfunction. Sepsis and septic shock are the causes of AKI and are known as Sepsis-Associated AKI (SA-AKI) and accounted for more than 50% of cases of AKI in the ICU, with poor prognosis. Acute Kidney Injury (AKI) is characterized by a sudden decline in kidney function for several hours/day, which results in the accumulation of creatinine, urea and other waste products. The most recent definition was formulated in the Kidney Disease consensus: Improving Global Outcome (KDIGO), published in 2012, where the AKI was established if the patient's current clinical manifestation met several criteria: an increase in serum creatinine levels ≥0.3 mg/dL (26.5 μmol/L) within 48 hours, an increase in serum creatinine for at least 1.5 times the baseline value within the previous 7 days; or urine volume ≤ 0.5 ml/kg body weight for 6 hours. The AKI pathophysiology includes ischemic vasodilation, endothelial leakage, necrosis in nephrons and microtrombus in capillaries. The management of sepsis associated with AKI consisted of fluid therapy, vasopressors, antibiotics and nephrotoxic substances, Renal Replacement Therapy (RRT) and diuretics. In the analysis of the BEST Kidney trial subgroup, the likelihood of hospital death was 50% higher in AKI sepsis compared to non-sepsis AKI. Understanding of sepsis and endotoxins that can cause SA-AKI is not yet fully known. Some evidence suggests that renal microcirculation hypoperfusion, lack of energy for cells, mitochondrial dysfunction, endothelial injury and cycle cell arrest can cause SA-AKI. Rapid identification of SA-AKI events, antibiotics and appropriate fluid therapy are crucial in the management of SA-AKI.

Keywords: Sepsis, Acute kidney injury

1. Introduction

Acute Kidney Injury is a syndrome that consists of several clinical conditions, due to sudden kidney dysfunction (within a few hours to several days) that causes retention of residual nitrogen (urea-creatinine) and non-nitrogenous metabolism, with or without oligouria, and is affected by some underlying disease. The most common causes of AKI in patients with critical illness are sepsis and septic shock, accounting for more than 50% of AKI cases in the ICU. The incidence of sepsis and AKI in critical patients increases gradually and both shows poor prognosis. In various epidemiological studies, it is said that AKI occurs in 11-60% of sepsis patients, 23% of severe sepsis patients and 51 – 64% in septic shock patients [1, 2]. Sepsis is one of the causes of Acute Kidney Injury (AKI) in critically ill patients treated in the ICU known as Sepsis-Associated AKI (SA-AKI). The morbidity and mortality

 IntechOpen

rate of SA-AKI is still quite high even though the development of supportive care technology has progressed. A good understanding of SA-AKI is expected to increase alertness and make appropriate decisions in initiating management so as to provide better outcomes for patients with SA-AKI in the ICU.

By definition, Sepsis is a life-threatening condition of organ dysfunction due to an uncontrolled body's response to a systemic infection. Meanwhile, septic shock is part of sepsis with higher mortality characterized by hypotension requiring vasoactive therapy to maintain an average arterial pressure of at least 65 mmHg and serum lactate above 2 mmol/L despite adequate fluid resuscitation with a mortality rate of>40% [2]. Organ dysfunction caused by inflammatory response can be used to distinguish infections with sepsis, using Sequential Organ Failure Assessment (SOFA) scoring where a minimum of 2 points is the most recent associated with a mortality rate of 10% [3–5]. Critically ill patients with sepsis when patients are undergoing treatment in the Intensive Care Unit (ICU) may experience organ failure, especially in the respiratory system (43%) and the renal system (36%) [6, 7].

2. Literature review

2.1 Definition

According to the latest definition, sepsis is characterized by suspicion or evidence of infection plus clinical signs and laboratory findings that indicate organ dysfunction (based on the SOFA/Sequential Organ Failure Assessment score) due to an immune response to the infection. The heart, liver, lungs and kidneys are organs that are often affected during this process [2]. For a longtime sepsis has been known as a cause of morbidity and mortality; the consensually agreed upon definition of sepsis has only been around for the last few decades [3]. The first consensual definition defined sepsis as a continuous physiological and serological disorder that causes progressive organ failure.

The consensual definition of Sepsis-3 is the response to the limitations of the old definition, where SIRS and severe sepsis are removed. Sepsis is defined as life-threatening organ dysfunction due to the body's uncontrolled response to infection. Organ dysfunction can be identified by a condition of acute changes associated with infection with at least 2 points on a Sequential Organ Failure Assessment (SOFA score), increasing the mortality rate by 10% [2]. The determination of the sepsis diagnosis in patients with infection can use the quick SOFA score, where two of the three criteria can meet the criteria of sepsis. Meanwhile, septic shock is sepsis with hypotension that requires a vasopressor to maintain a minimum MAP of 65 mmHg and serum lactate above 2 mmol/L despite adequate fluid resuscitation; this condition has a mortality rate of 40% [4]. Based on the European Society of Intensive Care Medicine and the Society of Critical Care Medicine's Third International Consensus Definition for Sepsis and Septic Shock in 2016, sepsis is defined as life-threatening organ dysfunction caused by dysregulation of the body's response to infection. So, the criteria for sepsis must also include the three elements, namely, infection, body response and organ dysfunction. The criterion for the diagnosis of sepsis is established through a SOFA (Sequential/Sepsis-related Organ Failure Assessment) score ≥ 2 [5].

Given the significantly high mortality rates, AKI as one of the most frequent complications of sepsis is considered an important issue in clinical practice and especially for hospitalized patients treated in the ICU. This may be due to the limited understanding of the pathogenesis of SA-AKI sepsis, the lack of ability to assess kidney function in early diagnosis of AKI, and the absence of specific treatments other than supportive care [3].

AKI is characterized by a sudden decline in kidney function for several hours to days, resulting in the accumulation of creatinine, urea and other waste products. The latest definition was formulated in the consensus of Kidney Disease: Improving Global Outcome (KDIGO) in 2012, where the AKI was established if it met the criteria: an increase in serum creatinine levels ≥0.3 mg/dL (26.5 μmol/L) within 48 hours, an increase in serum creatinine at least 1.5 times the baseline value within the previous 7 days, or urine volume ≤ 0.5 ml/kg body weight for 6 hours [6].

The initial definition of AKI was the result of the international consensus of the Acute Dialysis Quality Initiative (ADQI) in 2004 that produced RIFLE (Risk, Injury, Failure, Loss, End stage Kidney disease) criteria based on an assessment of increased serum creatinine, decreased Glumerular Filtration Rate (GFR) urine production, loss if AKI lasts >4 weeks and end stage Kidney disease if AKI continues >3 months [7]. Then in 2007, the Acute Kidney Injury Network (AKIN), an international nephrological network or community in the USA and Europe, issued a more specific measure on RIFLE criteria focusing on the condition of the injury, i.e. Risk, Injury, and Failure were changed into stages (stage 1, stage 2, stage 3); Loss and end stage Kidney disease was eliminated; and an increase in serum creatinine of 0.3 mg/dL within 48 hours was added [8].

In 2012, the KDIGO issued clinical guidelines for the management of AKI and made a classification of AKI by combining RIFLE and AKIN criteria. This KDIGO-based classification defines AKI based on an increase in serum creatinine of 0.3 mg/dL within 48 hours or an increase of 1.5 x serum creatinine from baseline or urine production <0.5 ml/kg/hour for 6-12 hours. Baseline serum creatinine is the examination value obtained in the last 7 days. KDIGO also introduced the definition of Acute Kidney Disease (AKD), where an increase in serum creatinine >7 days and < 3 months. This condition occurs due to injury to the kidney and it can also occur slowly, different from AKI with a significant decrease in kidney function occurring within 7 days after the cause of injury to the kidney [9].

In patients who meet both the criteria for sepsis and AKI, it is called SA-AKI [10, 11]. Sepsis can be associated with >50% of AKI cases, and > 60% of sepsis patients can experience AKI. SA-AKI can also be interpreted as AKI which is caused or worsened by sepsis, so that it can be classified as a different condition in AKI which is usually caused by nephrotoxic regimens and ischemic conditions. The inflammatory response is more prominent in SA-AKI compared to nephrotoxic and ischemic AKI [12, 13]. SA-AKI is a clinical syndrome due to acute damage to organ function and damage. It is related to long-term adverse outcomes depending on the severity of the underlying organ damage. In general, SA-AKI should be considered a syndrome, characterized by fulfilling the criteria for sepsis and AKI [6].

2.2 Epidemiology

Acute Kidney Injury (AKI) is a syndrome with a broad spectrum of etiology and various mechanisms; ischemia/hypoxia, nephrotoxics and inflammation play a role in the development of AKI. Among the various etiologies of AKI, sepsis is one of the main causes of AKI in the ICU. According to various reported data, 45-70% of all AKI cases are related to sepsis [8]. Among ICU patients in general, the incidence of AKI varies from 6–67% depending on the study population. The incidence of SA-AKI in patients treated in ICU varies from 13–78% depending on the severity of sepsis and the AKI criteria used. In patients with critical illness with AKI, as many as 20-67% also suffer from sepsis, severe sepsis or sepsis shock. Research conducted by Angus and others on 192,980 patients with severe sepsis from seven states in the United States found that AKI occurred in 22% of sepsis patients with a mortality rate of 38.2%. Whereas in the cohort study conducted by The Sepsis Occuring in Acutely Ill Patients (SOAP) on 3,147 patients treated in 198 ICUs throughout Europe, 37% of patients had sepsis and AKI occurred in 51% of them with a mortality rate in ICU of 41%. The FINNAKI study of 2,901 critically ill patients treated in ICU in Finland found that among 918 patients with severe sepsis, 53% met the KDIGO criteria for AKI [6].

SA-AKI is associated with a higher risk of death and mortality in hospitals. If the MMR has an overall mortality rate of 45%, the mortality rate of SA-AKI is much higher, which is above 70%. Bagshaw and others in their study found that mortality rates from SA-AKI cases in hospitals and intensive care units/ICUs had increased by 30% and 20% respectively, but it was also suggested that the severity of AKI had a positive correlation with morbidity and mortality rates of ICU patients, the higher the severity of AKI, the higher the mortality rate. Population at high risk for SA-AKI are elderly patients, females, and those with the presence of comorbidities such as diabetes mellitus, chronic kidney failure, congestive heart failure and malignancy. Sources of infection and side effects from treatment also contribute to risk factors for SA-AKI such as intra-abdominal infections, urosepsis, endocarditis and bloodstream infections [14, 15].

2.3 Etiology

Acute Kidney Injury (AKI) is a syndrome with a broad spectrum of etiology. Based on the mechanism of the cause, AKI can be divided into pre-renal, renal, and post-renal AKI.

1. The cause of pre-renal AKI is renal hypoperfusion, due to hypovolemia or a decrease in effective circulation volume, such as in the case of sepsis and heart failure, and intrarenal haemodynamic disorders, such as the use of non-steroidal anti-inflammatory drugs.

2. Renal AKI is caused by abnormalities in the vascular or tubular components of the kidney directly, such as vasculitis, malignant hypertension, acute glomerular nephritis, interstitial nephritis, nephrotoxic substances, etc., causing intrarenal vasoconstriction, ischemia and decreased renal filtration rate.

3. Post renal AKI is usually caused by intrarenal and extra renal obstruction problems that interfere with kidney blood flow [14].

2.4 Pathophysiology

The pathophysiology of the SA-AKI is not yet fully known, and so far it has only been known from the results of studies on animal models that may be of relevance only to specific conditions in humans. From studies in animals and humans, SA-AKI occurs due to an excessive inflammatory response that causes injury to the kidneys, injury to the tubular tight junction, cell cycle arrest, cellular apoptosis and others [4].

The immune response to sepsis will cause microcirculation dysfunction (in tubular and glomerular capillaries) due to the proinflammatory response resulting in injury to endothelial cells. Vascular permiability will increase and there will be a decrease in endothelial Nitric Oxide Synthase (eNOS) activity, which functions to inhibit platelet aggregation and leukocyte activation. Meanwhile, induction of Nitric Oxyde Synthase (iNOS), which works otherwise, will increase its activity. This condition will cause ischemia and hypoxia. Inflammatory reactions will also cause a cycle cell arrest and apoptosis as a form of protection so that the damage is not widespread. As a result of ischemic and hypoxia, cells will lack energy so that the mitochondria work abnormally, causing injury to the mitochondria, so that injury to the kidneys continues and kidney function will be disrupted.

In sepsis the pathophysiological process of AKI can be caused by the following process:

1. Ischemic vasodilation, causing a decrease in Renal Blood Flow (pre renal AKI) due to an increase in Nitrides Oxyde induced by iNOS.

2. Endothelial leakage, causing edema and increased renal interstitial hydrostatic pressure (glomerulus and tubules), thereby reducing kidney filtration.

3. Nephrosis of the nephron due to the release of neutralizing agents triggered by the release of mediators in sepsis (the formation of ROS or the ischemic process itself causes necrosis of the nephron).

4. Capillary microtrombus due to coagulopathy and platelet leukocyte activation in the kidney endothelium.

2.4.1 Early detection of SA-AKI

Sepsis and AKI can each increase morbidity and mortality, length of stay, and treatment costs, so early detection of SA-AKI is very important to be able to intervene earlier and provide better outcomes for patients. Especially for AKI, given the definition and classification generated from the consensus, it can actually be easier to diagnose AKI by the method of assessing the increase in serum creatinine and urine production. However, this method has limitations, where changes in serum creatinine run slowly and assessment of urine production is usually only routinely done in the ICU. Therefore, several bio-markers have begun to be investigated to be able to detect SA-AKI earlier. Biomarkers can be categorized into two groups: 1. Assessment of renal function, 2. Detection of injury to kidney cells. Biomarkers for detecting SA-AKI include: Cystatin C (Cys-C), Neutrophil Gelatinase-Associated Lipocalin (NGAL), Kidney Injury Molecule-1 (KIM-1), Interleukin-18 (IL-18), Liver Type Fatty Acid -Binding (L-FABP), soluble-triggering receptor Expressed on Myeloid cells-1 (sTREM-1) and Activating Transcriptional Factor-3 (ATF-3). The sensitivity and specificity of the biomarkers varies depending on the time of measurement and the type of sample used. In general, biomarkers from blood (serum) are lower in sensitivity compared to biomarkers from urine samples [16, 17].

Neutrophil Gelatinase-Associated Lipocalin (NGAL) is currently the chosen biomarker in AKI cases, because it can be a biomarker for proximal tubular function and for kidney injury. Below (**Table 1**) are some biomarker studies that assess the time, sensitivity and specificity of several biomarkers derived from serum and urine to detect SA-AKI from the last few years.

2.5 Clinical description

Signs and symptoms of sepsis vary not only with regard to organ involvement, but also from one individual to another because of the patient's special characteristics, vulnerability, and disease. Signs of sepsis reflect the phase of the disease and vary from symptoms confined to the main organ (e.g pneumonia) to severe multi-organ dysfunction syndrome (MODS) and septic shock. Health care workers must be alert for signs of infection, sepsis or septic shock when evaluating patients for kidney failure. Conversely, it is important to frequently monitor kidney

	Time	AUROC	Threshold value	Sensitivity	Specificity	References
Urine Biomarker						
NGAL (ng/mL)	12 hours after septic shock	0.86	>68	0.71	1.0	Martensson et al.
Cys-C (mg/L)	8 hours after patients have been treated	0.86	0.106	0.85	0.80	Aydogdu et al.
NGAL (ng/mL)	7 hours after onset of sepsis	0.86	402	0.89	0.74	Fan et al.
NGAL (ng/mL)	24 hours after patients have been treated	0.78	350	0.75	0.82	Matsa et al.
Serum Biomarker						
NGAL (ng/mL)	12 hours after septic shock	0.67	>120	0.83	0.50	Martensson et al.
Cys-C (mg/L)	8 hours after patients have been treated	0.82	1.5	0.73	0.68	Aydogdu et al.
NGAL (ng/mL)	24 hours after patients have been treated	0.88	400	0.79	0.75	Matsa et al.

From the above mention, it can be shown that both NGAL and Cyst C measurements from urine have higher sensitivity and specificity than serum and both of them can be detected earlier than creatinine. It can be also detected as urine biomarkers. *NGAL: Neutrophil Gelatinase-Associated Lipocalin.*
***Cys-C: Cystatine C.*

Table 1.
Research with NGAL and Cys-C biomarkers.

function (along with other organ involvement) in patients with documented or suspected sepsis.

Clinical studies based on physiological data and some postmortem reports have recently begun to define AKI caused by sepsis and how it differs from other types of kidney injury. Histologically, AKI induced by sepsis is characterized by heterogeneous tubular cell injury with apical vacuolization, but in the absence of tubular necrosis or even extensive apoptosis. All of these features can develop in the context of normal or increased renal blood flow (Renal Blood Flow/RBF) and represent a clinical phenotype characterized by decreased levels of glomerular filtration (GFR), creatininclearance, and uremia [18].

2.6 Diagnosis

A diagnosis of AKI caused by sepsis requires a diagnosis of sepsis and subsequent events of AKI. This is considered a PIRO (predisposition, infection, response, organ dysfunction) system. The diagnosis of sepsis is more complex than the original. In the new definition, several other important aspects of sepsis are included such as hemodynamics and organ dysfunction [18].

A 2016 task force organized by the national community including the Society of Critical Care Medicine (SCCM) and the European Society of Intensive Care Medicine (ESICM) proposed a new definition of sepsis, called Sepsis-3. This consensus defines sepsis as life-threatening organ dysfunction caused by dysregulation of the responhost to infection. The new definition does not use the Systemic Inflammatory Response Syndrome's (SIRS) criteria in the identification of sepsis and elimination of severe sepsis [18].

Sequential Organ Failure Assessment (SOFA) is a simple and objective score that allows for calculating both the number and severity of organ dysfunction in six organ systems (breathing, coagulation, liver, cardiovascular, kidney, and neurological), and the score can measure individual or aggregate organ dysfunction [19].

Early detection of AKI in ICU settings is very important. AKI has become a major issue with the increasing number of incidents, causing more than four million deaths per year worldwide. Also, the lack of a reliable initial biomarker for AKI causes a significant delay in starting an appropriate therapy. This is in contrast to the "biological revolution" in cardiology, which produces various markers (including troponin) for early diagnosis of heart damage that allows for early and effective treatments [19].

The diagnosis of AKI is based on an increase in serum creatinine and/or a decrease in urine output. The definition has evolved from the criteria of Risk, Injury, Failure, Loss, Endstage (RIFLE) (**Table 2**) in 2004 to the classification of the Acute Kidney Injury Network (AKIN) in 2007. In 2012, the two were merged, forming the Kidney Disease Improving Global Outcomes (KDIGO) classification [10].

Combined with evidence-based medicine, KDIGO published KDIGO guidelines in March 2012 and established diagnostic criteria for AKI (**Table 3**): increase in serum creatinine >0.3 mg/dl (26.5 μmol/L) within 48 hours; or an increase in serum creatinine to 1.5 times the baseline, which is known or thought to have occurred within 7 days; or urine output <0.5 ml/kg/hour for 6-12 hours. According to the severity, this condition is divided into stages 1, 2, and 3, similar to the classification of AKIN [10].

Categories	Serum Creatinine Criteria	Urine Output Criteria
RIFLE*		
Risk	↑ in SCr to 1.5 – < 2 x baseline	UO <0.5 mL/kg/hr. for 6 hrs
Injury	↑ in SCr to 2 – < 3 x baseline	UO <0.5 mL/kg/hr. for 12 hrs
Failure	↑ in SCr to ≥3 x baseline	UO <0.3 mL/kg/hr. for 24 hrs or Anuria for 12 hrs
Loss	Loss of Kidney function for >4 wks	
ESRD	Loss of Kidney function for >3 mos	
AKIN**		
Stage 1	↑ in SCr to 0.3 mg/dL or to 1.5 – 2 x baseline	UO <0.5 mL/kg/hr. for >8 hrs
Stage 2	↑ in SCr to >2 – 3 x baseline	UO <0.5 mL/kg/hr. for >12 hrs
Stage 3	↑ in SCR to >3 x baseline or	UO <0.5 mL/kg/hr. for >24 hrs
Stage 4	SCr ≥ 4 mg/dL with an acute increase of ≥0.5 mg/dL	or Anuria for 12 hrs

*There are little bit differences between RIFLE and AKIN Criteria, LOSS and ESRD in RIFLE criteria are included in Stage 4 in AKIN criteria. *RIFLE: Risk, Injury, Failure, Loss, ESRD (End Stage Renal Disease; AKIN: Acute Kidney Injury Network.*
***AKIN Criteria require the increase of serum creatinine to occur within 48 hrs; SCr: Serum Creatinine; UO: Urine Output.*

Table 2.
RIFLE and AKIN CRITERIA of AKI.

Stage	Serum Creatinine and urine output criteria
1	Serum creatinine increased 1.5 – 1.9 x baseline or increase ≥26.4 umol/L (0.3 mg/dL) or urinary output <0.5 ml/kg/h during a 6 hour block
2	Serum creatinine increased 2.0 – 2.9 x baseline or urinary output <0.5 ml/kg/h during two 6 blocks
3	Serum creatinine increased >3 x baseline or increased to ≥353 Umol/L (4 mg/dL) or initiation of renal replacement therapy or Urinary output <0.3 ml/kg/h during more than 24 hours or anuria For more than 12 hours

KDIGO: the Kidney Disease Improving Global Outcomes.
KDIGO criteria is most simple than RIFLE and AKIN, there are only 3 stages of AKI, but still using creatinine serum and urine output criteria.

Table 3.
KDIGO criteria of AKI.

The KDIGO guidelines highlight early diagnosis and treatment of AKI and diagnostic markers remain at serum creatinine levels. Because serum creatinine tests are convenient and inexpensive, they can be used as practical clinical indicators. However, there are some limitations. Renal hypoperfusion due to prerenal causes can cause an increase in creatinine, although there is no interference with the renal parenchyma. When the renal parenchyma is injured, renal compensation can cause lag in creatinine increase. Further, injury to 50% of the kidneys can occur without an increase in creatinine levels, so diagnosis and intervention are delayed. Thus, new markers with higher sensitivity and specificity are expected to help the initial diagnosis of AKI. At present, many studies report the presence of early diagnostic markers of AKI. Some of them are clinical trials that show good sensitivity and specificity, with initial diagnostic values for AKI. In addition, different biological markers have been shown to show various mechanisms of injury [20].

Evidently, AKI occurs through complex mechanisms often due to several factors. Different mechanisms cause injury in various parts of the kidney. It is difficult to establish a clear diagnosis and accurate localization of the injury using the same marker to diagnose injury to all kidney subregions caused by all diseases. Discrete studies of certain diseases and related kidney injuries will definitely improve diagnostic accuracy. About 45 – 70% of MMR is associated with sepsis, which is one of the most important causes of MMR. Furthermore, the proportion of septic patients with secondary kidney injury is 16 – 50%, whereas the mortality of sepsis associated with AKI is up to 50 – 60%. As such, pursuing focused studies of sepsis-induced AKI and searching for biomarkers associated with early diagnosis will help in solving important clinical problems of septic patients and AKI disease [20].

2.7 Management

As with sepsis management in general, the main therapy for SA-AKI is the provision of appropriate antibiotics and good supportive care. There are several things that must be considered in the management of SA-AKI:

2.7.1 Fluid therapy

Giving fluids is still fundamental in the treatment of sepsis. Patients who are responsive after being given fluids (fluid responder) can theoretically be interpreted as patients who have increased the stroke volume of 10-15% after giving a fluid challenge of 250-500 ml; in reality, there are less than 40% of sepsis patients who need fluids or fluid responder. Based on the Frank-Starling principle, if preload increases, the stroke volume will increase until it reaches the optimal preload volume. And if the preload given can no longer increase stroke volume, the volume of liquid given can be dangerous because it can increase arterial pressure, venous pressure, and ultimately pulmonary hydrostatic pressure. Further, the condition will stimulate the release of natriuretic peptide causing fluid transfer from the intravascular space to the interstitial space. Kidney function will also be affected by this condition where there is a decrease in GFR due to increased venous pressure, potentially increasing subcapsular pressure in the kidneys due to fluid transfer.

The "Fluid Expansion as Supportive Therapy" (FEAST) research can explain the dangers of giving fluid loading to patients with sepsis, where aggressive fluid therapy is associated with increased mortality.

In 2001, the concept of "early aggressive fluid resuscitation" was issued, known as the Early Goal Directed Therapy (EGDT). Following this, studies began using the EGDT protocol. It is interesting to find the reduction in mortality by reducing the volume of resuscitation fluid in the first 72 hours. Although the early sepsis phase shows an effective condition of circulating volume reduction, making it possible for fluid resuscitation to take place, the subsequent fluid therapy given can cause problems especially in the SA-AKI [21]. Besides being unable to improve septic shock, fluid therapy can also contribute to causing renal dysfunction through several mechanisms. The most rapid occurrence is an increase in venous pressure due to fluid therapy that directly increases the renal interstitial pressure and peritubular area in animal models [22]. Because the administration of large fluid boluses (20-30 ml/kg) is associated with the occurrence of fluid overload, it is currently recommended to use fluid volumes with lower volumes (200-500 ml) [22]. The 2014 Acute Dialysis Quality Initiative (ADQI) recommends giving fluid therapy to sepsis patients divided into 4 stages, namely using the rescue protocol, optimization, stabilization and de-escalation. A large liquid volume of 500 ml in a maximum of 15 minutes only at the rescue stage is given to overcome hypotension with close monitoring. At the optimization stage, a 100-200 ml fluid challenge for 5-10 minutes can be done. At the stage of stabilization, the patient is stable and fluid administration is a maintenance therapy of 1-2 ml/kg/hour.

The three stages above are followed by de-escalation, which is the stage to reduce total body fluids with the help of diuretics or Renal Replacement Therapy (RRT) with the target of negative cumulative fluid balance. Assessment of volume status during fluid therapy can proceed with the Passive Leg Raising method combined with measurement of stroke volume in real-time. This procedure is proven to be the most precise in assessing volume status clinically. The availability of ultrasound equipment in the ICU can prevent fluid overload by assessing the B-line on the Lung Ultrasound and the vena cava collapsibility index to assess the fluid responder. The MAP target of 65 – 75 mmHg is an adequate target for maintaining renal perfusion [22].

Fluid selection is also a consideration in the SA-AKI. Normal 0.9% saline is actually a non-physiological fluid and is less well administered to SA-AKI than other crystalloids. Normal saline can cause hyperchloremic metabolic acidosis, which can cause a decrease in Renal Blood Flow (RBF) by activating the mechanism of tubuloglumerular feedback and afferent vasoconstriction so as to increase the risk of further kidney injury. In a retrospective study involving 60734 adults with septic shock, normal single saline can increase mortality compared with crystalloid balance solution. Albumin has also been investigated for its use in sepsis patients with the risk of SA-AKI in the SAFE study, showing that albumin was not effective in reducing mortality and RRT requirements when compared with crystalloid fluids [23]. So that until now albumin cannot be recommended as a resuscitation fluid in SA-AKI. Hydroxyethyl Starches (HES) is not recommended and should not be used on SA-AKI.

2.7.2 Vasopressor

Norepinephrine is still the main therapy for septic shock and has been shown to increase MAP and improve perfusion to the kidneys. Norepinephrine itself is the first choice in various clinical studies and provides better outcomes and fewer side effects than other vasopressors. However, due to animal studies showing that norepinephrine can cause medullary hypoxia renal in SA-AKI, researchers have begun to look for other vasopressors in the condition of sepsis and SA-AKI. Vasopressin is the most desirable vasopressor to study; Vasopressin and Septic Shock (VAST) research tries to compare norepinephrine with vasopressin with the same results on the outcome and no side effects are obtained. Further, VANISH research proceeds, the results of which showing the absence of AKI events and side effects of both. Based on these data, vasopressin is the second-line choice of the current vasopressor and has been included in the latest sepsis guidelines. Angiotensin II is a hormone in the renin-angiotensin-aldosterone system which has also begun to be studied in shock conditions. Angiotensin II for the Treatment of High Output Shock (ATHOS) study in 344 patients with shock due to vasodilation (259 with sepsis) found that Angiotensin II significantly increased MAP. Improvements were also seen in SOFA cardiovascular scores. Another smaller study of patients who needed RRT showed that patients who received angiotensin II had a greater 28-day survival rate and were free of RRT on the seventh day more than placebo. If these results can be validated by larger studies, there is a possibility that angiotensin II can be a meaningful therapy for SA-AKI [23].

Levosimendan is a calcium sensitizing drug and has an inotropic effect that is often used in cord decompensation. One small study showed an increase in creatinine clearance and urine production compared to dobutamine. However, in a larger scale study comparing it with placebo (MAKE-28), there was no difference in outcomes in the kidney. So, there is no data to support its use in the SA-AKI [24].

2.7.3 Antibiotics and nephrotoxic substances

The survival rate in sepsis patients will decrease by 7.6% per hour if no appropriate antibiotic therapy is given. Regarding AKI, vancomycin antibiotics are reported to cause AKI even at the recommended dosage for infections caused by methicillin-resistance *Staphylococcus aureus* (MRSA) and it is also reported that vancomycin enhances the nephrotoxic effect of the antibiotic piperazilin-tazobactam. Then other nephrotoxic substances must also be avoided such as Amphotericin B, iodine contras substances, godalinium (a contrast agent for MRI) that can cause AKI [24].

2.7.4 Renal Replacement Therapy (RRT)

There are several aspects that must be considered in kidney replacement therapy, namely indication, time, modality and dosage given. Clinical indications that have been known so far, which are Acidosis, Electrolyte disturbances, Intoxication, O-fluid Overload and Uremia (A-E-I-O-U), can be applied to SA-AKI. Severe metabolic acidosis, fluid overload and uremia are the three most common indications of RRT in SA-AKI [24].

Criteria for Renal Replacement Therapy (hemodialysis) in critically ill patients with AKI include:

- Oligouria: urine output <2000 ml in 12 hours
- Anuria: urine production <50 ml in 12 hours

- Hyperkalemia: potassium levels>6.5 mmol/L
- Severe acidemia (acid poisoning): pH <7.0
- Azotemia: urea levels>30 mmol/L
- Uremic encephalopathy
- Uteric neuropathy/myopathy
- Uremic pericarditis
- Abnormalities of plasma sodium concentration > 155 mmol/L or < 120 mmol/L
- Hypertemia
- Drug poisoning

At the time of the RRT initiation, the available data give different answers. Although undesirable effects have been reported due to the late initiation of the RRT, leading to increased mortality and poor outcomes in the SA-AKI [25]. Up until this, the RRT initiation is still individual. Bouman et al. showed no significant difference in renal outcomes in early and late hemofiltration in patients who were able to survive. There are two large studies, with conflicting conclusions, specifically designed to determine the time of initiation of RRT in the condition of critically ill patients. The ELAIN study comparing early versus late initiation of the RRT shows the benefits of early strategy in reducing mortality. While in the AKIKI study, the results show the opposite, i.e. early strategy gives negative results. In both of these studies there were differences in inclusion criteria; in the ELAIN study, patients were in KDIGO stage 2 with a SOFA score of 15.6-16.0 while in the AKIKI study patients were in KDIGO stage 3 with a SOFA score of 10.8-10.9. Perhaps because of these different inclusion criteria, the opposite results were obtained. But at the moment there is an ongoing study, the STARRT-AKI study (standard vs. accelerated initiation of renal replacement therapy in acute kidney injury) that might reveal the best RRT initiation time. The most appropriate RRT modalities for SA-AKI are also still different. Some studies show the advantages of Continuous Renal Replacement Therapy (CRRT) compared to Intermittent Hemodialysis (IHD) on survival rates and time spent for the kidney function to improve. Although CRRT is superior to IHD based on its fluid removal ability, with a lack of hypotension in patients, it is more expensive than IHD.

The current CRRT dose is sourced from two large studies with sepsis patients but not specific to SA-AKI, which is 20-25 ml/kg/hour. In the condition of the SA-AKI, the dose given is 30–35 ml/kg/hour. Several studies have shown that increasing the CRRT dose does not provide benefits and improve patient survival.

2.7.5 Antimicrobials during CRRT

CRRT significantly influences the pharmacokinetics and pharmacodynamics of most antimicrobial agents. This is not sufficiently anticipated by the currently recommended dosage guidelines. Patients are significantly at risk of receiving lower doses (underdosing), potentially causing treatment failure and increasing resistance.

2.7.6 Diuretics

The use of diuretics to induce or increase urine production in the absence of hypervolemia is associated with increased mortality. KDIGO does not recommend the use of diuretics in the prevention or treatment of AKI. Conversely, diuretics can be used to improve outcomes when fluid balance remains positive or in the case of excess fluid (volume overload). Research by Ho and Power reviewed the use of furosemide in AKI and found no beneficial effect in reducing mortality.

2.8 Prognosis

Compared with other AKI etiologies, SA-AKI may have specific prognostic implications. In most reports, this is associated with higher short-term mortality rates. In the analysis of the BEST Kidney trial subgroup, the likelihood of hospital death is 50% higher in SA-AKI compared to non-SA-AKI. Obviously, the different prognosis between SA-AKI and non-SA-AKI is largely influenced by the composition of the non-sepsis group and its proportion from conditions with a poor prognosis (such as cardiogenic shock). In addition, the confusing role in the relationship between SA-AKI and mortality needs to be overcome because all studies consistently report higher disease severity at onset, with patients requiring RRT more frequently [6].

In contrast, for patients who survive in the hospital, SA-AKI has been associated with improved kidney improvement compared to other etiologies of AKI. In the BEST Kidney study, there was a tendency for lower serum creatinine and RRT dependence (9 vs. 14%, P = 0.052). Clearly, many other factors may play a role in kidney recovery such as RRT modality, RRT time, and further nephrotoxic or ischemic inhibition. Kidney recovery is also strongly influenced by premorbid conditions as illustrated by a French multicentric observational study, which shows that diabetic patients with SA-AKI who have survived going to the hospital tend to need more long-term RRT and have higher serum creatinine levels. Apart from short-term recovery, however, it is now clear that even one episode of AKI is associated with a greater risk of subsequent CKD and even end-stage renal disease [4].

3. Conclusion

SA-AKI is a clinical syndrome due to acute damage to function and organ damage associated with long-term adverse outcomes depending on the severity of the underlying organ damage. Generally clinical manifestations of AKI are more dominated by factors of precipitation or its main disease. The main purpose of managing AKI is to prevent further kidney damage and keep the patient alive until his kidney physiology returns to normal function. SA-AKI is a condition that is often faced by patients with sepsis in the ICU. Understanding of sepsis and endotoxins that can cause SA-AKI is not yet fully known. Some evidence suggests that renal microcirculation hypoperfusion, lack of energy for cells, mitochondrial dysfunction, endothelial injury and cycle cell arrest can cause SA-AKI. Rapid identification of SA-AKI events, antibiotics and appropriate fluid therapy are crucial actions in the management of SA-AKI. The availability of modality for organ support such as CRRT in ICU care can help patients with sepsis, due to kidney failure that often occurs, survive. Further studies related to SA-AKI are still continuing and are expected to be the basis for making a clinical guide in the management of SA-AKI.

Author details

Titik Setyawati, Ricky Aditya and Tinni Trihartini Maskoen*
Faculty of Medicine, Universitas Padjadjaran, Bandung, Indonesia

*Address all correspondence to: drtitiksetyawati73@gmail.com

References

[1] Hoste EAJ, Bagshaw SM, Bellomo R, Cely CM, Colman R, Cruz DN, et al. Epidemiology of acute kidney injury in critically ill patients: the multinational AKI-EPI study. Intensive Care Med. 2015; 41(7): 15p.

[2] Singer M, Deutschman CS, Seymour CW, et al. The Third International Consensus Definitions for Sepsis and Septic Shock (Sepsis-3). JAMA 2016;315:801-10.

[3] Gotts JE, Matthay MA. Sepsis: pathophysiology and clinical management. BMJ 2016;353:i1585.

[4] Shankar-Hari M, Phillips GS, Levy ML, et al. Sepsis Definitions Task Force. Developing a New Definition and Assessing New Clinical Criteria for Septic Shock: For the Third International Consensus Definitions for Sepsis and Septic Shock (Sepsis-3). JAMA 2016;315:775-87.

[5] Vincent JL, de Mendonça A, Cantraine F, et al. Use of the SOFA score to assess the incidence of organ dysfunction/failure in intensive care units: results of a multicenter, prospective study. Working group on "sepsis- related problems" of the European Society of Intensive Care Medicine. Crit Care Med 1998;26:1793-800.

[6] Bellomo R, Kellum JA, Ronco C, Wald R, Martensson J, Maiden M, et al. Acute Kidney Injury in Sepsis. Intensive Care Med. 2017; 43 :816-28.

[7] Bellomo R, Ronco C, Kellum JA, Mehta RL, Palevsky P. Acute Dialysis Quality Initiative workgroup. Acute renal failure - definition, outcome measures, animal models, fluid therapy and information technology needs: the Second International Consensus Conference of the Acute Dialysis Quality Initiative (ADQI) Group. Crit Care 2004;8:R204-12.

[8] Mehta RL, Kellum JA, Shah SV, et al. Acute Kidney Injury Network. Acute Kidney Injury Network: report of an initiative to improve outcomes in acute kidney injury. Crit Care 2007;11:R31.

[9] KDIGO. Kidney Disease: Improving Global Outcomes (KDIGO) Acute Kidney Injury Work Group. KDIGO Clinical Practice Guideline for Acute Kidney Injury. Kidney Int Suppl 2012;2:1-138. Melyda. Diagnosis dan Tatalaksana Acute Kidney Injury (AKI) pada Syok Septik.CKD- 259. 2017; 44(17): 907-11.

[10] Uchino S, Kellum JA, Bellomo R, et al. Beginning and Ending Supportive Therapy for the Kidney (BEST Kidney) Investigators. Acute renal failure in critically ill patients: a multinational, multicenter study. JAMA 2005;294: 813-8.

[11] Bagshaw SM, Lapinsky S, Dial S, et al. Cooperative Antimicrobial Therapy of Septic Shock (CATSS) Database Research Group. Acute kidney injury in septic shock: clinical outcomes and impact of duration of hypotension prior to initiation of antimicrobial therapy. Intensive Care Med 2009;35:871-81.

[12] Doi K. Role of kidney injury in sepsis. Journal of Intensive Care. 2016;4:17

[13] Rajapakse S, Rodrigo C, Wijewickrema E. Management of Sepsis-Induced Acute Kidney Injury. SLJCC. 2009; 1(1): 3-14.

[14] SharfuddinAA,MolitorisBA. Pathophysiology of ischemic acute kidney injury. Nature Review Nephrology. 2011;7(4):189-200

[15] Di Nardo M, Ficarella A, Ricci Z, Luciano R, Stoppa F, Picardo S, Picca S, Muraca M, Cogo P. Impact of severe sepsis on serum and urinary biomarkers

of acute kidney injury in critically ill children: An observational study. Blood Puri cation. 2013;35(1-3):172-176

[16] Aydogdu M, Gursel G, Sancak B, Yeni S, Sari G, Tasyurek S, Turk M, Yuksel S, Senes M, Ozis TN. The use of plasma and urine neutrophil gelatinase associated lipocalin (NGAL) and cystatin C in early diagnosis of septic acute kidney injury in critically ill patients. Disease Markers. 2013;34(4):237-246

[17] Zhang Z. Biomarkes, diagnosis and management of sepsis-induced acute kidney injury: a narrative review. Heart, Lung and Vessels. 2015; 7 (1): 64-73

[18] Marik P. E, Taeb A.M. SIRS, qSOFA and new ssepsis definition. J Thorac Dis. 2017; 9 (4): 943-5

[19] Wang K, Xie S, Xiao K, Yang P, He W, Xie L. Biomarkers of Sepsis-Induced Acute Kidney Injury. BioMed Research International. 2018; Article ID 6937947: 1-7

[20] Rivers E, Nguyen B, Havstad S, Ressler J, Muzzin A, Knoblich B, Peterson E, Tomlanovich M. Early goal-directed therapy in the treatment of severe sepsis and septic shock. New England Journal of Medicine. 2001;345(19):1368-1377

[21] Marik PE. Fluid therapy in 2015 and beyond: The mini- uid challenge and mini- fluid bolus approach. British Journal of Anaesthesiology. 2015;115(3):347-349

[22] Finfer S, McEvoy S, Bellomo R, McArthur C, Myburgh J, Norton R. SAFE Study Investigators. Impact of albumin compared to saline on organ function and mortality of patients with severe sepsis. Intensive Care Med 2011;37:86-96.

[23] Meaney CJ, Hynicka LM, Tsoukleris MG. Vancomycin-associated nephrotoxicity in adult medicine patients: Incidence, outcomes, and risk factors. Pharmacotherapy. 2014;34(7):653-661

[24] Liu KD, Himmelfarb J, Paganini E, Ikizler TA, Soroko SH, Mehta RL, Chertow GM. Timing of initiation of dialysis in critically ill patients with acute kidney injury. Clinical Journal of the American Society of Nephrology. 2006;1(5):915-919

[25] BoumanCS,Oudemans-Van Straaten HM, Tijssen JG, ZandstraDF, KesecioglulJ.E ects of early high-volume continuous venovenous hemo ltration on survival and recovery of renal function in intensive care patients with acute renal failure: A prospective, randomized trial. Critical Care Medicine. 2002;30(10):2205-2211

Chapter 18

Atrial Fibrillation during Septic Shock

Manuel Vélez-Gimón

Abstract

Atrial Fibrillation (AF) is an early and common occurrence during septic shock, accounting for 25–30% of admissions. Conventional cardiovascular risk factors do not generally increase its incidence, especially in cases of new-onset AF. Inflammation during the sepsis process has been postulated as a possible trigger. Detrimental effects of AF result in prognosis worsening, even when the probability for a negative outcome has been adjusted for severity of illness. New-onset AF (NOAF) has been associated with greater mortality rate than preexisting chronic AF. Early cardioversion has not uniformly improved hospital outcomes. In this review, the incidence, prognosis and management of AF in septic shock patients are summarized.

Keywords: atrial fibrillation, septic shock, sepsis, antiarrhythmic therapy, cardioversion, critical care

1. Introduction

The term sepsis derives from ancient Greek "sêpsis" ("putrefaction" or "decay of organic matter") and was first used in a medical context in Homer's Iliad more than 2700 years ago. Currently, sepsis is defined as a life-threatening organ dysfunction due to a dysregulated host response to infection [1]. Since 2016, the updated operative definition of sepsis no longer considers the presence of systemic inflammatory response syndrome, but requires an infection plus organ dysfunction indicated by an acute change in Sequential Organ Failure Assessment (SOFA) [2] of at least two points (see **Table 1**). Septic shock is defined as sepsis plus circulatory failure with increased risk of death, indicated by hypotension requiring vasopressor therapy to maintain a mean arterial pressure (MAP) 65 mmHg or greater and a serum lactate of greater than 2 mmol/L despite adequate fluid resuscitation [3]. Other indices of tissue hypoperfusion (e.g. altered mental status, oliguria, delayed capillary refill) are acceptable alternatives whenever serum lactate determination is not available.

In high-income countries, sepsis represents approximately 6% of adult hospitalizations and 10–37% of intensive care unit (ICU) admissions. Mortality estimates from sepsis and septic shock vary widely, rounding 15% and 22% respectively [4]. In low-income regions, sepsis and septic shock predictably carry an even higher mortality, up to 50% [5].

Generally speaking, atrial fibrillation (AF) is the most frequently found cardiac arrhythmia in the ICU setting. Previously known AF is significantly prevalent among older patients with chronic conditions who are at risk for critical illness. New-onset AF (NOAF), on the other hand, is frequently triggered by accelerated

IntechOpen

System	Score				
	0	1	2	3	4
Respiration PaO_2/FIO_2, mmHg (kPa)	≥400 (53.3)	<400 (53.3)	<300 (40)	<200 (26.7) with respiratory support	<100 (13.3) with respiratory support
Coagulation platelets, $\times 10^3$ μL^{-1}	≥150	<150	<100	<50	<20
Liver bilirubin, mg dL^{-1} ($\mu mol\ L^{-1}$)	<1.2 (20)	1.2–1.9 (20–32)	2.0–5.9 (33–101)	6.0–11.9 (102–204)	>120 (204)
Cardiovascular	MAP ≥70 mmHg	MAP<70 mmHg	Dopamine<5 or dobutamine (any dose)[a]	Dopamine 5.1–15 or epinephrine ≤0.1 or norepinephrine ≤0.1[a]	Dopamine >15 or epinephrine >0.1 or norepinephrine >0.1[a]
Central nervous system (CNS)					
Glasgow Coma Scale score[b]	15	13–14	10–12	6–9	<6
Renal creatinine, mg dL^{-1} ($\mu mol\ L^{-1}$) < 1.2 (110) 1.2–1.9 (110–170)	2.0–3.4 (171–299)	3.5–4.9 (300–440)	>5.0 (440)		
Urine output, mL per day				<500	<200

FIO_2, fraction of inspired oxygen; MAP, mean arterial pressure; PaO_2, partial pressure of oxygen.
[a]Catecholamine doses are given as $\mu g kg^{-1}\ min^{-1}$ for at least 1 h.
[b]Glasgow Coma Scale scores range from 3 to 15; higher score indicates belter neurological function.

Table 1.
Sequential organ failure assessment (SOFA) score [2].

atrial remodeling and by concomitant stressors during critical illness, such as electrolyte imbalances and use of vasopressor drugs [6].

In this narrative review, the pathogenesis, risk factors, incidence, prognosis and management of AF in septic shock patients are summarized.

2. Pathogenesis

The negative effects of sepsis on the heart are not limited to the contractile function and ventricular relaxation, but also affect the electric function. Although the precise mechanisms remain to be elucidated, inflammation seems to play an important role. The electrical instability of cardiomyocytes in patients with sepsis has been considered to be due to the use of vasopressor drugs and the presence of electrolyte disturbances. However, according to recent findings, atrial fibrillation (AF) could be the result of the necrosis and fibrosis induced by inflammation [7, 8]. These alterations are supposed to be able to trigger an arrhythmia due to a fluctuation in the myocardial cells' membrane potential [9].

The development of NOAF in septic shock patients depends upon the presence of an arrhythmogenic substrate, the trigger factors and the modulation factors such as autonomic nervous system or inflammation. Triggered activity has been shown in the musculature of the atrium. An imbalance between sympathetic and vagal tone leading to a reduction of heart rate variability has been proposed as an explanation for the development of NOAF in septic patients [10]. Vagal stimulation normally attenuates the inflammatory response [11]. In human atrial cardiomyocytes, partial blockage of the I(f) 'funny' pacemaker current has been observed after exposition to gram-negative bacteria endotoxin [12], which may contribute to a reduced responsiveness to both sympathetic and vagal autonomic stimuli (the name "funny current" arose because of its numerous unusual characteristics, including the mixed Na + and K+ current permeability, activation on hyperpolarization, and

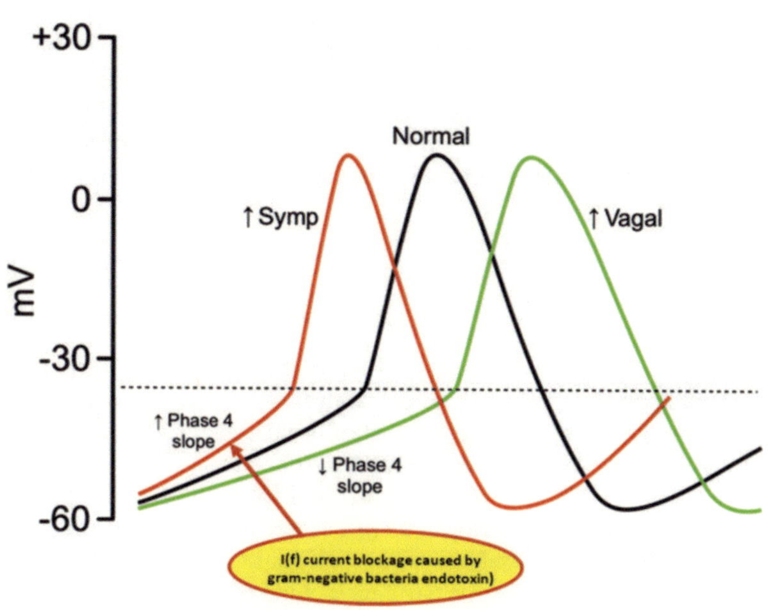

Figure 1.
Schematized transmembrane action potential of sinus node (pacemaker) cells. The black line shows normal slope in sinus rhythm. During gram-negative bacteria induced-sepsis, it has been shown I(f) current blockage, which results in an increased phase 4 slope, triggering sinus tachycardia and facilitating AF onset (red line) [12].

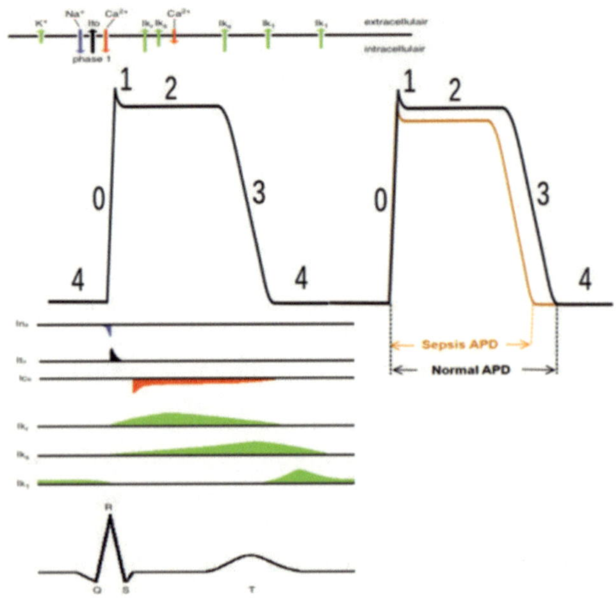

Figure 2.
Schematized transmembrane action potential of atrial myocytes in normal and septic animals. The orange line indicates how sepsis decrease phase 2 (plateau phase) duration and leads to decrease in APD (action potential duration). This is due to a decrease in influx of calcium through the voltage-dependent L-channels, which is at least in part caused by sepsis-induced tachycardia. The decrease in APD (and hence in the atrial refractory period) has been proposed to effectively trigger AF [15].

slow activation and deactivation kinetics [13]) (see **Figure 1**). This would result in a high heart rate output, which is commonly observed in septic patients. Unopposed sustained tachycardia during the will further increase calcium influx through L-type Ca2+ channels, which leads to marked shortening of the atrial refractory period and action potential duration (**Figure 1**) and elicit triggered activity, hence facilitating the onset of AF [14, 15] (see **Figure 2**). This process has been shown to be further enhanced due to beta-adrenergic stimulation after endotoxin application [16], which increases channel activity by prolonging the open time and shortening the close time of Ca2+ channel. These findings might explain the high sensitivity of cardiac pacemaker cells to positive inotropic effect of adrenergic stimulation and most likely development of new AF episode especially in the early stages of sepsis [17].

3. Risk factors

Sepsis itself is a strong risk factor for NOAF in the critical care setting. An extensive retrospective population-based cohort analysis by Walkey et al. revealed that compared to those without severe sepsis, patients with severe sepsis (n = 49,082) exhibited a significantly increased risk of NOAF (odds ratio (OR), 6.82; 95% confidence interval (CI), 6.54–7.11; $P < 0.001$) [18]. Multiple studies have been shown that the classic risk factors for the development of chronic atrial fibrillation in the general population may differ from those present in septic patients with NOAF. Risk factors for the occurrence of NOAF in septic patients include conditions that are not related to chronic cardiovascular disease, such as increased number of acute organ failures/dysfunction, mechanical ventilation, increased comorbidities, and use of pulmonary artery catheterization [18–22]. NOAF has been also associated with lower EF, older age, higher level of troponin-HS and NT-pro-BNP and longer QRS duration.

Sepsis due to bacterial pneumonia has been associated with a high risk of developing NOAF, while sepsis due to gastrointestinal infections has been related to AF recurrence with worse long-term prognosis [23]. It has been hypothesized that the type and severity of infection could have an impact on the atrial remodeling and the variety of cytokine expression during sepsis. Current evidence suggests that the severity of the inflammatory response in critically ill patients is associated with a higher risk of NOAF, and septic shock patients have in general a heightened probability of developing NOAF than patients with other acute critical illnesses after adjustment for underlying risk factors [21].

In a systematic review that included 11 studies, Kuipers et al. [19] identified independent risk factors with a high level of evidence for NOAF in septic patients. White race, organ failure and pulmonary catheter use were moderately associated with NOAF development, while there was a weak association with age and respiratory tract infection. On the other hand, history of diabetes and urinary tract infections were found to be weak protective factors. In other studies, markers of illness severity (such as the presence of organ failure and shock) as well as several critical care interventions were associated with an increased risk of NOAF in septic patients. Known risk factors for chronic or paroxysmal AF in the general population, such as advanced age, white race, male gender, obesity and (ischemic) heart failure, were in some studies also associated with the development of AF during sepsis [24, 25]. Specific electrocardiographic or echocardiographic features of AF such as P-wave duration or left atrial area, remain to be studied in septic shock patients, although both factors are known to predict the occurrence of AF in the general population [26, 27].

Data regarding risk factors for the occurrence of NOAF in septic shock patients is more limited. Guenancia et al. [26] found that NOAF patients were older and had higher levels of cardiac biomarkers (troponin ($p < 0.01$) and NT-pro-BNP ($p = 0.03$)), lower left ventricular ejection fraction (LVEF), longer duration of the QRS complex and more nonsustained supraventricular arrhythmias (< 30 seconds) on day 1 than patients who maintained sinus rhythm. Age (OR: 1.06; $p = 0.01$) and LVEF <45% (OR: 13.01, $p = 0.03$) were associated with NOAF in their multivariate analysis.

4. Incidence

Atrial fibrillation is a common occurrence in patients with sepsis and septic shock, and its incidence varies widely among investigators. This may be due to the different criteria used to define sepsis and septic shock, or the method used for the diagnosis of AF [28]. In the aforementioned systematic review, Kuipers et al. [19] showed that the mean incidence of new-onset AF was 8% in patients with sepsis and 23% in patients with septic shock. The authors of that study also observed a significant increase in ICU length of stay in this group of patients. In a large study conducted by Walkey et al. [21], which retrospectively analyzed data from over 60,000 patients admitted for sepsis, the investigators found an overall incidence of AF during sepsis of 25.5%. This number rose to 31.6% when considering only the ICU population.

To date, there have been relatively few published prospective investigations regarding the incidence of AF in septic shock patients, although there is more available information about the general topic of AF in septic patients. Seguin et al. [29] found AF developed in 24 patients (5.3%) of 460 patients admitted to the surgical intensive care unit and followed prospectively during a 6-month period. They reported that 29.2% (7 of 23 patients) of septic shock patients developed AF.

They concluded the presence of shock (especially septic shock) appeared to be an independent risk factor of AF in their cohort. It has to be recognized, however, that the operative definition of septic shock used at that time, the one proposed by Bone et al. [30], has since been substantially modified.

Steinberg et al. [28] published recently a one-year observational prospective study of 27 septic shock patients. Their aim was to evaluate the incidence of AF, and the mortality rate of patients with AF versus patients that maintained sinus rhythm. Nine (33%) patients developed AF during the first 72 hours. At admission and at 72 hours, SOFA was statistically higher in the patients with AF ($p = 0.012$ and $p = 0.002$, respectively).

In a single-center study, Meierhenrich et al. [31] prospectively studied all patients with NOAF and all patients suffering from septic shock in ICU during a 13 month period. Patients with preexisting chronic AF were excluded from their analysis. They found 23 out of the 50 patients with septic shock (46%) developed NOAF, compared to an overall incidence (septic and non-septic patients taken into account) of NOAF of 7.8% (49/629). The same aforementioned limitation in septic shock definition applies to this data.

Guenancia et al. [26] conducted a single-center prospective, observational study on patients with septic shock, and they found an incidence of new-onset AF of 44% (29 of 66 patients). Noteworthy, a 34% of new-onset AF would not be diagnosed without Holter ECG monitoring (silent AF).

More recently—and using an updated definition of septic shock—Rabie et al. [32] prospectively studied 100 septic shock patients, one of the largest series ever published. All patients were continuously monitored by three/five-lead monitor with arrhythmia detection algorithms, alarms, and Holter recording capabilities throughout the ICU stay. The investigators found the development of NOAF in 29 (29%), of which 22 (75,8%) patients had a single occurrence and 7 (24,2%) had recurrent AF during their ICU stay.

5. Prognosis

Whether NOAF acts as a surrogate marker for increased illness severity and subsequently poor prognosis in sepsis or whether it directly contributes to mortality and poor outcomes is not entirely clear. As stated before, the sepsis state can trigger AF mainly because of the combined mechanisms of inflammation, surge in catecholamines, and direct and indirect myocardial injury, and the poor prognosis noted whenever AF develop in critically ill patients may be the consequence of the presence of these factors.

In a retrospective analysis, Walkey et al. [33] found that patients with NOAF during a hospitalization for sepsis showed a higher five-year risk of hospitalization for heart failure (11.2% vs. 8.2%; HR, 1.25; 95% CI, 1.16–1.34), ischemic stroke (5.3% vs. 4.7%; HR, 1.22; 95% CI, 1.15–1.47), and death (74.8% vs. 72.1%; HR, 1.04; 95% CI, 1.01–1.07) than patients who did not develop NOAF.

Specific prospective data regarding the prognosis of NOAF in septic shock patients is also sparse. In a small series of 27 septic shock patients followed prospectively for one year, Steinberg et al. [28] reported that mortality was higher in AF patients (66%) than in patients in sinus ryhtm (11%) ($p = 0.006$). Age, rhythm and noradrenaline dosage were univariate predictors of total mortality. In the aforementioned study of Meierhenrich et al. [31], mortality in septic shock patients with NOAF was 44% compared with 22% in septic shock patients with maintained sinus rhythm ($p = 0.14$). The average length of ICU stay was shown to be increased in patients with NOAF (30 versus 17 days, $p = 0.017$). Failure to achieve sinus rhythm restoration was associated with greater ICU mortality (71.4% vs. 21.4%, p = 0.015). After two years, the investigators observed a statistically nonsignificant increase in mortality in septic shock patients with NOAF (p = 0.075).

In a larger prospective series, Rabie et al. [32] found that mortality in patients with single AF attacks were not statistically higher than non-AF patients (p = 0.143). However, recurrent attacks of AF had significantly higher mortality than non-AF or single AF attack (p < 0.05). Recurrent AF was associated with increased length of UCI stay (21.6 ± 7.2 vs. 12.9 ± 7.3 days, p = 0.004).

6. Management

When considering use of antiarrhythmic drugs or applying cardioversion in septic patients with atrial fibrillation and hemodynamic instability, causative factors must in parallel be addressed and corrected when feasible [34]. Since diastolic dysfunction is highly prevalent in ICU patients and is also an independent predictor of mortality [35], both excessive or insufficient fluid resuscitation should be avoided. For example, the so-called Early Goal Directed Therapy has shown marginal benefit [36] while heightening the risk of fluid overload and the overuse of betaadrenergic stimulant drugs to achieve central venous saturation above 65%. The resulting high cardiac output constitutes an arrhythmogenic setting. Interestingly, ceasing beta-stimulation and administering low-dose betablockers with concomitant preload correction has led to a dramatic decrease in mortality [37]. While the use of vasopressors in septic shock is recommended in early septic shock, preload assessment and timely administration of vasopressin can assist in diminishing the requirement of catecholaminergic drugs and consequently lower the risk of arrhythmia. Suboptimal volume replacement, on the other hand, carries the risk of higher sympathetic tone and consequent down-to regulation of adrenergic receptors which in turns leads to requirement of greater doses of vasopressor drugs. Hence, both conditions, namely fluid overload and hypovolaemia, are triggering factors for developing arrhythmias.

Electrolyte disturbances, which are commonplace in ICU patients, should be likewise identified and promptly corrected. Hypokalemia and hyperkalemia triggers supraventricular and ventricular arrhythmias. If the potassium level does not respond to adequate supplementation, magnesium levels must be assessed and corrected, since severe hypomagnesemia prevents the potassium level being corrected. It has been shown that septic patients tend to have lower serum magnesium levels when compared to nonseptic patients [38, 39]. Hypophosphatemia is associated with decreased myocardial contractility and a higher incidence of arrhythmia [40], and the correction of phosphorus level has been shown to prevent it [41]. Hypocalcemia may also be associated with arrhythmias [42, 43], although the data in septic patients is scarce.

Right ventricular dysfunction may cause acute cor pulmonale and supraventricular arrhythmias [44]. Instituting aggressive modalities of mechanical ventilation in septic patients with acute distress respiratory syndrome as an attempt to recruit consolidated lungs may trigger an increase in right ventricular afterload, with the consequent development of NOAF. Gradual opening of the consolidated lungs in a prone position [45] guided by periodic chest ultrasound and echocardiographic assessment may prevent the onset of supraventricular arrhythmias.

Guidelines for management of AF [46] do not usually apply readily to critically ill patients, since NOAF in patients treated on an ICU differs from AF in patients in the community in terms of causes of rhythm disturbance [47], and appropriate management [48].

6.1 Electrical therapy

Synchronized direct current cardioversion (SDCC) should be employed for patients with hemodynamic instability related to the arrhythmia, even though the probability of remaining in sinus rhythm may be low. In critically ill patients, SDCC has been investigated in few studies. The reported efficacy is generally low, ranging from 26.9% and 35.1% [49, 50]. Mayr et al. reported successful electrical cardioversion at one hour after the attempt in 13/37 (35.1%) ICU patients with NOAF. After 24 hours, six of these 37 patients (13.5%) remained in sinus rhythm. An additional study evaluating the efficacy of SDCC reported sinus rhythm restoration for at least 24 hours in 7/26 (26.9%) patients. Of note, 18 of these patients had received amiodarone prior to or during electrical cardioversion [49].

In septic shock patients with NOAF, there is lack of data on effectiveness. In a small series [28], SDCC was attempted in five patients due to hemodynamic instability. In three patients, the procedure was not effective, whereas, in one patient, sinus rhythm was restored. However, AF recurred shortly afterwards; and in one case, a stable sinus rhythm was obtained. The effectiveness of electrical therapy may be improved by concomitant antiarrhythmic medication. When electrically cardioverting 24% of septic shock patients on amiodarone and 36% on propafenone, the overall rate of sinus rhythm maintenance was significant (74% and 89%, respectively) [51]. After an initially successful cardioversion, failure to remain in sinus rhythm may signal a poor prognosis.

6.2 Antiarrhythmic pharmacological therapy

6.2.1 Amiodarone

Amiodarone is a Vaughan-Williams class III antiarrhythmic drug that is frequently used to treat atrial fibrillation, both in community and ICU settings. It is currently approved for cardioversion of atrial fibrillation (Class I, level of evidence A) [52]. It is a highly lipophilic compound with a long half life, and it is eliminated by hepatic metabolism and not by dialysis [53]. Being one of the few antiarrhythmic drugs that does not affect significantly the left ventricular ejection fraction (LVEF), its use is however limited by the occasional occurrence of systemic hypotension and because of its relatively highly toxic profile, including thyroid, lung and liver dysfunction among other detrimental effects (eg, corneal microdeposits, skin discoloration and neuropathies).

Amiodarone success in terms of rhythm control in sepsis patients varies widely, from 30% [54] to 95% [55], although rates of sustained sinus rhythm after cardioversion are substantially lower. Comparative observational studies in ICU septic patients have shown that amiodarone achieved lower rates of rhythm control than beta-blockers, magnesium and calcium channel blockers [51, 54, 56].

Specific data on amiodarone effectiveness in septic shock patients is scant. Balik et al. [51] showed in a recent study on septic shock and supraventricular arrhythmias (AF being the most frequent encountered) that amiodarone was the drug of choice in 76% of patients, likely due to the hemodynamic instability of patients in septic shock on vasoactive agents. Restoration to sinus rhythm was achieved in 74% patients while 23.7% of them required additional electrical cardioversion. The median total dose of amiodarone was 3.0 (1.8–4.6) g, given by infusion over 4 (2–6) days with a median of 1.4 (0.9–1.8) g during the first day. Due to its limited efficacy to cardiovert and to maintain sinus rhythm (74%), the patients with a persisting arrhythmia were often switched to propafenone. Interestingly, in this study, successfully cardioverted patients (with either amiodarone, propafenone or metoprolol) or those having chronic AF demonstrated not significantly lower ICU and 28-day, and 12-month mortalities compared to patients remaining in an acute onset arrhythmia.

In a retrospective review of adult medical or surgical ICU patients with septic shock and NOAF that received amiodarone (n = 239), Betthauser et al. [57] found that exposure to more than or equal to 2700 mg of amiodarone was positively correlated with longer ICU length of stay. The same investigators found that compared to non-septic shock patients, septic shock patients did not show significant difference in hemodynamic deterioration within 72 hours of intravenous amiodarone administration. Of 105 patients surviving hospital discharge, 29% continued receiving oral amiodarone at discharge.

6.2.2 Propafenone

Propafenone is a Vaughan-Williams class IC antiarrhythmic drug with some (but clinically limited) beta-blocking activity as a result of a structural similarity to beta-adrenoceptor antagonists [58]. Propafenone is currently approved and used frequently for cardioversion of atrial fibrillation (Class I, level of evidence A) [52]. However, since CAST (the Cardiac Arrhythmia Suppression Trial) [59] revealed that class IC antiarrhythmic drugs flecainide and encainide could increase the mortality risk when administered to patients with ventricular arrhythmias and coronary artery disease with significant left ventricular systolic dysfunction, current guidelines have restricted the recommendation of this class of drugs (including propafenone) to patients with NOAF who do not have structural heart disease [52].

The aforementioned study by Balik et al. [51], suggests that propafenone could be a drug of choice in septic shock patients with normal to moderately reduced LVEF. Propafenone was used in septic shock patients with NOAF as a primary antiarrhythmic in 17.5% of patients, but this figure rises to 33% if one takes into account the patients who were not able to cardiovert and maintain a sinus rhythm on amiodarone and then received propafenone. The observed cardioversion success rate was 86.1% at 24 h, although 35.5% needed additional SDCC to restore sinus rhythm. The success of cardioversion was significantly higher with propafenone than with amiodarone and almost the same as metoprolol (93%). The average propafenone dose was 670 (460–700) mg/day. Compared with amiodarone, propafenone use did not result in significantly lower ICU and 28-day mortalities, but was associated with a 12-month mortality benefit, although patients in propafenone group tended to have better LVFE at baseline and lower dose of vasopressor drugs (e.g., norepinephrine), likely reflecting more severe compromise of septic shock in the amiodarone group [34].

6.2.3 Beta-adrenergic blockers

Current guidelines recommend beta-blockers as first-choice drugs to control heart rate in AF patients with LVEF >40% (class I, level of evidence B) [52].

Autonomic dysfunction in septic shock may be accompanied by extreme tachycardia and high cardiac output. Tachycardia increases cardiac workload and myocardial oxygen consumption. In addition, shortening of diastolic relaxation time and impairment of diastolic function further affect coronary perfusion, contributing to a lower ischemic threshold. Although norepinephrine is the current recommended mainstay of treatment for sepsis-related hypotension, excessive adrenergic stress has multiple adverse effects including direct myocardial damage (e.g., takotsubo or stress cardiomyopathy and tachyarrhythmias), insulin resistance, thrombogenicity, immunosuppression, and enhanced bacterial growth [60].

Taken together, these mechanisms contribute to worsening of septic myocardial dysfunction and increased mortality [61].

The use of beta-adrenergic blockers has been proposed to mitigate the persistent sympathetic stimulation in septic shock patients, and this mechanism may in part be responsible of the observed improvement in prognosis. The production of cytokines may also be reduced with the consequent improvement in the metabolic dysregulation by means of reducing protein catabolism and by inhibiting gluconeogenesis [62]. On the other hand, using beta-blockers in septic shock patients is not without risks. Many patients with septic shock are already being treated with vasopressor and inotropic drugs, and treating them with beta-blockers can exacerbate hypotension and bradycardia promoting further hemodynamic instability [63].

In order to reduce the unnecessary load of catecholamines and the stimulation of their receptors, an easily titratable beta-blocker (e.g. esmolol or landiolol), may be safe in those patients who require vasopressor drugs in parallel for low systemic vascular resistance and hypotension. In an open-label, randomized single-center study ($n = 154$) by Morelli et al. [64], septic shock patients were assigned to receive a continuous infusion of esmolol titrated to maintain heart rate between 80/min and 94/min versus standard treatment. It was not specified how many of those patients had atrial fibrillation, so its main interest in this discussion relates to its tolerability, since traditionally it has been feared that betablockage in septic patients could result in hemodynamic deterioration. Nonetheless, the mean arterial pressure was maintained despite a marked reduction in norepinephrine requirements in the esmolol group. Also, stroke volume, systemic vascular resistance, and left ventricular stroke work indices were increased in the esmolol group. Noteworthy, it was shown that 28-day mortality was 49.4% in the esmolol group vs. 80.5% in the control group (adjusted hazard ratio, 0.39; 95% CI, 0.26 to 0.59; $p < 0.001$). These findings suggest that lowering of heart rate by esmolol allows better ventricular filling during diastole, hence improving stroke volume and thereby improving the efficiency of myocardial work and oxygen consumption.

Metoprolol is also well tolerated in septic shock patients with supraventricular arrhythmias. In septic shock patients with NOAF treated with intravenous metoprolol, Balik et al. [51] found that sinus rhythm was achieved in 92.3% patients with no additional electrical cardioversion. The median length of treatment was 5 (2–9) days, while the median intravenous metoprolol dose was 84 (48–120) mg/day.

A relatively new beta-blocker with high selectivity for beta1 receptors and a half-life of only 4 minutes, landiolol, has also been shown to be well tolerated in the critically ill for its limited negative inotropic effect and limited impact on blood pressure, as different Japanese teams of investigators have reported [65–67]. The use of low doses (5–10 mcg/kg/min) of landiolol is usually sufficient for the cardioversion of AF compared to controls. In sinus tachycardia, landiolol may prevent the occurrence of arrhythmias using an even lower dose (3–5 mcg/kg/min). In a multicenter, open-label, randomized controlled trial at 54 hospitals in Japan, in which 76 patients with sepsis or septic shock received intravenous landiolol and 75 patients were assigned to the control group, Kakihana et al. [68] found that Landiolol resulted in significantly more patients with sepsis-related tachyarrhythmia (55% vs. 33%, $p = 0.031$) achieving a heart rate of 60–94 bpm at 24 h and significantly reduced the incidence of new-onset arrhythmia. The investigators report that landiolol was also well tolerated, but should be used under appropriate monitoring of blood pressure and heart rate owing to the risk of hypotension in patients with sepsis and septic shock.

Balik et al. [34], based on studies on tachycardic patients with septic shock requiring catecholamine administration suggest the benefit of slowing heart rate by approximately 20%, but also warn that lowering heart rate below 100 per minute by means of betablockage may result in a cardiac output inadequate to meet the systemic oxygen demands in septic shock. Appropriately powered, randomized, controlled multicenter trials are required to further clarify the role of beta-blockers in septic shock patients with NOAF.

6.2.4 Digoxin

Digoxin and other cardiac glycosides have been long used to treat patients with heart failure and cardiac arrhythmias, atrial fibrillation among the latter. However, in the last couple of decades, various clinical trials have resulted in limiting the role of digoxin in the management of atrial fibrillation [52]. Digoxin acts at a cellular level by inhibiting the sodium-potassium pump, increasing the calcium availability to the contractile apparatus. This results in an increase in cardiac contractility and slowing of cardiac conduction through the atrioventricular node [69].

There is paucity of data regarding the use of digoxin in septic shock patients with NOAF. In a retrospective cohort study of ICU patients (n = 38,159) by Quian et al. [70], the investigators found an incidence of NOAF rounding 9%. After adjusting for multiple variables, they found that in patients with NOAF the use of digoxin was associated with an increased risk of 90-day mortality (hazard ratio 1.23, 95% CI 1.10–1.39, $p < 0.001$), although the proportion of sepsis patients in this population was not specified.

6.2.5 Anticoagulation therapy

While many clinical trials have shown that warfarin therapy reduces the risk of thromboembolic complications in patients with AF, it has not been unequivocally proved that oral anticoagulants provide similar benefits in critically ill septic patients with AF without carrying a significant bleeding risk. So, a common dilemma arises when deciding which septic patients with AF should receive anticoagulation therapy [71]. Walkey et al. [72] studied the practice patterns of anticoagulation in 38,582 septic patients with AF. They found that more than a third (35.3%) of the patients were anticoagulated with intravenous heparin or subcutaneous enoxaparin, while the rest of the patients did not receive anticoagulants. In those who did, significant bleeding was more frequently observed (8.6% vs. 7,2%, RR 1.21). Interestingly, there was no significant difference in the risk of ischemic stroke between anticoagulated and non-anticoagulated patients (1.4% vs. 1.3%, RR 0.94, CI 0.78–1.12). Furthermore, there was no difference in the risk of ischemic stroke between patients with preexistent AF and those with NOAF (RR, 1,12).

In a retrospective observational study to assess the incidence of stroke and anticoagulation-related complications (e.g., bleeding, heparin-induced thrombocytopenia) in AF patients with severe sepsis (n = 115), Darwish et al. [71] found no statistically significant difference in survival rates during their hospitalization (66.2% [53/80] in the non-anticoagulated group versus 74.3% (26/35) in the anticoagulated group, P = 0.392). There were no reports of strokes in either arm of the study, but this finding is at least in part explained by the small number of patients and the short period of time used for assessment. Up to date, prospective, comparative robust evidence for anticoagulation in septic shock patients is lacking.

6.2.6 Corticosteroid therapy

Due to its anti-inflammatory properties, low-dose hydrocortisone has been frequently used to achieve shock reversal and better outcomes in patients with septic shock [73]. However, after extensive review of the available evidence, the

Surviving Sepsis Campaign's guidelines restricted the use hydrocortisone in shock septic patients only when fluid resuscitation and vasopressor drugs failed to restore hemodynamic stability [74]. In a recent multicenter, prospective nonrandomized observational study in 261 septic shock patients, Launey et al. [75], a atrial fibrillation developed in 33 (24%) and 24 (19%) of no-hydrocortisone patients and hydrocortisone patients, respectively. In the weighted sample, the proportion of patients who developed AF was 28.8% in the nohydrocortisone group and 16.8% in the hydrocortisone group (difference: 11.9%; 95% confidence interval: 23.4% to 0.5%; $p = 0.04$), noting that patients who received hydrocortisone were more severely ill than those who did not receive hydrocortisone. Investigators conclude that low-dose hydrocortisone was associated with a lower risk of developing AF during the acute phase, although serious risk of bias due to missing covariates in the propensity score matching has to be taken into account.

7. Conclusions

AF during septic shock has been insufficiently studied. This has led to relevant uncertainties regarding its etiology, pathophysiology and appropriate management. Risk factors for chronic AF and NOAF frequently differ, and the unique pathophysiology of NOAF remains to be fully elucidated. Despite of a high probability of successful cardioversion achieved by pharmacological or electrical means, these treatment modalities have shown modest efficacy in affecting the medium and long-term prognosis of septic shock patients with AF. The benefits of anticoagulation in shock septic patients with AF have not been firmly established, while the risk of bleeding is increased in septic patients. Evidence-based guidelines and even expert consensus documents on the subject of NOAF management are lacking. Properly designed multicenter, prospective randomized trials are needed to clarify these questions.

Author details

Manuel Vélez-Gimón
Department of Cardiology, Caracas Medical Center, Caracas, Venezuela

*Address all correspondence to: hemodinamia@yahoo.com

References

[1] Singer M, Deutschman CS, Seymour CW, Shankar-Hari M, Annane D, Bauer M, et al. The third international consensus definitions for sepsis and septic shock (sepsis-3). JAMA 2016; 315: 801-810. DOI:10.1001/jama.2016.0287.

[2] Vincent JL, Moreno R, Takala J, Willatts S, De Mendonca A, Bruining H, et al. The SOFA (sepsis-related organ failure assessment) score to describe organ dysfunction/failure. On behalf of the working group on sepsis-related problems of the European Society of Intensive Care Medicine. Intensive Care Med 1996; 22: 707-710. DOI:10.1007/bf01709751.

[3] Thompson K, Venkatesh B, Finfer S. Sepsis and septic shock: current approaches to management. Int Med J 2019; 49: 160-170. DOI:10.1111/imj.14199.

[4] Fleischmann C, Scherag A, Adhikari NK, et al. Assessment of global incidence and mortality of hospital-treated sepsis: current estimates and limitations. Am J Respir Crit Care Med. 2016;193:259-272. DOI:10.1164/rccm.201504-0781oc.

[5] Machado FR, Cavalcanti AB, Bozza FA, et al. The epidemiology of sepsis in Brazilian intensive care units (the sepsis PREvalence assessment database, SPREAD): an observational study. Lancet Infect Dis. 2017;17:1180-1189. DOI:10.1016/S1473-3099(17)30322-5.

[6] Bosch NA, Cimini J, Walkey AJ. Atrial Fibrillation in the ICU. CHEST 2018; 154(6):1424-1434. DOI:10.1016/j.chest.2018.03.040.

[7] Harada M, Van Wagoner DR, Nattel S. Role of inflammation in atrial fibrillation pathophysiology and management. Circ J. 2015;79(3):495-502. DOI:10.1253/circj.CJ-15-0138.

[8] Hadi HA, Alsheikh-Ali AA, Mahmeed WA, Suwaidi JM. Inflammatory cytokines and atrial fibrillation: current and prospective views. J Inflamm Res. 2010;3:75-97. DOI:10.2147/JIR.S10095.

[9] Galea R, Cardillo MT, Caroli A, Marini MG, Sonnino C, Narducci ML, Biasucci LM. Inflammation and C-reactive protein in atrial fibrillation: cause or effect? Tex Heart Inst J. 2014 Oct 1;41(5):461-8. DOI:10.14503/THIJ-13-3466.

[10] Muller-Werdan U, Buerke M, Ebelt H, Heinroth KM, Herklotz A, Loppnow H, Ruß M, Schlegel F, Schlitt A, Schmidt HB, Söffker G, Werdan K. Septic cardiomyopathy – A not yet discovered cardiomyopathy? Exp Clin Cardiol. 2006 Fall;11(3):226-236.

[11] Tracey KJ. The inflammatory reflex. Nature. 2002 Dec 19-26;420(6917):853-9. DOI:10.1038/nature01321.

[12] Zorn-Pauly K, Pelzmann B, Lang P, Mächler H, Schmidt H, Ebelt H, Werdan K, Koidl B, Müller-Werdan U. Endotoxin impairs the human pacemaker current If. Shock. 2007 Dec;28(6):655-661.

[13] Mengesha HG, Tafesse TB, Bule MH. If Channel as an Emerging Therapeutic Target for Cardiovascular Diseases: A Review of Current Evidence and Controversies. Front Pharmacol. 2017 Nov 24;8:874. DOI:10.3389/fphar.2017.00874.

[14] Aldhoon B, Melenovský V, Peichl P, Kautzner J. New insights into mechanisms of atrial fibrillation. Physiol Res. 2010;59(1):1-12. DOI:10.33549/physiolres.931651.

[15] Greer J. Pathophysiology of cardiovascular dysfunction in sepsis. BJA Education 2015; 15(6):316-321. DOI:10.1093/bjaceaccp/mkv003

[16] Hung J, Lew WY. Cellular mechanisms of endotoxin-induced myocardial depression in rabbits. Circ Res. 1993 Jul;73(1):125-134. DOI:10.1161/01.res.73.1.125.

[17] Schwartz A, Brotfain E, Koyfman L, Klein M. Cardiac arrhythmias in a septic ICU population: a review. J Crit Care Med (Targu Mures). 2015 Nov 10;1(4):140-146. DOI:10.1515/jccm-2015-0027.

[18] Walkey AJ, Wiener RS, Ghobrial JM, Curtis LH, Benjamin EJ. Incident stroke and mortality associated with new-onset atrial fibrillation in patients hospitalized with severe sepsis. JAMA. 2011 Nov 23;306(20):2248-2254. DOI:10.1001/jama.2011.1615.

[19] Kuipers S, Klein Klouwenberg PM, Cremer OL. Incidence, risk factors and outcomes of new-onset atrial fibrillation in patients with sepsis: a systematic review. Crit Care. 2014 Dec 15;18(6):688. DOI:10.1186/s13054-014-0688-5.

[20] Klein Klouwenberg PM, Frencken JF, Kuipers S, Ong DS, Peelen LM, van Vught LA, Schultz MJ, van der Poll T, Bonten MJ, Cremer OL; MARS Consortium *. Incidence, Predictors, and Outcomes of New-Onset Atrial Fibrillation in Critically Ill Patients with Sepsis. A Cohort Study. Am J Respir Crit Care Med. 2017 Jan 15;195(2):205-211. DOI:10.1164/rccm.201603-0618OC.

[21] Walkey AJ, Greiner MA, Heckbert SR, Jensen PN, Piccini JP, Sinner MF, Curtis LH, Benjamin EJ. Atrial fibrillation among Medicare beneficiaries hospitalized with sepsis: incidence and risk factors. Am Heart J. 2013 Jun;165(6):949-955.e3. DOI:10.1016/j.ahj.2013.03.020.

[22] Christian SA, Schorr C, Ferchau L, Jarbrink ME, Parrillo JE, Gerber DR. Clinical characteristics and outcomes of septic patients with new-onset atrial fibrillation. J Crit Care. 2008 Dec;23(4):532-536. DOI:10.1016/j.jcrc.2007.09.005.

[23] Boos CJ. Infection and atrial fibrillation: inflammation begets AF. Eur Heart J. 2020 Mar 7;41(10):1120-1122. DOI:10.1093/eurheartj/ehz953.

[24] Schnabel RB, Sullivan LM, Levy D, Pencina MJ, Massaro JM, D'Agostino RB Sr, Newton-Cheh C, Yamamoto JF, Magnani JW, Tadros TM, Kannel WB, Wang TJ, Ellinor PT, Wolf PA, Vasan RS, Benjamin EJ. Development of a risk score for atrial fibrillation (Framingham Heart Study): a community-based cohort study. Lancet. 2009 Feb 28;373(9665):739-745. DOI:10.1016/S0140-6736(09)60443-8.

[25] Schnabel RB. Can we predict the occurrence of atrial fibrillation? Clin Cardiol. 2012 Jan;35 Suppl 1(Suppl 1): 5-9. DOI:10.1002/clc.20963.

[26] Guenancia C, Binquet C, Laurent G, Vinault S, Bruyère R, Prin S, Pavon A, Charles PE, Quenot JP. Incidence and Predictors of New-Onset Atrial Fibrillation in Septic Shock Patients in a Medical ICU: Data from 7-Day Holter ECG Monitoring. PLoS One. 2015 May 12;10(5):e0127168. DOI:10.1371/journal.pone.0127168.

[27] European Heart Rhythm Association; European Association for Cardio-Thoracic Surgery, Camm AJ, Kirchhof P, Lip GY, Schotten U, Savelieva I, Ernst S, Van Gelder IC, Al-Attar N, Hindricks G, Prendergast B, Heidbuchel H, Alfieri O, Angelini A, Atar D, Colonna P, De Caterina R, De Sutter J, Goette A, Gorenek B, Heldal M, Hohloser SH, Kolh P, Le Heuzey JY, Ponikowski P, Rutten FH. Guidelines for the management of atrial fibrillation: the Task Force for the Management of

Atrial Fibrillation of the European Society of Cardiology (ESC). Eur Heart J. 2010 Oct;31(19):2369-429. DOI:10.1093/eurheartj/ehq278.

[28] Steinberg I, Brogi E, Pratali L, Trunfio D, Giuliano G, Bignami E, Forfori F. Atrial Fibrillation in Patients with Septic Shock: A One-Year Observational Pilot Study. Turk J Anaesthesiol Reanim. 2019 Jun;47(3):213-219. DOI:10.5152/TJAR.2019.44789.

[29] Seguin P, Signouret T, Laviolle B, Branger B, Mallédant Y. Incidence and risk factors of atrial fibrillation in a surgical intensive care unit. Crit Care Med. 2004 Mar;32(3):722-726. DOI:10.1097/01.ccm.0000114579.56430.e0.

[30] Bone RC, Balk RA, Cerra FB, Dellinger RP, Fein AM, Knaus WA, Schein RM, Sibbald WJ. Definitions for sepsis and organ failure and guidelines for the use of innovative therapies in sepsis. The ACCP/SCCM Consensus Conference Committee. American College of Chest Physicians/Society of Critical Care Medicine. Chest. 1992 Jun;101(6):1644-1655. DOI:10.1378/chest.101.6.1644.

[31] Meierhenrich R, Steinhilber E, Eggermann C, Weiss M, Voglic S, Bögelein D, Gauss A, Georgieff M, Stahl W. Incidence and prognostic impact of new-onset atrial fibrillation in patients with septic shock: a prospective observational study. Crit Care. 2010;14(3):R108. DOI:10.1186/cc9057.

[32] Rabie A, Fahmy TS, Aal A, El-Hadiyi A. EJICT 2017;7(1):1-12. Prognostic value of new-onset atrial fibrillation in patients with septic shock.

[33] Walkey AJ, Hammill BG, Curtis LH, Benjamin EJ. Long-term outcomes following development of new-onset atrial fibrillation during sepsis. Chest. 2014 Nov;146(5):1187-1195. DOI:10.1378/chest.14-0003.

[34] Balik M, Matousek V, Maly M, Brozek T. Management of arrhythmia in sepsis and septic shock. Anaesthesiol Intensive Ther. 2017;49(5):419-429. DOI:10.5603/ait.a2017.0061.

[35] Sanfilippo F, Corredor C, Fletcher N, et al. Diastolic dysfunction and mortality in septic patients: a systematic review and meta-analysis. Intensive Care Med. 2015; 41(6): 1004-1013. DOI:10.1007/s00134-015-3748-7.

[36] Xu JY, Chen QH, Liu SQ, et al. The effect of early goal-directed therapy on outcome in adult severe sepsis and septic shock patients: a meta-analysis of randomized clinical trials. Anesth Analg. 2016; 123(2): 371-381. DOI:10.1213/ane.0000000000001278.

[37] Morelli A, Ertmer C, Westphal M, et al. Effect of heart rate control with esmolol on hemodynamic and clinical outcomes in patients with septic shock: a randomized clinical trial. JAMA. 2013; 310(16): 1683-1691. DOI:10.1001/jama.2013.278477.

[38] Velissaris D, Karamouzos V, Pierrakos C, Aretha D, Karanikolas M. Hypomagnesemia in critically ill sepsis patients. J Clin Med Res. 2015;7(12):911-918. DOI:10.14740/jocmr2351w.

[39] Cojocaru IM, Cojocaru M, Tanasescu R, Iacob SA, Iliescu I. Changes of magnesium serum levels in patients with acute ischemic stroke and acute infections. Rom J Intern Med. 2009;47(2):169-171.

[40] Bugg NC, Jones JA. Hypophosphataemia. Pathophysiology, effects and management on the intensive care unit. Anaesthesia. 1998; 53(9): 895-902. DOI:10.1046/j.1365-2044.1998.00463.x.

[41] Schwartz A, Brotfain E, Koyfman L, et al. Association between hypophosphatemia and cardiac

arrhythmias in the early stage of sepsis: could phosphorus replacement treatment reduce the incidence of arrhythmias? Electrolyte Blood Press. 2014; 12(1): 19-25. DOI:10.5049/ebp.2014.12.1.19.

[42] Lee JW. Fluid and electrolyte disturbances in critically ill patients. Electrolyte Blood Press. 2010; 8(2): 72-81. DOI:10.5049/ebp.2010.8.2.72.

[43] Hypocalcemia: a pervasive metabolic abnormality in the critically ill. Am J Kidney Dis. 2001; 37(4): 689-698. DOI:10.1016/s0272-6386(01)80116-5.

[44] Jardin F,Vieillard-Baron A. Isthere a safe plateau pressure in ARDS? The right heart only knows. Intensive Care Med. 2007; 33(3): 444-447. DOI:10.1007/s00134-007-0552-z.

[45] Vieillard-Baron A, Charron C, Caille V, et al. Prone positioning unloads the right ventricle in severe ARDS. Chest. 2007; 132(5): 1440-1446. DOI:10.1378/chest.07-1013.

[46] Hindricks G, Potpara T, Dagres N, Arbelo E, Bax JJ, Blomström-Lundqvist C, et al. 2020 ESC Guidelines for the diagnosis and management of atrial fbrillation developed in collaboration with the European Association for Cardio-Thoracic Surgery (EACTS): The Task Force for the diagnosis and management of atrial fbrillation of the European Society of Cardiology (ESC) Developed with the special contribution of the European Heart Rhythm Association (EHRA) of the ESC. Eur Heart J. 2020;42(5):373-498. DOI:10.1093/eurheartj/ehaa612.

[47] Walkey AJ, Hogarth DK, Lip GYH. Optimizing atrial fbrillation management: from ICU and beyond. Chest. 2015;148(4):859-864. DOI:10.1378/chest.15-0358.

[48] Drikite L, Bedford JP, O'Bryan L, Petrinic T, Rajappan K, Doidge J, Harrison DA, Rowan KM, Mouncey PR, Young D, Watkinson PJ, Corbett M. Treatment strategies for new onset atrial fibrillation in patients treated on an intensive care unit: a systematic scoping review. Crit Care. 2021 Jul 21;25(1):257. DOI:10.1186/s13054-021-03684-5.

[49] Kanji S, Williamson DR, Yaghchi BM, Albert M, McIntyre L; Canadian Critical Care Trials Group. Epidemiology and management of atrial fibrillation in medical and noncardiac surgical adult intensive care unit patients. J Crit Care. 2012 Jun;27(3):326.e1-8. DOI:10.1016/j.jcrc.2011.10.011.

[50] Mayr A, Ritsch N, Knotzer H, Dünser M, Schobersberger W, Ulmer H, Mutz N, Hasibeder W. Effectiveness of direct-current cardioversion for treatment of supraventricular tachyarrhythmias, in particular atrial fibrillation, in surgical intensive care patients. Crit Care Med, 2003 Feb;31(2):401-405. DOI:10.1097/01.CCM.0000048627.39686.79.

[51] Balik M, Kolnikova I, Maly M, Waldauf P, Tavazzi G, Kristof J. Propafenone for supraventricular arrhythmias in septic shock-Comparison to amiodarone and metoprolol. J Crit Care. 2017 Oct;41:16-23. DOI:10.1016/j.jcrc.2017.04.02.

[52] Hindricks G, Potpara T, Dagres N, Arbelo E, Bax JJ, Blomström-Lundqvist C, Boriani G, Castella M, Dan GA, Dilaveris PE, Fauchier L, Filippatos G, Kalman JM, La Meir M, Lane DA, Lebeau JP, Lettino M, Lip GYH, Pinto FJ, Thomas GN, Valgimigli M, Van Gelder IC, Van Putte BP, Watkins CL; ESC Scientific Document Group. 2020 ESC Guidelines for the diagnosis and management of atrial fibrillation developed in collaboration with the European Association for Cardio-Thoracic Surgery (EACTS): The Task Force for the

diagnosis and management of atrial fibrillation of the European Society of Cardiology (ESC) Developed with the special contribution of the European Heart Rhythm Association (EHRA) of the ESC. Eur Heart J. 2021 Feb 1;42(5):373-498. DOI:10.1093/eurheartj/ehaa612.

[53] Hughes M, Binning A. Intravenous amiodarone in intensive care. Time for a reappraisal? Intensive Care Med. 2000 Dec;26(12):1730-1739. DOI:10.1007/s001340000668.

[54] Yoshida T, Uchino S, Yokota T, Fujii T, Uezono S, Takinami M. The impact of sustained new-onset atrial fibrillation on mortality and stroke incidence in critically ill patients: A retrospective cohort study. J Crit Care. 2018 Apr;44:267-272. DOI:10.1016/j.jcrc.2017.11.040.

[55] Sleeswijk ME, Tulleken JE, Van Noord T, Meertens JH, Ligtenberg JJ, Zijlstra JG. Efficacy of magnesium-amiodarone step-up scheme in critically ill patients with new-onset atrial fibrillation: a prospective observational study. J Intensive Care Med. 2008 Jan-Feb;23(1):61-66. DOI:10.1177/0885066607310181.

[56] Liu WC, Lin WY, Lin CS, Huang HB, Lin TC, Cheng SM, Yang SP, Lin JC, Lin WS. Prognostic impact of restored sinus rhythm in patients with sepsis and new-onset atrial fibrillation. Crit Care. 2016 Nov 18;20(1):373. DOI:10.1186/s13054-016-1548-2.

[57] Betthauser KD, Gibson GA, Piche SL, Pope HE. Evaluation of Amiodarone Use for New-Onset Atrial Fibrillation in Critically Ill Patients With Septic Shock. Hosp Pharm. 2021 Apr;56(2):116-123. DOI:10.1177/0018578719868405.

[58] Stoschitzky K, Stoschitzky G, Lercher P, Brussee H, Lamprecht G, Lindner W. Propafenone shows class Ic and class II antiarrhythmic effects. Europace. 2016 Apr;18(4):568-571. DOI:10.1093/europace/euv195

[59] Cardiac Arrhythmia Suppression Trial (CAST) Investigators. Preliminary report: effect of encainide and flecainide on mortality in a randomized trial of arrhythmia suppression after myocardial infarction. N Engl J Med. 1989 Aug 10;321(6):406-412. DOI:10.1056/NEJM198908103210629.

[60] Dünser MW, Hasibeder WR. Sympathetic overstimulation during critical illness: adverse effects of adrenergic stress. J Intensive Care Med. 2009 Sep-Oct;24(5):293-316. DOI:10.1177/0885066609340519.

[61] Schmittinger CA, Torgersen C, Luckner G, Schröder DC, Lorenz I, Dünser MW. Adverse cardiac events during catecholamine vasopressor therapy: a prospective observational study. Intensive Care Med. 2012 Jun;38(6):950-958. DOI:10.1007/s00134-012-2531-2.

[62] Gadallah, R.R., Aboseif, E.M.K., Ibrahim, D.A. et al. Evaluation of the safety and efficacy of beta blockers in septic patients: a randomized control trial. Ain-Shams J Anesthesiol 2020;12(1):57. DOI:10.1186/s42077-020-00107-5.

[63] Sanfilippo F, Santonocito C, Morelli A, Foex P. Beta-blocker use in severe sepsis and septic shock: a systematic review. Curr Med Res Opin. 2015;31(10):1817-1825. DOI:10.1185/03007995.2015.1062357.

[64] Morelli A, Ertmer C, Westphal M, Rehberg S, Kampmeier T, Ligges S, Orecchioni A, D'Egidio A, D'Ippoliti F, Raffone C, Venditti M, Guarracino F, Girardis M, Tritapepe L, Pietropaoli P, Mebazaa A, Singer M. Effect of heart rate control with esmolol on hemodynamic and clinical outcomes in patients with septic shock: a randomized

clinical trial. JAMA. 2013 Oct 23;310(16):1683-1691. DOI:10.1001/jama.2013.278477.

[65] Ojima T, Nakamori M, Nakamura M, Katsuda M, Hayata K, Kato T, Kitadani J, Tabata H, Takeuchi A, Yamaue H. Randomized clinical trial of landiolol hydrochloride for the prevention of atrial fibrillation and postoperative complications after oesophagectomy for cancer. Br J Surg. 2017 Jul;104(8):1003-1009. DOI:10.1002/bjs.10548.

[66] Nojiri T, Yamamoto K, Maeda H, Takeuchi Y, Funakoshi Y, Maekura R, Okumura M. Efficacy of low-dose landiolol, an ultrashort-acting β-blocker, on postoperative atrial fibrillation in patients undergoing pulmonary resection for lung cancer. Gen Thorac Cardiovasc Surg. 2011 Dec;59(12):799-805. DOI:10.1007/s11748-011-0841-x.

[67] Nakano T, Shimizu K, Kawashima O, Kamiyoshihara M, Nagashima T, Ibe T, Takeyoshi I. Effect of landiolol hydrochloride, an ultra-short-acting beta 1-selective blocker, on supraventricular tachycardia, atrial fibrillation and flutter after pulmonary resection. J Clin Pharm Ther. 2012 Aug;37(4):431-435. DOI:10.1111/j.1365-2710.2011.01315.x.

[68] Kakihana Y, Nishida O, Taniguchi T, Okajima M, Morimatsu H, Ogura H, Yamada Y, Nagano T, Morishima E, Matsuda N; J-Land 3S Study Group. Efficacy and safety of landiolol, an ultra-short-acting β1-selective antagonist, for treatment of sepsis-related tachyarrhythmia (J-Land 3S): a multicentre, open-label, randomised controlled trial. Lancet Respir Med. 2020 Sep;8(9):863-872. DOI:10.1016/S2213-2600(20)30037-0.

[69] Yang EH, Shah S, Criley JM. Digitalis toxicity: a fading but crucial complication to recognize. Am J Med. 2012 Apr;125(4):337-343. DOI:10.1016/j.amjmed.2011.09.019.

[70] Qian J, Kuang L, Chen F, Liu X, Che L. Prognosis and management of new-onset atrial fibrillation in critically ill patients. BMC Cardiovasc Disord. 2021 May 5;21(1):231. DOI:10.1186/s12872-021-02039-w.

[71] Darwish OS, Strube S, Nguyen HM, Tanios MA. Challenges of anticoagulation for atrial fibrillation in patients with severe sepsis. Ann Pharmacother. 2013 Oct;47(10):1266-1271. DOI:10.1177/1060028013500938.

[72] Walkey AJ, Quinn EK, Winter MR, McManus DD, Benjamin EJ. Practice Patterns and Outcomes Associated With Use of Anticoagulation Among Patients With Atrial Fibrillation During Sepsis. JAMA Cardiol. 2016 Sep 1;1(6):682-690. DOI:10.1001/jamacardio.2016.2181.

[73] Annane D, Sébille V, Charpentier C, Bollaert PE, François B, Korach JM, Capellier G, Cohen Y, Azoulay E, Troché G, Chaumet-Riffaud P, Bellissant E. Effect of treatment with low doses of hydrocortisone and fludrocortisone on mortality in patients with septic shock. JAMA. 2002 Aug 21;288(7):862-871. DOI:10.1001/jama.288.7.862.

[74] Dellinger RP, Levy MM, Carlet JM, Bion J, Parker MM, Jaeschke R, Reinhart K, Angus DC, Brun-Buisson C, Beale R, Calandra T, Dhainaut JF, Gerlach H, Harvey M, Marini JJ, Marshall J, Ranieri M, Ramsay G, Sevransky J, Thompson BT, Townsend S, Vender JS, Zimmerman JL, Vincent JL; International Surviving Sepsis Campaign Guidelines Committee; American Association of Critical-Care Nurses; American College of Chest Physicians; American College of Emergency Physicians; Canadian Critical Care Society; European Society of Clinical Microbiology and Infectious Diseases; European Society of Intensive

Care Medicine; European Respiratory Society; International Sepsis Forum; Japanese Association for Acute Medicine; Japanese Society of Intensive Care Medicine; Society of Critical Care Medicine; Society of Hospital Medicine; Surgical Infection Society; World Federation of Societies of Intensive and Critical Care Medicine. Surviving Sepsis Campaign: international guidelines for management of severe sepsis and septic shock: 2008. Crit Care Med. 2008 Jan;36(1):296-327. DOI:10.1097/01.CCM.0000298158.12101.41.

[75] Launey Y, Lasocki S, Asehnoune K, Gaudriot B, Chassier C, Cinotti R, Maguet PL, Laksiri L, Mimoz O, Tawa A, Nesseler N, Malledant Y, Perrot B, Seguin P. Impact of Low-Dose Hydrocortisone on the Incidence of Atrial Fibrillation in Patients With Septic Shock: A Propensity Score-Inverse Probability of Treatment Weighting Cohort Study. J Intensive Care Med. 2019 Mar;34(3):238-244. DOI:10.1177/0885066617696847.